WORLD HEART RESEARCH YEARBOOK

VOLUME 1

World Heart Research Yearbook

Additional books in this series can be found on Nova's website
under the Series tab.

Additional e-books in this series can be found on Nova's website
under the e-books tab.

WORLD HEART RESEARCH YEARBOOK

VOLUME 1

FRANZ HALBERG
AND
R. B. SINGH
EDITORS

Nova Science Publishers, Inc.
New York

Library of Congress Cataloging-in-Publication Data

ISSN: 2167-2873
ISBN: 978-1-60741-881-8

Published by Nova Science Publishers, Inc. † New York

CONTENTS

PREFACE

This new yearbook presents important research in the field of cardiovascular research from around the world. Particular emphasis is placed on circadian medicine and its relationship to cardiovascular events as well as other new areas such as gene therapy in heart disease.

In: World Heart Research Yearbook. Volume 1
Editors: Franz Halberg and R. B. Singh
ISBN: 978-1-60741-881-8

INTRODUCING A JOURNAL AND ITS EDITOR-IN-CHIEF

Franz Halberg and Germaine Cornélissen
Halberg Chronobiology Center, University of Minnesota, Minneapolis, MN, US

In the issues to follow, a World Heart Journal could usher in a new health care. It can live up to the "new" in this "world". With respect to content, it could deal with new vascular variability disorders, e.g., Figure 1, Sections IIA-C, and Figure 2. As to scope, altered dynamics in blood pressure (BP) and heart rate (HR) constitute a worldwide problem as pre-hypertension and pre-diabetes, as a pre-metabolic syndrome [1-8], occurring in the currently neglected, and hence, to many, "new" normal range, that can be split chronomically, that is time-structurally. The journal can draw attention to predictable rhythms in everyday physiology with treatable alterations that represent risks greater than hypertension, Figure 1. About-daily and about-yearly rhythms, photic and thermic signatures of day and night and of the seasons, are modulated by and, with advancing age, in part replaced by non-photic competing signatures of the sun and the earth, a concern linked to weather in extra-terrestrial space [9-13].

By teaching automated self-surveillance, a new World Heart Journal can serve the care provider and, directly, the care recipient. All it has to do is help 1) replace the question "What is the ('true', or rather imaginary) BP, HR, ...?" by a question regarding variabilities of these and other body functions that are rightly called variables, and 2) provide the means to assess alterations of variability, in the light of gender, age and preferably ethnicity-specified reference values, Figures 1-3. Everyone can benefit from the mapping of chronomes (time structures) in us and around us, by diagnosing chronomically abnormal patterns in a person's BP and/or HR and by restoring healthy chronomes with timed treatment (chronotherapy). By assessing, in populations, the wide spectrum of rhythms in morbidity and mortality that are influenced by space weather as well as by local climate, prophylactic interventions on a population basis may become possible [12].

Chronomics complements chronobiology, the study of the mechanisms of biological time structures, Figure 4. For this purpose, chronomics also maps environmental along with biological rhythms. By extending the perspective from an organism as such to its ambiance near and far, chronomics adds a figurative telescopy in time to chronobiology's figurative microscopy in time. The opportunity to treat an elevated risk of developing cardiovascular disease, such as circadian BP overswinging, while all data are in the "normal range" is an immediate benefit documented worldwide in Figures 1-3.

The treatment as well as the detection of risk, called prehabilitation, can be made known for care providers, notably upstream, in medical schools. Everybody interested in self-care could also be informed and motivated by this journal to implement prehabilitation him/herself. Chronomics is a practicable cost-effective complement to investments into rehabilitation after end-organ damage or after an adverse event, such as a myocardial infarction (MI) or brain stroke has occurred. The treatment of high BP also needs more than spotchecks during waking, when, in a given patient, unknown to his care provider, during 11 consecutive days the diastolic BP can reach about 120 mm Hg each night, while values during office hours remain within conventional limits, as it did in a documented case, Figure 1, Section I. Much more important for primary prevention is the availability of special time-microscopic methods to quantify earliest alterations of variability, opportunities that cannot be obtained by the unaided eye alone or by day-night ratios [4, 6, 8].

The journal welcomes reports of public as well as professional education to motivate patients to survey their everyday routines by emphasis on nutrition, exercise and other behaviors, notably if they are optimized by timing. BP and HR monitoring for the detection (and treatment) of risk elevation is also important in medicated patients with high BP. By simply changing the timing of conventional medication, monitoring helps adjust the treatment to maximize the hypotensive effect and to minimize risks associated with BP overswinging or other alterations of the BP and/or HR chronomes [1-3, 5, 6]. The journal also addresses the timing of nutriceuticals as well as chronobiologic aspects of gene therapy. Reference to imaginary setpoints is best replaced by measurable changes in chronome characteristics. The journal's topics will include findings on laboratory animals [14], suggesting the possible use of chronomics for rehabilitation, e.g., by considering the role of timing in stem cell collection for cellular cardiomyoplasty and, in the same context, for manipulating, again by timing, various aspects of scar formation. The use of modern telemetry, ongoing routinely in laboratory animals and only in research as yet on humans, may lead to the recognition of the etiology of BP disorders, including overswinging, and thus to the specification of refined treatment options. Chronomics detects not only prehypertension but also a broader premetabolic syndrome, including glucose sensitivity [7, 8]. Calling attention to the accumulating evidence in various aspects of chronomics and motivating the population for self-help is a raison d'être of this journal.

Prof. Ram Bahadur (R.B.) Singh of Moradabad, India, the editor-in-chief, plays a key role in the BIOCOS project (on The BIOsphere and the COSmos) [15; cf. 9-11], which collects reference values for the foregoing aims, also studying how biological processes are affected by the environment near and far, whenever possible before the dynamics exceed the range of everyday physiology.

Major activities of BIOCOS are the around the clock monitoring and special analyses of BP and HR. Longitudinal studies over decades (in one case for 40 years of manual measurements about 5 times a day or in another case automatically collected half-hourly data for up to 20 years) are routinely complemented by half-hourly around-the-clock surveillance for up to 7 days in various geographical locations, Figure 3, now also including Australia and South America. The records are interpreted in the light of reference standards specified as a function of a broad time structure (including the usually present, often prominent circadian variation), gender and age. For the past several years, in collaboration with BIOCOS, Prof. Singh uncovered associations of circadian characteristics with respect to prayer [15] and nutrition. Some of his other findings, notably in the detection of disorders of BP variabilities [16], are reproduced independently in other BIOCOS centers and have been readily aligned with them, Figure 3.

Chronomics Detects Nocturnal Escape from Treatment (I), Risk of Stroke and Nephropathy Greater than Hypertension (IIA-B), even in MESOR-Normotension (IIC) and Monitors Transient and/or Lasting Success of Treatment (IIIA-C)*

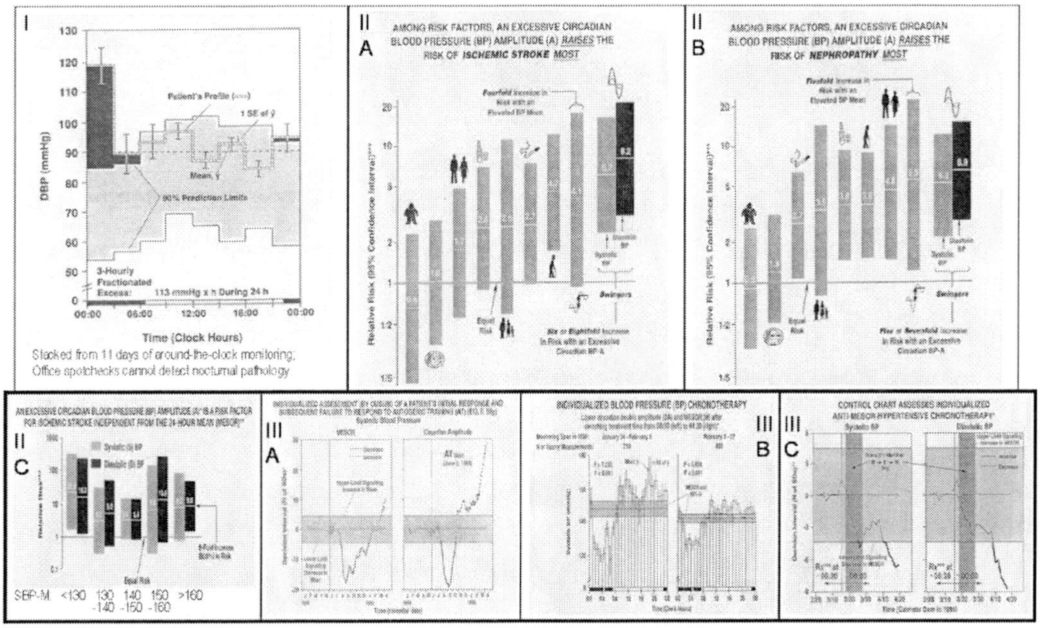

* During span examined, demonstrating the desirability of lifetime monitoring once abnormality in the normal range is detected (IIC).

Figure 1. Results supporting need for continued surveillance and for chronomic data analysis. Merits are:

- Detection of abnormality during the night when medication happens to be no longer effective, not seen during office visits in the afternoon when measurements can be acceptable (I; 5, 6);
- Detection of abnormal circadian pattern of blood pressure (CHAT, "overswinging") associated with a risk of cerebral ischemia and nephropathy larger than a number of other risks (including "hypertension") assessed concomitantly (IIA and B);
- CHAT carries a very high risk even among MESOR-normotensives who do not need anti-hypertensive medication (IIC);
- Statistical procedures such as a self-starting cumulative sum (CUSUM), applicable to the individual patient, determine whether an intervention such as autogenic training is effective and for how long the intervention remains effective (IIIA);
- N-of-1 designs for the optimization of treatment timing: the same dose of the same medication can further lower the same subject's blood pressure MESOR and circadian amplitude when the timing of daily administration is changed (IIIB and C), as ascertained by as-one-goes (sequential) testing and parameter tests, procedures applicable to the given individual [3; cf. 39]. © Halberg.

In cooperating with Prof. Singh, we learned about the many hurdles to be overcome in doing research with relatively limited means. BP and HR records do not always cover 7 days and have interruptions due to problems such as the failure to recharge batteries, as well as to other technical problems with the use of the monitors. Ways to solve problems are invariably sought and a solution is often found eventually. Prof. Singh is involved in many activities, often delegating tasks to his associates or colleagues locally and around the world. In the case of our recent collaboration in BIOCOS, the data are retrieved directly from the monitors electronically and the files are coded, being decoded in our center in Minnesota, where numerical analyses are also carried out. Whenever a question arises, Prof. Singh answers by return mail to our complete satisfaction.

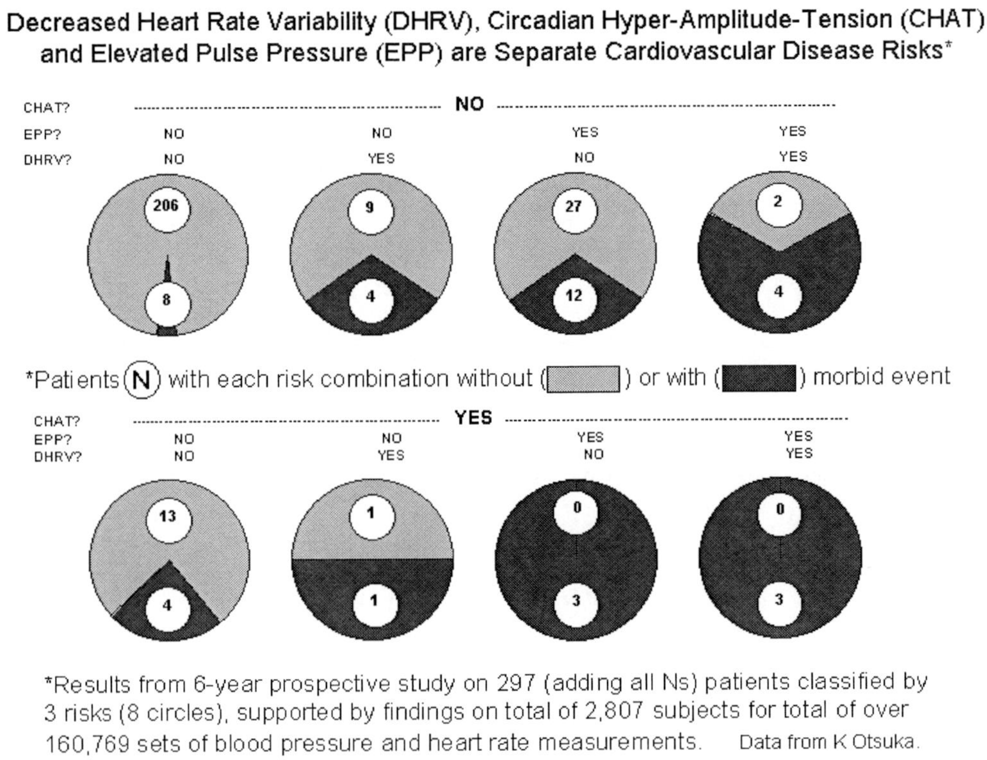

Figure 2. Several conditions related to the variability in blood pressure (BP) and/or heart rate (HR) are each associated with a separate increase in vascular disease risk: a decreased heart rate variability (DHRV), circadian hyper-amplitude-tension (CHAT) and an elevated pulse pressure (EPP). The circadian (or preferably circaseptan) profile gauges EPP as too large a pulse pressure (the difference between systolic [S] BP and diastolic [D] BP, i.e., between the heart's contraction or relaxation, or the extent of change in BP during a cardiac cycle) and DHRV by the standard deviation of HR, in relation to a threshold, (eventually all) in gender- and age-matched clinically healthy peers. Not shown is an abnormal circadian timing of BP but not of HR, circadian BP ecphasia, yet another vascular variability disorder, VVD [4]. Vascular disease risk is elevated in the presence of any one of these risk factors, and is elevated further when more than a single risk factor (VVD) is present, suggesting that these abnormalities in variability of BP and HR are mostly independent and additive, becoming a vascular variability syndrome, VVS. Abnormalities in the variability of BP and HR, impossible to find in a conventional office visit (the latter aiming at the fiction of a "true" BP), can raise cardiovascular disease risk (gauged by the occurrence of a morbid event like a stroke in the next six years) from 4% to 100%. By comparison to subjects with acceptable BP and HR variability, the relative cardiovascular disease risk associated with DHRV, EPP and/or CHAT is greatly and statistically significantly increased. These risks, silent to the person involved and to the care provider, notably the risk of CHAT, can usually be reversed by chronobiologic self-help, also with a non-pharmacologic approach in the absence of MESOR-hypertension [2]. © Halberg.

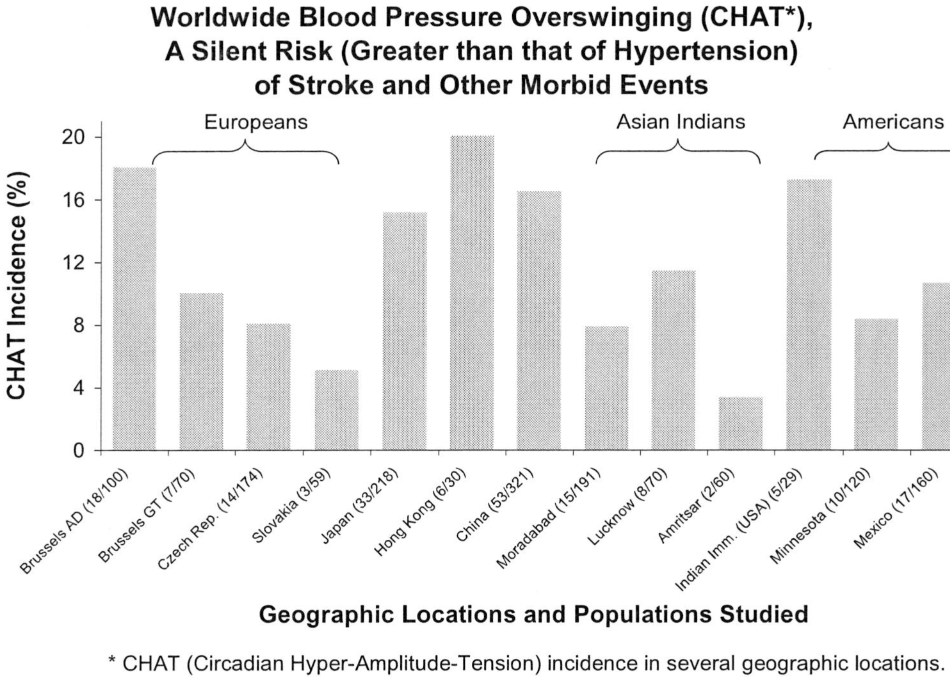

Figure 3. First summary of 191 cases of CHAT in 1602 profiles (many of them covering 7 days) aims at indicating that CHAT is present under various conditions in various populations in many geographic and geomagnetic locations, in the presence or absence of MESOR-hypertension [44]. © Halberg.

The late V. (Vulimiri) Ramalingaswami, known as Rama (as head of the All-India Institute for Medical Research in New Delhi), and the late B.R. (Bagepalli Ramachandrachar) Seshachar, former presidents of one of India's two national academies of science, both wanted to bring chronobiology to health care in India, and Rama, later in his life, represented India at the World Health Organization and thus had broader scope. Prof. Singh, by dint of hundreds of already summarized BP and HR profiles, succeeded in implementing what opinion leaders and others sought. Should his recent findings of associations of prayer and diet with desirable aspects of variability be confirmed longitudinally rather than only by a group comparison [15, 16], these non-pharmacological approaches could serve to reduce high vascular disease risk factors, a deficient HR variability and an elevated HR, respectively. The findings on risk are based on a large number of subjects and a large number of data [5, 6]. Prof. Singh adds to these findings data from the Indian subcontinent, Figure 3, thus implementing in Moradabad what we achieved neither in Old and New Delhi nor in many developed areas with many more resources. It remains common practice in most research elsewhere to rely on single measurements of BP as a start [17] or at best on 1- or 2-day around-the-clock profiles [18]. Prof. Singh's investigations target routine 7-day half-hourly profiles and by computer analyses of the data, at least in his research and, we trust, soon in practice, he picks up otherwise undetected variability disorders, that are not recognized by most others.

CHRONOBIOLOGY (CENTER)-SPAWNED TRANSDISCIPLINARY SCIENCES,
CHRONOMICS AND YET-TO-BE-DEVELOPED CHRONOBIOETHICS,
AIMING TO SERVE
INDIVIDUALS' HEALTH, NATIONS' WELL-BEING AND COSMOS' INTEGRITY

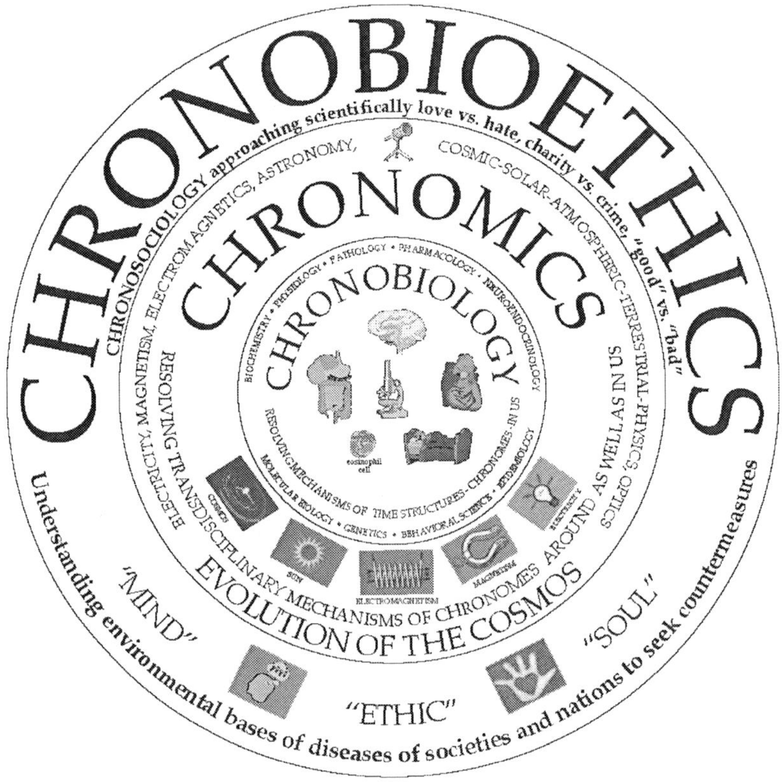

Figure 4. Chronobiology (microscopy in time, inner circle) uncovered mechanisms underlying the ubiquity, importance, and genetics of circadians and their synchronization with daily routines [3, 43]. Chronomics (telescopy in time) reveals many other wobbly cycles not only in us, but also cycles around us, uncovering rhythms in the "good" and "bad", in religious motivation vs. crime and war. Monitoring blood pressure and heart rate as a start and mental functions, among others, is advocated, to start with for stroke prevention, but with the added aim of using the same approach for a rhythmometry focused on societal disease. Most recent findings reveal matching transyearly cycles of ~1.3 year length and other nonphotics in terrorism, heliogeomagnetics, systolic blood pressure, heart rate, and the self-rating of mood. Moreover, when a given spectral band in the satellite-measured speed of the solar wind or in terrestrial magnetism is (naturally) amplified or dampened (by the sun), so are corresponding spectral bands in the incidence of terrorism in the last four decades [49, 50], and so is human 1-minute estimation. Removal of a broad transyearly spectral band in the solar wind's speed is accompanied by the partial loss and damping of the remaining corresponding band in the systolic blood pressure of an elderly man [12]. The World Heart Journal could broaden the perspective (from "flying blind" between office visits or from a circadian bitemporal hemianopsia) to the spectrum in Figure 6 that shows many corresponding periods in and around us. Some of these cycles are associated with dying suddenly [12, 52] or by one's own hand [51] or being killed [49, 50]. Chronobioethics serves as a basis for eventually developing timely and timed countermeasures to diseases not only of individuals but also of societies and civilizations [1-3], all within the broader scope of a new journal. © Halberg.

Prof. Singh's endeavors along chronobiologic lines are not new. He follows the late Frederic C. Bartter of Bartter syndrome fame, head of the then Hypertension and Endocrine Branch at the U.S. National Institutes of Health (NIH). As to BP, Bartter, who eventually became chief of the clinical center at NIH, wrote, about a patient whose BP was diagnosed differently by two other physicians who saw him at different times of day [19]: "By conventional standards, this patient is clearly normotensive every morning. But the blood pressure determined each day at 6 in the afternoon provides especially convincing evidence that this patient is a hypertensive. ... My plea today [in 1974 !] is that information contained in [data curves compiled under differing circumstances, such as 24 hours a day/7 days a week] become a *routine minimal amount* of information accepted for the description of a patient's blood pressure. *The analysis of this information by cosinor should become a routine.* It is essential that enough information be collected to allow objective characterization of a periodic phenomenon, to wit, an estimate of M [the time structure or chronome-adjusted mean, or MESOR] ... an estimate of [the amplitude] A itself, and finally an estimate of acrophase, ϕ [a measure of timing]. In this way, a patient can be compared with himself at another time, or under another treatment, and the patient can be compared with a normal or with another patient" [19].Bartter then introduced the chronotherapy of hypertension [20], but his suggestion regarding diagnosis is also not new. Rather, it is in keeping with the insights of Theodore C. Janeway of Johns Hopkins Medical School, an opinion leader from the turn of the 20th century, who in 1904 wrote: "... *it is essential* that a record of the pressure be made at frequent intervals *at some time previous* [presumably to an examination], to establish the *normal level* and the *extent of the periodic variations.* When this is done, it may be possible to demonstrate changes of small extent, which, lacking this standard for comparison, would be considered within the limits of normal variation" [21].

Prof. Singh goes several important steps further, beyond spotchecks at the (putative "true", yet only instantaneous and fictitious if extrapolated beyond the moment of measurement) BP. He assesses the variability of this variable (sic). Instead of reference values applicable to everybody above 18 years, male or female [17], he uses reference standards specified by age and gender. As compared to Janeway, who looked for periodicity with his unaided eyes, Prof. Singh uses time microscopy, with special computer methodology [22, 23], including the cosinor procedure that Bartter had recommended [19]. Prof. Singh now collects reference standards specified for a broader than circadian time structure, realizing that to assess circadians, as some do on the basis of 24- or 48-hour records is equivalent to taking the pulse for one or two cycles (seconds!) [24-26].

Activities as a clinician, educator, epidemiologist and nutritionist, with basic contributions to the role of magnesium in heart health, were augmented when Prof. Singh founded and presided over the International College of Cardiology, with repeated, successful meetings [27, 28]. Should a spotcheck "evidence"-based health care be supplanted with an instrumented self-surveillance (by his impact in the footsteps of the late Bartter in the US and the late Seshachar and the late Ramalingaswami in India), credit will go to Prof. R.B. Singh for many things *(multa).* Carl Friedrich Gauss, the titan of science, wanted much, but not many things *(multum sed non multa).* He wanted to be *in*tensive, not *ex*tensive. Prof. Singh tries to do both. He brings much (chronobiologic tools and concepts) into the service of many things that are all pertinent to individual and international health and could thus lead to *multum.* To realize this goal, and by reference to a series of concerns discussed elsewhere [3], we suggest:

1. In the future, all authors in this new journal should be requested to provide data (whenever possible and pertinent) together with a manuscript before it is accepted for publication. Referees could thus see firsthand whether the conclusions stated in the paper are warranted. One of us heard in his student days that Justus von Liebig in the original Liebig's Annalen [29] in the 1830s did not publish a paper in his then prestigious journal before he did not successfully repeat the author's claim in his laboratory.
2. Mistakes as to new claims are an unpleasant fact and do occur. It is part of the referees' task to make sure that a paper is as sound as possible before it is accepted for publication. Yet the best referees can err. Gauss, the king of mathematicians, erred in a judgement of a colleague's contribution in his own field. So will most of us who are shouldering more than we can carry. The refereeing process is sometimes problematic, insofar as it can be subjective, and some journals have adopted the policy to hide the authors' names to assure better objectivity in the review, a highly recommended procedure.
3. Mistakes are often committed in the choice of methodology used to analyze a given set of data. Some years ago, our laboratory reported substantial benefit from timing ara-C to treat leukemia in experimental animals [30-32], at variance with other researchers [33]. The apparent discrepancy between the results of the two teams was readily resolved after it was found that the contenders [33] had not used the surviving (cured!) mice to calculate the average survival time, and thus ignored the merit of any cures [32]! The results were published in reputable journals [30-33]. The contenders' results [33], to our knowledge, were never retracted.

The NIH, as does the profession at large, continue to disregard the benefit from chrono-chemotherapy or -radiotherapy [34-37]. Radiation, when timed at the peak of the patient's tumor temperature, has doubled the 2-year disease free survival rate of patients with perioral cancers in India in the hands of Dr. B.D. Gupta and Dr. Akhil Deka, another Indian achievement [34, 38].

Chronobiology has also been largely ignored in cardiology, recommendations by several international consensus meetings [e.g., 39] based on the documented risks associated with abnormal dynamics within the normal range and the demonstrated benefits from chronotherapy notwithstanding. If the already-available information is disseminated, thanks to Prof. R.B. Singh, many strokes and other hard events may be prevented in his setting in Moradabad and in neighboring settings, as a model for the world as a whole, yet with modest local resources. We wish him success as chief editor in seeing to it that health care does not "fly blind", as another journal's leader put it in a spontaneous editorial [40].

EPILOGUE

This editorial is dedicated to the memory of Kozo OKAMOTO, to whom we owe the spontaneously hypertensive rat (SHR), in particular the stroke-prone SHR (SHR-SP). Thanks to him, the diagnosis of essential or idiopathic hypertension, implying the absence of a known cause for high BP, can be scrutinized in its time course in the light of a model amenable to scrutiny in terms of its genetics and of the role played by environmental loads. In the pre-telemetry era, under the burdens of repeated 4-hourly measurements, with the animal in a wire mesh screen under a gooseneck lamp, circadian BP overswinging was first documented and led us to intensify focus on BP variability [41]. Kozo Okamoto was well aware of the importance of doing this with due regard for rhythms: When a pharmaceutical company offered him a round trip ticket from Japan to the U.S. National Institutes of Health (NIH) (to which he was invited for lectures by a friend who was director of the NIH clinical center) and to the pharmaceutical company's headquarters, but the company would not pay for a side trip to Minnesota in their offering, Dr. Okamoto cancelled his visits to the NIH and to the pharmaceutical company, bought his own ticket to Minnesota, along with that of a colleague, and graced us with his and his colleague' presence as houseguests, and with the greatest gift, i.a., of the SHR-SP rats that led to the finding of circadian hyper-amplitude-tension under a load of handling for measurement by immobilization and heating for tail blood sphygmomanometry, but not in the absence of these acute burdens, albeit with a permanently implanted catheter [41].

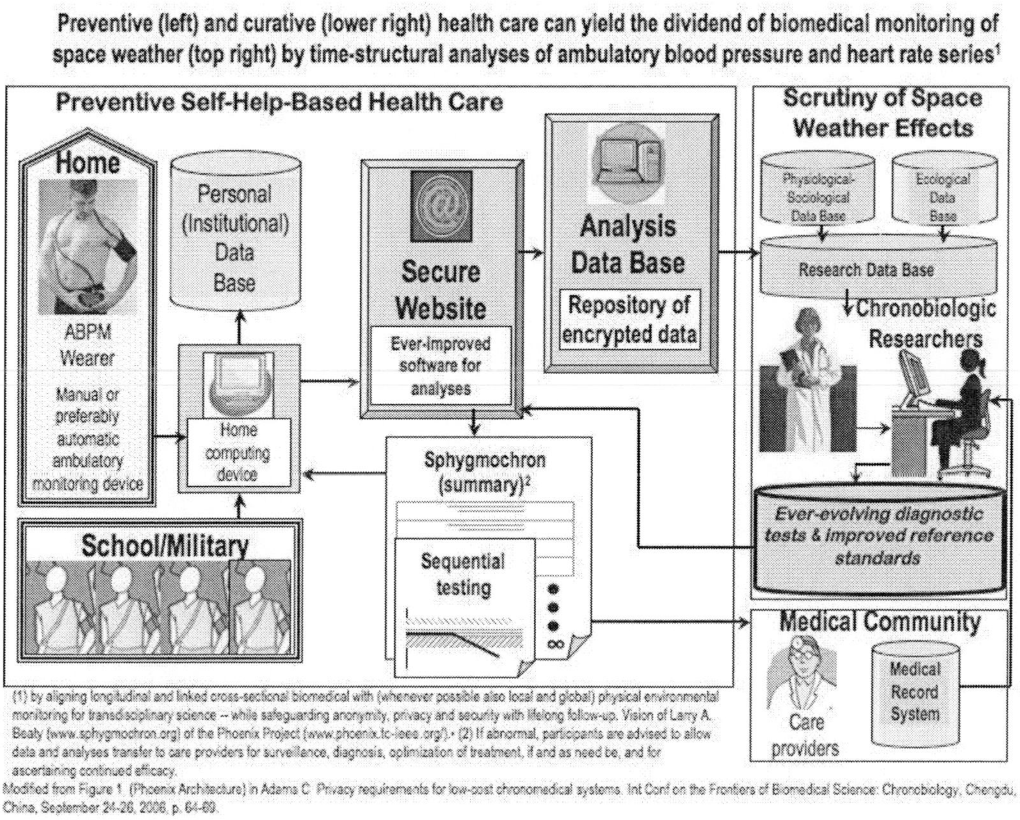

Figure 5. The Phoenix Project of volunteering members of the Twin Cities chapter of the Institute of Electrical and Electronics Engineers (http://www.phoenix.tc-ieee.org/) is planning on developing an inexpensive, cuffless automatic monitor of blood pressure and on implementing the concept of a website (www.sphygmochron.org/) for a service in exchange for the data that in turn are to be used for refining methods and for monitoring psychophysiological effects of the variability in space weather. © Halberg.

We have much to learn about the mechanisms involved in a worldwide hypertension and prehypertension [42-48], in the first model for prehypertension validated in humans. Telemetry is now available for rodents and, we trust, will someday become available for humans as well. Manual measurements can also serve [16, 42], if they are chronomically assessed. In advocating time-microscopy, the new World Heart Journal could open many eyes, just as in diagnosing a malignant tumor, we no longer rely on tumor, rubor, calor, and dolor, but use microscopy. By the same token, a microscopy in time is needed for hypertension and prehypertension not to remain silent to the care receiver and care provider. A multilingual website, Figure 5 (http://www.sphygmochron.org/), now planned by the Phoenix Project of the Twin Cities chapter of the Institute of Electrical and Electronics Engineers (IEEE) (http://www.phoenix.tc-ieee.org), may serve for both self-help in health care and research, which has most recently revealed associations of terrorism [49, 50] as well as suicides [51] and tachyarrhythmias [52] with heliogeo-magnetics. Figure 6 broadens the perspective from circadian hemianopsia to a wide spectrum of novel components that relate to dying suddenly [52] or by one's own hand [51] or being killed [49, 50].

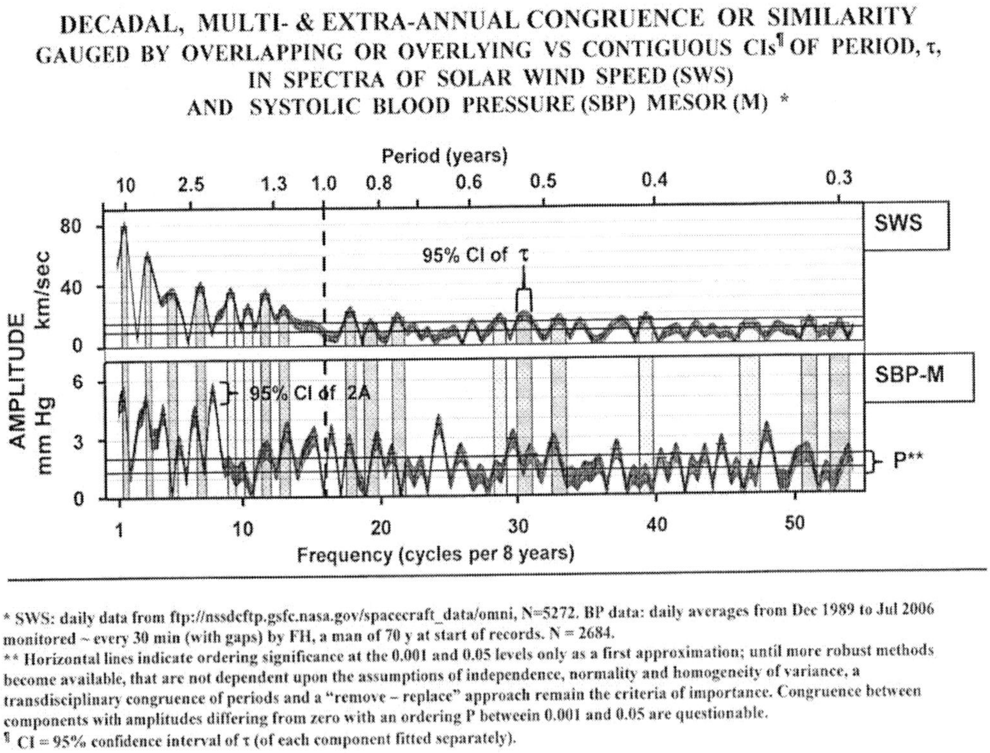

Figure 6. Congruent periods, τ, in the biosphere and around us [52] point to associations between the human circulation (as a gauge of biospheric response) and its cosmos (read: space weather). While no causal relations are implied by the findings as such of periods with overlapping if not overlying 95% confidence intervals, the subtraction and addition approach [12] provides evidence of interactions, awaiting associations with photic and nonphotic cycles on the one hand and morbidity and mortality cycles in solar activity on the other hand. Just as are the photic and thermal, now also societal cycles of the day and night and of the seasons, so may nonphotic cycles also be coded in our genes. © Halberg.

REFERENCES

[1] Otsuka K, Cornélissen G, Schwartzkopff O, Bakken EE, Halberg F, Burioka N, Katinas GS, Kane R, Regal PJ, Schaffer E, Sonkowsky R, Patterson R, Engebretson M, Brockway B, Wang ZR, Delmore P, Halpin C, Sarkozy S, Wall D, Halberg J. Clinical chronobiology and chronome-geriatrics: At variance with recommendations of subsequent guidelines, yet focusing indeed on pre-hypertension in the physiological range. *Biomed Pharmacother* 2003; 57 (Suppl 1): 164s-198s.

[2] Cornélissen G, Halberg F, Bakken EE, Singh RB, Otsuka K, Tomlinson B, Delcourt A, Toussaint G, Bathina S, Schwartzkopff O, Wang ZR, Tarquini R, Perfetto F, Pantaleoni GC, Jozsa R, Delmore PA, Nolley E. 100 or 30 years after Janeway or Bartter, Healthwatch helps avoid "flying blind". *Biomed Pharmacother* 2004; 58 (Suppl 1): S69-S86.

[3] Halberg F, Cornélissen G, Katinas G, Tvildiani L, Gigolashvili M, Janashia K, Toba T, Revilla M, Regal P, Sothern RB, Wendt HW, Wang ZR, Zeman M, Jozsa R, Singh RB, Mitsutake G, Chibisov SM, Lee J, Holley D, Holte JE, Sonkowsky RP, Schwartzkopff O, Delmore P, Otsuka K, Bakken EE, Czaplicki J, International BIOCOS Group. Chronobiology's progress: Part II, chronomics for an immediately applicable biomedicine. *J Applied Biomedicine* 2006; 4: 73-86. *http://www.zsf.jcu.cz/vyzkum /jab/4_2/halberg 2.pdf.*

[4] Cornélissen G, Chen CH, Halberg F. Predictive value of blood pressure variability: merits of circadian parameters versus dipping patterns. *N Engl J Med* 2006 [Aug 14]; 355; 8: 850.

[5] Halberg F, Cornélissen G, Halberg J, Schwartzkopff O. Pre-hypertensive and other variabilities also await treatment. *Am J Medicine* 2007; 120: e19-e20. doi:10.1016 /j.amjmed.2006.02.045.

[6] Cornélissen G, Halberg F, Otsuka K, Singh RB, Chen CH. Chronobiology predicts actual and proxy outcomes when dipping fails. *Hypertension* 2007; 49: 237-239. doi:10.1161/01.HYP.0000250392.51418.64.

[7] Sanchez de la Pena S, Gonzalez C, Cornélissen G, Halberg F. Blood pressure (BP), heart rate (HR) and non-insulin-dependent diabetes mellitus (NIDDM) chronobiology. Abstract S8-06, 3rd Int Congress on Cardiovascular Disease, Taipei, Taiwan, 26-28 Nov 2004. *Int J Cardiol* 2004; 97 (Suppl 2): S14.

[8] Halberg F, Cornélissen G, Sothern RB, Hillman D, Katinas GS, Nolley ES, Beaty LA, Otsuka K, Siegelova J, Greenway F, Gupta A, Revilla M, Masalov M, Syutkina EV, Malkova I, Chibisov SM, Schwartzkopff O, Bakken EE. Global challenges of monitoring vascular variability and space weather. In: Halberg F, Kenner T, Fiser B, Siegelova J, eds. *Proceedings, Noninvasive Methods in Cardiology* 2007, Brno, Czech Republic, November 11-14, 2007. Brno: Department of Functional Diagnostics and Rehabilitation, Faculty of Medicine, Masaryk University (ISBN 978 80 7018 463 4); 2007. p. 10-27.

[9] Halberg F, Cornélissen G, Otsuka K, Watanabe Y, Katinas GS, Burioka N, Delyukov A, Gorgo Y, Zhao ZY, Weydahl A, Sothern RB, Siegelova J, Fiser B, Dusek J, Syutkina EV, Perfetto F, Tarquini R, Singh RB, Rhees B, Lofstrom D, Lofstrom P, Johnson PWC, Schwartzkopff O, International BIOCOS Study Group. Cross-spectrally

coherent ~10.5- and 21-year biological and physical cycles, magnetic storms and myocardial infarctions. *Neuroendocrinol Lett* 2000; 21: 233-258.

[10] Cornélissen G, Halberg F, Breus T, Syutkina EV, Baevsky R, Weydahl A, Watanabe Y, Otsuka K, Siegelova J, Fiser B, Bakken EE. Non-photic solar associations of heart rate variability and myocardial infarction. *J Atmos Solar-Terr Phys* 2002; 64: 707-720.

[11] Halberg F, Cornélissen G, Regal P, Otsuka K, Wang ZR, Katinas GS, Siegelova J, Homolka P, Prikryl P, Chibisov SM, Holley DC, Wendt HW, Bingham C, Palm SL, Sonkowsky RP, Sothern RB, Pales E, Mikulecky M, Tarquini R, Perfetto F, Salti R, Maggioni C, Jozsa R, Konradov AA, Kharlitskaya EV, Revilla M, Wan CM, Herold M, Syutkina EV, Masalov AV, Faraone P, Singh RB, Singh RK, Kumar A, Singh R, Sundaram S, Sarabandi T, Pantaleoni GC, Watanabe Y, Kumagai Y, Gubin D, Uezono K, Olah A, Borer K, Kanabrocki EA, Bathina S, Haus E, Hillman D, Schwartzkopff O, Bakken EE, Zeman M. Chronoastrobiology: proposal, nine conferences, heliogeomagnetics, transyears, near-weeks, near-decades, phylogenetic and ontogenetic memories. *Biomed Pharmacother* 2004; 58 (Suppl 1): S150-S187.

[12] Halberg F, Cornélissen G, Katinas G, Tvildiani L, Gigolashvili M, Janashia K, Toba T, Revilla M, Regal P, Sothern RB, Wendt HW, Wang ZR, Zeman M, Jozsa R, Singh RB, Mitsutake G, Chibisov SM, Lee J, Holley D, Holte JE, Sonkowsky RP, Schwartzkopff O, Delmore P, Otsuka K, Bakken EE, Czaplicki J, International BIOCOS Group. Chronobiology's progress: Part I, season's appreciations 2004-2005. Time-, frequency-, phase-, variable-, individual-, age- and site-specific chronomics. *J Applied Biomedicine* 2006; 4: 1-38. *http://www.zsf.jcu.cz/vyzkum/jab/4_1/ halberg.pdf.*

[13] Cornélissen G, Halberg F, Singh RB, International BIOCOS Group. Editorial: unseen space weather also relates to cardiac events. This volume.

[14] Nozawa M, Sugimoto K-i, Ohmori M, Ando H, Fujimura A. Dosing time-dependent effect of temocapril on the mortality of stroke-prone spontaneously hypertensive rats. *J Pharmacol Exp Ther* 2006; 316: 176-181.

[15] Singh RB, Cornélissen G, Kumar A, Bathina S, Halberg F. Active prayer lowering heart rate variability along the scale of 168 hours in Asian Indians. *Proceedings, International Conference on the Frontiers of Biomedical Science: Chronobiology*, Chengdu, China, September 24-26, 2006, p. 193-195.

[16] Singh RB, Cornélissen G, Siegelova J, Homolka P, Halberg F. About half-weekly (circasemiseptan) pattern of blood pressure and heart rate in men and women of India. *Scripta medica (Brno)* 2002; 75: 125-128.

[17] Hagen P (ed.) *Mayo Clinic Guide to Self-Care: Answers for Everyday Health Problems.* Rochester, MN / Jacksonville, FL / Scottsdale, AZ: Mayo Clinic; 2003. p. 180-181.

[18] Pickering TG, Shimbo D, Haas D. Ambulatory blood pressure monitoring. *N Engl J Med* 2006; 354: 2368-2374.

[19] Bartter FC. Periodicity and medicine. In: Scheving LE, Halberg F, Pauly JE, eds. *Chronobiology*. Tokyo: Igaku Shoin Ltd., 1974: 6-13.

[20] Güllner HG, Bartter FC, Halberg F. Timing antihypertensive medication. *The Lancet*, September 8, 1979: 527.

[21] Janeway TC. *The clinical study of blood pressure*. New York: D. Appleton & Co., 1904, 300 pp.

[22] Halberg F. Chronobiology. *Annu Rev Physiol* 1969; 31: 675-725.

[23] Cornélissen G, Halberg F. Chronomedicine. In: Armitage P, Colton T, editors. *Encyclopedia of Biostatistics*, 2nd ed. Chichester, UK: John Wiley & Sons Ltd; 2005. p. 796-812.

[24] Cornélissen G, Bakken E, Delmore P, Orth-Gomer K, Akerstedt T, Carandente O, Carandente F, Halberg F. From various kinds of heart rate variability to chronocardiology. *Am J Cardiol* 1990; 66: 863-868.

[25] Wood MA, Simpson PM, London WB, Stambler BS, Herre JM, Bernstein RC, Ellenbogen KA. Circadian pattern of ventricular tachyarrhythmias in patients with implantable cardioverter-defibrillators. *J Am Coll Cardiol* 1995; 25: 901-907.

[26] Halberg F, Cornélissen G, Otsuka K, Watanabe Y, Wood MA, Lambert CR, Zaslavskaya R, Gubin D, Petukhova EY, Delmore P, Bakken E. Rewards in practice from recycling heart rate, ectopy, ischemia, and blood pressure information. *J Medical Engineering & Technology* 1997; 21: 174-184.

[27] Mitro P, Pella D, Rybar R, Valocik G, editors. *Proceedings, 2nd Congress on Cardiovascular Diseases*, Kosice, Slovakia, 25-27 April 2002. Bologna: Monduzzi Editore; 2002.

[28] Abstracts of the 3rd International Congress on Cardiovascular Disease, Taipei, Taiwan, 26-28 Nov 2004. *Int J Cardiol* 2004; 97 (Suppl 2): S1-S81.

[29] Liebigs Annalen/Recueil: Aims and Scope. *http://www.interscience.wiley.com/jpages/0947-3440/aims.html. (c) 2003.*

[30] Haus E, Halberg F, Scheving L, Pauly JE, Cardoso S, Kuehl JFW, Sothern R, Shiotsuka RN, Hwang DS. Increased tolerance of leukemic mice to arabinosyl cytosine given on schedule adjusted to circadian system. *Science* 1972; 177: 80-82.

[31] Halberg F, Haus E, Cardoso SS, Scheving LE, Kuehl JFW, Shiotsuka R, Rosene G, Pauly JE, Runge W, Spalding JF, Lee JK, Good RA. Toward a chronotherapy of neoplasia: Tolerance of treatment depends upon host rhythms. *Experientia (Basel)* 1973; 29: 909-934.

[32] Halberg F, Nelson W, Cornélissen G, Haus E, Scheving LE, Good RA. On methods for testing and achieving cancer chronotherapy. *Cancer Treatment Rep* 1979; 63: 1428-1430.

[33] Rose WC, Trader MW, Laster WR Jr, Schabel FM Jr. Chronochemotherapy of L1210 leukemic mice with cytosine arabinoside or cyclophosphamide. *Cancer Treatment Reports* 1978; 62(9): 1337-1349.

[34] Halberg F. Biological as well as physical parameters relate to radiology. Guest Lecture, *Proc. 30th Ann. Cong. Rad.*, January 1977, Post-Graduate Institute of Medical Education and Research, Chandigarh, India, 8 pp.

[35] Halberg F, Gupta BD, Haus E, Halberg E, Deka AC, Nelson W, Sothern RB, Cornélissen G, Lee JK, Lakatua DJ, Scheving LE, Burns ER. Steps toward a cancer chronopolytherapy. In: *Proc. XIV International Congress of Therapeutics*. Montpellier, France: L'Expansion Scientifique Française; 1977. p. 151-196.

[36] Halberg Francine, Halberg J, Halberg E, Halberg Franz. Chronobiology, radiobiology and steps toward the timing of cancer radiotherapy. In: Goldson AL (vol ed.) *Cancer Growth and Progression*, vol. 9, ch. 19, Kaiser H (series ed.) Dordrecht: Kluwer Academic Publ.; 1989. p. 227-253.

[37] Cornélissen G, Halberg F. The chronobiologic pilot study with special reference to cancer research: Is chronobiology or, rather, its neglect wasteful? In: Goldson AL (vol

ed.) *Cancer Growth and Progression*, vol. 9, ch. 9, Kaiser H (series ed.) Dordrecht: Kluwer Academic Publ.; 1989. p. 103-133.

[38] Halberg F, Cornélissen G, Wang ZR, Wan C, Ulmer W, Katinas G, Singh Ranjana, Singh RK, Singh Rajesh, Gupta BD, Singh RB, Kumar A, Kanabrocki E, Sothern RB, Rao G, Bhatt MLBD, Srivastava M, Rai G, Singh S, Pati AK, Nath P, Halberg Francine, Halberg J, Schwartzkopff O, Bakken E, Shastri VK. Chronomics: circadian and circaseptan timing of radiotherapy, drugs, calories, perhaps nutriceuticals and beyond. *J Exp Therapeutics Oncol* 2003; 3: 223-260.

[39] Halberg F, Cornélissen G, International Womb-to-Tomb Chronome Initiative Group: Resolution from a meeting of the International Society for Research on Civilization Diseases and the Environment (New SIRMCE Confederation), Brussels, Belgium, March 17-18, 1995: Fairy tale or reality? *Medtronic Chronobiology Seminar* #8, April 1995, 12 pp. text, 18 figures. *http://www.msi.umn.edu/~halberg/*

[40] Fossel M. Editor's Note [to Halberg F, Cornélissen G, Halberg J, Fink H, Chen C-H, Otsuka K, Watanabe Y, Kumagai Y, Syutkina EV, Kawasaki T, Uezono K, Zhao ZY, Schwartzkopff O. Circadian Hyper-Amplitude-Tension, CHAT: a disease risk syndrome of anti-aging medicine]. *J Anti-Aging Med* 1998; 1: 239.

[41] Halberg J, Halberg E, Hayes DK, Smith RD, Halberg F, Delea CS, Danielson RS, Bartter FC. Schedule shifts, life quality and quantity modeled by murine blood pressure elevation and arthropod lifespan. *Int J Chronobiol* 1980; 7: 17-64.

[42] Stinson SM, Cornélissen G, Scarpelli PT, Halberg F. Self-measurement and ambulatory monitoring of blood pressure: a subject's chronobiological perspective. *Biomed Pharmacother* 2002; 56 (Suppl 2): 333s-338s.

[43] Halberg Franz, Cornélissen G, Katinas G, Syutkina EV, Sothern RB, Zaslavskaya R, Halberg Francine, Watanabe Y, Schwartzkopff O, Otsuka K, Tarquini R, Perfetto P, Siegelova J. Transdisciplinary unifying implications of circadian findings in the 1950s. *J Circadian Rhythms* 2003; 1: 2. 61 pp. *www.JCircadianRhythms.com /content/pdf/1740-3391/1/2.pdf*

[44] Cornélissen G, Delcourt A, Toussaint G, Otsuka K, Watanabe Y, Siegelova J, Fiser B, Dusek J, Homolka P, Singh RB, Kumar A, Singh RK, Sanchez S, Gonzalez C, Holley D, Sundaram B, Zhao Z, Tomlinson B, Fok B, Zeman M, Dulkova K, Halberg F. Opportunity of detecting pre-hypertension: worldwide data on blood pressure overswinging. *Biomed Pharmacother* 2005; 59 (Suppl 1): S152-S157.

[45] Kumagai Y, Shiga T, Sunaga K, Cornélissen G, Ebihara A, Halberg F. Usefulness of circadian amplitude of blood pressure in predicting hypertensive cardiac involvement. *Chronobiologia* 1992; 19: 43-58.

[46] Watanabe Y, Cornélissen G, Halberg F, Bingham C, Siegelova J, Otsuka K, Kikuchi T. Incidence pattern and treatment of a clinical entity, overswinging or circadian hyperamplitudetension (CHAT). *Scripta medica (Brno)* 1997; 70: 245-261.

[47] Kumagai Y, Cornélissen G, Halberg F, Watanabe Y, Otsuka K, Schwartzkopff O, Singh RB. Kumagai's, Cugini's and other vascular variability disorders, detected chronobiologically, misdiagnosed by dipping. PS-050, *Proceedings, 2nd World Congress of Chronobiology*, November 4-6, 2007, Tokyo, Japan, p. 86.

[48] Cornélissen G, Cugini P, Siegelova J, Fiser B, Halberg F. Cugini's minimal change hypertensive retinopathy, resolved chronobiologically while dipping fails, supports the concept of 'pre-hypertension'. In: Halberg F, Kenner T, Fiser B, Siegelova J, eds.

Proceedings, Noninvasive Methods in Cardiology 2007, Brno, Czech Republic, November 11-14, 2007. Brno: Department of Functional Diagnostics and Rehabilitation, Faculty of Medicine, Masaryk University (ISBN 978 80 7018 463 4); 2007. p. 55-61.

[49] Halberg F, Cornélissen G, Sothern RB, Chibisov SM, Wendt H. Do unseen, very weak magnetic mechanisms contribute to terrorism in wobbly spectral windows? *8th Int Cong "Health and education millennium"*, People's Friendship University of Russia, Moscow, Russia, November 14-17, 2007, in press.

[50] Cornélissen G, Halberg F, Wendt H, Chibisov SM. Human violence-terrorism characterized by Aeolian weak magnetoperiodism, an ~1.3-year (transyear) cycle, rather than an annual socio-photo-thermoperiodism. *8th Int Cong "Health and education millennium",* People's Friendship University of Russia, Moscow, Russia, November 14-17, 2007, in press.

[51] Cornélissen G, Halberg F. Chronomics of suicides and the solar wind. *Br J Psychiatry* 2006; 189: 567-568.

[52] Cornélissen G, Benser M, Halberg F. Patterns of incidence of tachyarrhythmias recorded in implantable cardioverter-defibrillators during 2001-2005. PS-004, *Proceedings, 2nd World Congress of Chronobiology*, November 4-6, 2007, Tokyo, Japan, p. 63.

In: World Heart Research Yearbook. Volume 1
Editors: Franz Halberg and R. B. Singh
ISBN: 978-1-60741-881-8

UNSEEN SPACE WEATHER ALSO RELATES TO CARDIAC EVENTS

Germaine Cornélissen[1], Franz Halberg[1], R. B. Singh[2] and the International BIOCOS (The BIOsphere and the COSmos) Project
[1] University of Minnesota, Minneapolis, MN, US
[2] Halberg Hospital and Research Institute, Moradabad, India

MEMBERS OF THE INTERNATIONAL PROJECT ON THE BIOSPHERE AND THE COSMOS (BIOCOS)

Armenia: Nubar Aslanyan, Institute of Cardiology, Yerevan.

Belgium: Jean De Prins, Université Libre de Bruxelles, Brussels; Christian Muller, Olga Quadens, Aerospace Institute, Brussels; Alain Delcourt and Guy Toussaint, private practice physicians, Brussels.

Brazil: Nelson Marques, Luiz Menna Barreto, University of São Paulo.

China: Zhengrong Wang and Jinyi Wu, West China University of Medical Sciences, Chengdu; Ziyan Zhao, Shandong Academy of Medical Sciences, Jinan.

Czech Republic: Bohumil Fiser, Jarmila Siegelova, Jiri Dusek, Pavel Homolka, Muhammad Al-Kubati, Pavel Prikryl, Masaryk University, Brno; Jaroslav Strestik, Geophysical Institute, Academy of Sciences of the Czech Republic, Prague.

Germany: John Komlos, Department of Economics, University of Munich; Sigrid Berger, University of Heidelberg; Karl Hecht, Charité Hospital, Humboldt University, Berlin.

Hungary: Rita Jozsa, University Pécs.

India: R.B. Singh, Medical Hospital and Research Centre, Centre for Nutrition and Heart Research, Moradabad; R.K. Singh, Department of Biochemistry, King George's Medical College, Lucknow; Atanu Kumar Pati, Pandit Ravishankar Shukla University, Raipur.

Italy: Franca Carandente, Department of Chronobiology, and Cristina Maggioni, Department of Obstetrics, University of Milan; Giacomo Laffi, Federico Perfetto, Roberto Tarquini, Carlo Rostagno, Department of Medicine; Roberto Salti, Mayer Pediatric Hospital, University of Florence.

Japan: Kuniaki Otsuka, Yoshihiko Watanabe and Gen Mitsutake, Department of Medicine, Tokyo Women's Medical University, Medical Center East, Tokyo; Terukazu Kawasaki and Keiko Uezono, Institute of Health Sciences, Kyushu University, Fukuoka; Yuji

Kumagai, Jichi Medical School, Tochigi; Naoto Burioka, 3rd Department of Internal Medicine, Tottori University, Yonago.

Mexico: Salvador Sánchez de la Peña, Instituto Mexicano del Seguro Social, Mexico City.

Norway: Andi Weydahl, Finnmark College, Alta.

Russia: Mikhail Blank and Olga Denisova, N.N. Petrov Oncology Research Institute, Ministry of Health; Tamara K. Breus, Space Research Institute, Moscow; Semyon I. Rapoport, Moscow Medical Academy, Moscow; Maria Mitish, Elena V. Syutkina, Tatiana Turti, Galina V. Yatsyk, Institute of Pediatrics, Academy of Medical Sciences, Moscow; Anatoly Masalov, Lebedev Physics Institute, Moscow; Rina M. Zaslavskaya, Moscow Hospital #60, Moscow; Sergey M. Chibisov, Russian People's Friendship University, Moscow.

Slovakia: Anna Gvozdjakova, Miroslav Mikulecky Sr, and Michal Zeman, Comenius University, Bratislava.

Spain: Miguel Revilla, Department of Mathematics and Computer Science, University of Valladolid.

Switzerland: Waldemar Ulmer, Varian International, Zug.

UK: Douglas Wilson, ADAS Bioengineering Unit, Cheltenham, England; Hugh Simpson, Department of Surgery, University of Glasgow, Scotland.

USA: Germaine Cornélissen, Franz Halberg, Chronobiology Laboratories; Dana Johnson, Department of Pediatrics; Christopher Bingham, Douglas Hawkins, Department of Applied Statistics; Jim Holte, Department of Electrical Engineering; Mark Engebretson, Department of Space Physics, Augsburg College, Minneapolis, Minnesota; Earl Bakken, Medtronic Inc, Minneapolis, Minnesota; Dan Holley, Department of Biological Sciences, San Jose State University, San Jose, California; Sasikumar Sundaram, United Medical Center, Cheyenne, Wyoming.

Relationships between coronary disease and meteorology were documented in 10-year data as a 13% increase in event rates of all age groups ($P<0.0001$) (18% for the 55- to 64-year olds) with a 10°C decrease in temperature [1], a finding in keeping with the highest fatality from acute myocardial infarction (MI) on the coldest days reported from Helsinki in 1977 [2] and other meteorological analyses in relation to MI [3]. The effect of cold weather is also documented in the laboratory on days when ECG was monitored after ligation of the descending coronary artery in dogs: more sudden deaths occurred in November-February (42%) vs. July-August (6%) [4]. Contradictory reports from subtropical climates claim that the seasons do not [5] or do [6] affect the frequency of acute MI. In cold cities, both high and low temperatures were associated with increased cardiovascular mortality [7].

As to hot temperatures acting specifically upon hospital admissions for heart disease, much of the effect has been interpreted as an increase with average temperature constituting a short-term displacement of pattern [8]. Other preliminary data also suggest that atrial fibrillation-related mortality extends beyond colder climates to hotter climates (with sufficiently large relative changes in ambient temperature during the year) [9].

This finding is in keeping with the number of deaths in patients with congestive heart failure after prior MI in cold- and warm-weather months being higher than that in spring and fall months [10].

Against this background, Pella et al. [11], based on a paper by the chief editor [12], review the role of hot, not only of cold climate in the genesis of MI. Apart from focus only upon the extremes of weather on earth triggering cardiac events, even the usual change of the seasons corresponding to the calendar year suffices to show, among other temporal factors, an association with MI, as seen in the middle of Figure 1 for Minnesota, USA [13]. By comparison to the role of the photic and thermic and now also societal changes in the earth's proximate climate, any association of MI with unseen space weather seems relatively small, although it is present, as shown in part by a circadecadal component (Figure 1, left) [13, 14]. A far-transyear [15, 16] with a period of about 1.23 years and a CI (95% confidence interval) from 1.20 to 1.26 years and a near-transyear [17] of about 1.05 years with a CI not overlapping the precise calendar year are also present in MI in Minnesota (1968-1996). The far-transyear's amplitude is just 17% of that of the calendar year, Figure 2.

The 10.7-year amplitude is 95% of that of the half-year, which also constitutes a geomagnetic signature [18]. In keeping with Pella et al. [11] and Singh et al. [12] and others [1-4, 6-10], however, photic and thermic components predominate in the spectrum of MI. Non-photics include a heliomagnetic circadecadal, a transyearly and a cis-half-yearly component [19, 20; cf. 21], all having a smaller amplitude. The half-year is also prominent, whether it accounts for a nonsinusoidal circannual component, or whether it represents in part a non-photic geomagnetic effect [18].

With the separation by the 10th revision of the International Classification of Diseases (ICD10) of MI from sudden cardiac death (SCD), space weather gains in importance in certain geographic, geomagnetic or dip-magnetic location. By contrast to MI, the latter electrical incidents of the heart (ICD10 code I46.1), at least in some specific localities and at certain times thus far (and not overall) have patterns that correspond to features of unseen space weather, Figure 3. A far-transyear, with a period longer than a year by a few months, characterizes the incidence of SCD in Arkansas, Minnesota, Tokyo (Japan), and the Czech Republic. A cis-half-year, with a period of about 5 months, is detected in Minnesota, Tokyo (Japan), Austria and the Czech Republic, among others.

These spectral components resemble cycles seen in the speed of the ionized particles ejected by the sun, called the solar wind [22, 23], or in cosmic rays [24], and also found in geomagnetics [25]. The prevalence in Minnesota solely of a transyear, longer than a calendar year by several months, with no calendar-yearly component in SCD contrasts with both a calendar-year component and a transyear found in Arkansas, USA, and in the Czech Republic, and only a calendar-year component in North Carolina, USA, in Hungary, the Republic of Georgia, Latvia, Lithuania and Hong Kong, Figure 3 [21, 26-29].

In addition to transyears, a signature of hard solar flares [19, 20] is also seen in SCD in Minnesota, Hungary and Lithuania, and part of the time in the Czech Republic [21]. The contrast in Minnesota between SCD (Figure 3) and MI (Figure 2) awaits scrutiny on longer-than-available time series on both conditions in the same localities.

Clinical implications are:

1. The decision to separate MI from electrical accidents of the heart in ICD10 is supported in some geographic locations by drastically different patterns in spectra of their incidences, based on MI that exclude SCD vs. the spectra (of the non-photic solar signatures) of SCD.

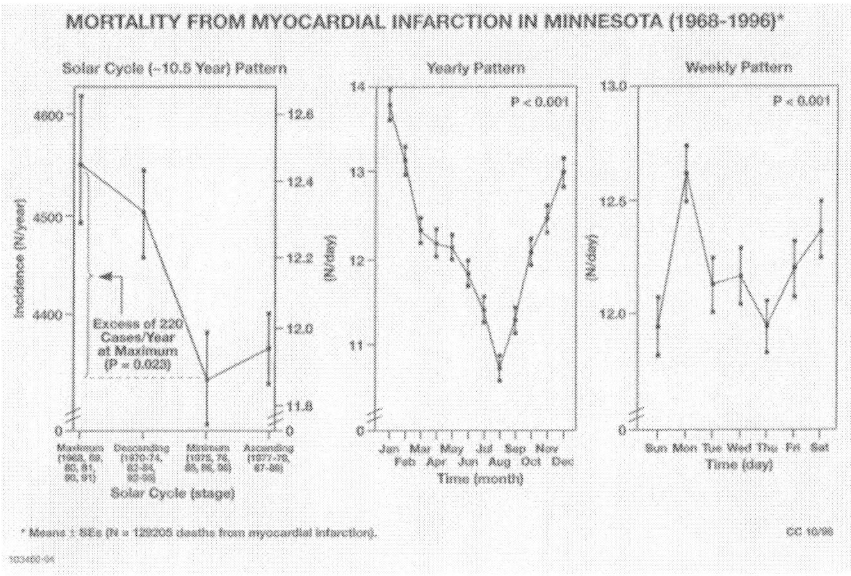

Figure 1. Non-random patterns of incidence of 129,205 deaths from myocardial infarction in Minnesota (1968-1996) along the scales of the photic and thermic year (middle), of the non-photic helio- and geomagnetic about 6.75-day but socially synchronized week (right), and of Schwabe's about 10.5-year sunspot activity cycle (left). Data shown as means ± SEs. As compared to times of solar minimum, there is an excess of 220 deaths/year at times of solar maximum [13,14]. © Halberg.

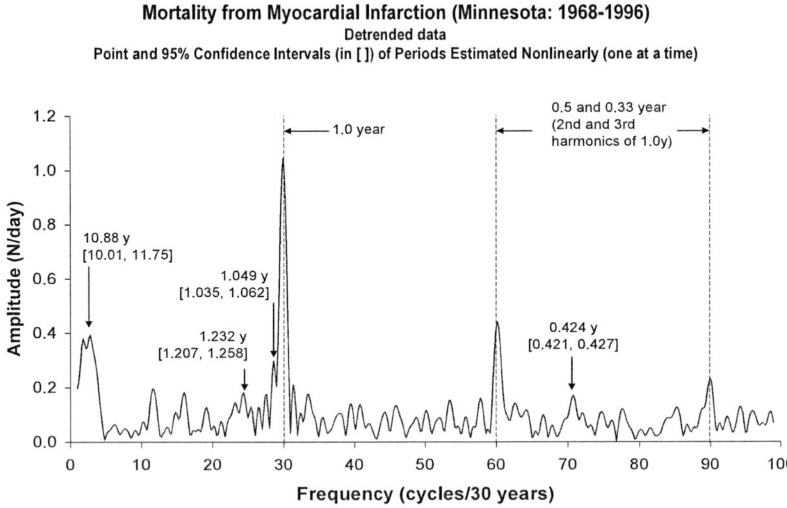

Figure 2. Spectral visualization of the importance of the photic circannual feature in mortality from myocardial infarction (vertical dashed lines and horizontal arrows at first 3 harmonics of 1 year). The vertical arrows emphasize separate peaks of probable non-photic origin, with amplitudes much smaller than that of the photic yearly component. A near-transyear of about 1.05 years (in biology, beyond MI) is also found in other variables and has a 95% confidence interval (CI) not overlapping precisely one year. So does a far-transyear of about 1.23 years, corresponding roughly to a component often found in solar wind speed. The about 0.42-year cis-halfyear has a CI not overlapping the precise half-year, which could represent the waveform of the yearly component or could also be contributed by geomagnetics [18]. By contrast, the cis-halfyear corresponds to a periodicity in hard solar flares [19, 20; cf. 21]. © Halberg.

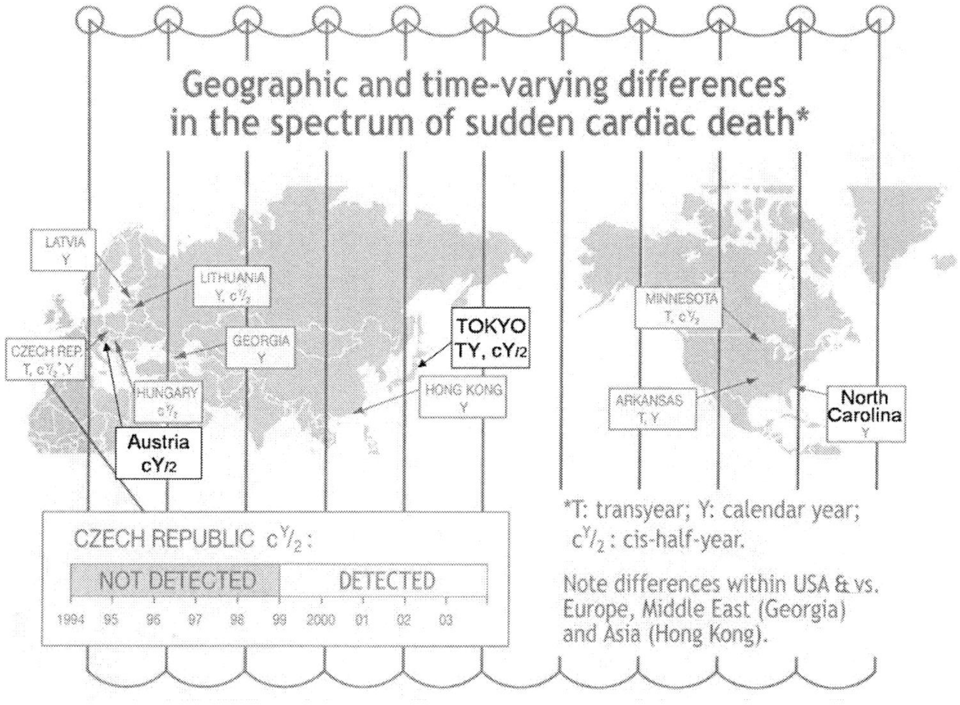

Figure 3. A curtain of uncertainty, because of limited available data, hides any time- and geographic (geomagnetic or dip-magnetic) site-specificity of various spectral aspects of sudden cardiac death (SCD). Thus, we find a transyear in Minnesota with a cis-half-year (cY/2) and both a calendar year and a transyear in Arkansas and the Czech Republic: at the latter site, a cis-half-year, corresponding to an also-transient cycle in hard solar flares [19, 20], is detected after but not before 1999 [21]. In 1998, Minorsky [30] re-evaluated latitudinal differences in coconut palms' foliar spiral direction (FSD). He hypothesized that latitude-dependent biases in FSD, a non-Mendelian trait, will be associated with a temporally varying component of the earth's magnetic field. Earth currents, which are measurable in trees, bias the difference of auxin (or auxin transport proteins) in young embryos, such that left-handed palm trees (LHP) are produced preferentially in the Northern Hemisphere and right-handed ones (RHP) in the Southern Hemisphere. He built his observations on a previously collected data base by Davis and Davis, revealing that the ratio of LHP – RHP / total was better correlated with magnetic (dip) latitude than with geographic or geomagnetic (centered dipole) latitude. Minorsky and Bronstein [32] referred to this classical case of morphological antisymmetry in which dextral and sinistral forms are not inherited and are equally common within a species, proposing that Pc1-induced earth currents may bias the diffusion of morphogens in coconut palm embryos, thereby giving rise in asymmetries of FSD. Whether other geographic differences in SCD may also relate to any magnetic latitude deserves scrutiny, notably since cardiac arrhythmias can also transiently reveal a transyear or a cishalfyear, each in a different solar Schwabe cycle stage [21]. © Halberg.

2. The signatures in SCD of transyears of the solar wind and cosmic rays and of cis-halfyears of hard solar flares are modulated by telluric factors that underlie the unequal geographic/geomagnetic/dip-magnetic distribution of non-photic cyclic patterns and may provide clues to physical environmental influences associated with SCD.
3. To the extent that a weak correlation with geomagnetics of SCD [28] can be confirmed and the mechanisms of solar-terrestrial interaction in SCD are identified, improvements may be undertaken in devices such as cardiac pacemaker-cardioverter-

defibrillators, notably since the incidence of tachyarrhythmia recorded by such devices may mimic the pattern of SCD [31].

4. The systematic recording of health statistics in different geographic locations [21, 30, cf. 32, 33] and their associations with environmental variables may help our understanding of underlying risks and may help design preventive countermeasures.
5. As the care recipient and caregiver learn about effects of space weather, a report on earth weather should gradually include also events occurring beyond our protective magnetosphere.

References

[1] Danet S, Richard F, Montaye M, Beauchant S, Lemaire B, Graux C, Cottel D, Marécaux N, Amouyel P. Unhealthy effects of atmospheric temperature and pressure on the occurrence of myocardial infarction and coronary deaths. A 10-year survey: the Lille-World Health Organization MONICA Project (Monitoring Trends and Determinants in Cardiovascular Disease). *Circulation* 1999; 100: e1-e7.

[2] Sarna S, Romo M, Siltanen P. Myocardial infarction and weather. *Annals of Clinical Research* 1977; 9: 222-232.

[3] Cohen JC, der Megreditchian G, Gerbier N, Choisnel E, Pezzi-Giraud D, Pasteyer J, Poisvert M, Besancon F. Prévision des recrudescences d'infarctus du myocarde, fondée sur une analyse météorologique multivariée. *Semaine des Hôpitaux* 1984; 60 (9): 598-601.

[4] Scherlag BJ, Patterson E, Lazzara R. Seasonal variation in sudden cardiac death after experimental myocardial infarction. *J Electrocardiology* 1990; 23: 223-230.

[5] Ku CS, Yang CY, Lee WJ, Chiang HT, Liu CP, Lin SL. Absence of a seasonal variation in myocardial infarction onset in a region without temperature extremes. *Cardiology* 1998; 89: 277-282.

[6] Sharovsky R, Cesar LA, Ramires JA. Temperature, air pollution, and mortality from myocardial infarction in Sao Paulo, Brazil. *Brazilian J Med Biol Res* 2004; 37: 1651-1657.

[7] Braga AL, Zanobetti A, Schwartz J. The effect of weather on respiratory and cardiovascular deaths in 12 U.S. cities. *Environmental Health Perspectives* 2002; 110: 859-863.

[8] Schwartz J, Samet JM, Patz JA. Hospital admissions for heart disease: the effects of temperature and humidity. *Epidemiology* 2004; 15: 755-761.

[9] Kiu A, Horowitz JD, Stewart S. Seasonal variation in AF-related admissions to a coronary care unit in a "hot" climate: fact or fiction? *J Cardiovascular Nursing* 2004; 19: 138-141.

[10] Aronow WS, Ahn C. Elderly nursing home patients with congestive heart failure after myocardial infarction living in New York City have a higher prevalence of mortality in cold weather and warm weather months. *J Gerontology Series A: Biological Sciences & Medical Sciences* 2004; 59: 146-147.

[11] Pella D, Dudova D, Kumar R, Gupta SB. Not only a cold climate but also a hot climate can trigger cardiac events. *World Heart J* 2007; 1: [PRINTER: Please insert page numbers].

[12] Singh RB, Pella D, Sharma JP, Rastogi S, Kartikey K, Goel VK, Sharma R, Neki NS, Kumar A, Otsuka K. Increased concentrations of lipoprotein(a), circadian rhythms and metabolic reactions evoked by acute myocardial infarction associated with acute reactions in relation to large breakfasts. *Biomed Pharmacother* 2004; 58 (Suppl 1): S111-S115.

[13] Cornélissen G, Halberg F, Schwartzkopff O, Delmore P, Katinas G, Hunter D, Tarquini B, Tarquini R, Perfetto F, Watanabe Y, Otsuka K. Chronomes, time structures, for chronobioengineering for "a full life". *Biomed Instrum Technol* 1999; 33: 152-187.

[14] Cornélissen G, Halberg F, Breus T, Syutkina EV, Baevsky R, Weydahl A, Watanabe Y, Otsuka K, Siegelova J, Fiser B, Bakken EE. Non-photic solar associations of heart rate variability and myocardial infarction. *J Atmos Solar-Terr Phys* 2002; 64: 707-720.

[15] Halberg F, Cornélissen G, Schack B, Wendt HW, Minne H, Sothern RB, Watanabe Y, Katinas G, Otsuka K, Bakken EE. Blood pressure self-surveillance for health also reflects 1.3-year Richardson solar wind variation: spin-off from chronomics. *Biomed Pharmacother* 2003; 57 (Suppl 1): 58s-76s.

[16] Cornélissen G, Masalov A, Halberg F, Richardson JD, Katinas GS, Sothern RB, Watanabe Y, Syutkina EV, Wendt HW, Bakken EE, Romanov Y. Multiple resonances among time structures, chronomes, around and in us. Is an about 1.3-year periodicity in solar wind built into the human cardiovascular chronome? *Human Physiology* 2004; 30 (2): 86-92.

[17] Halberg F, Cornélissen G, Katinas G, Sampson M, Schwartzkopff O, members of the BIOCOS project, Spector NH, Faraone P, Tomescu S, Hriscu M. In memoriam: Ion Baciu. Mutually supporting neartransyears in solar and terrestrial magnetics, microbial and cell biology, physiology and pathology. In: Cornélissen G, Kenner R, Fiser B, Siegelova J (eds.) *Proceedings, Symposium: Chronobiology in Medicine.* Dedicated to the 85th Anniversary of Professor Franz Halberg. Brno: Masaryk University; 2004. p. 78-86.

[18] Cornélissen G, Halberg F, Pöllmann L, Pöllman B, Katinas GS, Minne H, Breus T, Sothern RB, Watanabe Y, Tarquini R, Perfetto F, Maggioni C, Wilson D, Gubin D, Otsuka K, Bakken EE. Circasemiannual chronomics: half-yearly biospheric changes in their own right and as a circannual waveform. *Biomed Pharmacother* 2003; 57 (Suppl 1): 45s-54s.

[19] Rieger A, Share GH, Forrest DJ, Kanbach G, Reppin C, Chupp EL. A 154-day periodicity in the occurrence of hard solar flares? *Nature* 1984; 312: 623-625.

[20] Ballester JL, Oliver R, Carbonell M. The near 160-day periodicity in the photospheric magnetic flux. *Astrophys J* 2002; 566: 505-511.

[21] Halberg F, Cornélissen G, Katinas G, Tvildiani L, Gigolashvili M, Janashia K, Toba T, Revilla M, Regal P, Sothern RB, Wendt HW, Wang ZR, Zeman M, Jozsa R, Singh RB, Mitsutake G, Chibisov SM, Lee J, Holley D, Holte JE, Sonkowsky RP, Schwartzkopff O, Delmore P, Otsuka K, Bakken EE, Czaplicki J, International BIOCOS Group. Chronobiology's progress: Part I, season's appreciations 2004-2005. Time-, frequency-, phase-, variable-, individual-, age- and site-specific chronomics. *J Applied Biomedicine* 2006a; 4: 1-38. *http://www.zsf.jcu.cz/vyzkum/jab/4_1/ halberg.pdf.*

[22] Richardson JD, Paularena KI, Belcher JW, Lazarus AJ. Solar wind oscillations with a 1.3-year period. *Geophys Res Lett* 1994; 21: 1559-1560.

[23] Mursula K, Zieger B. The 1.3-year variation in solar wind speed and geomagnetic activity. *Adv Space Res* 2000; 25: 1939-1942.

[24] Valdés-Galicia JF, Pérez-Enriquez R, Otaola JA. The cosmic-ray 1.68-year variation: a clue to understand the nature of the solar cycle? *Solar Physics* 1996; 167: 409-417.

[25] Halberg F, Cornélissen G, Panksepp J, Otsuka K, Johnson D. Chronomics of autism and suicide. *Biomed Pharmacother* 2005; 59 (Suppl 1): S100-S108.

[26] Halberg F, Cornélissen G, Schwartzkopff O, Bakken EE. Cycles in the biosphere in the service of solar-terrestrial physics? In: Schroeder W (ed.) *Case studies in physics and geophysics*. Bremen: Wilfried Schroeder/Science Edition, 2006, p. 39-87.

[27] Halberg F, Cornélissen G, Gigolashvili M, Katinas G, Sothern RB, Schwartzkopff O, Otsuka K, Bakken EE. Chronomics and sudden cardiac death: a geographic challenge? In: *Proceedings, 59th Annual Meeting, Japan Society of Neurovegetative Research*, Tokyo, November 1-3, 2006, p. 33-36.

[28] Cornélissen G, Halberg F, Rostagno C, Otsuka K. A chronomic approach to cardiac arrhythmia and sudden cardiac death. In: *Proceedings, 59th Annual Meeting, Japan Society of Neurovegetative Research*, Tokyo, November 1-3, 2006, p. 56-59.

[29] Halberg F, Cornélissen G, Otsuka K, Fiser B, Mitsutake G, Wendt HW, Johnson P, Gigolashvili M, Breus T, Sonkowsky R, Chibisov SM, Katinas G, Siegelova J, Dusek J, Singh RB, Berri BL, Schwartzkopff O. Incidence of sudden cardiac death, myocardial infarction and far- and near-transyears. *Biomed Pharmacother* 2005; 59 (Suppl 1): S239-S261.

[30] Minorsky PV. Latitudinal differences in coconut foliar spiral direction: a re-evaluation and hypothesis. *Annals of Botany* 1998; 82: 133-140.

[31] Cornélissen G, Benser M, Halberg F. Patterns of incidence of tachyarrhythmias recorded in implantable cardioverter-defibrillators during 2001-2005. PS-004, *Proceedings, 2nd World Congress of Chronobiology*, November 4-6, 2007, Tokyo, Japan, p.63.

[32] Minorsky PV, Bronstein NB. Do geomagnetic variations affect the foliar spiral direction of coconut palms? *Eos Trans. AGU* 2005; 86 (52), *Fall Meeting Suppl.*, Abstract GP33A-0103.

[33] Crawford VLS, Cornélissen G, Fiser B, Dusek J, Siegelova J, Halberg F. Infrannual changes in the incidence of myocardial infarctions and strokes in Northern Ireland. Abstract, *Noninvasive methods in cardiology*, 2.11.2004, Congress MEFA, Brno, Czech Republic, 2.-4.11.2004, p. 9.

In: World Heart Research Yearbook. Volume 1
Editors: Franz Halberg and R. B. Singh
ISBN: 978-1-60741-881-8

MYOCARDIAL VIABILITY EVALUATION BY DELAYED CONTRAST MRI

***Rakesh Sharma*[1,*] *and Ram B. Singh*[2]**

[1] Department of Medicine and Radiology, Columbia University, New York, NY, US
[2] International College of Cardiology, Slovakia

Ischemic injury causes loss of myocardial viability at injury sites. Revascularization intervention has become state of the art method of choice to heal up the evolving myocardial infarctions. With growing potentials and newer developments of the noninvasive imaging methods the attention was diverted to measure and identify the myocardial viability in subendocardial inferior wall and apex along with possibility of hibernating myocardium and revascularization benefits on LV function [1,2,3,4]. Myocardial viability quantitation depends on the success of various imaging methods such as delayed Magnetic Resonance Imaging (MRI), ^{201}Tl SPECT, Dobutamine stress echocardiography (DSE) in measurement of wall thickness, transmural extent with high predictive value of functional recovery after revascularization or other cardiac intervention. The recent trend indicates that evaluation of myocardial viability of dysfunctional myocardium by delayed contrast MRI has the potential to predict the functional recovery after revascularization in ischemic heart disease [5]. Scintigraphic techniques and DSE were routinely used to identify high-risk patients who could benefit from revascularization but inconclusive [5,6,7,8]. It is too early to say due to very limited data is available comparing cardiac MRI, ^{201}Tl SPECT and DSE. Moreover, there is paucity in information on the sensitivity, specificity, reproducibility, predictability, diagnostic accuracy, cost-effect reliability and precision of delayed contrast-enhanced cardiac MRI in comparison with ^{201}Tl SPECT and DSE to assess myocardial viability in predicting functional recovery after revascularization in patients with chronic ischemic heart failure. The current opinion is focused on the evaluation of myocardial viability by delayed contrast MRI with its advantages over other imaging ^{201}Tl SPECT and DSE techniques in prediction of functional recovery, efficacy of revascularization and limitations of existing imaging techniques. In this issue, Wu et al. have attempted remarkably to address these issues with novelty of delayed contrast MRI method in 40 chronic patients.

In recent years, the value of cardiac MRI was highlighted to assess myocardial fibrosis and scar burden, coronary perfusion and contractile reserve with excellent image quality [9,10,11,12]. Different approaches using intravenous administration of a gadolinium-chelate (such as Gd-DTPA) were reported such as inversion-recovery prepared T_1-weighted gradient-

---

* Correspondence to Rakesh Sharma, Ph.D, W181 Street, 736, Broadway, New York, NY 11032 E-mail rs2010@columbia.edu.

echo sequence, delayed enhancement to visualize regions of old infarction appearing nonviable by ^{201}Tl scintigraphy. High resolution MRI further improved the sensitivity for non-transmural infarction in evaluation of possible functional recovery after revascularization of dysfunctional myocardium [12, 13]. Recovery of regional and global LV function was reported unpredictable in the group of patients with residual MRI contrast [13, 14, 15]. However, the value of myocardial MRI in predicting functional recovery after revascularization in patients with chronic LV dysfunction, in comparison with well-established ^{201}Tl SPECT and DSE is lacking and remains to be established. MRI and DSE of tissue perfusion after coronary revascularization reflect the severity of microvascular disruption, occlusion, or extra-vascular compression by edema or hemorrhage. Thus, the revascularization patterns serve as surrogates of myocardial injury rather than a direct indicator of myocardial cellular viability [16,17,18]. A potential advantage of the MRI approach over other imaging methods is that MRI provides quantitative edge definition of the endocardial and epicardial surface for precise measurement of systolic wall thickening, end-diastolic wall thickness as morphological indicator of likely viability of an ischemically impaired region.

Application of delayed MRI techniques for myocardial viability in a region of ischemic injury can be grouped into 3 categories:

1. MRI evaluation of myocardial perfusion after revascularization,
2. comparison of MRI with ^{201}Tl SPECT and DSE response of myocardial contractile reserve, and
3. use of MRI contrast in morphological characterization of myocardial functional recovery.

The first MRI approach by Rogers et al. established the myocardial contrast enhancement on both first-pass and delayed MRI images[17]. The contrast enhancement identified that hypoenhancement on first-pass imaging was an indictor of poor functional recovery after the acute event. Hyperenhancement was observed in the periphery of the infarction or entire infarction in these patients. MRI also demonstrated the hypoenhancement regions within the infarct zone in patients with microvascular obstruction in the core of the infarction with severe LV remodeling[13,17]. It indicated that MRI hyperenhancement in the core of acute infarctions after revascularization either on first-pass or delayed MRI is predictive of more severe injury with possible poor functional recovery and poor outcome.

The second MRI approach may predict both myocardial viability and contractile reserve. It can measure the subendocardial wall thickness comparable with dobutamine echocardiography demonstrating residual contractile response in an ischemically injured or chronically ischemic region[19]. Quantitative assessment of dobutamine-induced systolic wall thickening on cine MRI serves as a reliable indicator of regional LV function improvement and ejection function after revascularization. ^{19}F-fluorodeoxyglucose PET for residual viability, dobutamine transesophageal echocardiography (TEE) and dobutamine cine MRI for prior myocardial infarction suggested the sensitivity and specificity of both dobutamine TEE and cine MRI for PET-defined viability [19]. An end-diastolic wall thickness measured by cine MRI in ischemic dysfunction segments appeared indicative of myocardial viability by ^{201}Tl SPECT radionuclide imaging or favorable response to revascularization.

A third MRI approach for determining myocardial viability in a region of ischemic injury uses dysprosium Dy-DTPA or GdDTPA as MRI contrast agents to probe cellular membrane integrity. Both of these contrast agents display extracellular distribution and are excluded by myocardial cell membranes. Dy-DTPA attenuates the intracellular signal due to its distribution in extracellular space and tissue microheterogeneity. A series of rapid inversion-recovery echo-planar images measured the precise in vivo measurement of T1 relaxation constants of myocardium using optimized inversion time at which T1 signal was nulled in both normal and ischemic myocardium on its pre-contrast and post-contrast MRI scans [20]. T1 relaxation constants of Gd MRI contrast media determined the distribution volume of Gd chelates in normal and ischemically injured myocardium. Contrast distribution volume may provide an index of the percentage of necrotic myocardial cells within a zone of ischemic injury [20]. The relative concentration of Gd chelate contrast media in myocardium and blood can be determined by its relative distribution volume in the myocardium. The distribution volume in ischemic injured myocardium may be observed slightly expanded by interstitial edema but significantly increased by loss of myocardial cellular membrane integrity. The distribution volume of MRI contrast media might be used to estimate the percentage of nonviable cells in a region of revascularized ischemic injury. At equilibration, the relative concentration of Gd DTPA-BMA in myocardium and blood can be determined by the relative distribution volume in the acute myocardial infarction[1]. During the past decade, high-molecular-weight MRI contrast agents were used to keep the contrast agents in the blood pool for several hours to improve coronary MRA [21]. Blood pool contrast media showed enhancement of the infarct periphery zone and demarcated a less enhanced central core in reperfused ischemic injury of graded severity [17,18,21]. It seems that delivery of the blood pool contrast agent to the core of the infarction depends on the duration of contrast media and intact microvasculature. However, low-molecular-size extracellular contrast agents can easily reach the infarction core by diffusion even in case of microvascular damage.

In recent years, the well known major problems were identified as *in vivo* assessment of myocardial viability, inferior heart wall, scars and evaluating their relationship with functional recovery after revascularization and contractile reserve to make the decision of myocardial intervention or heart transplantation. Delayed contrast enhancement on MRI and reduced uptake by ^{201}Tl SPECT suggested the efficacy of heart transplantation based on the myocardial viability index in percutaneous coronary intervention (PCI) and coronary bypass surgery (CABG) patients with or without scars and their functional recovery after revascularization and restored contractile reserve by dobutamine response [1,7,14,20,21]. MRI and ^{201}Tl SPECT both may indicate new hyperenhancement segments in their post-revascularization scan in CABG and PCI groups to evaluate the LVEF, total LV mass, LV end-diastolic volume index, LV end-systolic volume index. As of today, the use of both MRI and ^{201}Tl SPECT methods is in infancy to use them as clinical The increased subendocardial wall thickening, at inferior apex and systolic wall thickening determined by MRI may not be conclusive to show functional recovery but depends on its transmural scar extent. The delayed MRI displayed better diagnostic accuracy, sensitivity, specificity, positive predictive value and negative predictive value of viability over ^{201}Tl SPECT. Myocardial contrast echocardiography determines myocardial reperfusion in acutely occluded epicardial coronary arteries [22]. Myocardial viability assessment by ^{18}F-FDG PET is limited due to its high cost.

In the current view, delayed MRI contrast enhancement analysis may be considered better than reduced radionuclide uptake ^{201}Tl SPECT or DSE response. However, contractile reserve detection by DSE and myocardial viability with scar detection in the proportion of transmural extent of delayed enhancement on MRI may provide better clue but observations are inconclusive. Chronic CAD patients with LV dysfunction undergoing revascularization indicated the functional recovery with both the extent and severity of nonviable tissue by MRI due to relationship of chronic CAD and severe LV dysfunction [22,23]. Contractile reserve may be observed as impaired with no scar or minor scar detected on MRI. Extensive scar on MRI and/or SPECT can have contractile function at rest. A clear advantage of MRI over ^{201}Tl SPECT is its better capability to distinguish the myocardial recovered function with viable myocardium from the visible scar without recovery after revascularization. In a recent study, MRI identified the subendocardial infarcts but missed by ^{201}Tl SPECT [22,23]. ^{201}Tl SPECT might overestimate the scar tissue, especially in the inferior wall and apex. The inferior wall is one of the most severely attenuated regions in the heart. So, greater attenuation of ^{201}Tl in the inferior segments is commonly observed in ^{201}Tl SPECT. Another limitation of dysfunctional myocardium viable on ^{201}Tl SPECT and not on MRI can be due to the presence of a thin rim of viable tissue. Myocardial viability detected by MRI may be valuable on the clinical evaluation of potential benefits from high-risk revascularization procedures. However, several factors should be considered affecting the functional recovery such as intervention procedures, completeness of revascularization, and perioperative myocardial infarctions [24]. Other limitations in the evaluation of myocardial viability may be small and limited patients with revascularization receiving simultaneous DSE and ^{201}Tl imaging or receiving no revascularization at all. So, it complicates the MRI prediction of functional recovery.

In consideration of the time-series evaluation of myocardial viability, delayed contrast MRI and ^{201}Tl SPECT are reported in this issue as a possible index of potential myocardial viability in patients with revascularized myocardial infarctions. Using delayed MRI, the first-pass distribution of MRI contrast media indicated that the reperfusion at the myocardium tissue level was impeded in more than half of the injured regions. The cause of impeded perfusion was predictive of poorer contractile recovery 7 weeks after the acute event. This study demonstrated good correlations among DSE, ^{201}Tl SPECT and MRI in the detection of myocardial viability. These observations as mentioned in the paper by Wu et al. corroborated with earlier reports [25,26,27].

In conclusion, use of MRI for the evaluation of ischemic heart disease was proposed two decades ago. However, ^{201}Tl SPECT radionuclide imaging and echocardiography DSE have been considered useful in diagnosis of ischemic heart disease due to easy accessibility. Recently, non-invasive MRI imaging modality has emerged as cost-effective promising technique with lot of new imaging options in ischemic heart disease in prediction of myocardial viability after ischemic injury. The present view on myocardial viability and functional recovery evaluation by using radionuclide imaging, MRI and DSE will certainly open new opportunities of predicting the viability index and limitations of each technique in morphological, interventional assessment of ischemic heart disease in clinical decision making. The success of MRI multiple capabilities in ischemic heart disease will also depend on robust and fast techniques developed for coronary artery MRA angiographic methods. Presently, the coupled noninvasive coronary MRA with flow measurement appears as method of choice in the diagnosis of coronary artery disease. Cardiovascular MRI may provide a unique tool to assess cardiac structure and function in a single study session. The correlation among DSE, ^{201}Tl SPECT and MRI in the detection of myocardial viability, MRI detects viability better than ^{201}Tl SPECT, especially in the inferior wall and apex. Cardiac MRI certainly has higher predictive value of predicting functional recovery. In severe ischemic cardiomyopathy, MRI may provide valuable clinical decisions regarding high-risk revascularization procedures.

REFERENCES

[1] Huang PJ, Lin LC, Yen RF, et al. Accuracy of biphasic response, sustained improvement and worsening during dobutamine echocardiography in predicting recovery of myocardial dysfunction after revascularization: comparison with simultaneous thallium-201 reinjection SPECT. *Ultrasound Med Biol* 2001; 27:925-931.

[2] Allman KC, Shaw LJ, Hachamovitch R, et al. Myocardial viability testing and impact of revascularization on prognosis in patients with coronary artery disease and left ventricular dysfunction: a meta-analysis. *J Am Coll Cardiol* 2002; 39:151-158.

[3] Underwood SR, Bax JJ, vom Dahl J, et al. Imaging techniques for the assessment of myocardial hibernation: report of a study group of the European Society of Cardiology. *Eur Heart J* 2004; 25:815-836.

[4] Bax JJ, Poldermans D, Schinkel AF, et al. Perfusion and contractile reserve in chronic dysfunctional myocardium: relation to functional outcome after surgical revascularization. *Circulation* 2002; 106:114-118.

[5] Baer FM, Voth E, Schenider CA, Theissen P, Schicha H, Sechtem U. Dobutamine gradient echo MR: a functional and morphologic approach to the detection of residual myocardial viability. *Circulation.* 1995;91:1006–1015.

[6] Shan K, Constatine G, Sivananthan M, Flamm S. Role of cardiac magnetic resonance imaging in the assessment of myocardial viability. *Circulation* 2004; 109:1328-1334.

[7] Mahrholdt H, Wagner A, Holly TA, et al. Reproducibility of chronic infarct size measurement by contrast-enhanced magnetic resonance imaging. *Circulation* 2002; 39:1151-1158.

[8] Wagner A, Mahrholdt H, Regenfus M, et al. Contrast-enhanced MR and routine single photon emission computed tomography (SPECT) perfusion imaging for detection of subendocardial myocardial infarcts: an imaging study. *Lancet* 2003; 361:364-379.

[9] Kim RJ, Wu E, Rafael A, et al. The use of contrast-enhanced magnetic resonance imaging to identify reversible myocardial dysfunction. *N Engl J Med* 2000; 343:1445-1453.

[10] Cerqueira MD, Weissman NJ, Dilsizian V, et al. Standardized myocardial segmentation and nomenclature for tomographic imaging of the heart. *Circulation* 2002; 105:539-542.

[11] Mahrholdt H, Wagner A, Holly TA, et al. Reproducibility of chronic infarct size measurement by contrast-enhanced magnetic resonance imaging. *Circulation* 2002; 106:2322-2327.

[12] Knuesel PR, Nanz D, Wyss C, et al. Characterization of dysfunctional myocardium by positron emission tomography and magnetic resonance: relation to functional outcome after revascularization. *Circulation* 2003; 108:1095-1100.

[13] Tseng WY, Liao TY, Wang JL. Normal systolic and diastolic functions of the left ventricle and left atrium by cine magnetic resonance imaging. *J Cardiovasc Magn Reson* 2002; 4:443-457.

[14] Nelson C, McCrohon J, Khafagi F, et al. Impact of scar thickness on the assessment of viability using dobutamine echocardiography and thallium single photon emission computed tomography: a comparison with contrast-enhancement magnetic resonance imaging. *J Am Coll Cardiol* 2004; 43: 1248-1256.

[15] Klein C, Nekolla SG, Bengel FM, et al. Assessment of myocardial viability with contrast-enhanced magnetic resonance imaging: comparison with positron emission tomography. *Circulation* 2002; 105:162-167.

[16] Zamorano J, Delgado J, Almeria C, et al. Reason for discrepancies in identifying myocardial viability by thallium-201 redistribution, magnetic resonance imaging and dobutamine echocardiography. *Am J Cardiol* 2002; 90:455-459.

[17] Rogers WJ, Kramer CM, Geskin G, Hu Y-L, Theobald TM, Vido DA, Petruolo S, Reichek N. Early contrast-enhanced MRI predicts late functional recovery after reperfused myocardial infarction. *Circulation.* 1999;99:744–750.

[18] Wu KC, Zerhouni EA, Judd RM, Lugo-Olivieri CH, Barouch LA, Schulman SP, Blumenthal RS, Lima JAC. Prognostic significance of microvascular obstruction by magnetic resonance imaging in patients with acute myocardial infarction. *Circulation.* 1998;97:765–772.

[19] Baer FM, Theissen P, Schneider CA, Voth E, Sechtem U, Schicha H, Erdmann E. Dobutamine magnetic resonance imaging predicts contractile recovery of chronically dysfunctional myocardium after successful revascularization. *J Am Coll Cardiol.* 1998;31:5:1040–1048.

[20] Wendland MF, Saeed M, Arheden H, Gao D-W, Canet E, Bremerich MD, Dae MW, Higgins CB. Toward necrotic cell fraction measurement by contrast-enhanced MRI of reperfused ischemically injured myocardium. *Acad Radiol.* 1998;5(suppl):S45–S46.

[21] Sharma R, Sharma A. Advances in Magnetic Resonance Angiography, Chapter 3, 2004: pp 119-187 in: A Hand Book in Medical Imaging, Editors: Suri, Wilson and Laxminarayana, Springer Science, USA.

[22] Sakuma H, Blake LM, Amidon TM, OíSullivan M, Szolar DH, Furber AP, Bernstein MA, Foo MKF, Higgins CB. Coronary flow reserve: noninvasive measurement in humans with breath-hold velocity-encoded cine MR imaging. *Radiology.* 1996;198:745–750.

[23] Hundley WG, Lange RA, Clarke G, Meshack BM, Payne J, Landau C, McColl R, Sayad DE, Willet DWL, Willard JE, Hillis LD, Peshock RM. Assessment of coronary arterial flow and flow reserve in humans with magnetic resonance imaging. *Circulation.* 1996;93:1502–1508.

[24] Selvanayagam JB, Petersen SE, Francis JM, et al. Effects of off-pump versus on-pump coronary surgery on reversible and irreversible myocardial injury. A randomized trail using cardiovascular magnetic resonance imaging and biochemical markers. *Circulation* 2004; 109:345-350.

[25] Wu YW, Huang PJ, Su MY, Lin LC, Yen RF, Chen YS, Lee CM, Yu HY, Ting Y, Tzen KY, Tseng WYI. Myocardium Viability Assessed by Late Enhancement Magnetic Resonance in Patients with Severe Ischemic Heart Failure: A Comparison with Thallium SPECT and Dobutamine Echocardiography. *World Heart J.* 2005; ------.

[26] Duerinckx AJ. Myocardial Viability Using MR Imaging: Is It Ready for Clinical Use? *Am. J. Roentgenol.,* June 1, 2000; 174(6): 1741 - 1743.

[27] Higgins CB. Prediction of myocardial viability by MRI *Circulation.* 1999;99:727-729.

In: World Heart Research Yearbook. Volume 1
Editors: Franz Halberg and R. B. Singh

ISBN: 978-1-60741-881-8

GENE THERAPY FOR HEART DISEASE

Anjali Mohan
Independent Consultant in Internal Medicine, India

Insights into the molecular basis of cardiac disease have led to the development of gene therapy as a possible treatment mode. The genetic understanding of some disorders such as vascular disease, including atherosclerosis, hypertrophic cardiomyopathy, prolonged Q-T interval, and heart failure has rendered them to gene manipulation to improve both structure and function. Direct gene transfer for hepatic regulation of lipoprotein metabolism holds promise for human gene therapy in familial hypercholesterolaemia.

Cardiovascular disorders are not single gene diseases. Multiple genes appear to be associated in cardiovascular disease, but not all studies of associated genes can be replicated. [1] As compared with hereditary single-gene disorders, cancers, or AIDS, the risk-to-benefit for cardiovascular patients is higher. Identification of candidate genes for treatment has been difficult. However, potential candidate genes have, and are still being, identified. There have been improvements in catheter design and delivery, gene expression, and vector pharmacokinetics, so that gene therapy now appears to be on the way to becoming a therapeutic option for cardiovascular patients. [2]

Whereas clinical cardiology earlier focused on angiographically demonstrable stenotic lesions for addressing myocardial infarction and unstable angina, basic research is now highlighting the role of inflammatory mediators in these disease states. Some of the cytokines may be amenable to genetic manipulation. Genetic understanding of atherosclerosis can help modify this process also. Further, myocardial damage following infarction is free-radical mediated. Genes and proteins involved have been identified giving hope of a favourable outcome by their manipulation.

Coronary restenosis following balloon angioplasty is well known. The insertion of drug-eluting stents has improved outcomes, but restenosis still occurs. Gene therapy may be a useful approach here, [3] as also for cardiac pacemaking disorders, despite the advancements in implantable pacemakers/defibrillators. [4]

The identification of candidate genes is only the first step. Vectors are needed to deliver the genetic material to the target cells. The ideal vector should be synthetic, non-immunogenic, and capable of targeting the desired cell. Plasmid liposomes have limited efficiency for gene transfer. Retroviruses not only have limited gene transfer efficiency, but also have the associated risk of transformation. Adenoviruses are highly efficient at gene transfer and can transduce quiescent cells. However, even second-generation adenoviruses provoke a local inflammatory response, and the transgene expression is only transient. In humans who have been preimmunised with native adenoviruses, this method of delivering gene therapy may be ineffective. Further, the safety of gene therapy using adenoviral vectors has been questioned, particularly in diseases such as coronary restenosis, which are, by and large, rarely lethal. [5]

Recently interventional magnetic resonance imaging (MRI) has been used for providing real time guidance for gene and cell delivery into the heart, and for assessing heart modeling. Genes, proteins, and cells for tissue engineering can be accurately delivered by intramyocardial injection. [6] This may be a significant advance in the delivery of genes into the cardiac myocytes. The vascular smooth muscle and endothelial cells are more easily accessible through the percutaneous intra-arterial route, and with improvements in design of delivery catheters targeting these cells may be facilitated further.

The problem that remains after this is how long will the gene expression last in the relevant cells? As of now, the duration does not exceed a few weeks, which leads to the question—what next? Also, many of the studies have been done mainly on animals. Would the results in humans be the same?

It appears that, whereas we may not have actually "arrived" there, we are probably well on our way to developing gene therapy into a useful therapeutic option in the practice of cardiovascular medicine.

REFERENCES

[1] Sturm A.C.: Cardiovascular genetics: are we there yet? *Journal of Medical Genetics 2004*; 41:321-323.

[2] Nabel E.G.: Gene therapy for cardiovascular disease. *Circulation* 1995; 91:541-548.

[3] O'Sullivan M.J.; Bennet M.R.: Gene therapy for coronary restenosis: is the enthusiasm justified? *Heart* 2001; 86: 491-493.

[4] Edelberg J.M.; Huang D.T.; Josephson M. E. et al: Molecular enhancement of porcine cardiac chronotropy. Heart 2003; 86: 559-562.

[5] O'Sullivan M.J.; Bennet M.R.: Gene therapy for coronary restenosis: is the enthusiasm justified? *Heart* 2001; 86: 491-493.

[6] Barbash I.M.; Leor J.; Feinberg M.S.: Interventional magnetic resonance imaging for guiding gene and cell transfer in the heart. *Heart* 2004; 90: 87-91.

In: World Heart Research Yearbook. Volume 1
Editors: Franz Halberg and R. B. Singh
ISBN: 978-1-60741-881-8

Dietary/Blood Cholesterol and Coronary Heart Disease

F. De Meester[1], C. Gopalan[2] and A. P. Simopoulos[3]
[1] Belovo S.A., Z.I. 1, 31, 6600 Bastogne, Belgium
[2] Nutrition Foundation of India, New Dehli, India
[3] The Centre for Genetics, Nutrition and Health, Washington DC, US

In some individuals, dietary cholesterol influences blood cholesterol when tested clinically and, therefore, it has long been perceived as a causal factor in the development of atherosclerosis and CHD. The time has come when this long-held perception is scientifically examined in the light of emerging knowledge.

Dietary and blood cholesterols are identical interchangeable molecules and dietary cholesterol is not essential for homeostasis and health in young healthy men and women. In omnivorous men and women, it is estimated that, on average, ± $2/3^{rd}$ of plasma cholesterol is produced by the liver and ± $1/3^{rd}$ is derived from the diet and biliary salts. There also seems to be a daily intake threshold (± 500 mg) above which dietary cholesterol has no more clinically observable influence on blood cholesterol.

The clinically established dietary-blood cholesterol relationship does not survive the test of time. Epidemiological surveys conclude to a null relationship between dietary and blood cholesterol and, therefore, to a null relationship between dietary cholesterol and coronary heart disease (CHD) (Dawber et al., 1982). This epidemiological observation comes in strong support to the otherwise undisputed scientifically established evidence that dietary cholesterol efficiently suppresses – just as efficiently as blood cholesterol – the body's own synthesis.

The way the overall dietary pattern affects blood cholesterol is phenotype-driven. It depends on genetic, environmental/constitutional, and developmental factors, which basically influence cholesterol's absorption, circulation/distribution, and excretion. Re-analyzing clinical and epidemiological studies carried out in the last quarter of the last century for confounding factors, McNamara (2002) has provided evidence that dietary saturated fatty acids and blood cholesterol could well be leading factors in CHD; however, Okuyama (2000) has raised the interesting point which saturated fatty acid intake and high blood cholesterol in western industrialized countries are associated with high intake of vegetable and animal fats abnormally rich in omega-6 fatty acids. At the same time, the diet of Inuits, known to have high cholesterol-saturated fats index (CSI), but also to contain high amount of omega-3 fatty acids, has been reported to protect against CHD.

It, therefore, seems reasonable to suggest that the blood cholesterol-dietary saturated fats index is a marker for CHD in western industrialized civilizations for the main reason that their dietary lipid patterns are characterized by artificially high omega-6:omega-3 fatty acids ratios.

Epidemiological Evidence

As a result of the last 40-years of generally extended phobia around the classical dietary cholesterol-saturated fats index (CSI), animal fat has become synonymous with CHD. This is at least the present perception that the consumer and, to a large extent, health authorities, medical doctors, dieticians and opinion leaders have of the dietary lipids/heart diseases relationship. Classic recommendations for the prevention of these diseases, apparently established in the sixties, were that the intake of cholesterol should be reduced and the polyunsatured:saturated (P:S) ratio of dietary fatty acids should be increased. Basically, a decrease intake of animal fats was advised, whereas increased intake of hydrogenated vegetable margarine and high-linoleic acid vegetable oils was recommended.

Despite a failure to demonstrate the effectiveness of this recommendation, the recommendation has continued until very recently in all industrialized countries, in the hope that a long-term follow-up trial would prove the effectiveness of such recommendations (Okuyama, 2000). However, long-term follow-up studies performed in the West and in Japan conclusively demonstrate the following two facts:

- Those with higher blood cholesterol survive longer, possibly due to decreased cancer mortality, decreased mortality from infectious diseases and/or decreased apoplexy
- Blood cholesterol is not an independent risk factor for atherosclerosis and CHD.

Dietary Cholesterol – A Beneficial Nutrient?

The ingestion of dietary cholesterol translates into a parallel increased synthesis of apo E in the body's tissues, starting with the intestinal enterocytes. The increased apo E level concomitantly increases cholesterol secondary circulation (reverse cholesterol transport) throughout the body through participation of HDL-1 and HDLc while, at the same time, it reduces the body's own cholesterol synthesis in the liver.

Cholesterol is an important component of cell membranes. It is well known that macrophages synthesize and excrete large amounts of apo E at sites of injury as chemo-attractants for tissue- and cell-repairing cholesterol.

On the other hand, this sterol is so crucial to life and cell-functioning that man's brain has developed an almost independent biological manufacturing process for the cholesterol it requires in a typical omega-3 rich environment.

The body's own synthesis of cholesterol is hormone-sensitive and energy-demanding. To some extent, it shares common features with other animal-derived nutrients such as long chain polyunsaturated fatty acids or LC-PUFAs. Therefore, there are scientific reasons to support the hypothesis that dietary cholesterol might be needed for normal metabolism and more so infants and aging adults.

We can therefore conclude that dietary cholesterol has all the potential of being beneficial to human health – protecting it against infection, cancer, and degenerative diseases – and that it is the individual phenotype that defines how dietary/blood cholesterol circulates and is distributed in and excreted out of the body. The classical clinical blood cholesterol profile (TC, LDL, HDL) is just an in-print of this individual specific phenotype-dietary/blood cholesterol interaction at a certain time of our life. In no such case, can this temporary signature be assimilated to a risk factor for CHD and degenerative diseases per se.

There is epidemiological evidence to support the view that dietary cholesterol might be beneficial to nascent life and longevity, and that it is not related, per se, to health diseases in normal adults:

- Mother's milk provides 18-mg cholesterol per 100-ml milk or 27-mg cholesterol per kg body weight (150-ml) to the breast-fed infant, in association with essential and conditionally essential fatty acids
- Among those highest in age followed for 10 years in the Netherlands (Weverling-Rijnsburger et al., 1997), no significant correlation was found between serum cholesterol level and CHD mortality. Instead, both cancer mortality and mortality from infectious diseases were higher when serum CHL was lower, and all causes of mortality were negatively correlated with serum cholesterol level. A similar conclusion was obtained when people older than 70 years were followed for 10 years in the USA (Krumholz et al., 1994)
- The 24-industrialized countries' epidemiological data suggest that countries where egg consumption is the highest are those where the risk of fatal cardiovascular diseases is the lowest (McNamara, 2000). Interestingly, the four countries (France, Spain, Japan, Mexico) with the highest egg consumption and the lowest rate of CVD-mortality are also those where the average dietary lipid profile is the most perfectly balanced (ideal dietary ω6:ω3 ratio from greens and game) and where the average consumption of antioxidant-rich foods (wine, fruits, vegetables, spices,...) is the highest. The Japanese consume more than 340 eggs per capital per year, twice the amount reported for the United Kingdom, but the incidence of heart disease in Japan is one of the lowest in the world (Simopoulos, 1991).

These observations run counter to the long held perception that dietary/blood cholesterol is a causal factor in the genesis of CHD.

Based on "Common Statement" emerging from the International Congress on the Columbus® Concept; edited by Artemis P. Simopoulos.

References

Dawber TR, Nickerson RJ, Brand FN, Pool J. Eggs, serum cholesterol, and coronary heart disease.*Am J Clin Nutr* 1982,36:617-25.

Krumholz HM, Seeman TE, Merrill SS, et al. Lack of association between cholesterol and coronary heart disease mortality and morbidity and all-cause mortality in persons older than 70 years. *JAMA* 1994,272:1335-1340.

McNamara DJ. Dietary cholesterol and atherosclerosis. *Biochim Acta* 2000,1529:310.

McNamara DJ. Egg, plasma cholesterol and heart disease risk. Eggs and Health Promotion. Watson RR(ed), Iowa State Press 2002,8,p71-81.

Okuyama H, Fuyii Y, Ikemoto A.n-6/n-3 ratio of dietary fatty acids rather than hypercholesterolemia as the major risk factor for atherosclerosis and coronary heart disease. *J Health Sci* 2000,46(3):157-177.

Simopoulos AP. Omega-3 fatty acids in health and disease and in growth and development. *Am J Clin Nutr* 1991, 54:438-463.

Weverling-Rijnsburger AW, Blauw GJ, Lagaay AM, Knook DL, Meinders AE, Westendorp RG.Total cholesterol and risk of mortality in the oldest old. *Lancet* 1997,350:1119-1123.

In: World Heart Research Yearbook. Volume 1
Editors: Franz Halberg and R. B. Singh
ISBN: 978-1-60741-881-8

REVASCULARIZATION IN ACUTE MYOCARDIAL INFARCTION USING PERCUSURGE IN DISTAL PROTECTION ACRONYM: RAPID

Keyur H. Parikh[2], Hetal D. Shah[1], Milan C. Chag[2], Urmil G. Shah [2], Hemang A. Baxi[2], Anish H. Chandarana[2], Ajay M. Naik[2], Gunvant T. Patel[2], Joyal N. Shah[2] and Ramesh K. Goyal[1,*]

[1] Department of Pharmacology, L. M. College of Pharmacy Navrangpura, Gujarat, India
[2] Care Cardiovascular Consultants Pvt Ltd, Parimal Garden, Gujarat, India

ABSTRACT

Background: The PercuSurge Guardwire Plus Temporary Occlusion And Aspiration System is underused due to the misconceptions that it is less user-friendly and makes PCI in AMI complicated and time consuming. This prospective study evaluates the efficacy of the PercuSurge device in primary/rescue PCI and focuses on the actual procedural time involved with or without its use.

Methods: It is a single center prospective study in 67 AMI patients undergoing PCI for thrombotic lesions. The patients were divided randomly into two groups, one where PercuSurge was used during PCI (n=30) and the other where it was not (n=37). In addition to the conventional demographic and angiographic parameters including TIMI flow and TMP grade, the time involved in various steps of the PCI were recorded. We considered the total procedural time as the time involved after the engagement of the guide catheter to the attainment of the desired end point.

Results: PercuSurge use showed a significantly greater achievement of TIMI III flow and TMP III grade ($p<0.01$). The total procedural time for PCI was significantly reduced with PercuSurge use (25.01 ± 2.17 min vs. 31.98 ± 2.52 min without its use, $p<0.05$). The time required after wire crossing to reach stent placement and to achieve TIMI III flow was also significantly less with PercuSurge use. Further, use of PercuSurge significantly reduced the time after PTCA balloon inflation / stent placement till optimal TIMI flow achievement (17.37 ± 2.21 min vs. 24.41 ± 2.5 min without its use, $p<0.05$). The incidences of no/slow reflow were significantly reduced ($p<0.001$) with use of PercuSurge, thus requiring less administration of intracoronary vasodilators and GP IIb/IIIa receptor inhibitors.

* Address for Correspondence and Reprints: Professor Ramesh K Goyal, Department of Pharmacology, L. M. College of Pharmacy Navrangpura, Ahmedabad 380 006. Gujarat, INDIA. Phone: 91-79-26302746 Email: goyalrk@hotmail.com.

Conclusions: Recent results of EMERALD trial have shown that PercuSurge increases the procedural time. However, our experience seems to have shown significant time and TMP advantage (as seen in the RUBY registry). More studies need to be done in focused and experienced centres.

Keywords: PercuSurge, Distal protection, acute myocardial infarction, procedural time

ABBREVIATIONS

MACE	Major Adverse Cardiac Events
SVG	Saphenous Vein Graft
NTG	Nitroglycerin OR Glyceryl Trinitrate
ACC	American College of Cardiology
Re MI	Recurrent Myocardial Infarction

INTRODUCTION

The efficacy of primary angioplasty in acute myocardial infarction (AMI) has been well proven by randomized clinical trials [1]. Increasing evidence has suggested that microvascular debris and/or platelet–thrombus plays a crucial role in embolization to the microvasculature [2, 3], which subsequently leads to the no reflow phenomenon [2, 4] during elective or primary percutaneous coronary interventions (PCI). This distal embolization of plaque or thrombotic debris during angioplasty in AMI results in infarct extension and high periprocedural mortality [5]. Recently, some studies demonstrated that infarct related arteries (IRAs) usually contain high burden thrombus formation (HBTF) [6, 7] and lipid pool like contents [8, 9]. Several distal protection devices have been developed to prevent distal embolization during angioplasty, [10-14] and their effectiveness has been reported [15-17]. The PercuSurge Guardwire Plus Temporary Occlusion and Aspiration System (Medtronic AVE, Santa Rosa, CA) is one such device designed to provide protection of the distal microcirculation during percutaneous intervention by temporarily occluding the distal vessel, thereby facilitating aspiration of dislodged atheromatous and thrombotic material before it can reach the arteriolar and capillary beds. Some studies have reported favorable results with this device as an adjunct to percutaneous intervention in saphenous vein graft, [18-20] carotid artery, [21-23] and the coronaries. Trials like SAFE and SAFER have already proven the efficacy of this device with reduction in MACE, MI and mortality in patients with SVG lesions [19, 20].

Large-scale trials like EMRALD and RUBY registry have investigated the efficacy of the device in patients with AMI. Interim conclusions from RUBY registry have shown that the device has a high delivery success rate and a large number of patients were found to achieve TIMI III after the procedure. However, the results from EMERALD trial, which is the largest one in AMI, failed to show a beneficial effect from the use of distal embolic protection devices. On the contrary, it showed that the Guardwire device was not associated with an improvement in the primary endpoints of post-procedure ST resolution or final infarct size. Further, it concluded that the procedural duration was significantly longer in the Guardwire arm of the study than without its use. Thus, there is a possibility that using these devices makes the intervention more complicated and time consuming as compared with conventional PCI. In this study we investigated the efficacy of this device in the setting of primary / rescue PCI in AMI. Also, the time required in the procedure with and without the use of PercuSurge was compared.

MATERIALS AND METHODS

Study Population

67 consecutive AMI patients with angiographically detected thrombotic lesions who were to undergo primary/rescue PCI within 24hrs of the onset of chest pain were enrolled for the study from September 2003 to December 2003. The patients were randomly divided into two groups depending on whether PercuSurge was used or not during PCI. In all, Guardwire was used in 30 patients. The remaining 37 patients formed the control group.

Study Protocol

It was a single centered, random, open clinical trial. It was non-blind and based on parallel group design. Informed consent was obtained from all the patients. After recording the baseline demographic and hemodynamic parameters, the angiographic parameters were also assessed. PCI was performed according to the conventional methods. An angiographic criteria of <30% residual stenosis was used to determine the end point of PCI. The incidences of no/slow reflow as well as the use of intracoronary vasodilators like adenosine, sodium nitroprusside, NTG, and GP IIb/IIIa receptor antagonists were also recorded. TIMI flow and TMP grade after PCI were assessed and the total procedural time and the time for individual steps of the PCI were recorded.

Device Description

The description of the Guardwire system has been well elaborated in a recent article.[24] It consists of four principal components: the Guardwire Plus Temporary Occlusion Catheter, the Micro Seal Adaptor, the Export Catheter, and the EZ flator inflation device (Figure 1). The Guardwire catheter is a novel 0.014 inches balloon-on-a-hypotube-wire catheter with a distal elastomeric occlusion balloon.

Procedure Description

The femoral arterial approach was used in all cases. After a proper guiding catheter was engaged to the target vessel, the Guardwire (or conventional soft guidewire in cases where the device was not used) was first attempted to cross the culprit lesion. If there was difficulty passing the Guardwire, a conventional guidewire was passed over which the Guardwire was crossed using the buddy wire technique. The Guardwire was advanced till the distal balloon was positioned a few centimeters beyond the target lesion. To protect the side branches it was important not to push the Guardwire too far distal from the lesion. The Guardwire catheter then served as an adequate guidewire for delivery of dilatation balloons and a multitude of stents. After inflating the Guardwire distal balloon, PCI was performed according to the conventional methods. The distal balloon was kept inflated during the treatment of the culprit lesion. Before deflating this balloon, the liberated debris (after PTCA balloon inflation and stent implantation) was aspirated through the Export aspiration catheter.

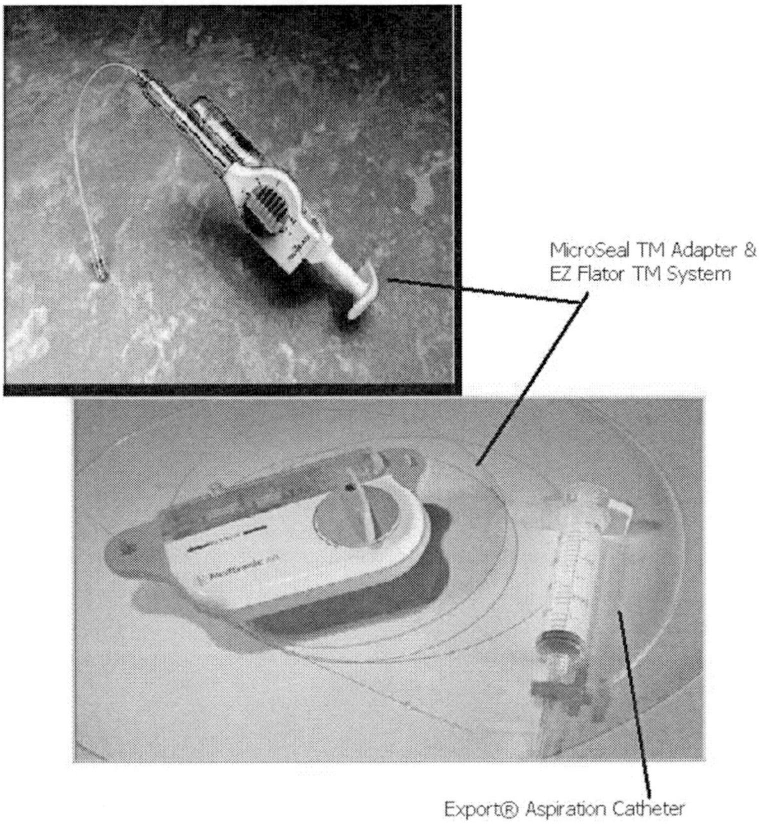

Figure 1. Components of PercuSurge device.

Angiographic Analysis

2 independent cardiologists unaware of the patients' medical histories and details reviewed coronary angiograms separately, to avoid inter observer bias. The degree of perfusion was evaluated according to Thrombolysis in Myocardial Ischemia (TIMI) criteria. Good collateral flow was defined as grade 2 or 3 (discussed below). Angiographic thrombus was defined as a filling defect seen in multiple projections surrounded by contrast and in the absence of calcification. Angiographic distal embolization was defined as the angiographic cut-off of a distal branch or vessel at any point during the procedure.

Procedural Time

Time in minutes required for various steps of the PCI procedure was recorded. The time count was started after the guiding catheter was engaged and viewed under fluoroscopy to ensure that it was in place. The rest of the time frames were calculated considering the guiding catheter time as zero or start time of the procedure. Various time periods like time for crossing of the lesion by the wire; time required to achieve PTCA balloon inflations; time to reach stent implantation, and time to achieve optimal TIMI flow were recorded separately in addition to the total procedural time. The *total procedural time*, in our trial, consists precisely of the time period from the first cinefilm of guide catheter engagement to the last one when the final TIMI flow is achieved.

Study Endpoints

The primary endpoint of this study was to evaluate the presence of distal embolization, which was demonstrated by Thrombolysis in Myocardial Infarction (TIMI) flow and Myocardial Blush grade. A secondary endpoint was to evaluate the clinical performance of the Guard- wire system combined with Plain-old balloon angioplasty (POBA) and/or stenting in AMI patients during emergency PCI. This included immediate technical device success, angiographic success and procedural success.

Assessment of Blood Flow

Thrombolysis in Myocardial Infarction (TIMI) Flow Grades

The culprit lesion was determined by its anatomical location and its perfusion characteristics according to Thrombolysis in Myocardial Infarction (TIMI) classification for flow through the infarct related vessel:[25]

TIMI flow 0 was assigned if there was no anterograde flow beyond the point of occlusion or there was no visible filling of any collateral channel.

TIMI I flow was designated if there was penetration, but without perfusion, or only minor perfusion, i.e., contrast material passed beyond the area of obstruction, but "hung up" and failed to opacify the entire coronary bed distal to the obstruction for the duration of the cineangiographic filming sequence. There was filling by means of collateral channels of side branches of the vessel but without any dye reaching the epicardial segment of that vessel.

Blood flow was graded as TIMI II when there was partial or mild perfusion. The passing of the obstruction by the contrast material or its rate of clearance from the distal bed (or both) was perceptibly slower than its entry into or clearance from comparable areas not perfused by previously occluded vessels. Partial filling occurred via collateral channels of the epicardial segment of the vessel.

TIMI III flow was assigned for complete and good perfusion as visualized by complete filling of the vessel. Anterograde flow into the bed distal to the obstruction occurred as promptly as anterograde flow into the bed proximal to the obstruction, and clearance of contrast material from the involved bed was as rapid as clearance from an uninvolved bed in the same vessel or an opposite artery.

Myocardial Blush Grade/ TIMI Myocardial Perfusion (TMP)

Perfusion can be defined as tissue blood flow at the capillary level. Perfusion of the myocardium can be categorized using the TIMI myocardial perfusion (TMP) classification described below: [26]

Myocardial blush was graded as 0 when there was failure of the dye to enter the microvasculature. There was either minimal or no ground-glass appearance ("blush") or opacification of the myocardium in the distribution of the culprit artery, indicating lack of tissue-level perfusion.

TMP grade 1 was assigned when the dye slowly entered but failed to exit the microvasculature. There was ground-glass appearance ("blush") or opacification of the myocardium in the distribution of the culprit lesion that failed to clear from the microvasculature, and dye staining was present on the next injection.

TMP grade was considered as 2 when there was delayed entry and exit of dye from the microvasculature. There was ground-glass appearance ("blush") or opacification of the myocardium in the distribution of the culprit lesion that was strongly persistent at the end of the washout phase (i.e., dye was strongly persistent after 3 cardiac cycles of the washout phase and either did not, or only minimally, diminished in intensity during washout).

TMP grade 3 was designated when there was normal entry and exit of dye from the microvasculature. There was ground-glass appearance ("blush") or opacification of the myocardium in the distribution of the culprit lesion that cleared normally. It was either gone or only mildly/moderately persistent at the end of the washout phase (i.e., the dye was gone or mildly/moderately persistent after 3 cardiac cycles of the washout phase and diminished noticeably in intensity during this phase), similar to that in an uninvolved artery. Blush that was only of mild intensity throughout the washout phase but faded minimally was also classified as grade 3.

Device Success

Device success was defined as successful deployment of the Guardwire catheter, occlusion of the distal flow and performance of aspiration.

Angiographic Success

Angiographic success was defined as residual lumen diameter (stenosis) < 30% and TIMI flow grade 3 after the intervention.

Procedural Success

Procedural success was defined as angiographic success without the occurrence of periprocedural adverse events.

Periprocedural Adverse Events

Periprocedural adverse events were defined as distal embolization; spasm; no/slow reflow during the procedure, and all causes of death, including new Q wave or non Q wave AMI, emergent CABG, or repeat percutaneous target vessel revascularization within 3 days of the index procedure.

No Reflow

Coronary occlusion leads to cellular necrosis and myocardial damage. During a short period of occlusion, a variable number of myocytes may become necrotic while the microvascular network is still intact. If coronary occlusion is prolonged, the microvasculature shows loss of its anatomic integrity. [27]. At the time of coronary reopening, myocardial reperfusion is achieved only in areas with anatomically preserved microvasculature, where as reflow does not occur in myocardium with extensive microvascular damage. The no reflow phenomenon is therefore associated with relatively more extensive necrosis and, as a consequence, is a predictor of poor regional and global contractile function. Angiographic 'no reflow' was defined as the cessation of flow into the distal coronary circulation of the treated vessel with a to and fro contrast movement after intervention (TIMI grade 0 or 1 flow in patients with prior TIMI grade 2 or 3, or TMP grade 0 or 1) not attributable to high grade stenosis or spasm of the original target vessel.

Statistical Analysis

Values have been expressed as mean ± SEM (standard error of mean). Continuous data were compared using unpaired Student's t test. Independent variables included were age, sex, classic coronary risk factors, angiographic lesion characteristics and interventional strategies and were compared by non-parametric test. A p value <0.05 was considered to be statistically significant.

RESULTS

Baseline Demographic, Hemodynamic and Biochemical Characteristics

Out of the 67 patients undergoing primary/rescue PCI, Guardwire system was used in 30 patients. Baseline demographic, hemodynamic characteristics, and risk factor presentation (Table 1) were nearly identical in both the arms indicating symmetry in the study design. *However, group II had more diabetic patients (41%) as compared to group I (20%).* The Guardwire system was successfully deployed, distal balloon occlusion established and aspiration completed in all the cases in which PercuSurge was used (100% device success) without any complications. Group I consisted of 30 patients in which PercuSurge was used and Group II consisted of 37 patients in which PercuSurge was not used.

Angiographic and Lesion Characteristics and PCI Details

Most of the patients in both the groups had single vessel disease (80% in group I and 68% in group II). Left anterior Descending artery (LAD) was found to be the culprit coronary in maximum number of cases (53% in group I and 62% in group II). 23% of patients in group I and 27% in group II had a type B1 lesion whereas 70% in group I and 54% in group II depicted type B2 lesion. Type C lesion was present in 7% of group I and 19% of group II patients. Thrombus was present in all the cases and the culprit artery was totally occluded in 73% and 65% patients in groups I and II respectively. Predilatation was done before stenting of the artery in 47% and 57%of cases in groups I and II respectively. However, plain old balloon angioplasty (POBA) as well as direct stenting were also performed in rest of the cases at the cardiologist's discretion (Table 2). Angiographic and procedural success was achieved in 100% of patients in whom Guardwire was used.

Table 1. Baseline Demographic and Hemodynamic Characteristics of patients

	Group I (n=30)	Group II (n=37)
Demographic Characteristics		
Age	55.17 ± 2.19	56.16 ± 1.86
% Males	90%	95%
% Females	10%	5%
Risk Factors		
Smoking	17%	19%
Tobacco Consumption	7%	27%
Diabetes	20%	41%
Hypertension	20%	28%
Hyperlipidemia	3%	8%
Significant Family History	23%	27%
Vital Signs		
Systolic BP (mm Hg)	117 ± 4	118 ± 3
Diastolic BP (mm Hg)	75 ± 3	72 ± 2
Heart Rate (beats/min)	84 ± 4	87 ± 3
Haematological & Biochemical investigations		
Hb (Gm %)	13.05 ± 0.43	13.37 ± 0.26
TC (counts x 10^9/L)	11.740 ± 0.736	11.281 ± 0.678
PC (counts x 10^9/L)	257.522 ± 15.938	267.939 ± 11.949
Random blood sugar (mmol/L)	6.69 ± 0.89	10.89 ± 0.96
Urea (mg/dl)	34.85 ± 4.64	29.83 ± 2.13
Creatinine (μmol/L)	106.08 ± 9.72	96.35 ± 3.53
Na+ (mmol/L)	138.2 ± 0.99	137.63 ± 0.74
K+ (mmol /L)	4.23 ± 0.13	4.13 ± 0.09

Data expressed as Mean ± SEM; % patients.
Group I: PCI with use of PercuSurge device.
Group II: PCI without use of PercuSurge device.

Table 2. Lesion Characteristics and Procedure Details

Parameters		Group I (n=30)	Group II (n=37)
Angiographic Characteristics			
LVEF (%)		33.44 ± 4.69	41.22 ± 4.79
Single Vessel Disease (SVD)		80%	68%
Double Vessel Disease (DVD)		13%	19%
Triple Vessel Disease (TVD)		7%	13%
Culprit Coronaries	LAD	53%	62%
	RCA	43%	24%
	LCX	4%	14%
Area of the artery having the lesion	Proximal	70%	62%
	Mid	10%	3%
	Distal	10%	5%

Parameters		Group I (n=30)	Group II (n=37)
	Prox. / Mid	7%	8%
	Ostial	4%	-
Lesion Details			
Lesion Type	A	-	-
	B1	23%	27%
	B2	70%	54%
	C	7%	19%
Lesion Characteristics	Thrombus	100%	100%
	Total Occlusion	73%	65%
	Calcification	-	8%
	Ulcerated	3%	3%
Procedure Details			
Plain Balloon PTCA		20%	35%
Predilatation		47%	57%
Direct Stenting		33%	8%
Type of Stents Used	Cypher	17%	19%
	Driver	26%	8%
	S7	13%	19%
	S670	10%	8%
	BE2	10%	5%
	Others	-	5%
Incidences of No Reflow (p<0.001)		30% (9)	84%(31)
% patients in whom TIMI III achieved (p=0.003)		87% (26)	49% (18)
% patients in whom TMP III achieved (p<0.001)		80% (24)	14% (5)
% patients in whom GP IIb/IIIa inhibitors used (p=0.048)		43% (13)	70% (26)
% patients with use of IC drugs	Adenosine	53 %(16)	86% (32)(p=0.007)
	SNP	53% (16)	76% (28) (p=0.098)
	NTG	20% (6)	40% (15) (p=0.124)

Data expressed as Mean ± SEM; % patients.
Group I: PCI with use of PercuSurge device; Group II: PCI without use of PercuSurge device.

Periprocedural Adverse Event, Intracoronary Agents and Myocardial Flow Assessment

Incidence of no/slow reflow occurred in 30% of cases in group I and in 84% in group II after predilatation / direct stenting or POBA (Table 2). The higher incidences of no reflow may be due to the higher thrombotic burden in group II. This debris was aspirated in group I by the PercuSurge device, leading to fewer incidences of no/slow reflow and other periprocedural events in this group. 87% of patients achieved TIMI III and 80% TMP III in group I whereas only 49% achieved TIMI III and 14% achieved TMP III in group II without the use of PercuSurge (Table 2).

Figure 2 (a, b, c, d) and Figure 3(a and b) show the angiographic views of PCI done with and without the use of PercuSurge and depict the improvement in TIMI flow and TMP grade achieved with the use of Guardwire system as compared to PCI without its use. Figure 2(a) and Figure 3(a) shows the LAD artery with stenosis before PCI was done. In figure 2(b), the distal balloon of PercuSurge device is shown inflated. Figure 2(c and d) show the artery after PCI was done. TIMI flow III and TMP grade 3 were obtained with use of PercuSurge as seen in these figures.

Figure 3(b) shows that adequate TIMI and TMP flow were not obtained after PCI wherein PercuSurge was not used. In order to optimize the TIMI flow and the myocardial perfusion when no reflow occurred, intracoronary (IC) boluses of vasodilators that included adenosine, sodium nitroprusside as well as NTG were administered.

Further, a concomitant use of GP IIb/IIIa antagonists was required in significantly less patients if PercuSurge was used, based on the ACC guidelines (Class II indication) (43% patients in group I vs. 70% in group II, $p<0.05$, Table 2). It was observed that such simultaneous administration of drugs was minimal in the Guardwire arm as compared to the other arm.

Further, no major periprocedural adverse events including death, new Q wave or non Q wave AMI, emergent CABG, or repeat target vessel revascularization within 3 days of the index procedure were observed in the PercuSurge arm. In group I, one patient had Re MI and died in hospital while death occurred in one patient within 1 month of the PCI in group II.

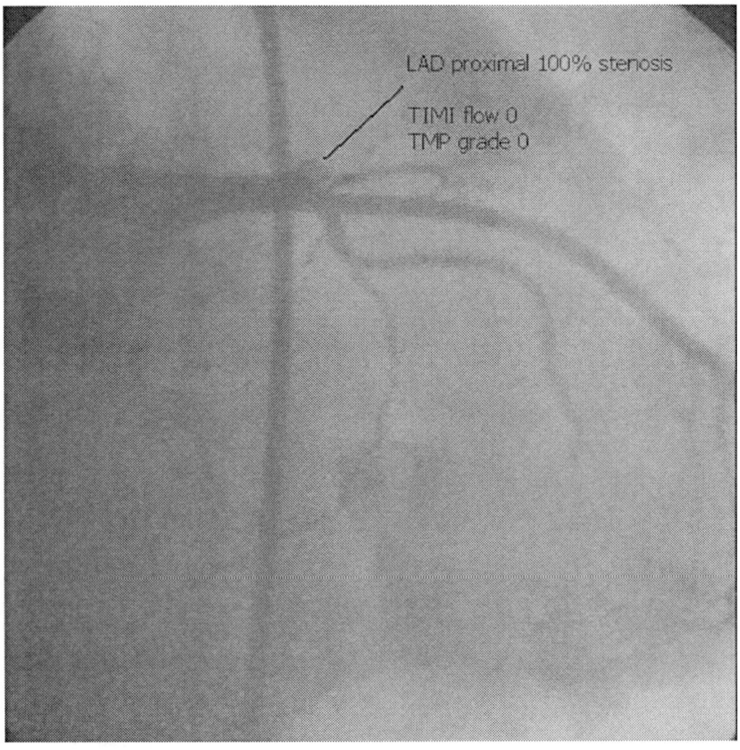

a

2 (a) Figure shows LAD proximal segment 100 % blocked TIMI flow as well as TMP grade was 0 before PCI.

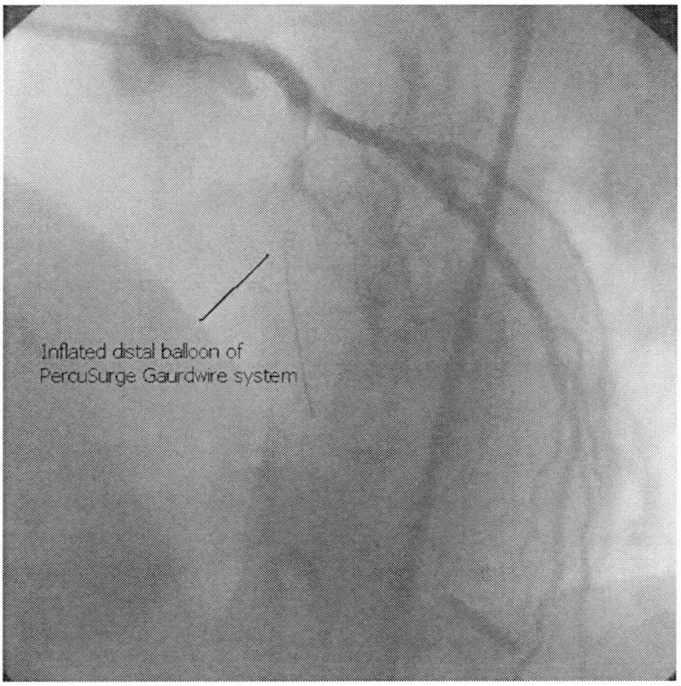

b

(b) Figure shows the inflated distal balloon of PercuSurge device

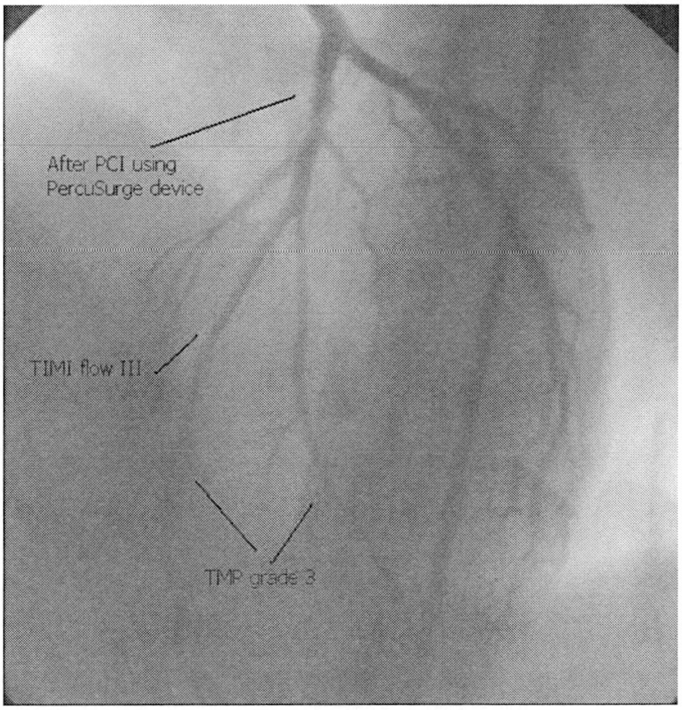

c

Figure 2. (Continued).

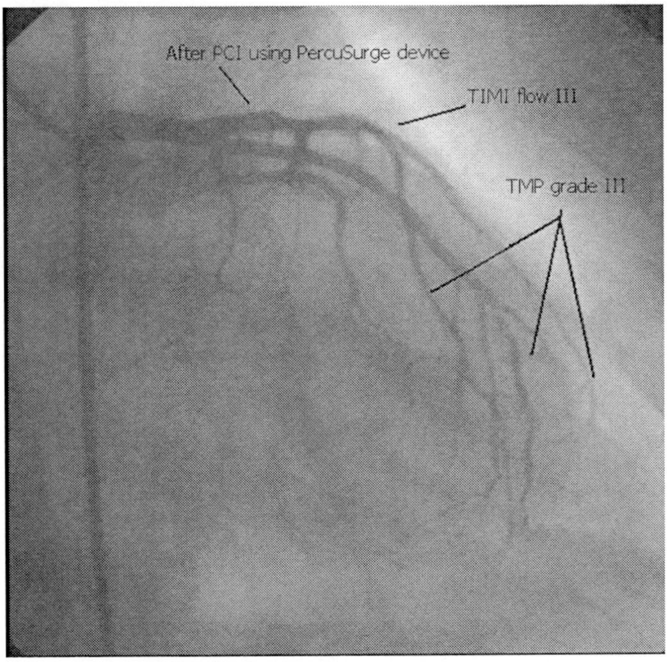

d

Figure 2. Angiograms of a patient treated with PCI using PercuSurge Guardwire system. (c) and (d) LAD Proximal segment shown in fig 2(a) treated with PCI with use of PercuSurge "No reflow" did not occur and the final TIMI flow III and TMP grade 3 was achieved. Figures 2(c) and 1(d) depict blood flow and myocardial blush.

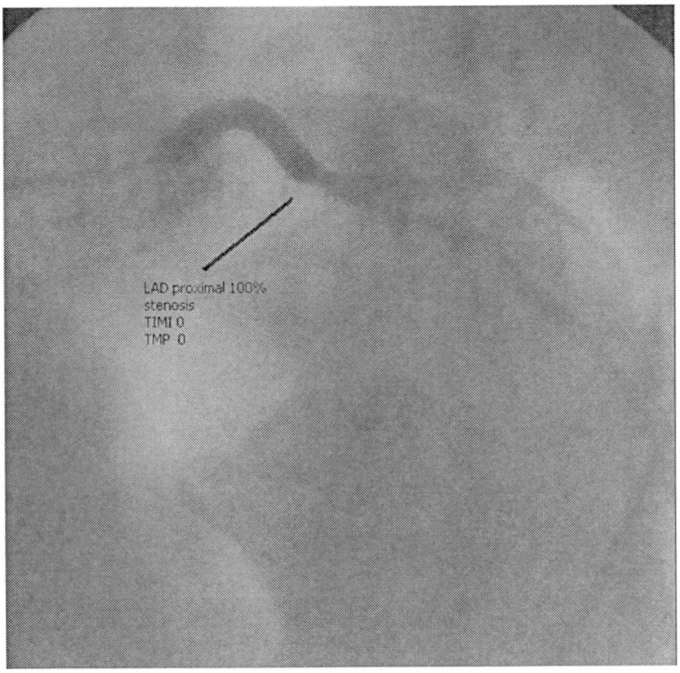

a

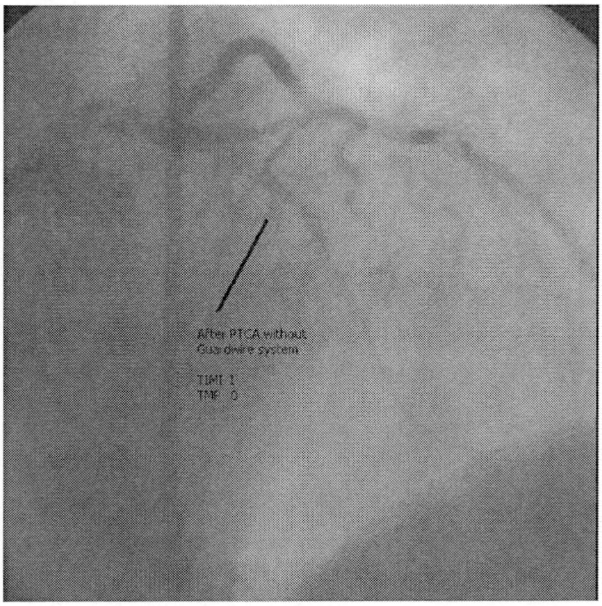

b

Figure 3. Angiogram of a patient treated with PCI without using PercuSurge Guardwire system. (a) Figure shows LAD proximal segment 100 % blocked TIMI flow as well as TMP grade was 0 before PCI. (b) LAD Proximal segment in fig 1(a) treated with PCI without use of PercuSurge. "No reflow" occurred and the final TIMI flow achieved was 1 and TMP grade was not improved.

Time in Minutes Involved in Different Steps of the Procedure

The total procedural time as well as time involved in individual steps of the PCI were recorded and compared (Table 3). It was observed that the time consumed in crossing the lesion by the wire was similar in both the groups (2.84 ± 0.65 minutes in group I vs. 2.89 ± 0.38 minutes in group II). An additional time of 3.04 ± 0.57 minutes was consumed in the PercuSurge arm to inflate the distal balloon. Inspite of this, the time consumed to reach PTCA balloon inflation after the wire crossing was identical in both the arms. Similarly, the total fluoroscopy time was also identical in both the groups (Table 3). The time to reach stent placement after wire crossing was significantly less ($p<0.05$) in group I (9.26 ± 1.25 minutes) as compared to that in group II (14.55 ± 2.27 minutes).

We also calculated the time required after lesion crossing by wire till achievement of TIMI III / optimal TIMI flow (in case of PCI without use of PercuSurge). This was found to be significantly less in Guardwire system group (21.04 ± 2.19 minutes) as compared to group II (28.58 ± 2.52 minutes, $p=0.017$). The time frame from PTCA balloon inflation/stent placement (in case of direct stenting) till attainment of TIMI III / optimal TIMI flow was also significantly less in procedures with Guardwire use (17.37 ± 2.21 minutes in group I vs. 24.41 ± 2.5 minutes in group II, $p=0.025$). During this time frame the periprocedural adverse events like no reflow and distal embolization take place. The total procedural time consumed in PCI was found to be significantly less with use of PercuSurge as compared to PCI without its use (25.01 ± 2.17 minutes in group I vs. 31.98 ± 2.52 minutes in group II, $p=0.027$). The longest procedure in the PercuSurge group lasted 53.9 minutes where the shortest procedure was of

8.3 minutes whereas in group II, where PercuSurge was not used, the longest PCI lasted 69.1 minutes and the shortest procedure lasted 11.9 minutes.

Table 3. Time involved in the different stages of the PTCA procedure

Parameters	Group I (DPD) (n=30) Time in minutes	Group II (without DPD) (n=37) Time in minutes	p value
Individual time frame for each step of the Procedure			
Time for lesion crossing by wire	2.84 ± 0.65	2.89 ± 0.38	0.947
Time to inflate Distal balloon of Guardwire System	3.04 ± 0.57	-	
Total Time required for various steps of the procedure			
Total time after wire crossing until PTCA balloon inflation	4.4± 0.67	4.17 ± 0.61	0.779
Total time after wire crossing until stent placement	9.26 ± 1.25	14.55 ± 2.27	0.037 *
Total time after wire crossing to achievement of TIMI III flow	*21.04* ± 2.19	*28.58* ± 2.52	*0.017**
Total time from PTCA balloon inflation (in POB) OR final stent Placement to TIMI III flow	*17.37* ± 2.21	*24.41* ± 2.5	*0.025**
Total Fluoroscopy time	10.07 ± 1.01	10.78 ± 0.68	0.507
Total PROCEDURAL TIME	25.01 ± 2.17	31.98 ± 2.52	0.027 *

Data expressed as Mean (time in minutes) ± SEM.
* Unpaired Student's t test, Significantly less as compared to group II, $p<0.05$.
Group I: PCI with use of PercuSurge device.
Group II: PCI without use of PercuSurge device.

DISCUSSION

Microembolization may be a relatively frequent event among patients with acute coronary syndromes or after PCI. The benefit of primary PCI is limited by a 5% to 20% incidence of no reflow [28, 29]. The 'no reflow' phenomenon has been documented in ≥ 30% of patients after thrombolysis or PCI for AMI [4, 30], characterized by profound reduction in epicardial anterograde coronary flow without evidence of vessel dissection, thrombosis, or embolization.

Mechanical devices have recently emerged as an attractive tool to prevent both embolization in the microvasculature and no reflow [15, 20, 31]. Muller et al.[18] have shown that the PercuSurge system is a safe and effective device for the protection of distal embolization during interventions in degenerated aorto-coronary saphenous vein grafts. The study showed that the TIMI flow was significantly improved by the use of PercuSurge Guardwire system. Our study also shows that the number of patients achieving TIMI III flow was significantly higher with the use of PercuSurge as compared to PCI without its use. Even achievement of TMP III was significantly greater in patients with use of PercuSurge whereas PCI without its use could not result in optimal TIMI and TMP flow in all the cases. *The % of diabetics was significantly higher in group II (41%) as compared to group I (20%). This may be one of the factors responsible for the comparatively poorer outcome in group II. However, there are several other reports that support the contention that the use of PercuSurge is beneficial in preventing no-reflow as well as embolization in the distal microvasculature.* Huang et al.[24] have reported that no patient developed angiographic evidence of no reflow or distal embolization with the use of PercuSurge. In our study, also, we observed that the incidences of no/slow reflow were significantly less with use of PercuSurge as compared to PCI without its use, irrespective of the indications. Our study also showed that the use of PercuSurge significantly reduced the requirement of GP IIb/IIIa inhibitors and intracoronary administration of vasodilators like adenosine, sodium nitroprusside, etc. that were employed to overcome the no/slow reflow and distal embolization in the thrombotic lesions. In our study myocardial blush grade 3 was achieved in 85% of patients, which is similar to that shown by Huang et al., i.e. 86.7% of patients.

Preliminary encouraging results with PercuSurge have been confirmed in the SAFER (Saphenous Vein Graft Angioplasty Free of emboli randomized) trial [20]. A significant reduction in MACE, MI and no reflow was reported in degenerated SV grafts. SAFE study[19] has also proved the efficacy of PercuSurge in patients with degenerated SVGs. However, very few studies have been done in AMI involving native coronaries. The preliminary results of RUBY (Revascularization Utilizing Balloon protection in acute coronarY ischemic syndrome) registry have shown the efficacy of this Guardwire in the setting of AMI. The interim conclusions of RUBY registry suggest a high number of patients with TIMI III and low 30-day mortality in AMI patients using PercuSurge for distal protection. Our study also supports the above results along with a significant finding of less time consumed in the procedure.

The results of the single, large scale, Guardwire trial in AMI patients, EMERALD (Enhanced Myocardial Efficacy and Recovery by Aspiration of Liberated Debris) have been recently released. It has shown that the Guardwire was not associated with an improvement in the primary endpoints of post procedure ST resolution or infarct size. Also, the procedure duration was significantly longer in the Guardwire arm in this trial. Contrary to these results of EMERALD study, our results show that the total procedural time is in fact significantly less with the use of Guardwire system. In our trial, however, we have considered the precise period after the guide catheter engagement till the last cinefilm as the end of procedure to determine the total procedural time. This stringent time slot consideration may be responsible for our results, contrary to the EMERALD trial.

Pershad et al [32] has, in fact, in a case, reported thrombus at the site of the distal occlusive balloon of PercuSurge. However, no large-scale data is available in the line of this finding. In fact, in our study no procedural complication was observed. The device success and procedural success achieved were 100%. We also report for the first time that the total time required after lesion crossing by wire till achievement of TIMI III was significantly less as compared to PCI without its use. This time represents the slot when the atherothrombotic plaque is ruptured leading to distal micro- embolization and no reflow, thus complicating the procedure. Various agents including GP IIb/IIIa inhibitors and intracoronary vasodilators like adenosine, sodium nitroprusside; NTG, etc. are thus employed to overcome this complication that then prolongs the time of PCI if PercuSurge is not used. We found in our study that using PercuSurge provides distal protection against microembolization and aspiration of the thrombotic debris, thus reducing the incidences of no reflow. Even the total procedural time was significantly less in PCI using the PercuSurge system by experienced operators.

Significance and Limitations of Our Study

Unlike the EMERALD trial, our study did show lesser time consumed to achieve TIMI III flow using distal protection device and also better TIMI flow and TMP grade. This single centered study is limited by small size and the lack of a randomized set up. However, this will certainly be one of the important aspects for any future study using this protective device in native coronary arteries.

Our experience shows that at least 10 cases using the PercuSurge device have to be done before the operator and nurses develop proficiency in its use. The speed of the procedure is related to the "learning curve". It is our opinion that centers with higher usage of Guardwire system takes lesser time, which has a direct and clinically relevant impact on the outcome.

Conclusion

These preliminary results suggest the efficacy and time saving aspect of the PercuSurge Guardwire system for distal protection against embolization during urgent coronary intervention in AMI. It is effective in reducing the risk of intraprocedual embolization and no reflow phenomenon without increasing the procedural time. These findings are contrary to the large, multi-centered EMERALD trial. We suggest that interventional cardiologists get experience with distal protection devices, which are efficient and time saving.

References

[1] Keeley EC, Boura JA, Grines CL. Primary angioplasty vs. intravenous thrombolytic therapy for acute myocardial infarction: a quantitative review of 23 randomized trials. *Lancet* 2003; 361: 13-20.

[2] Topol EJ, Yadav JS. Recognition of the importance of embolization in atherosclerotic vascular disease. *Circ* 2000; 101:570-80.

[3] Prati F, Pawlowski T, Gil R, Labellarte A, Gziut A, Caradonna E, Manzoli A, Pappalardo A, Burzotta F, Boccanelli A. Stenting of culprit lesions in unstable angina leads to marked reduction in plaque burden: a major role of plaque embolization? A serial intravascular ultrasound study. *Circ* 2003; 107:2320-25.

[4] Ito H, Maruyama A, Iwakura K, Takiuchi S, Masuyama T, Hori M, Higashino Y, Fujii K, Minamino T. Clinical implications of "no reflow" phenomenon: a predictor of complications and left ventricular remodeling in reperfused anterior wall myocardial infarction. *Circ* 1996; 93: 223-8.

[5] Saber R.S, Edwards WD, Bailey KR, McGovern TW, Schwartz RS, Holmes DR Jr. Coronary embolization after balloon angioplasty or thrombolytic therapy: an autopsy study of 32 cases. *J Amer Coll Cardiol* 1993; 22: 1283-8.

[6] Yip HK, Wu CJ, Chang HW, Chen MC, Hang CL, Fang CY, Hsieh YK, Yang CH, Yeh KH, Fu M. Comparison of impact of primary percutaneous transluminal coronary angioplasty and primary stenting on short term mortality in patients with cardiogenic shock and evaluation of prognostic determinants. *Amer J Cardiol* 2001; 87: 1184-8.

[7] Yip HK, Chen MC, Chang HW, Hang CL, Hsieh YK, Fang CY, Wu CJ, Yang CH. Angiographic morphologic features of infarct-related arteries and timely reperfusion in acute myocardial infarction: predictors of slow-flow and no-reflow. *Chest* 2002; 122: 1322-32.

[8] Tanaka A, Kawarabayashi T, Nishibori Y, Sano T, Nishida Y, Fukuda D, Shimada K, Yoshikawa J. No-reflow phenomenon and lesion morphology in patients with acute myocardial infarction. *Circ* 2002; 105: 2148-52.

[9] Gibson CM, de Lemos JA, Murphy SA, Marble SJ, McCable CH, Cannon P, Antman EM, Braunwald E. Combination therapy with abciximab reduces angiographically evident thrombus in acute myocardial infarction: a TIMI 14 substudy. *Circ* 2001; 103: 2550-4.

[10] Singh M, Berger PB, Ting HH, Rihal CS, Wilson SH, Lennon RJ, Reeder GS, Bresnahan JF, Holmes DR Jr. Influence of coronay thrombus on outcome of percutaneous coronary angioplasty in the current era (the Mayo Clinic experience). *Amer J Cardiol* 2001; 88: 1091-96.

[11] Macdonald RG, Feldman RL, Conti CR, Pepine CJ. Thromboembolic complications of coronary angioplasty. *Amer J Cardiol* 1984; 54:916-7.

[12] Weyne AE, H3eyndrickx GR, Vandekerckhove YR, Clement DL. Embolization of complicating coronary angioplasty in the presence of an intracoronary thrombus. *Clin Cardiol* 1986; 9:463-5.

[13] Cameron J, Buchbinder M, Wexler L, Oesterle SN. Thromboembolic complications of percutaneous transluminal coronary angioplasty for myocardial infarction. *Cathet Cardiovasc Diagn* 1987; 13:100-6.

[14] Arora RR, Platko WP, Bhadwar K, Simpfendorfer C. Role of intracoronary thrombus in acute complications during percutaneous transluminal coronary angioplasty. *Cathet Cardiovasc Diagn* 1989; 16:226-9.

[15] Grube e, Gerckens U, Yeung AC, Rowold S, Kirchhof N, Sedgewick J, Yadav JS, Stertzer S. Prevention of distal embolization during coronary angioplasty in saphenous vein grafts and native vessels using porous filter protection. *Circ* 2001; 104:2436-41.

[16] Van Ommen V, Michels R, Heymen E, Van Asseldonk J, Bonnier H, Nainer J, De Swart H, Koolen J. Usefulness of the rescue PT catheter to remove fresh thrombus from coronary arteries and bypass grafts in acute myocardial infarction. *Amer J Cardiol* 2001; 88: 306-8.

[17] Beran G, Lang I, Schreiber W, Denk S, Stefenelli T, Syeda B, Maurer G, Glogar D, Siostrzonek P. Intracoronary thrombectomy with the X-sizer catheter system improves epicardial flow and accelerates ST segment resolution in patients with acute coronary syndrome: a prospective, randomized, controlled study. *Circ* 2002; 105: 2355-60.

[18] Muller R, Gerckens U, Staberock M, Grube E. Clinical experiences with the PercuSurge Guardwire: a new system for prevention of peripheral embolisms in catheter interventions on degenerated coronary artery venous bypasses. *Z Kario*l 2000; 89: 316-22.

[19] Grube E, Schofer JJ, Webb J, Schuler G, Colombo A, Sievert H, Gerckens U, Stone GW, Saphenous Venin Graft angioplasty free of emboli (SAFE) trial study group. Evaluation of a balloon occlusion and aspiration system for protection from distal embolization during stenting in saphenous vein grafts. *Amer J Cardiol* 2002; 89: 941-945.

[20] Baim DS, Wahr D, George B. on behalf of the Saphenous vein graft angioplasty free of Emboli Randomized (SAFER) trial investigators. Randomized trial of a distal embolic protection device during percutaneous intervention of saphenous vein aorto-coronary grafts. *Circ* 2002; 105: 1285-90.

[21] Henry M, Amor M, Henry I, Klonaris C, Chati Z, Masson I, Kownator S, Luizy F, Hugel M. Carotid stenting with cererbral protection: first clinical experience using the PercuSurge Guardwire system. *J Endovasc Surg* 1999; 6: 321-31.

[22] Al-Mubarak N, Roubin GS, Vitek JJ, Lyer SS, New G, Leon MB. Effect of the distal balloon protection system on microembolization during carotid stenting. *Circ* 2001; 104: 1999-2002.

[23] Henry M, Henry I, Klonaris C, Masson I, Hugel M, Tzvetanov K, Ethevenot G, Le BE, Kownator S, Luizi F, Folliguet B. Benefits of cerebral protection during carotid stenting with the PercuSurge Guardwire system: midterm results. *J Endovasc Ther* 2002; 9: 1-13.

[24] Huang Z, Katoh O, Nakamura s, Negoro S, Kobayashi T, Tanigawa J. Evaluation of the PercuSurge Guardwire Plus Temporary Occlusion and aspiration system during primary angioplasty in acute myocardial infarction. *Cathet Cardiovasc Interv* 2003; 60: 443-51.

[25] Sutsch G, Kiowski W, Bossard A, Luscher TF, Maier W, Vogt P, Amann FW. Use of an emboli containment and retrieval system during Percutaneous coronary angioplasty in native coronary arteries. *Schweiz Med Wochenschr* 2000; 130:1135-45.

[26] Gibson Mc, Cannon CP, Murphy SA, Ryan KA, Mesley R, Marble SJ, McCabe CH, Van de Werf F, Braunwald E for the TIMI study group. *Circ* 2000; 101: 125-30.

[27] Van't hof AWJ, Liem A, Suryapranata H, Hoorntji JCA, Jan de Boer M, Zijlstra F. Angiographic assessment of myocardial reperfusion in patients treated with primary angioplasty for acute myocardial infarction. *Circ* 1998; 97: 2302-6.

[28] Cura Fa, L'Allier PL, Kapadia SR, Houghtaling PL, Dipaola LM, Ellis SG, Topol EJ, Brener SJ. Predictors and prognosis of suboptimal coronary blood flow after primary coronary angioplasty in patients with acute myocardial infarction. *Amer J Cardiol* 2001; 88: 124-8.

[29] Yip HK, Wu CJ, Chang HW, Fang CY, Yang CH, Chen SM, Hung WC, Chen CJ, Cheng CI, Hsieh YK. Effect of the PercuSurge Guardwire Device on the Integrity of Microvascular and clinical outcomes during primary transradial coronary intervention in acute myocardial infarction. *Amer J Cardiol* 2003; 92: 1331-5.

[30] Eeckhout E, Kern MJ. The coronary no-reflow phenomenon: a review of mechanisms and therapies *Eur Heart J* 2001; 22: 729-39.

[31] Belli g, Pezzano A, De Biase AM, Baonacina E, Silva P, Salvade P, Piccalo G, Klugmann S. Adjunctive thrombus aspiration and mechanical protection from distal embolization in primary percutaneous intervention for acute myocardial infarction. *Cathet Cardiovasc Intervent* 2000; 50:362-70.

[32] Pershad A, Cherukiri G, Kirby A. PercuSurge guardwire balloon associated thrombus—a limitation of the PercuSurge distal protection system. *J Invasive Cardiol* 2002; 630-2.

In: World Heart Research Yearbook. Volume 1
Editors: Franz Halberg and R. B. Singh
ISBN: 978-1-60741-881-8

THE EFFECT OF AN ALPHA-LINOLENIC-ACID-RICH DIET ON THE CIRCADIAN RHYTHM OF CARDIAC EVENTS

Gal Dubnov, Daniel Pella[1] and Ram B. Singh[2,*]
Department of Human Nutrition & Metabolism,
Hebrew University- Hadassah Medical School, Jerusalem, Israel
[1] Faculty of Medicine, Safaric University, Kosice, Slovakia
[2] Centre of Nutrition and Heart, Medical Hospital and Research Centre, Moradabad, India

ABSTRACT

Objective: Coronary artery disease events have a circadian rhythmicity, clustering more in the second quartile of the day. n-3 fatty acid supplementation reduces the rate of cardiac events, but its effect on their circadian rhythmicity has not been tested.

Design: The Indo-Mediterranean Diet Heart Study was a single blind randomized study that assessed the effect of a diet rich in alpha-linolenic acid, the parent n-3 fatty acid, on the occurrence of myocardial infarction and sudden cardiac death.

Subjects: One thousand subjects of the Indo-Mediterranean Diet Heart Study, focusing on the 115 patients from both control and intervention groups in which cardiac events occurred.

Intervention: The timing of cardiac events throughout the day was compared between the intervention and control groups. The distribution of cardiac events along the four quartiles of the day was compared between groups as well as against equal distribution.

Results: The risk ratio for a cardiac event was lowest between 4:00 and 8:00 in the morning for the intervention group. The control group had a higher, rate of events in the second quartile of the day, which deviated from an equal distribution, as expected ($P=0.013$). In the intervention group events were equally distributed along the day. No statistically significant difference was found in daily event distribution between the groups.

Conclusion: A diet rich in alpha-linolenic acid may abolish the higher rate of cardiac events, normally seen in the second quartile of the day. Additional studies are needed to identify the underlying mechanism.

* Corresponding author: Ram B. Singh, MD. Centre of Nutrition and Heart, Medical Hospital and Research Centre, Moradabad-10 (UP)244001, India. E-mail: icn2005@mickyonline.com.

Introduction

The classical manifestations of coronary artery disease (CAD), such as angina pectoris, silent ischemia, myocardial infarction (MI) and sudden cardiac death, have a pronounced circadian rhythmicity, tending to cluster in the second quartile of the day [1-10]. This increase in the rate of cardiovascular events in the morning may be due to a hypercoagulable state, consisted of increased platelet aggregation, increased tPA inhibitor levels, and rapid metabolism of heparin in the morning [11-13]. In addition, the morning hours are associated with a decrease in vagal tone and increase in sympathetic activity, resulting in lower levels of acetylecholine and melatonin and increased concentrations of cortisol, aldosterone, catecholamines and angiotensin, which make the atherosclerotic plaques more vulnerable to rupture and thrombosis [14-16]. These circadian manifestations are associated with a decreased heart rate variability (HRV), which is an independent risk factor for cardiovascular events [13-16].

Recent studies indicate that n-3 fatty acids may have a beneficial effect on HRV, platelet aggregation, and endothelial function, and that they are neuroprotectors and may enhance hippocampal acetylecholine levels [15-26]. In randomized controlled trials, treatment with n-3 fatty acids led to a significant reduction in cardiac events, in both patients after a MI and those with risk factors only [27-30]. To our knowledge, no study has examined the effect of n-3 fatty acids on the timing of cardiovascular events. The aim of the present study is to examine the influence of a diet rich in alpha-linolenic acid, the parent n-3 fatty acid, on the circadian rhythm of cardiac events.

Methods

Subjects and Study Design

The Indo-Mediterranean Diet Heart Study was a randomized, single-blind study designed to assess the effect of a diet rich in n-3 fatty acids from plant sources on the occurrence of myocardial infarction and sudden cardiac death [29]. One thousand subjects were randomized to either an intervention or a control group by selection of a card from a pile. The intervention group consisted of 499 patients, and the control group 501. The ethics committee of the Medical Hospital and Research Centre at Moradabad approved the study, and written informed consent was obtained from all participants.

Participants in both groups were advised to eat food elements that would provide a dietary intake similar to that recommended at the time by the National Cholesterol Education Program (NCEP) step I prudent diet [31], wherein less than 30% of energy comes from total fat, less than 10% from saturated fat, and less than 300 mg of cholesterol is consumed per day. Patients in the intervention group were advised to verify the intake of at least 250–300 g of fruit, 125–150 g of vegetables, and 25–50 g of nuts. They were also encouraged to eat 400–500 g of whole grains (legumes, rice, maize, wheat) daily, as well as to use mustard seed or soy bean oil in 3 to 4 servings per day, in order to ensure a high intake of alpha-linolenic acid.

Both groups were advised to exercise daily and practice yoga meditation techniques, to abstain from smoking and alcohol consumption, and to continue the use of their regular medications.

Food intake and physical activity were monitored by self-report diaries, first weekly, then monthly, and then every 3 months. Nutrient intakes were calculated using Indian foods composition tables and other sources [32,33].and reinforce adherence. Height, weight, and blood pressure were monitored by standard methods. Blood concentrations of glucose, total cholesterol (TC), high-density lipoprotein (HDL) cholesterol, low-density lipoprotein (LDL) cholesterol and triglycerides were also measured. Clinical data, drug intake, adverse events, blood pressure, blood glucose levels, blood lipid levels, hospital admission and coronary events were recorded by physicians blinded to patient grouping.

At the 2-year follow up in the original study, cardiac events had occurred in 39 subjects from the intervention group and in 76 subjects from the control group.

Cardiac Events

The principal endpoints of the original study were fatal or nonfatal MI, sudden cardiac deaths, and the combined total of these events. Owing to the relatively small number of events in each category, we did not attempt a subgroup analysis and focused only on the combined end-point of total cardiac events.

In hospitalized patients, a diagnosis of nonfatal MI was based on a diagnostic electrocardiograph at the time of the event, or the presence of ischaemic cardiac pain and diagnostic enzyme levels of at least twice the upper limit of normal, or the presence of ischaemic cardiac pain and equivocal enzyme levels and an equivocal electrocardiograph. In patients who had not been admitted to the hospital, the diagnosis of MI was considered if they complained of chest pain, breathlessness, or syncope, combined with a diagnostic electrocardiograph at the time of event or new electrocardiographic changes consistent with MI at routine check-up. The electrocardiographic coding and analysis were performed by a cardiologist blinded to patient grouping.

Fatal MI was diagnosed when a hospital record was consistent with cause of death, and there was either a preterminal hospital admission with a definite MI, or official documentation of a myocardial infarction.

Sudden cardiac death was diagnosed when coronary heart disease had been noted, and death occurred within one hour of symptom onset.

Statistical Analysis

Analyses were performed in two ways. One was determining the risk for cardiac events in specific time frames among the whole study population. Second, we determined the number of events in the four quartiles of the day among only those subjects with events in both groups.

In order to assess the effect of the ALA-rich diet on the timing of cardiac event, we constructed a Cox multivariate model, with cardiac event as outcome variable, stratified into six 4-hour periods (0:01-4:00, 4:01-8:00, 8:01-12:00, 12:01-16:00, 16:01-20:00, and 20:01-

24:00). In each model, we examined the risk ratio associated with the intervention diet, with patient's age, gender and BMI as covariates. The last available values served as the final risk factors data for the subjects who had fatal events. The analyses were held using standard statistical package (SPSS 11.0).

When comparing only the subgroups in which events occurred, Student's *t* test with a Bonferroni adjustment was used to analyze between-group differences of the continuous variables; P values less than 0.005 were considered statistically significant. The distribution of the number of events in each quartile of the day was compared by the chi-square test. Event rates were compared between the control and intervention groups, as well as for each group against equal distribution. Thus, for the latter, the observed event rates in the control group were compared with an expected rate of 19 (76 divided by 4) events in each quartile of the day, and the observed events in the intervention group were compared with an expected rate of 9.75 (39 divided by 4) in each quartile of the day. A two-tailed P value less than 0.05 was considered statistically significant for the parametric variables.

RESULTS

Timing of Events in Total Study Population

Baseline characteristics of the Indo-Mediterranean Diet Heart study population was presented elsewhere [29]. In all strata, the ALA-rich diet was associated with protective effect for cardiac events. The lowest risk ratio (RR=0.05; 95%CI: 0.01-0.24) was calculated for cardiac events between 4:01 and 8:00, while the highest was for events between 0:01 to 4:00 (RR=0.15 (95% CI:0.03 – 0.87) as shown in Figure 1. However, differences between strata did not reach statistical significance.

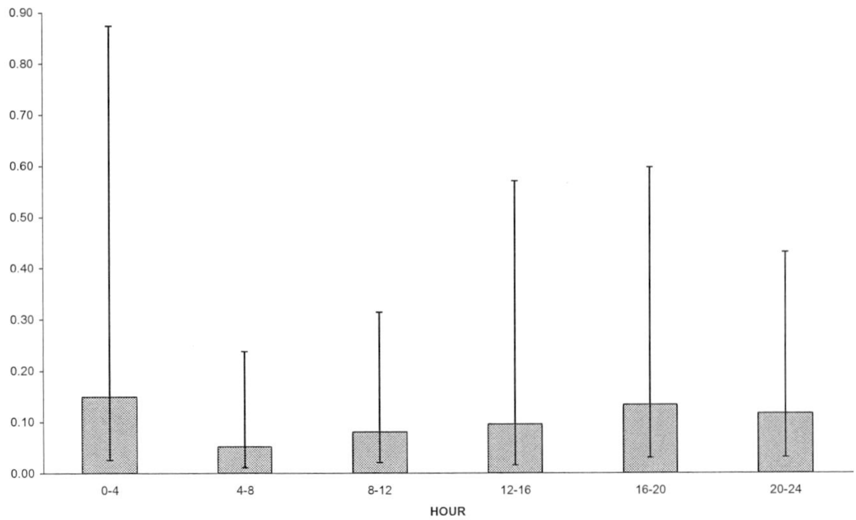

Figure 1. The risk ratio for cardiac events in the intervention group (n=499) compared with the control group (n=501) distributed into 4-hour intervals of the day.

Dispersion of Events Along Quartiles of the Day

Baseline characteristics of the subjects with cardiac events from both groups is presented in Table 1. Subjects in both groups were comparable for all major baseline variables except for body weight (borderline significance, P=0.006), yet BMIs were comparable between groups. At 2 years, only TC and LDL levels differed significantly between groups, with lower values noted in the intervention group. Nutritional data are presented in Table 2. At baseline, values of all nutrients, including fatty acids, were similar in the two groups. At 2 years, n-3 fatty acid intake was significantly higher in the intervention group, and the n-6/n-3 fatty acid ratio was lower. The number of cardiovascular events of each type in both groups is given in Table 3.

The dispersion of cardiac events along the quartiles of the day is presented in Table 4. In the control group, there was an increased rate of cardiac events clustered in the second quartile of the day, which deviated from an equal distribution (P=0.013). In the intervention group, the events were distributed equally along the day (P=0.49 when comparing observed rates and equal distribution). There was no statistically significant difference in the rate of events in each quartile of the day between the two groups (P=0.54).

Table 1. Cardiovascular risk factors at baseline and after 2 years in the intervention and control groups. Data presented as means ± SD. BMI- body mass index, BP- blood pressure, TC- total cholesterol, TG- triglyceride, FBG- fasting blood glucose

	Intervention Group A, n = 39			Control Group B, n = 76			P value at 2 years between groups
	Baseline	2 years	P value	Baseline	2 years	P value	
Age (years)	51 ± 10	-	-	49 ± 8	-	-	-
Weight, kg	65 ± 5	62 ± 7	0.0002	68 ± 6	67 ± 6	0.0004	<0.0001
BMI, kg/m^2	24 ± 3	23 ± 3	0.0005	25 ± 2	24 ± 2	0.0005	0.0172
Systolic BP	134 ± 15	129 ± 15	0.0064	133 ± 19	132 ± 17	0.0040	0.2051
Diastolic BP	86 ± 6	84 ± 10	0.0931	88 ± 10	87 ± 10	0.0063	0.0532
Cigarettes / day	18 ± 9	19 ± 9	0.0961	21 ± 8	16 ± 5	0.0001	0.1608
TC, mmol/L	232 ± 43	220 ± 39	0.0029	245 ± 34	245 ± 32	0.7507	0.0001
LDL, mmol/L	150 ± 26	137 ± 30	0.0001	156 ± 32	157 ± 31	0.9745	0.0005
HDL, mmol/L	45 ± 15	44 ± 11	0.1319	44 ± 6	43 ± 11	0.3524	0.4414
TG, mmol/L	181 ± 51	169 ± 43	0.0259	176 ± 33	175 ± 35	0.8080	0.1881
FBG, mmol/L	112 ± 28	106 ± 25	0.0001	115 ± 33	109 ± 27	0.0029	0.2661

Table 2. Nutrient data at baseline and after 2 years in the intervention and control groups. Data presented as means ± SD

	Intervention Group A, n = 39			**Control Group B, n = 76**			**P value at 2 years between groups**
	Baseline	**2 years**	**P value**	**Baseline**	**2 years**	**P value**	0.2589
Energy (kcal.day)	2116 ± 175	2098 241	0.3279	2167 ± 183	2123 ± 163	0.0099	<0.0001
CHO (%en)	57 ± 2	58 ± 3	0.0007	56 ± 2	55 ± 1	<0.0001	<0.0001

Table 2. (Continued)

	Intervention Group A, n = 39			**Control Group B, n = 76**			**P value at 2 years between groups**
	Baseline	**2 years**	**P value**	**Baseline**	**2 years**	**P value**	0.2589
Protein (%en)	14 ± 1.7	14 ± 1.3	0.0112	14 ± 1.5	15 ± 0.8	0.1862	0.0241
Fat (%en)	27 ± 3	28 ± 3	0.0206	28 ± 2	30 ± 1.5	<0.0001	<0.0001
Saturated fat (%en)	13 ± 1.8	11 ± 2.3	0.0017	12 ± 1.4	13 ± 1.6	0.0003	<0.0001
MUFA (%en)	7.3 ± 1.6	9.0 ± 2.2	<0.0001	8.1 ± 2.1	8.8 ± 1.3	0.3857	0.01929
PUFA (%en)	7.0 ± 1.0	7.5±1.0	<0.0001	7.5 ± 1.0	7.9 ± 0.8	0.0111	0.0052
n-6 (%en)	6.8 ± 0.9	6.9 ± 1.0	0.4042	7.3 ± 1.0	7.6 ± 0.8	0.0001	<0.0001
n-3 (%en)	0.2 ± 0.1	0.5 ± 0.2	<0.0001	0.2 ± 0.1	0.3 ± 0.1	0.0003	<0.0001

Table 3. Distribution of cardiac events in intervention and control groups. MI – myocardial infarction

	Intervention group (n=39)	Control group (n=76)
Nonfatal MI	21	43
Fatal MI	12	17
Sudden cardiac death	6	16

Table 4. Distribution of cardiac events along the quartiles of the day in the intervention and control groups. In the intervention group, events are near-equally distributed along the day. In the control group, quartile 2 has more events than would be expected assuming equal distribution

Quartile (time range)	Intervention group (n=39) n (% within group)	Control group (n=76) n (% within group)
1 (00:01 – 06:00)	10 (26%)	15 (20%)
2 (06:01 – 12:00)	11 (28%)	29 (38%)
3 (12:01 – 18:00)	8 (21%)	10 (13%)
4 (18:01 – 00:00)	10 (26%)	22 (29%)

DISCUSSION

This study is the first to assess the effect of an ALA-rich diet on the circadian rhythm of cardiac events. We have found that although the intervention diet dramatically lowered the risk for events throughout the day, it nearly abolished it in the early morning hours. The increased rate of events known to occur in the second quartile of the day was eliminated by the diet.

Although n-3-rich diets have been found to be cardioprotective in several randomized controlled trials [27-30], their exact mode of action is still unknown. Our results suggest that dietary supplementation of alpha-linolenic acid may lead to a change in the circadian occurrence of cardiac events. The only major risk factors that differed significantly between the groups at the end of the trial along the trial were the lower levels of total cholesterol and LDL. However, we would expect this change to influence the total rate of events, and not just their distribution during the day, which was the focus of this study.

We are unaware of any other large-scale study that has examined the effect of n-3 fatty acids on the circadian rhythmicity of cardiac events. The Physicians Health Study recorded the number of myocardial infarctions in patients treated with aspirin or not, and found a significant decrease in the rhythmicity of myocardial infarctions in the aspirin group [34]. It is possible that this reduction was the result of the inhibitory effect of aspirin on platelet aggregation, a quality also possessed by n-3 fatty acids [25]. When these findings are combined, it appears that one of the triggers for MI in the morning hours is the increased tendency of platelets to aggregate.

Christensen and coworkers [17] reported a positive correlation between HRV and the platelet content of n-3 fatty acids (docosahexaenoic acid, DHA) in patients with post-MI left ventricular dysfunction. The increase in HRV occurred even after intake of only one fish meal per week, with an increase in standard deviation of normal-normal (SDNN) from 103 to 122ms. Further analysis revealed a negative correlation between the ratio of arachidonic acid/ DHA and the SDNN interval [18], consistent with earlier findings. In a more recent study, of 291 patients referred for coronary angiography that completed a food frequency questionnaire, researchers measured the n-3 fatty acid composition of granulocyte membranes and adipose tissue along with 24-hour HRV analysis [19]. Significant positive correlations were found between HRV indices and the levels of n-3 fatty acids in granulocytes. The positive influence of n-3 fatty acids on HRV suggests that this is indeed a major mechanism of CAD event reduction, as seen even after a few months of treatment [28].

HRV is a manifestation of sympathetic and parasympathetic activity of the heart, and a decreased HRV enhances the risk of circadian rhythmicity of cardiac events. This may well be another mechanism by which n-3 fatty acids reduce coronary events in the morning hours. In one randomized, controlled trial, of 81 patients after MI [17], treatment with n-3 fatty acids was associated with significant increase in HRV compared with controls, indicating an increased vagal cardiac tone. A retrospective analysis of a randomized, controlled intervention trial among 118 (fish oil group) and 122 (control group) patients with acute MI showed that treatment with fish oil (rich in EPA and DHA) was associated with a significant reduction in cardiac events (30% vs 56%, $P<0.02$) [27]. While the majority of cardiac events in the control group were reported in the second quartile of the day compared to first and third quartiles (35.7% vs 16.0%, 19.6%, respectively, $P<0.01$), no such association was observed in the fish oil group (unpublished data). These results are consistent with the view that fish oil administration may have a beneficial effect on circadian rhythmicity of cardiac events.

Alpha-linolenic acid is the parent n-3 fatty acid which is converted into long-chain fatty acids such as EPA and DHA in the body, to be later incorporated among phospholipids in cell membranes and adipose tissue. By using a control group which was also given dietary and exercise advice, we were able to isolate and highlight the role of the n-3 fatty acids. A detailed analysis of the role of specific nutrients in our Indo- Mediterranean diet is currently underway. Interim calculations show that the dietary intake of n-3 fatty acids had a major impact on the risk for cardiac events in the intervention group. The main sources of n-3 fatty acids in our diet were plants: walnuts, green leafy vegetables, whole grains, soy bean oil, and mustard oil. Thus, it is not necessary to consume the fish-derived long chain acids, DHA and EPA, in order to reap the benefits of n-3 fatty acids.

The exact mechanism underlying the circadian rhythmicity of cardiac events and its regulation by n-3 fatty acids remains unknown. There is consistent evidence that this rhythmicity is controlled by the suprachiasmatic nucleus [35], a tiny clump of cells in the brain which works as a biological clock and is influenced by daily changes in light and darkness. Brain neurons are rich in n-3 fatty acids, as are cell membranes of cardiomyocytes, endothelial cells and arterial smooth muscle cells. It is therefore possible that a relative deficiency of n-3 fatty acids in these cells enhances their susceptibility to excitation, causing greater neurohumoral and cardiovascular dysfunction, and resulting in a marked increase in the rhythmicity of cardiac events [36]. Increased vagal tone decreases the synthesis of tumor necrosis factor-alpha (TNF-alpha) in the liver and inhibits the release of proinflammatory cytokines such as IL-6 [20-22]. It is possible that low levels of n-3 fatty acids decrease the vagal tone, leading to increased synthesis of TNF-alpha and a greater release of proinflammatory cytokines by increased sympathetic activity. Treatment with n-3 fatty acids may break this cycle, decreasing inflammation and excitation of neurons, cardiomyocytes, endothelial and smooth muscle cells, bringing about a decreased vulnerability for cardiac events. Furthermore, n-3 fatty acids may also enhance brain acetylecholine level and parasympathetic tone, resulting in increased HRV, and hence, protection from pronounced rhythmicity of cardiac events [17-22]. One major limitation of our study is the relatively small number of events both overall and in each quartile of the day, owing to both the concomitant primary prevention arm of our original study (about half of the 1000 subjects had only risk factors for CAD, and were not post-MI patients), and the large reduction in event rate in the intervention group, brought about by the n-3 supplementation. Thus, the statistical analyses cannot definitely rule out this factor as the reason for the fairly equal distribution of events in the n-3 group. Given the measured proportion of events in the high risk hours (28%), a power of 80% and 39 participants in the intervention group, allowed the minimal detection of 17% difference compared to the control group; the difference observed was 10%. Nevertheless, the many mechanisms by which n-3 fatty acids may influence the circadian rhythm of CAD events cannot be overlooked, and we therefore believe that a biological explanation is plausible. A larger interventional study with more events is needed to confirm our findings.

In summary, our study suggests that an Indo-Mediterranean diet, which is rich in fruits, vegetables, nuts, whole grains, soy and mustard oils, can provide sufficient alpha-linolenic acid, to result in a modulation in the rhythmicity of cardiac events by n-3 fatty acids. Since a high n-6/n-3 ratio may blunt the beneficial effects of n-3 fatty acids, soybean oil should be replaced by more mustard oil. The exact nature of the cardioprotective action of n-3 fatty acids, whether by influencing platelet function or HRV through brain-heart connections, remains to be elucidated.

References

[1] Pell S, D'Alonzo CA. Acute myocardial infarction in a large industrial population. *JAMA* 1963;185:831-8.

[2] Arntz HR, Willich SN, Schreiber C, et al. Diurnal, weekly and seasonal variation of sudden death. *Eur Heart J* 2000;21:315-20.

[3] Willich SN. European survey on circadian variation of angina pectoris (ESCVA): design and preliminary results. *J Cardiovasc Pharmacol* 1999;34(suppl 2):s9-13.

[4] Singh RB, Pella D, Neki NS, et al. Mechanism of acute myocardial infarction study (MAMY Study). *Biomed Pharmacother* 2004;57:in press.

[5] Rocco MB, Barry J, Campbell BAS, et al. Circadian variation of transient myocardial ischemia in patients with coronary artery disease. *Circulation* 1987;75:395-400.

[6] Muller JE, Stone PH, Turi ZG, et al. Circadian variation in the frequency of onset of acute myocardial infarction. *N Engl J Med* 1985;313:1315-22.

[7] Goldberg R, Brady P, Chen J, et al. Time of onset of acute myocardial infarction after awakening. *J Am Coll Cardiol* 1989;13:133A [abstract].

[8] Davies MJ, Thomas A. Thrombosis and acute coronary artery lesions in sudden cardiac ischemic death. *N Engl J Med* 1984;310:1137-41.

[9] Muller JE, Ludmer PL, Willich SN, et al. Circadian variation in the frequency of sudden cardiac death. *Circulation* 1987;75:131-8

[10] International Study of Infarct Survival-2 (ISIS-2) Collaborative Group. Morning peak in the incidence of myocardial infarction: experience in the ISIS-2 trial. *Eur Heart J* 1992;13:594-608.

[11] Toffler GH, Brezinski D, Schaefer A, et al. Concurrent morning increase in platelet aggregability and the risk of myocardial infarction and sudden cardiac death. *N Engl J Med* 1987;316:1514-8.

[12] Chasen C, Muller JE. Cardiovascular triggers and morning events. *Blood Pressure Monit* 1998;3:35-42.

[13] Deedwania PC. Hemodynamic changes as triggers of cardiovascular events. *Cardiol Clin* 1996;14:229-38.

[14] Singh RB, Cornelissen G, Siegelova J, et al. About half-weekly (circasemiseptan) pattern of blood pressure and heart rate in men and women of India. *Scripta Medica* (Brno) 2002;75:125-8.

[15] Singh RB, Weydahl A, Otsuka K, et al. Can nutrition influence circadian rhythm and heart rate variability? *Biomed Pharmacother* 2001;55 (suppl 11):s115-24.

[16] Singh RB, Niaz MA, Cornelissen GS, et al. Circadian rhythmicity of circulating vitamin concentrations. *Scripta Medica* (Brno) 2001;74:93-6.

[17] Christensen JH, Gustenhoff P, Komp E, et al. Effect of fish oil on heart rate variability in survivors of myocardial infarction. *Br Med J* 1996;312:677-8.

[18] Christensen JH, Komp E, Aaroe J, et al. Fish consumption, n-3 fatty acids in cell membranes and heart rate variability in survivors of myocardial infarction with left ventricular dysfunction. *Am J Cardiol* 1997;79:1670-2.

[19] Christensen JH, Skou HA, Fog L, et al. Marine n-3 fatty acids, wine intake, and heart rate variability in patients referred for coronary angiography. *Circulation* 2001;103:651-7.

[20] Chin JPF. Marine oils and cardiovascular reactivity. *Prostaglandins Leukot Essent Fatty Acids* 1994;50:211-22.

[21] Borovikova LV, Ivanova S, Zhang M, et al. Vagus nerve stimulation attenuates the systemic inflammatory response to endotoxin. *Nature* 2000;405:458-62.

[22] Das UN. The brain-lipid-heart connection. *Nutrition* 2001;17:260-3.

[23] Lauritzen I, Blondeau N, Heurteaux C, et al. Polyunsaturated fatty acids are potent neuroprotectors. *EMBO J* 2000;19:1784-93.
[24] Minami M, Kimura S, Endo T, et al. Dietary docosahexaenoic acid increases cerebral acetylcholine levels and improves passive avoidance performance in stroke-prone spontaneously hypertensive rates. *Pharmacol Biochem Behav* 1997;58:1123-9.
[25] Goodnight SH Jr, Harris WS, Connor WE. The effects of dietary omega-3 fatty acids upon platelet composition and function in man: a prospective controlled study. *Blood* 1981;58:880-5.
[26] Pella D, Singh RB, Otsuka K, et al. Nutritional predictors and modulators of insulin resistance. *J Nutr Environ Med* 2004;14:3-16
[27] Singh RB, Niaz MA, Sharma JP, et al. Randomized, double blind, placebo controlled trial of fish oil and mustard oil in patients with suspected acute myocardial infarction. The Indian Experiment of Infarct Survival. *Cardiovasc Drug Ther* 1997;11:485-91.
[28] Marchioli R, Barzi F, Bobma E, et al. Early protection against sudden death by n-3 polyunsaturated fatty acids after myocardial infarction. time-course analysis of the results of the Gruppo Italiano per lo Studio della Sopravvivenza nell'Infarto Miocardico (GISSI)-Prevenzione. *Circulation* 2002;105:1897-903.
[29] Singh RB, Dubnov G, Niaz MA, et al. Effect of an Indo-Mediterranean diet on progression of coronary artery disease in high risk patients (Indo-Mediterranean Diet Heart Study): a randomised single-blind trial. *Lancet* 2002;360:1455-61.
[30] de Lorgeril M, Salen P, Martin JL, et al. Mediterranean diet, traditional risk factors and the rate of cardiovascular complications after myocardial infarction. Final report of the Lyon Diet Heart Study. *Circulation* 1999; 99: 779–85.
[31] National Cholesterol Education Program. Second report of the expert panel on detection, evaluation, and treatment of high blood cholesterol in adults (adult treatment panel II). *Circulation* 1994;89:1333-445.
[32] Narasinga Rao BS, Deosthale YG, Pant KC. Nutrient composition of Indian foods. Hyderbad, India: National Institute of Nutrition, Indian Council of Medical Research. 1989.
[33] Goodhart RS, Shils ME, eds. Modern nutrition in health and disease. Philadelphia, PA: *Lea & Febiger,* 1980.
[34] Ridker PM, Manson JE, Buring JE, et al. Circadian variation of acute myocardial *infarction* and the effect of low dose aspirin in a randomized trial of physicians. Circulation 1990;82:897-902.
[35] Ralph MR, Foster RG, Davis FC, et al. Transplanted suprachiasmatic nucleus determines circadian period. *Science* 1990;247:975-8.
[36] Yehuda S. Omega-6/omega-3 ratio and brain related functions. *World Rev Nutr Diet* 2003;92:37-56.

In: World Heart Research Yearbook. Volume 1
Editors: Franz Halberg and R. B. Singh
ISBN: 978-1-60741-881-8

MYOCARDIUM VIABILITY ASSESSED BY DELAYED CONTRAST-ENHANCED MAGNETIC RESONANCE IMAGING IN PATIENTS WITH SEVERE ISCHEMIC HEART FAILURE: A COMPARISON WITH THALLIUM SPECT AND DOBUTAMINE ECHOCARDIOGRAPHY

Yen-Wen Wu,[1,2] Por-Jau Huang,[2] Mao-Yuan Su,[3] Lung-Chun Lin,[2] Ruoh-Fang Yen,[1] Yih-Sharng Chen,[4] Chii-Ming Lee,[2] Hsi-Yu Yu,[4] Yi-Ting Wang,[3] Kai-Yuan Tzen[1] and Wen-Yih I. Tseng[3,*]

[1] Department of Nuclear Medicine, Taipei, Taiwan
[2] Department of Internal Medicine, Taipei, Taiwan
[3] Department of Medical Imaging, Taipei, Taiwan
[4] Department of Surgery, National Taiwan University Hospital and National Taiwan University College of Medicine, Taipei, Taiwan

ABSTRACT

Purpose: Functional recovery of ischemic cardiomyopathy depends on accurate identification of viable myocardium. We evaluated the value of delayed contrast-enhanced magnetic resonance imaging (MRI) in the assessment of myocardial viability.

Materials and Methods: Forty patients with significant coronary artery disease and severe left ventricular (LV) dysfunction received delayed contrast-enhanced MRI and ^{201}Tl single-photon emission computed tomography (SPECT) within one month. Ten of them received simultaneous ^{201}Tl SPECT and dobutamine stress echocardiography (DSE). Three imaging modalities were compared based on a standardized 17-segment model. Improved regional wall thickening on follow-up MRI was used as an index of functional recovery in patients received revascularization.

Results: Of 680 segments, MRI hyperenhancement showed positive correlation with ^{201}Tl reduction (r =0.61, $p < 0.0001$). The viability concordance was 75.3% between DSE and MRI, 80.5% between ^{201}Tl SPECT and MRI, and 66.5% among all tests. Contrast-

*Reprints requests: Wen-Yih I. Tseng, MD, PhD. Department of Medical Imaging, National Taiwan University Hospital and Center of Optoelectronic Biomedicine, National Taiwan University College of Medicine. No.7, Chung-Shan South Road, Taipei, Taiwan. Tel: 886-2-23123456, ext 8758; Fax: 886-2-23926922; E-mail: wytseng@ha.mc.ntu.edu.tw.

enhanced MRI detected more myocardial viability than ^{201}Tl SPECT, especially in the inferior wall and apex ($p < 0.0001$). Eight patients underwent revascularization. Comparing with functional recovery in the follow-up results, the diagnostic accuracy, sensitivity, specificity, positive predictive value, and negative predictive value of delayed contrast-enhanced MRI were 64%, 95%, 24%, 62% and 77%, respectively. For ^{201}Tl SPECT, these values were 55%, 75%, 29%, 58% and 54%, respectively.

Areas under the ROC curves by MRI and ^{201}Tl SPECT were 0.59 ± 0.04, 0.52 ± 0.05, respectively (p=0.07). Of 16 segments viable on MRI but nonviable on ^{201}Tl SPECT, 12 (75%) recovered function after revascularization, while only one of 3 segments classified as nonviable on MRI but viable on ^{201}Tl SPECT recovered function ($p < 0.05$). Of 10 segments classified as scar by both tests, none recovered function after revascularization.

Conclusion: Delayed contrast-enhanced MRI detects viability better than ^{201}Tl SPECT, especially in the inferior wall and apex. Myocardial viability detected by MRI may predict functional recovery after revascularization in ischemic cardiomyopathy, even in patients with severe LV dysfunction.

Keywords: Myocardial viability, magnetic resonance imaging, ^{201}Tl SPECT, dobutamine stress, echocardiography

INTRODUCTION

Improved ejection fraction (EF) after revascularization shows positive impact on prognosis in chronic ischemic cardiomyopathy [1,2]. Measurement of regional wall thickening of dysfunctional myocardium offers quantitative assessment of functional recovery after revascularization [3-5]. Determination of the viability of dysfunctional myocardium, however, remains a problem. The sensitivity of the dobutamine stress echo (DSE) is poor. Although the positron-emitting and single photon-emitting scintigraphic imaging techniques are known to assess myocardial viability, these modalities display rather lower specificity [1,2,5-8]. Cardiac MRI was reported to offer reliable and accurate assessment of myocardial scar burden [9], coronary perfusion [10] and contractile reserve [11].

The technique of delayed contrast-enhanced MRI using an inversion-recovery prepared T_1-weighted gradient-echo sequence was shown to provide exquisite contrast and spatial resolution of myocardial fibrosis [12,13]. While the infarct areas in the myocardium appeared cold regions on ^{201}Tl single-photon emission tomography (^{201}Tl SPECT) [12], it was vividly enhanced on MRI [13]. In addition, superior resolution of MRI made it more sensitive than other techniques to differentiate transmural from non-transmural infarction [14]. Larger transmural extent of contrast enhancement was found to correlate with less functional recovery after revascularization of dysfunctional myocardium [15].

To date, reports on comparing cardiac MRI, ^{201}Tl SPECT and DSE in the assessment of chronic ischemic cardiomyopathy are limited. The present study aimed to compare the delayed contrast-enhanced MRI with ^{201}Tl SPECT and DSE in the assessment of myocardial viability, and to evaluate its predictive power of functional recovery after revascularization in patients with chronic ischemic heart failure.

Materials and Methods

Patients

Between February, 2002 and September, 2004, forty consecutive patients (36 male; age, 59.4 ± 12.5 years) with angiographically significant coronary artery disease (CAD) (≥ 70% diameter stenosis) and symptoms of heart failure (New York Heart Association functional class ≥ II) for more than three months were prospectively enrolled for the evaluation of myocardial viability as shown in Table 1. All patients had a LVEF ≤ 40% and dysfunctional myocardium identified by resting echocardiography. All patients were excluded for recent myocardial infarction (MI) or unstable angina pectoris for < six weeks, valvular disease or contraindications to MRI as criteria laid down elsewhere.

All patients consented under the approval of the Institutional Review Board of the National Taiwan University Hospital. All the imaging studies on myocardial viability received by each patient were performed within the duration of one month. Eight patients underwent revascularization within one month after viability study, and another cardiac MRI study was followed at least 3 months after the intervention. A flow chart of viability study and treatment of these patients is shown in the Figure 1.

Table 1. Patient Demographics

	Patients	N = 40
Male gender	36	90 %
Age, yrs	59.4 ± 12.5	37 – 83
Risk factors		
Hypertension	25	63%
Diabetes	14	35%
Hyperlipidemia	14	35%
History of MI (> 6 weeks)	20	50%
Previous interventions	23	58%
PCI	20	
CABG	3	
NYHA functional class		
II	20	50%
III	14	35%
IV	6	15%
Mean	2.7 ± 0.7	
CAD		
1-VD	4	10%
2-VD	12	30%
3-VD	24	60%

Values are mean ± SD. MI = myocardial infarction; PCI = percutaneous coronary intervention; CABG = coronary artery bypass surgery; NYHA = New York Heart Association; CAD = coronary artery disease; VD = vessel-disease.

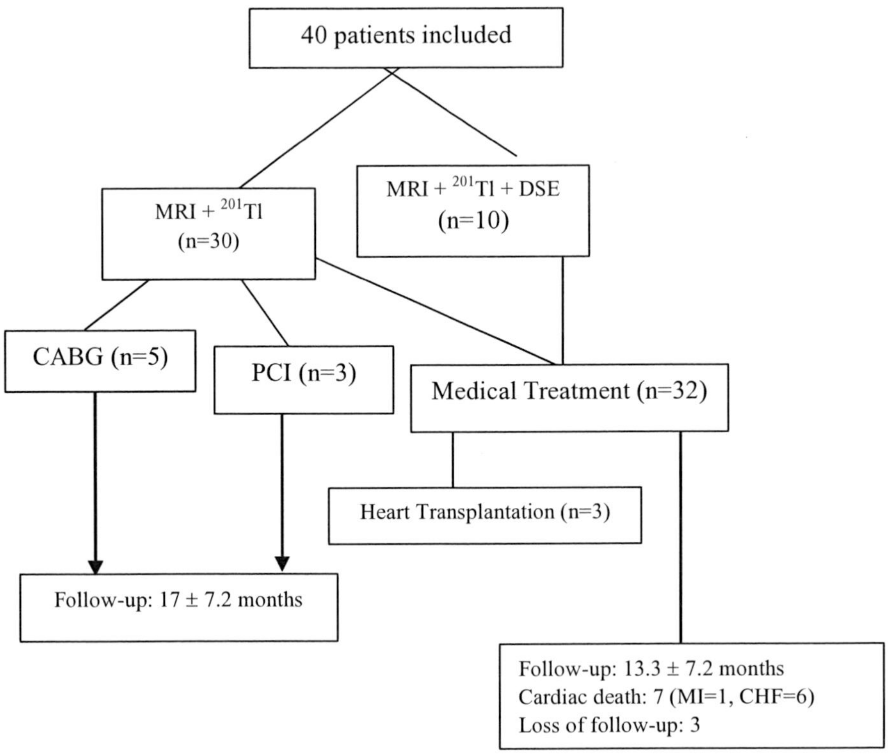

Figure 1. The flow chart of viability studies and treatments of patients included in this study. (DSE = dobutamine stress echocardiography; PCI = percutaneous coronary intervention; CABG = coronary artery bypass surgery; MI = myocardial infarction; CHF = congestive heart failure).

Echocardiography

M-mode and 2D echocardiography data were received at the echo lab using a Sonos-4500/5500 imaging system (Hewlett Packard, Palo Alto, CA) to assess contractile function and measure left atrial and LV dimensions according to standard criteria [16].

^{201}Tl SPECT Protocols

Eight patients were studied under the exercise stress test. For the rest who were unable to exercise adequately, we used the pharmacological stress test: dipyridamole for 14 patients and simultaneous DSE and ^{201}Tl SPECT for the remaining 10 patents. The exercise stress test was performed using a modified Bruce protocol [17]. The injection of ^{201}Tl (2-3 mCi) was timed at peak exercise. After the injection, exercise was continued for another minute. For the dipyridamole stress test, intravenous dipyridamole (0.56 mg/kg in 4 minutes) was infused to induce coronary hyperemia and ^{201}Tl was injected 3 minutes after the completion of the infusion [18]. Simultaneous DSE and ^{201}Tl imaging was performed as described previously [5, 19]. In brief, dobutamine was intravenously infused at rates of 5, 10, 20, 30 and 40 μg/kg/min in 3-minute stages. Atropine was given if the patient's heart rate was lower than

85% of age-predicted maximum heart rate. ^{201}Tl was injected one minute before the termination of dobutamine infusion. Stress SPECT imaging was started within 5 minutes after the injection of ^{201}Tl and the redistribution imaging was acquired 4 hours later. If images showed irreversible defects, additional 1 mCi ^{201}Tl was injected and a third set of images was obtained 15 minutes after the reinjection.

Rest-Redistribution ^{201}Tl SPECT (n=8)

Eight patients underwent rest-redistribution ^{201}Tl SPECT imaging because of their severe heart failure. The ^{201}Tl SPECT images were acquired 15 minutes and 4 hours after administration of 2-3 mCi ^{201}Tl. The post-processing and reconstruction of ^{201}Tl images was performed as described elsewhere [5, 17-20].

Cardiac MRI

Electrocardiographic-gated MRI was performed on a 1.5-T scanner (Sonata, Siemens, Erlangen, Germany) using a phased-array coil (CP Body Array Flex, Siemens, Erlangen, Germany) attached with respiratory and cardiac gating during repeated breath holds. Using steady-state free precession, MRI cine images were acquired as multiple short-axis views (every 1 cm throughout the entire LV) and 2 perpendicular long-axis planes. In another session, gadolinium contrast (Gd-DTPA, 0.15 mmol/kg) was administered intravenously, and contrast-enhanced images were acquired 10 minutes after administration using a segmented inversion-recovery prepared turbo gradient echo technique [15] in the identical planes. The imaging parameters were as follows: TR/TE/flip angle = 750 ms/4.18 ms/25°; FOV/matrix size/spatial resolution = 290×340 mm/216×256/0.75 mm; and the inversion time (TI) = 250 ms optimized to null the signal intensities of normal myocardium.

Image Processing and Analysis

The MRI images were interpreted by two independent blinded radiologists. If two interpretations did not agree with one another, the images were reviewed by the two physicians to reach a consensus. The LV myocardium was divided into 17 segments for analysis as AHA criteria recommendation [21].

Echocardiographic Analysis

Segmental wall motion and contractile reserve were defined by echocardiography before and after low-dose infusion of dobutamine as described earlier with accuracy of interobserver agreement 94% (κ=0.85) [17,22].

SPECT Image Analysis

SPECT images were normalized to peak myocardial activity as 100%. ^{201}Tl activity in each segment was scored as 0 = normal perfusion, 1 = mild decrease of photon counts, 2 = moderate decrease of photon counts, 3 = severe decrease of photon counts, and 4 = absent photon counts [23]. Each segment in SPECT images was scored for viability by perfusion photon counts normalized to peak myocardial activity as 100% based on the methods used previously [23, 24]. Our interobserver agreement for ^{201}Tl SPECT interpretations was 96% as previously reported [17].

MR Image Analysis

LV function parameters were assessed in a standard way using computing software (Matlab®, MathWorks Inc., MA, USA). The planimeter method was used to determine LV volumes, LVEF and cardiac mass and endocardial and epicardial borders on all short-axis cine images [25]. Wall thickening on cine MR images was measured as the percentage of systolic wall thickening (SWT) according to the following formula: (end-systolic wall thickness – end-diastolic wall thickness)/end-diastolic wall thickness × 100%. The delayed contrast enhancement (DC) in each segment was quantified using computing software (Mathematica®, Wolfram Research, Inc., IL, USA), following the criteria as described elsewhere [26]. The percentage of pixels showing hyperintensities out of the total myocardial pixels was determined by a 4-score grading: grade 0, no DC; grade 1, 1% to 25% DC; grade 2, 26% to 50% DC; grade 3, 51% to 75% DC; grade 4, > 75% DC. To compare MRI with SPECT and DSE data, grade 3 defined as non-viable myocardium. In the follow-up study, an increase of ≥ 15% SWT change was used to define improvement of post-revascularization contractile function [27].

Statistical Analysis

Data were collected as mean ± SD showing comparisons between groups by use of 2-sample *t* test and chi-square analysis for continuous and categorical variables, respectively. ANOVA (analysis of variance) with Bonferroni's post hoc test was performed to detect any associations between two or more variables. Agreement between the diagnostic tests was evaluated using κappa index. Correlations between the extent of DC on MRI and ^{201}Tl uptake on SPECT were analyzed using linear regression analyses. Changes between baseline and follow-up measurements were assessed by paired *t* tests. ROC curves were used to compare predictive accuracy of both MRI and ^{201}Tl SPECT to predict an increase of ≥ 15% SWT change at follow-up. Areas under the ROC curves were compared by use of the z test. A p value < 0.05 (two-sided) was predetermined to be statistically significant. All statistical analyses were done using scientific statistical software packages (Stata 8, Texas, USA).

RESULTS

Forty patients with demography as shown in Table 1, were studied at baseline by MRI and ^{201}Tl SPECT. Ten of them underwent simultaneous DSE and ^{201}Tl studies. Of these patients, eight underwent revascularization after viability studies, including percutaneous coronary intervention (PCI) in three (left anterior descending artery in two patients and left circumflex artery in one patient) and coronary bypass surgery (CABG) in five patients. Follow-up MRI studies were performed 5.0 ± 4.3 months after the revascularization procedures. One patient had non-ST elevation myocardial infarction during PCI. No other patient had clinical events between two MRI studies.

Of patients who were treated medically, three received heart transplantation within one month after viability studies. Seven patients died during the follow-up periods, including acute MI in one and intractable heart failure in another six patients as shown in Figure 1.

Comparison of Viability Data

The results of myocardial viability assessed by MRI and ^{201}Tl SPECT are shown in Table 2 (A, B). Viable myocardium detected on MRI had positive relationship with ^{201}Tl activity. The concordant rate of viability was 80.5% between ^{201}Tl SPECT and MRI (κ=0.52), and overall concordant rate was 66.5% among DSE, ^{201}Tl SPECT and MRI tests (κ=0.51).

The contractile reserve detected by late enhancement on MRI showed higher proportion of transmural extent of DC on MRI (Table 2C). In some cases, contractile reserve was impaired resulting with invisible or minor scar detected on MRI (21/102, 21%). All segments with extensive scar on MRI and or SPECT showed no contractile function at rest (Figure 2), although almost all segments with > 50% DC showed marked impairment of resting function.

Table 2. Comparison of Myocardial Viability Using Different Diagnostic Modalities

(A) Relationship between viability detected by dobutamine stress echocardiography, MRI and ^{201}Tl SPECT

170 segments	DSE +		DSE -	
	Tl +	Tl -	Tl +	Tl -
MRI +	79	12	23	14
MRI -	3	2	3	34

(B) Concordance between viability detected by MRI and ^{201}Tl SPECT

680 segments		MRI	
		+	-
Tl	+	411	33
	-	93	109

(C) Relationship between transmural extent of DC on MRI and contractile reserve detected by dobutamine stress echocardiography

170 segments	Transmural Extent of DC on MRI			
	0 - 25%	26 - 50%	51 - 75%	76 - 100%
DSE +	81	10	5	0
DSE −	21	17	17	9

DSE = dobutamine stress echocardiography; Tl = ^{201}Tl SPECT; + = viable; - = scar, DC = delayed contrast enhancement.

(A)

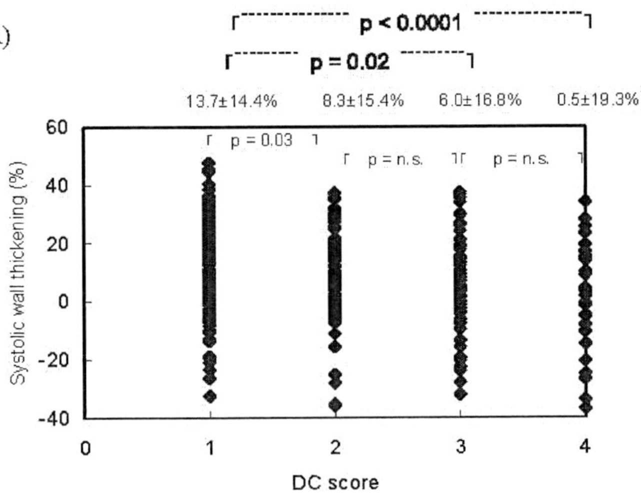

(B)

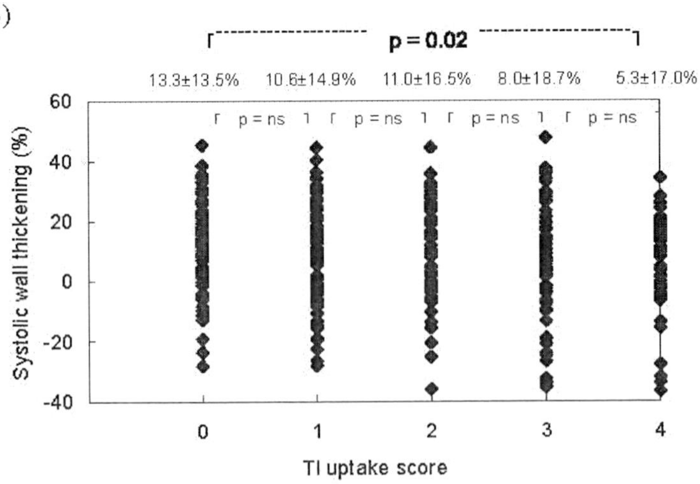

Figure 2. Relationship between (A) delayed contrast enhancement on MRI, (B) ^{201}Tl uptake on SPECT and percentage of systolic wall thickening on MRI (ns = non-significant, DC = delayed contrast enhancement).

In 680 segments from 40 patients, the amount of viable tissue on MRI correlated positively with ^{201}Tl uptake (^{201}Tl uptake score = 0.67 DC score − 0.69, r=0.61, $p < 0.0001$). The extent of DC enhancement on MRI and the reduction of ^{201}Tl uptake both showed agreement (κ=0.51, Figure 3). The MRI detected more myocardial viability than ^{201}Tl SPECT in the inferior wall (92/120 vs. 63/120, $p < 0.0001$), and apex (23/40 vs. 15/40, $p < 0.0001$). The discrepancy between viability determined by ^{201}Tl SPECT and MRI is shown in Table 3.

The representative examples of concordant and disconcordant myocardial viability detected by MRI and ^{201}Tl SPECT are shown in Figure 4 and 5.

Follow-up Data

A total of 106 segments (97 dysfunctional) in eight patients were revascularized after viability tests. Among 97 dysfunctional segments, 84 (87%) were viable on MRI and 71 (73%) were viable on ^{201}Tl SPECT. Two of the eight patients had evidence of new delayed enhanced segments in their post-revascularization scan (one patient in CABG group had three and the other patient in PCI group had two new delayed enhanced segments). The LVEF in the eight patients at baseline was 26.3 ± 8.1% and increased significantly to 38.6 ± 16.8% at follow-up (p=0.04). Total LV mass (217.5 ± 54.5 to 183.0 ± 47.9 g), LV end-diastolic volume index (110.5 ± 38.7 to 86.6 ± 36.0 mL/m^2), LV end-systolic volume index (82.3 ± 37.4 to 55.9 ± 36.9 mL/m^2) were also decreased postoperatively, but statistically insignificant.

In terms of regional function change, the SWT measured by MRI was used as the parameter of myocardial viability. Of the 97 dysfunctional segments, 55 (57%) showed functional recovery (increase of segmental SWT ≥ 15%). The overall diagnostic accuracy, sensitivity, specificity, positive predictive value and negative predictive value of viability detected by MRI were, respectively, 64%, 95%, 24%, 62% and 77%, whereas they were 55%, 75%, 29%, 58% and 54% by ^{201}Tl SPECT. Moreover, the SWT improvement after revascularization in dysfunctional segments was dependent on its transmural extent shown in Table 4. However, there was no significant difference in areas under the ROC curves by MRI and ^{201}Tl SPECT, respectively (0.59 ± 0.04 vs. 0.52 ± 0.05, p=0.07).

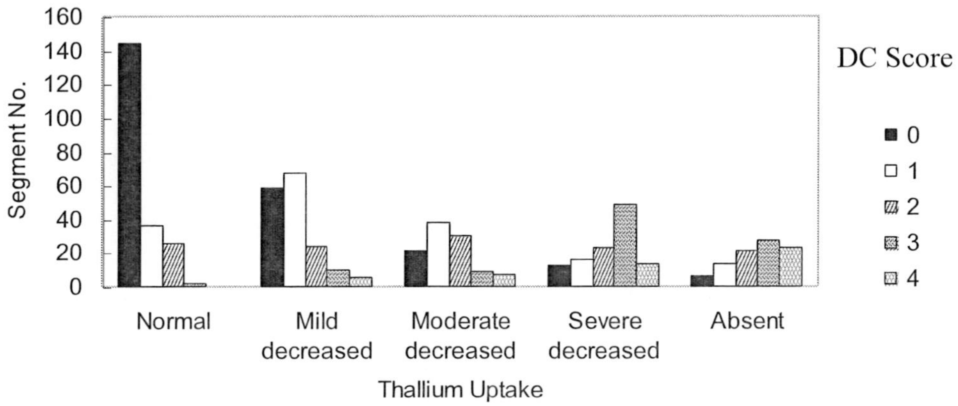

Figure 3. Relationship between thallium uptake and delayed contrast enhancement in MRI. (DC = delayed contrast enhancement).

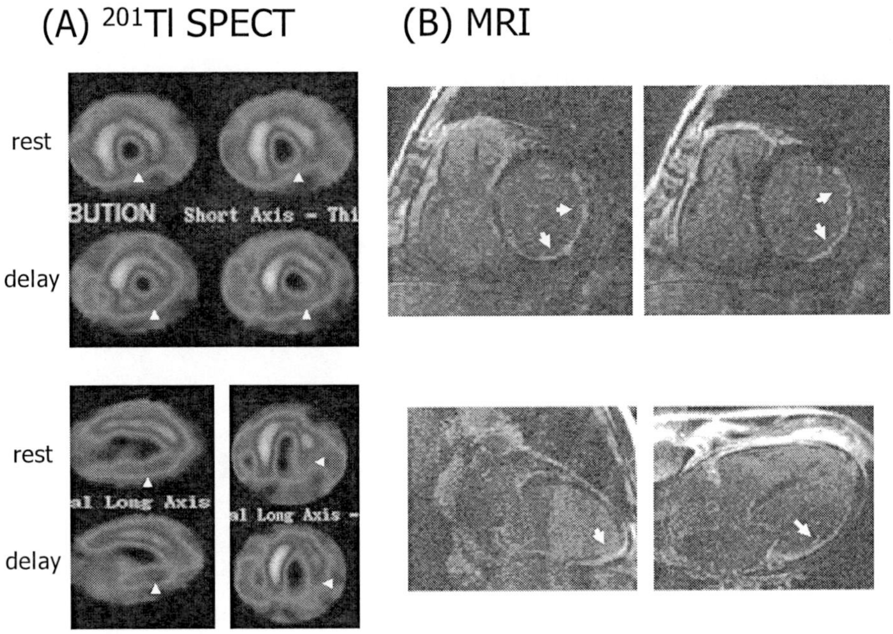

Figure 4. A 64-year-old patients with old inferior myocardial infarction (LVEF 17%) showed concordant scars in the inferior and inferolateral walls on the rest-redistribution ^{201}Tl SPECT (A, arrow heads) and delayed contrast-enhanced MRI (B, arrows).

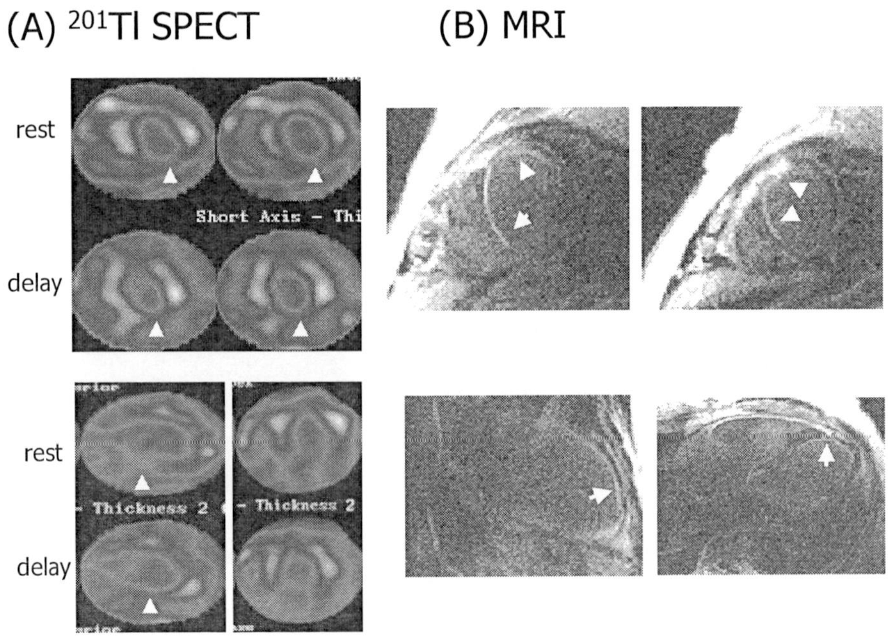

Figure 5. A 43-year-old man with 3-vessel disease (LVEF 8%) showed scar in the inferior wall (arrow heads) on the rest-redistribution ^{201}Tl SPECT (A), which is discordant with contrast-enhanced MRI (B) showing delayed enhancement in the anterior and septal walls (arrows).

Table 3. Distribution of Discrepancies in Identifying Myocardial Viability by 201Tl SPECT and MRI

(A) Scar detected by MRI but viable by ^{201}Tl SPECT (n = 33 segments)

	Anterior	Anteroseptal	Inferoseptal	Inferior	Inferolateral	Lateral	Apex
Basal	1	1	4	0	0	2	
Mid-ventricular	2	3	4	1	3	2	2
Apical	1	4		2	2		

(B) Scar detected by ^{201}Tl SPECT but viable by MRI (n = 93 segments)

	Anterior	Anteroseptal	Inferoseptal	Inferior	Inferolateral	Lateral	Apex
Basal	3	4	5	10	9	0	
Mid-ventricular	3	4	1	11	5	1	9
Apical	6	6		11	5		

Table 4. Influence of Transmural Extent of Delayed Contrast Enhancement on Recovery of Regional Function in 97 Dysfunctional Segments at Baseline

	Systolic Wall Thickening Ratio (%)			
Transmurality	**Baseline**	**Follow-Up**	**Difference**	***P***
0 - 25% (n=52)	9.7 ± 14.8	28.0 ± 12.9	17.9 ± 15.6	< 0.0001
26 - 50% (n=32)	6.2 ± 13.9	15.2 ± 15.3	9.0 ± 18.6	0.01
51 - 75% (n=9)	0.1 ± 6.0	3.7 ± 19.0	3.6 ± 17.9	0.56
76 -100% (n=4)	-11.9 ± 17.1%	-1.8 ± 22.8	10.2 ± 29.7	0.56

Of sixteen segments viable on MRI but nonviable on ^{201}Tl SPECT, twelve (75%) segments showed function recovery after revascularization, while only one of three segments classified as nonviable on MRI but viable on ^{201}Tl SPECT recovered function ($p < 0.05$). Out of ten segments classified as scar by both tests, no segment showed the function improvement after revascularization.

Out of five new segments with hyperenhancement after the interventions, four segments indicated unrecovered regional wall function with transmural involvement (SWT change, – 0.19 ± 8.9%). However, improvement was seen in the only segment with hyperenhancement confined to the subendocardial layer (SWT change, 33.75%).

DISCUSSION

The identification of hibernating myocardium in patients with chronic heart failure is becoming state of the art in cardiovascular science. Previous studies have shown great potentials in terms of outcome and recovery of LV function after revascularization [1-5]. Myocardial viability assessment by ^{18}F-fluorodeoxyglucose (^{18}F-FDG) positron emission tomography (PET) is clinically important in these patients, but high costs and limited availability of PET cameras and radiotracers hamper the clinical applications. Recent advance in cardiac MRI allows imaging myocardial viability with excellent imaging quality [9-15]. However, reports on its value in predicting functional recovery after revascularization in patients with chronic severe LV dysfunction, in comparison with well-established ^{201}Tl SPECT and DSE, are still lacking.

Our results are in agreement with previous works [28,29] that dobutamine response depends on the transmural scar extent shown on DC. Our data corroborated with previous reports [1,6-8,29] and highlighted that DSE detected less viable myocardium in comparison with both ^{201}Tl SPECT and MRI imaging methods. However, the concordance between DSE and MRI (75.3%) or between DSE and ^{201}Tl SPECT (76.5%) was similar.

In the present study, we observed that the amount of viable myocardial tissue on cardiac MRI was positively correlated with ^{201}Tl uptake. Similar findings were reported to assess by ^{18}F-FDG PET and MRI techniques [27,30].

Our data were consistent with previous findings that MRI identified subendocardial infarcts but missed by SPECT [14,29]. We also observed that ^{201}Tl SPECT might overestimate the scar tissue, especially in the inferior wall and apex. These discrepancies may be explained in part by the low-energy X-ray emission and soft tissue attenuation. The inferior wall is one of the most sensitive to ^{201}Tl attenuation region in the heart, thus greater attenuation of ^{201}Tl in the inferior segments could be anticipated. However, limited success was reported by using infarct location adjusted thresholds for viability assessment [31-34]. The regions of dysfunctional myocardium seen as viable on ^{201}Tl SPECT but MRI invisible can be attributed to the fact that ^{201}Tl scan could become positive in the presence of a thin rim of viable tissue as previously reported [35,36].

Earlier reports showed that in patients with LV dysfunction undergoing revascularization, the extent and severity of nonviable tissue defined by MRI correlates was well correlated with the likelihood of functional recovery assessed by LVEF [16,27].

Our study extends the information further showing relationship of chronic CAD and severe LV dysfunction in our research volunteers (most patients with LVEF $\leq$ 25%). Our results further suggest that the myocardial viability detected by MRI may be valuable on the clinical evaluation of potential benefits from high-risk revascularization procedures.

The functional recovery assessment shown in our study after intervention was not homogeneous. Several factors affect the functional recovery including different intervention procedures, completeness of revascularization, and peri- and post-operative MI events [37,38]. Furthermore, the degree and duration of pre-procedural cellular structure change may influence the functional recovery.

However, there are some recognized limitations. Our sample size was relatively small, and limited patients underwent revascularization. Neither of patients who received simultaneous DSE and ^{201}Tl imaging received the revascularization, so the comparison between DSE and MRI in predicting functional recovery is still lacking.

The ^{201}Tl imaging method in this study reflected our routine clinical protocol, no additional correction algorithm or prone position imaging was applied, which has been proposed to decrease the false-positive rate [39,40].

Conclusion

Cardiovascular MRI provides a unique tool to assess cardiac structure and function in a single study session. The present study demonstrates the good correlations among DSE, ^{201}Tl SPECT and MRI in the detection of myocardial viability. MRI detects better viability than ^{201}Tl SPECT, especially in the inferior wall and apex. MRI has marginally higher predictive value in predicting functional recovery. For patients with severe ischemic cardiomyopathy, noninvasive MRI may provide better clinical decision on using high-risk revascularization procedures.

Acknowledgments

The work was supported in part by grant NSC-91-2314-B002-272 from the National Science Council, Taiwan.

References

[1] Allman KC, Shaw LJ, Hachamovitch R, et al. Myocardial viability testing and impact of revascularization on prognosis in patients with coronary artery disease and left ventricular dysfunction: a meta-analysis. *J Am Coll Cardiol* 2002; 39:151-158.

[2] Underwood SR, Bax JJ, vom Dahl J, et al. Imaging techniques for the assessment of myocardial hibernation: report of a study group of the European Society of Cardiology. *Eur Heart J* 2004; 25:815-836.

[3] Rahimtoola SH. A perspective on the three large multicenter randomized clinical trials of coronary bypass surgery for chronic stable angina. *Circulation* 1985; 72(6 pt 2) V-123-V-135.

[4] Van-den-Berg EK Jr, Popma JJ, Dehmer GJ, et al. Reversible segmental left ventricular dysfunction after coronary angioplasty. *Circulation* 1990; 81:1210-6.

[5] Huang PJ, Lin LC, Yen RF, et al. Accuracy of biphasic response, sustained improvement and worsening during dobutamine echocardiography in predicting recovery of myocardial dysfunction after revascularization: comparison with simultaneous thallium-201 reinjection SPECT. *Ultrasound Med Biol* 2001; 27:925-931.

[6] Shan K, Constatine G, Sivananthan M, Flamm S. Role of cardiac magnetic resonance imaging in the assessment of myocardial viability. *Circulation* 2004; 109:1328-1334.

[7] Dilsizian V, Rocco TP, Freedman NMT, Leon MB, Bonow RO. Enhanced detection ischemic but viable myocardium by the reinjection of thallium after stress-redistribution imaging. *N Engl J Med* 1990; 323:141-146.

[8] Cigarroa C, De Fillipi C, Brickner ME, Alvarez L, Wait MA, Grayburn PA. Dobutamine stress echocardiography identifies hibernating myocardium and predicts recovery of left ventricular function after coronary revascularization. *Circulation* 1993; 88:430-436.

[9] Mahrholdt H, Wagner A, Holly TA, et al. Reproducibility of chronic infarct size measurement by contrast-enhanced magnetic resonance imaging. *Circulation* 2002; 39:1151-1158.

[10] Al Saadi N, Nagel E, Gross M, et al. Noninvasive detection of myocardial ischemia perfusion reserve based on cardiovascular magnetic resonance. *Circulation* 2000; 101:1379-1383.

[11] Baer FM, Theissen P, Schneider CA, et al. Dobutamine magnetic resonance imaging predicts contractile recovery of chronically dysfunctional myocardium after successful revascularization. *J Am Coll Cardiol* 1998; 31:1040-1048.

[12] Ramani K, Judd RM, Holly TA, et al. Contrast magnetic resonance imaging in the assessment of myocardial viability in patients with stable coronary artery and left ventricular dysfunction. *Circulation* 1998; 98:2687-2694.

[13] Kim RJ, Fieno DS, Parrish TB, et al. Relationship of MRI delayed contrast enhancement to irreversible injury, infarct age, and contractile function. Circulation 1999; 100:1992-2002.

[14] Wagner A, Mahrholdt H, Regenfus M, et al. Contrast-enhanced MR and routine single photon emission computed tomography (SPECT) perfusion imaging for detection of subendocardial myocardial infarcts: an imaging study. *Lancet* 2003; 361:364-379.

[15] Kim RJ, Wu E, Rafael A, et al. The use of contrast-enhanced magnetic resonance imaging to identify reversible myocardial dysfunction. *N Engl J Med* 2000; 343:1445-1453.

[16] Oh JK, Seward JB, Tajik J. The echo manual. 2nd ed. Philadelphia, *Lippincott Williams and Wilkins*, 1999; 7-43.

[17] Huang PJ, Chieng PU, Lee YT,, et al. Exercise thallium-201 tomographic scintigraphy in the diagnosis of coronary artery disease: emphasis on the effect of exercise level. *J Formos Med Assoc* 1992; 91:1096-1101.

[18] Ho FM, Huang PJ, Liau CS, Lee FK, Chieng PU, Su CT. Dobutamine stress echocardiography compared with dipyridamole thallium-201 single-photon emission computed tomography in detecting coronary artery disease. *Eur Heart J* 1995; 16:570-575.

[19] Huang PJ, Ho YL, Wu CC, et al. Simultaneous dobutamine stress echocardiography and thallium-201 perfusion imaging for the detection of coronary artery disease. *Cardiology* 1997; 88:556-562.

[20] Lomboy CT, Schulman DS, Grill HP, et al. Rest-redistribution thallium-201 scintigraphy to determine myocardial viability early after myocardial infarction. *J Am Coll Cardiol* 1995; 25:210-217.

[21] Cerqueira MD, Weissman NJ, Dilsizian V, et al. Standardized myocardial segmentation and nomclature for tomographic imaging of the heart. *Circulation* 2002; 105:539-542.

[22] American Society of Echocardiography Committee on Standards: Recommendations for quantitation of the left ventricle by two-dimensional echocardiography. *J Am Soc Echocardiogr* 1989; 2:358-267.

[23] Kiat H, Maddahi J, Roy LT, Van Train K, Friedman J, Resser K, et al. Comparison of technetium-99m methoxy-isobutyteryle and thallium-201 evaluation of coronary artery disease by planar and tomographic methods. *Am Heart J* 1989; 117:1-11.

[24] Dilsizian V, Freedman NMT, Bacharach SL, Perrone-Filardi P, Bonow RO. Regional thallium uptake in irreversible defects: magnitude of change in thallium activity after

reinjection distinguishes viable from nonviable myocardium. *Circulation* 1992; 85:627-634.

[25] Tseng WY, Liao TY, Wang JL. Normal systolic and diastolic functions of the left ventricle and left atrium by cine magnetic resonance imaging. *J Cardiovasc Magn Reson* 2002; 4:443-457.

[26] Mahrholdt H, Wagner A, Holly TA, et al. Reproducibility of chronic infarct size measurement by contrast-enhanced magnetic resonance imaging. *Circulation* 2002; 106:2322-2327.

[27] Knuesel PR, Nanz D, Wyss C, et al. Characterization of dysfunctional myocardium by positron emission tomography and magnetic resonance: relation to functional outcome after revascularization. *Circulation* 2003; 108:1095-1100.

[28] Shan K, Bick RJ, Poindexter BJ, et al. Altered adrenergic receptor density in myocardial hibernations in humans: a possible mechanism of depressed myocardial function. *J Am Coll Cardiol* 1996; 28:432-442.

[29] Nelson C, McCrohon J, Khafagi F, et al. Impact of scar thickness on the assessment of viability using dobutamine echocardiography and thallium single photon emission computed tomography: a comparison with contrast-enhancement magnetic resonance imaging. *J Am Coll Cardiol* 2004; 43: 1248-1256.

[30] Klein C, Nekolla SG, Bengel FM, et al. Assessment of myocardial viability with contrast-enhanced magnetic resonance imaging: comparison with positron emission tomography. *Circulation* 2002; 105:162-167.

[31] Vanoverschelde J-LJ, DeHondt A-M, Marwick T, et al. Head-to-head comparison of exercise-redistribution-reinjection thallium single photon emission computed tomography and low dose dobutamine echocardiography for prediction of reversibility of chronic left ventricular ischemic dysfunction. *J Am Coll Cardiol* 1996; 28:432-442.

[32] Gunnung MG, Anagnostopoulous C, Knight CJ, et al. Comparison of Tl-201, technetium-99m tetrafosmin and dobutamine magnetic resonance imaging in idenfying hibernating myocardium. *Circulation* 1998; 98:1869-1874.

[33] Udelson JE, Coleman PS, Metherall J, et al. Predicting recovery of severe regional ventricular dysfunction. Comparison of resting scintigraphy with 201 Tl and 99m-Tc-sestamibi. *Circulation* 1994; 89:2552-2561.

[34] Schneider CA, Voth E, Gawlich S, et al. Significance of rest technetium-99m sestamibi imaging for the prediction of improvement of left ventricular dysfunction after Q wave myocardial infarction: importance of infarct location adjusted thresholds. *J Am Coll Cardiol* 1998; 32:648-654.

[35] Zamorano J, Delgado J, Almeria C, et al. Reason for discrepancies in identifying myocardial viability by thallium-201 redistribution, magnetic resonance imaging and dobutamine echocardiography. *Am J Cardiol* 2002; 90:455-459.

[36] Baumgartner H, Porenta G, Lau YK, et al. Assessment of myocardial viability by dobutamine echocardiography, positron emission tomography and thallium-201 SPECT. Correlation with histopathology in explanted hearts. *J Am Coll Cardiol* 1998;32: 1701-1708.

[37] Ricciardi MJ, Wu E, Davidson CJ, et al. Visualization of discrete microinfarction after percutaneous coronary intervention associated with mild creatine kinase-MB elevation. *Circulation* 2001; 103:2780-2783.

[38] Selvanayagam JB, Petersen SE, Francis JM, et al. Effects of off-pump versus on-pump coronary surgery on reversible and irreversible myocardial injury. A randomized trail using cardiovascular magnetic resonance imaging and biochemical markers. *Circulation* 2004; 109:345-350.

[39] Esquerre JP, Coca FJ, Martinez SJ, et al. Prone decubitus: a solution to inferior wall attenuation in thallium-201 myocardial tomography. *J Nucl Med* 1989; 30:398-401.

[40] Hendel RC, Berman DS, Cullom SJ, et al. Multicenter clinical trial to evaluate the efficacy of correction for photon attenuation and scatter in SPECT myocardial perfusion imaging. *Circulation* 1999; 99:2742-2749.

In: World Heart Research Yearbook. Volume 1
Editors: Franz Halberg and R. B. Singh
ISBN: 978-1-60741-881-8

BENEFICIAL EFFECTS OF ADDITION OF FENOFIBRATE TO STATIN THERAPY IN PATIENTS WITH ACUTE CORONARY SYNDROME AFTER PERCUTANEOUS CORONARY INTERVENTIONS

Hetal D. Shah[1], Keyur H. Parikh[2], Milan C. Chag[2], Urmil G. Shah[2], Hemang A. Baxi[2], Anish H. Chandarana[2], Ajay M. Naik[2], Joyal N. Shah[2], Kanan J. Shah[1] and Ramesh K. Goyal[1,*]

[1] Department of Pharmacology, L. M. College of Pharmacy Navrangpura, Gujarat, India
[2]The Heart Care Clinic, Care Cardiology Consultants Pvt Ltd, Gujarat, India

ABSTRACT

Objective: The objective of the present investigation was to find out whether the addition of fenofibrate to statin monotherapy produced any synergistic or additive beneficial effects in reducing risk factors, especially plasma fibrinogen, in patients of Acute Coronary Syndromes (ACS) requiring Percutaneous Coronary Interventions (PCI).

Methods: This was a randomized, non-blind, prospective study with parallel group design, conducted in 102 patients who had angiographically documented Coronary Artery Disease (CAD). All had undergone angioplasty. The patients were randomized to atorvastatin (20mg/day, n=25), simvastatin (40mg/day, n=27), atorvastatin(10mg/day)-fenofibrate (200mg/day) combination (n=25) and simvastatin (20mg/day)-fenofibrate(200mg/day) combination (n=25). The serum lipid profile and plasma fibrinogen were recorded before initiation of therapy and after 3 months of the respective treatments.

Results: All the patients already had desirable lipid levels as per the NCEP ATP III guidelines. The addition of fenofibrate to statin monotherapy produced additional benefits on reduction in triglyceride (TG) and very low density lipoprotein (VLDL) levels, and an increase in high density lipoprotein (HDL) levels. All the treatment groups showed a significant decrease in the plasma fibrinogen levels. This did not correlate with any of the study parameters like age, body weight, hemodynamic characteristics and lipoprotein levels. Statin monotherapy produced a significant decrease in the fibrinogen levels and the addition of fenofibrate further enhanced the reduction.

Conclusions: Addition of fenofibrate to statins seems to be beneficial in patients with ACS. Statins, contrary to various reports, were found to decrease plasma fibrinogen

* Address for Correspondence and Reprints: Professor Ramesh K Goyal, Department of Pharmacology, L. M. College of Pharmacy Navrangpura, Ahmedabad 380 006 Gujarat, INDIA. Phone: 91-79-26302746. Email: goyalrk@hotmail.com, hetald_shah@yahoo.com.

significantly. Further, in combination with fenofibrate there was enhanced reduction of the novel risk factor, fibrinogen.

Keywords: Acute coronary syndromes, statins, fenofibrate, plasma fibrinogen

INTRODUCTION

The last century has seen a rapid increase in the global prevalence of Coronary artery disease (CAD). Estimates from the Global Burden of Disease Study have predicted that India faces the greatest health burden due to Coronary Artery Disease.[1] A number of inflammatory markers have been studied for their ability to predict future cardiovascular events in asymptomatic individuals and patients with established atherosclerotic disease.[2] Among the emerging novel cardiac markers, plasma fibrinogen has been identified as an important risk factor for cardiovascular diseases. Many cross-sectional, case controlled, and numerous prospective cohort studies have identified elevated plasma fibrinogen levels as an independent risk factor for coronary heart disease, stroke, and peripheral vascular disease [3]

Fibrinogen is an acute phase protein that is directly involved in coagulation. The transcription of fibrinogen is stimulated by IL-6; its synthesis is suppressed by IL-1β and TNF-α. [4,5] Fibrinogen and its metabolites strongly affect hemostasis, hemorheology, platelet aggregation and endothelial function. Infact, fibrinogen's association with increased mortality lies probably in its ability to promote thromboses, or clots, by causing platelet aggregation in blood vessels. The recognition that fibrinogen is an important factor in the promotion of various disease states has led to the search for specific therapies intended to reduce plasma fibrinogen levels.

The use of statins in the prevention of primary [6] and secondary [7,8] CAD has been demonstrated to significantly reduce cardiovascular events and total mortality. Nevertheless, the majority of patients on statin treatment still experience coronary events. [9] It is clear that a more effective reduction in the incidences of coronary events is needed. This could probably be accomplished by a further reduction in the conventional as well as novel risk factors like plasma fibrinogen, homocysteine, and C-reactive protein. Multiple small studies have reported changes in fibrinogen levels with different statins. [10, 11] While atorvastatin is claimed to increase plasma fibrinogen, simvastatin is reported to either increase or have a neutral effect. Although many different pharmacologic approaches and strategies for therapeutic modulation of fibrinogen have been tested, the efficacy of different treatments to lower plasma fibrinogen in humans is limited and the mode of action unidentified. [12, 13] Among the few compounds known to lower circulating fibrinogen levels in humans are certain fibrates.

Fibrates reportedly lower plasma fibrinogen in humans, but the regulatory mechanism of this effect remains to be clarified. Activation of the nuclear hormone receptor PPARα mediates the suppression of fibrinogen gene transcription by fibrates in rodents.[3] This establishes PPARα as a key regulatory factor in fibrinogen gene expression in rodents and may explain the suppressive effect of fibrates on plasma fibrinogen levels in humans. The fibrinogen molecule is arranged as a dimer, with each monomer composed of 3 nonidentical polypeptide chains: Aα, Bβ and γ. [14] The 3 fibrinogen chains are encoded by 3 separate, closely linked genes situated on the same chromosome and located in the sequence γ, Aα, and

Bβ, with the last one in opposite transcriptional orientation to the first one.[15] Binsack et al [16] reported that in the human hepatoma cell line, HepG2, bezafibrate suppressed Aα-, Bβ- and γ- chain mRNA levels.[17] The genes encoding the 3 fibrinogen chains are negatively regulated by PPARα and since fibrates act through these receptors, it helps to explain the benefits of fibrate therapy to target a reduction in fibrinogen levels. Maison et al[18] showed that fibrinogen concentration decreased after fibrate therapy, while it increased after statin treatment. Thus this study was conducted to investigate the controversial role of statins in modifying fibrinogen levels and to study the benefits of addition of fenofibrate to statin therapy in modifying levels of plasma fibrinogen.

Research Design and Methods

The study was a controlled clinical trial. It was randomized, non blind and based on parallel group design. The protocol of the study received approval from the Institutional Review Board of the Sterling Hospital, Ahmedabad. Patients of ACS of either sex who had undergone Percutaneous Transluminal Coronary Angioplasty (PTCA) procedure irrespective of the presence of diabetes mellitus were included in the study after taking their consent. Patients with second or third degree AV (atrioventricular) block, renal or hepatic failure, recent cerebrovascular events, valve replacement surgery, or Balloon Mitral Valvuloplasty (BMV) and patients on lipid lowering therapy other than statins were excluded from the study. 102 consecutive patients meeting the eligibility criteria were randomized into four treatment groups, consisting of patients given atorvastatin, simvastatin, atorvastatin-fenofibrate combination and simvastatin-fenofibrate combination. Treatment was started after the PTCA and was continued for 3 months. Atorvastatin was given in a single dose of 20mg per day (if alone) and 10mg per day (in combination with fenofibrate), simvastatin was given in a single dose of 40mg per day (if alone) and 20mg per day (in combination with fenofibrate) and fenofibrate was given in a single dose of 200mg per day. The first blood samples were collected before the onset of the treatment and were analyzed for total cholesterol, triglycerides(TG), LDL, HDL, VLDL and plasma fibrinogen. The second blood samples were collected after 3 months of treatment for total cholesterol, triglycerides, HDL, LDL, VLDL, plasma fibrinogen and liver function tests that included SGPT, SGOT, total bilirubin and alkaline phosphatase. Total cholesterol, TG, HDL-C, SGPT, SGOT, total bilirubin and alkaline phosphatase were analyzed on automated VITROS 250 analyzer using enzymatic assay methods. LDL-C was analyzed by enzymatic method. VLDL-C was calculated using Friedewald's formula.

Plasma fibrinogen was assayed using Immunoprecipitation method using the RANDOX® kits. Many studies measure fibrinogen by the Clauss Method. However, data from the Framingham Heart Study [19] suggest that levels determined by the immunoprecipitation test have a stronger association with cardiovascular disease than those obtained by Clauss method. The results were analyzed by applying Student's t test, ANOVA and linear regression to find out degree of correlation between parameters. The probability value of less than 5% ($p<0.05$) was considered to be statistically significant.

RESULTS

We included in our study, 102 patients from the cardiology unit of Sterling hospital. All of them had angiographically documented CAD and had undergone PTCA. 25 patients each were enrolled in atorvastatin, atorvastatin-fenofibrate combination and simvastatin-fenofibrate combination treatment groups and 27 patients were enrolled in simvastatin treatment group. We had 4 dropouts in atorvastatin-fenofibrate group as well as in simvastatin monotherapy group and 3 dropouts in simvastatin-fenofibrate group, all due to non-technical reasons. So, the analysis is based on a total of 91 patients who completed the follow-up successfully. The baseline, demographic characteristics like age, sex, BMI, smoking/tobacco/ alcohol habits, past history of diabetes, hypertension, family history etc. and other hemodynamic parameters like hemoglobin, urea, creatinine, etc were recorded (Table 1). These parameters were found to be identical in all the four treatment groups indicating a symmetric study design and population.

Table 1. Baseline Demographic and Haemodynamic characteristics of the Patients

Characteristics	**Atorvastatin (n=25)**	**Atorvastatin + Fenofibrate (n=25)**	**Simvastatin (n=27)**	**Simvastatin + Fenofibrate (n=25)**
Age(years)	56.76 ± 9.4	56.44 ± 9.95	58.44 ± 11.4	58.35 ± 11.35
Females (%)	4%	12 %	7.4%	20%
Males (%)	96%	88%	92.6 %	80%
Body Mass Index(BMI)	25.79 ± 3.5	23.62 ± 1.95	25.3 ± 3.90	25.44 ± 4.25
Smokers	12%	20%	14.81 %	8%
Tobacco Chewers	12%	12%	7.4 %	4%
Diabetics	24%	36%	29.62%	48%
Hypertensives	28%	28%	51.85 %	40%
Haemoglobin (gm%)	12.61± 1.6	12.17 ± 1.75	13.16 ± 1.76	13.07 ± 1.65
Urea (mg/dl)	30.7± 18.9	26.81 ± 11.95	26.93 ± 15.46	26.91 ± 13.2
Creatinine (mg/dl)	1.23± 0.5	1.28 ± 1.1	1.10 ± 0.31	1.10 ± 0.3
Random bl. Sugar (mg/dl)	130.33± 39.25	146.73± 65.45	137.8 ± 57.45	137.48 ± 56.6
Systolic BP (mm Hg)	126.54 ± 16.05	129.52 ± 24.25	128.22 ± 22.47	128.84 ± 22.8
Diastolic BP (mm Hg)	81.29 ± 8.75	78.35 ± 9.00	80.55 ± 11.31	80.96 ± 11.55
Pulse	77.09 ± 15.4	80.55 ± 10.9	75.02 ± 15.46	75.29 ± 15.65
LVEF (%)	46.8 ± 12.35	50.94 ± 16.25	52.44 ± 12.79	52.51 ± 5.76
Single Vessel disease	68%	56%	55.55%	44%
Double vessel disease	28%	28%	29.62 %	36%
Triple vessel disease	4%	16%	14.81%	20%

Data expressed as mean ± SD; % of patients.

The effects of all the treatments on lipid parameters are given in Table 2. Atorvastatin and simvastatin monotherapy reduced serum LDL-C and interestingly increased serum HDL-C significantly ($p<0.05$). Atorvastatin-fenofibrate combination produced a significant decrease in TG, VLDL ($p<0.05$) and also increased HDL-C significantly as compared to atorvastatin alone ($p<0.05$). Similar to simvastatin monotherapy, simvastatin-fenofibrate combination produced a significant increase in HDL and decrease in LDL levels ($p<0.05$). It, however, did not reduce TG significantly. All the four treatments significantly reduced total cholesterol/HDL ratio and LDL/HDL ratio ($p<0.05$). ANOVA test was applied to find if there was any difference in the effects between the four groups. The results however, indicated that the percentage change in lipoprotein levels obtained were not significantly different from each other between the four treatment groups (Figure 1).

Table 2. Effect of treatments of serum lipoprotein levels

Parameters	Time interval	Atorvastatin[1] (n=25)	Atorvastatin + Fenofibrate [2] (n=21)	Simvastatin[3] (n=23)	Simvastatin + fenofibrate [4] (n=22)
		Mean ± SD	**Mean ± SD**	**Mean ± SD**	**Mean ± SD**
Total cholesterol mg/dl	baseline	156.6 ± 34.15	150.9± 46.39	150.44 ± 31.1	148.9 ± 31.98
	3 months	149.68 ± 42.8	155.76± 25.42	146.42±53.65	139.74 ± 30.67
TG mg/dl	baseline	144.85±76.65	155.1±112.12	138.5 ± 78.55	136.43 ± 78.97
	3 months	133.86±61.85	108.5±47.63*	123.5±100.7	110.12±47.5
HDL-C mg/dl	baseline	37.69 ±9.1	35.34 ± 9.25	34.91 ± 8.57	34.88 ± 8.67
	3 months	41.55 ±9.2*	46.61±8.38*	43.74 ± 12.9*	43.74 ± 13.27*
LDL-C mg/dl	baseline	101.44 ± 33.5	91.11 ± 33.06	93.39± 23.33	92.10 ± 24.10
	3 months	82.49 ±34.5*	86.74 ± 18.64	76.48 ± 26.3*	76.48 ± 26.35*
VLDL-C mg/dl	baseline	28.96 ±15.2	31.0 ± 22.39	27.68 ± 15.71	27.78 ± 15.85
	3 months	26.87 ± 12.35	21.71±9.66*	24.27 ± 19.97	24.17 ± 20.02
LDL- C/HDL-C	baseline	2.87 ± 1.35	2.66 ± 0.82	2.89 ± 1.05	3.13 ± 1.92
	3 months	2.06 ±0.95*	1.91 ± 0.50*	1.92 ± 0.81*	1.92 ± 0.79*
total cholesterol/ HDL-C	baseline	4.33 ± 1.25	4.41 ± 1.42	4.42 ± 1.29	4.37 ± 1.31
	3 months	3.71 ± 1.2 *	3.42 ± 0.69	3.66 ± 1.77*	3.66 ± 1.78*

Baseline: before starting of treatment
3 months: after 3 months of treatment
* Significant change from baseline values; student's t test, $p<0.05$;
$df^1=24$, $df^2=20$, $df^3=22$, $df^4=21$ (degree of freedom).

Table 3. Effect of treatments on plasma fibrinogen levels

Plasma Fibrinogen Gm/Lt	Atorvastatin [1] (n=25)	Atorvastatin + Fenofibrate [2] (n=21)	Simvastatin[3] (n=23)	Simvastatin + fenofibrate [4] (n=22)
Initial Levels	4.44 ± 0.26	4.29 ± 0.4	4.25 ± 0.25	4.21 ± 0.27
After 3 months	3.47 ±0.18 *	3.10 ± 0.28*	3.12 ± 0.14*	3.12 ± 0.15 *

*significant change from baseline values; Paired Student's t test, $p<0.05$
$df^1 = 24$, $df^2 = 20$, $df^3 = 22$, $df^4 = 21$.

The effect of the treatments on plasma fibrinogen are given in Table 3. Atorvastatin as well as simvastatin was found to decrease plasma fibrinogen significantly ($p<0.01$). Combination of statins with fenofibrate also showed a significant decrease in plasma fibrinogen ($p<0.01$). However, the treatment groups were not significantly different from each other when analyzed by ANOVA test. Thus, contrary to reports, statins in our study decreased plasma fibrinogen significantly while addition of fenofibrate enhanced this effect, however significantly. No correlation was found between fibrinogen levels and various demographical, haemodynamic and biochemical parameters (Table 4). Thus, plasma fibrinogen was found to be an independent risk factor for CAD and was lowered significantly by atorvastatin and simvastatin alone and in combination with fenofibrate. No significant elevations in the serum bilirubin concentration, transaminases (SGPT, SGOT) and alkaline phosphatase levels were observed in any treatment group (Table 5). It thus appeared that all the treatments were safely tolerated in the given doses without any adverse hepatotoxic effects.

Table 4. Correlation coefficient between fibrinogen and other study parameters

Parameters	**Correlation coefficient (r)**
Body Mass Index (BMI)	-0.02
Haemoglobin	-0.21
Urea	0.18
Creatinine	-0.21
Blood Glucose	-0.14
Cholesterol	0.05
Triglycerides	0.01
HDL-C	-0.10
LDL-C	0.07
VLDL-C	-0.02
LDL-C/HDL-C	0.10
CHO/HDL-C	0.10

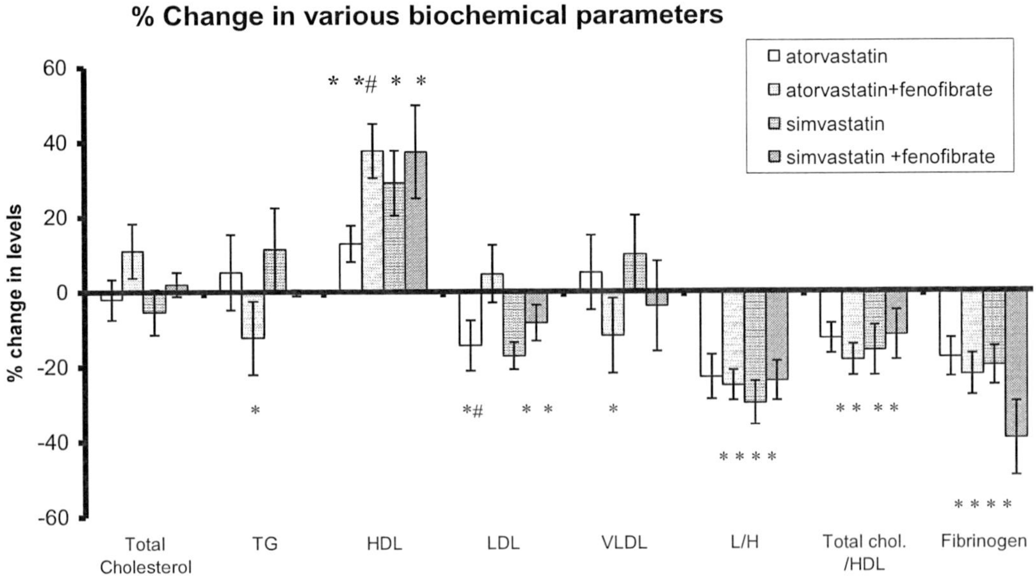

*Significant change from baseline values, Student's t test, p<0.05.
Significant change as compared to the respective statin monotherapy or combination, Unpaired Student's t test, p<0.05
ANOVA test applied on % change in levels, P>0.05, Changes are not significantly different from each other between the groups

Figure 1. % change in lipid levels between both the treatment group.

Table 5. Effect of treatments of Liver Function Parameters at the end of three months

Parameters	Atorvastatin[1] (n=25)	Atorvastatin + Fenofibrate [2] (n=21)	Simvastatin[3] (n=23)	Simvastatin + fenofibrate [4] (n=22)
		Mean ± SD	Mean ± SD	Mean ± SD
Total bilirubin mg/dl	0.7 ± 0.25	0.67 ± 0.18	0.71 ± 0.28	0.71 ± 0.28
SGPT U/Lt	28.16 ± 10.9	29.62 ± 7.19	31.67 ± 7.99	31.48 ± 1.72
SGOT U/Lt	24.46 ±7.1	29.14 ± 6.59	27.62 ± 7.28	27.55 ± 1.56
Alk.Phosph-atase U/Lt	94.04 ±23.05	69.00 ± 16.48	74.51 ± 26.25	73.80 ± 5.42

Data expressed as Mean ± SD
*Significant change from baseline values; student's t test, $p<0.05$;
$df^1=24$, $df^2=20$, $df^3=22$, $df^4=21$ (degree of freedom).

DISCUSSION

Statins alone as well as in combination with fenofibrate were found to produce beneficial effects in CAD patients after PTCA. Statins are potent inhibitors of HMG Co-A reductase, which decreases LDL-C by upregulating LDL receptor activity in the liver and reducing the secretion of apolipoprotein B containing lipoprotein. The latter is believed to be responsible for the TG lowering effect of atorvastatin and is profound at higher doses.[20] Various reports have indicated that atorvastatin lowers LDL-C and increases HDL.[21,22,23] The effects of atorvastatin in our study comply with such reports. On the other hand, simvastatin is reported to produce a decrease in LDL-C from 26% to 50% in various doses.[24, 25] Also, reports from Hunninghake et al [26] showed that simvastatin consistently produces a larger increase in HDL-C as compared to atorvastatin. Results from our study comply with the above findings as simvastatin in our study too produced a significant decrease in LDL-C and increase in HDL-C as compared to atorvastatin. Fibrates activate PPAR-α which ultimately leads to their HDL raising and TG lowering effects.[27,28] Certain previous studies have suggested increased benefits of a combination of fenofibrate with statins. [29,30] Reports are available that show benefits of combining fenofibrate and simvastatin. [30, 31] A study of the literature also shows that a greater change in HDL and TG levels is obtained with fenofibrate - atorvastatin combination as compared to monotherapy [32] with either drug. Our results comply with reported findings. We observed that combining fenofibrate with statins offered a greater benefit in reducing TG and VLDL levels as well as increasing HDL levels. Thus, the combination therapy proved both safe and beneficial in our patients with ACS. In prospective studies, plasma fibrinogen has been found to be an independent predictor of myocardial infarction in both genders. It provides information on CAD risk over and beyond that supplied by established risk factors. [33] The Framingham study has shown that for both sexes, the risk of cardiovascular diseases was correlated positively to antecedent fibrinogen values higher than 1.3 to 7.0 gm/L.[34] We found that fibrinogen in our study did not correlate with any of our study parameters including demographic characters and lipid levels. Thus, fibrinogen does appear to be an independent risk factor for CAD. Reports from large-scale trials consistently show statins to have a neutral effect on fibrinogen. [35,36] Various studies on plasma fibrinogen indicate that fenofibrate lowers fibrinogen levels but the effects of atorvastatin and simvastatin have been variable and controversial, particularly that of atorvastatin. Wierzbicki et al [37] showed that atorvastatin increases plasma fibrinogen by 22%. Song et al. [38] also found a significant increase in fibrinogen with atorvastatin treatment where as simvastatin was reported to have a neutral effect. Various reports indicated that fenofibrate decreased plasma fibrinogen significantly whereas atorvastatin produced an increase in fibrinogen levels.[39, 40,41] Otto et al [42] showed that plasma fibrinogen and other hemorheologic parameters were unchanged during atorvastatin treatment in comparison to simvastatin treatment. Athyros et al. [43] reported that plasma fibrinogen was unaffected by atorvastatin and was significantly reduced by fenofibrate and combination of both. Ceska et al [44] showed that fenofibrate is a potent hypolipidemic drug with only rare side effects and reduces fibrinogen significantly. In our study, however, contrary to all above reports for statins, we observed that atorvastatin as well as simvastatin produced a significant decrease in plasma fibrinogen levels. However, our results comply with some recent findings by Kadikoylu and co- workers that show a decrease in plasma fibrinogen by atorvastatin and simvastatin. [45] Another study by Leibovitz et al. [47] proved that atorvastatin reduces fibrinogen levels in patients with severe hypercholesterolemia. fibrinogen levels dropped by almost 18% in this study. Tekin et al [48] has also shown a reduction in plasma fibrinogen levels by atorvastatin in hyperlipidemic patients with angiographically proved CAD. These findings with atorvastatin are consistent with such recent data. The combination of statins with fenofibrate also produced a further decrease in fibrinogen, though not significant. These results are in agreement with the reported claims of fenofibrate to decrease plasma fibrinogen. Previous studies have indicated an increased risk of myopathy with statin-fibrate combination. [29,46] However, no cessation of therapy was required in any patient due to such complications in our study. Liver function tests of all patients were also normal at the end of 3 months of treatments indicating no adverse hepatotoxic effects. These findings suggest that it may be safe to use fenofibrate and statins in combination contrary to reported contra- indications for the combined use of these two classes of drugs. However, we have not looked into the long-term toxicity associated with the use of these drugs in combination. Moreover, the strategy appears to be distinctly beneficial in lowering the risk factor plasma fibrinogen. Thus, the therapy offers a new method to treat patients with acute coronary syndromes.

Conclusion

Addition of fenofibrate to statins seems to be beneficial in patients with ACS. Statins, contrary to various reports, were found to decrease plasma fibrinogen significantly. Also, in combination with fenofibrate there was enhanced reduction of the novel risk factor, fibrinogen.

References

[1] Murray JL, Lopez AL. Alternative projections of mortality and disability by cause 1990-2020. Global Burden of Disease Study. *Lancet* 1997; 349:1498-1504.

[2] Tsimihodimos V, Kostoula A, Kakafika A, Bairaktari E, Tselepis AD, Mikhailidis DP, Elisaf M. Effect of fenofibrate on serum inflammatory markers in patients with high triglyceride values. *J Cardiovasc Pharmacol Ther* 2004; 9:27-33.

[3] Kockx M, Gervois PP, Poulain P, Derudas B, Peters JM, Gonzalez FJ, Princen HM, Kooistra T, Staels B. Fibrates suppress fibrinogen gene expression in rodents via activation of the peroxisome proliferators-activated receptor-alpha. *Blood* 1999; 93: 2991-8.

[4] Green F, Humphries S. Control of plasma fibrinogen levels. *Baillieres Clin Haematol* 1989;2: 945-59.

[5] Woods A, Brull DJ, Humphries SE, Montgomery HE. Genetics of inflammation and risk of coronary artery disease: the central role of interleukin-6. *Eur Heart J* 2002; 21: 1574-83.

[6] Shepherd, J., Cobbe, S. M., Ford, I. Prevention of coronary heart disease with pravastatin in men with hypercholesterolemia. *N Engl J Med* 1995; 333: 1301-7.

[7] Sacks, F. M., Pfeffer, M. A., Moye, L. A. The effect of pravastatin on coronary events after myocardial infarction in patients with average cholesterol levels. *N Engl J Med* 1996 335:1001-9

[8] The Scandinavian Simvastatin Survival Group. Randomized trial of cholesterol lowering in 4444 patients with coronary heart disease: The Scandinavian Simvastatin Survival Study (4S*)*. *Lancet* 1994; 344: 1383-9.

[9] Athyros, V. G., Papageorgiou, A. A., Hatzikonstandinou, H. A., Athyrou, V. V., Kontopoulos, A. G.Effect of atorvastatin versus simvastatin on lipid profile and plasma fibrinogen in patients with hypercholesterolemia. *Clin Drug Inves* 1998; 16: 219-27.

[10] Rosenson RS, Tangney CC, Casey LC. Inhibition of proinflammatory cytokine production by pravastatin. *Lancet* 1999; 353: 983-4.

[11] Rosenson RS, Tangney CC. Anti-atherothrombotic properties of statins: implications for cardiovascular event reduction. *JAMA* 1998; 279:1643-50.

[12] Handley DA, Hughes TE. Pharmacological approaches and strategies for therapeutic modulation of fibrinogen. *Thromb Res* 1997: 87:1-5.

[13] Ernst E, Resch KL. Therapeutic interventions to lower plasma fibrinogen concentration. *Eur Heart J* 1995; 16:47-51.

[14] Fuller GM. Fibrinogen: a multifunctional acute phase protein, in Mackiewicz A, Kushner I, Baumann H (eds): Acute phase proteins: Molecular Biology, biochemistry and clinical applications, New York, NY, Doubleday, 1993,p 169.

[15] Kant JA, Fornace AJ, Saxe D, Simon MI, McBride OW, Crabtree GR. Evolution and organization of the fibrinogen locus on chromosome 4: Gene duplication accompanied by transposition and inversion. *Proc Natl Acad Sci* USA 1985: 82: 2344-50

[16] Binsack R, Stegmeier K, Dorge L, Volkl A. Bezafibrate down-regulates fibrinogen biosynthesis in human hepatoma HepG2 cells. *Eur J Clin Invest* 1998; 28:151-5.

[17] Roy SN, Mukhopadhyay G, Redman CM. Regulation of fibrinogen assembly. Transfection of Hep G2 cells with B beta cDNA specifically enhances synthesis of the 3 component chains of fibrinogen. *J Biol Chem* 1990; 265:6389-93.

[18] Maison, P., Mennon, L., Sapinho, D., Balkau, B., Sigalas, J., Chesnier, M. C., Eschwege, E. D.E.S.I.R. Study group. A pharmacoepidemiological assessment of the effect of statins and fibrates on fibrinogen concentration. *Atheroscler* 2002; 160:155-60

[19] Stec JJ, Silbershatz H, Tofler GH, Matheney TH, Sutherland P,Lipinska I, Massaro JM, Wilson PF, Muller JE, D'Agostino RB Sr. Association of fibrinogen with cardiovascular risk factors and cardiovascular disease in the Framingham Offspring Population. *Circ* 2000; 102: 1634-8.

[20] Burnett JR, Wilcox LT, Telford DE, Kleinstiver SJ, Barrett PHR, Newton RS, Huff MW. Inhibition of HMG Co A reductase by atorvastatin decreases both VLDL and LDL, apoB productionin miniature pigs. *Arterioscler Thromb Vasc Biol* 1997;17:2489-2500.

[21] Haw N, Fowler G, Patel H, Eminton Z, Maton S. An assessment of the efficacy of atorvastatin in achieving LDL cholesterol target levels in patients with coronary heart disease: a general practice study. *Int J Clin Prac* 1999;53:422-6.

[22] Marais AD, Firth JC, Bateman M, Jones J, Mountney J. Atorvastatin is a powerful and safe agent for lowering plasma cholesterol concentration in heterozygous familial hypercholesterolemia. *Atheroscler* 1994;109:316-20.

[23] Frost R, Otto C, Geiss C, Schwandt P, Parhofer KG. Effects of atorvastatin versus fenofibrate on lipoprotein profiles, low density lipoprotein subfraction distribution, and hemorheologic parameters in type 2 diabetes mellitus with mixed hyperlipoproteinemia. *Am J Cardiol* 2001;87:44-8.

[24] Jones, P., Kafonek, S., Laurova, I. Comparative dose efficacy study of atorvastatin versus simvastatin, pravastatin, lovastatin and fluvastatin in patients with hypercholesterolemia. (The CURVES Study). *Am J Cardiol* 1998; 81: 582-7.

[25] Crouse JR III, Frolich J, Ose L, Mercuri M, Tobert JA. Effects of high doses of simvastatin and atorvastatin on high-density lipoprotein cholesterol and apolipoprotein A-1. *Am J Cardiol* 1999;83:1476-7.

[26] Hunninghake DB, Ballantyne CM, Maccubbin DL, Shah AK, Gumbiner B, Mitchel YB. Comparative effects of simvastatin and atorvastatin in hypercholesterolemic patients with characteristics of metabolic syndrome. *Clin Ther* 2003;25:1670-86.

[27] Staels B, Dallongvile J, Auwerx J, Schoonjans K, Leitersdorf E, Fruchart JC. Mechanism of action of fibrates on lipid and lipoprotein metabolism. *Circ* 1998;98:2088-93.

[28] Watts GF, Dimmit SB. Fibrates, dyslipoproteinemia and cardiovascular disease. *Curr Opin Lipid* 1999;10:561-74.

[29] Athyros VG, Papageorgiou AA, Hatziknonstandinou HA, Didangelos TP, Carina MV, Kranitsas DF, Kontupoulos AG. Safety and efficacy of long term statin-fibrate combination in patients with refractory familial combined hyperlipidemia. *Amer J Cardiol* 1997; 80: 608-13.

[30] Ruth LBE and Ruth McPherson. Long term efficacy and safety of fenofibrate and statin in treatment of combined hyperlipidemia. *Amer J Cardiol* 1998; 81: 60B-65B.

[31] Vega GL, Ma PT, Cater NB, Fillipchuk N, Megura S, Garcia AB, Grundy SM. Effects of adding fenofibrate (200mg/day) in patients with combined hyperlipidemia and metabolic syndrome. *Amer J Cardiol* 2003; 91: 956-60.

[32] Keating GM, Ormod D. Micronised fenofibrate: an updated review of its clinical efficacy in the management of dyslipidaemia. *Drugs* 2002; 62:1909-44.

[33] Heinrich, J., Assmann, G. Fibrinogen and cardiovascular risk. *J Cardiovasc Risk* 1995;2: 197-205.

[34] Kannel, W. B., Neaton, J. D., Wentworth, D., Thomas, H. E., Stamler, J., Hulley, S. B. For the MRFIT Research group. Overall and coronary heart disease mortality rates in relation to major risk factors in 325,348 men screened for the MRFIT trial. Multiple Risk Factor Intervention Trial. *Am Heart J* 1987; 112:825-36.

[35] Rosenson RS, Koenig W. Utility of inflammatory markers in the management of Coronary artery disease. *Amer J Cardiol* 2003; 92:10i-18i.

[36] Lowe G, Rumley A, Norrie J, Ford I, Shepherd J, Cobbe S, Macfarlane P, Packard C, on behalf of the West of Scotland Coronary Prevention Study Group. Blood Rheology, cardiovascular risk factors and cardiovascular disease: the west of Scotland Coronary Prevention Study. *Thromb Haemost* 2000; 84: 553-8.

[37] Wierzbicki, A. S., Lumb, P. J., Semra, Y. K. Effect of atorvastatin on plasma fibrinogen. *Lancet* 1998; 351:569-70.

[38] Song, J. C., White, C. M. Do HMG CoA reductase inhibitors affect fibrinogen? *Ann Pharmacother* 2001; 35:236-41.

[39] Bairaktari, E. T., Tzallas, C. S., Tsimihodimos, V. K., Liberopoulos, E. N., Miltiadous, G. A., Elisaf, M. S. Comparison of the efficacy of atorvastatin and micronized fenofibrate in the treatment of mixed hyperlipidemia. *J Cardiovasc Risk* 1999; 6:113-6.

[40] Frost, R., Otto, C., Geiss, C., Schwandt, P., Parhofer, K. G. Effects of atorvastatin versus fenofibrate on lipoprotein profiles, low density lipoprotein subfraction distribution, and hemorheologic parameters in type 2 diabetes mellitus with mixed hyperlipoproteinemia. *Am J Cardiol* 2001; 87:44-8.

[41] Serna, G., Cadarso, C. Fenofibrate decreases plasma fibrinogen, improves lipid profile, and reduces uricemia. *Clin Pharmacol Ther* 1999; 66:166-72.

[42] Otto, C., Geiss, H. C., Donner, M. G., Parhofer, K. G., Schwandt, P. Influence of atorvastatin versus simvastatin on fibrinogen and other hemorheological parameters in patients with severe hypercholesterolemia treated with regular low density lipoprotein immunoadsorption apheresis. *Ther Apher* 2000; 4:244-8.

[43] Athyros, V. G., Papageorgiou, A. A., Athyrou, V. V., Demitriadis, D. S., Kontopoulos, A. G. Atorvastatin and micronized fenofibrate alone and in combination in type 2 diabetes with combined hyperlipidemia. *Diab Care* 2002; 25:1198-1202.

[44] Ceska R, Sobra J, Kvasnicka J, Prochazkova R, Kvasilova M, Haas T. The effect of micronized fenofibrate on lipid parameters and fibrinogen in heterozygous familial hypercholesterolemia and familial combined hyperlipidemia. *Cas Lek Cesk* 1996;135: 413-6.

[45] Kadikoylu, G., Yukselen, V., Yavasoglu, I., Bolaman, Z. Hemostatic effects of atorvastatin versus simvastatin. *Ann Pharmacother* 2003; 37:478-84.

[46] Tikkanen MJ. Statins within-group comparisons, statin escape and combination therapy. *Curr Opin Lipidol* 1996; 7: 385-8.

[47] Leibovitz E, Hazanov N, Frieman A, Elly I, Gavish D. Atorvastatin reduces fibrinogen levels in patients with severe hypercholesterolemia: additional evidence to support the anti-inflammatory effects of statins. *Isr Med Assoc J* 2004;6:456-9.

[48] Tekin A, Tekin G, Guzelsoy D, Kaya A, Gurel CV, Yigit Z, Ulutin T. Effects of atorvastatin (10 mg) on hemostatic and inflammatory parameters in hyperlipidemic patients with angiographically proven coronary artery disease. *Am J Cardiol.* 2004;94:206-9.

In: World Heart Research Yearbook. Volume 1
Editors: Franz Halberg and R. B. Singh
ISBN: 978-1-60741-881-8

EFFECTS OF SILDENAFIL IN CARDIOVASCULAR DISEASE

Ram B. Singh*[1,*], *Dasa Dudova*[2], *Daniel Pella*[2], *Shashi B. Gupta*[3] and *Rakesh C. Kukreja*[4]
[1] Halberg Hospital and Research Institute and
Subharti Medical College, Moradabad, India
[2] Safaric University, Slovakia
[3] Kosice, Slovakia, Railway Hospital, Mumbai, India
[4] VCU Medical Centre, Richmond, VA, US

ABSTRACT

Recent studies indicate that sildenafil is cardioprotective by preconditioning of the myocardial and endothelial cells. In the present review, we examine the available evidence regarding this beneficial effect. Experimental studies indicate that sildenafil can provide beneficial effects to the myocardium and endothelium by enhancing preconditioning. There are a few clinical studies among healthy subjects and a few observational studies indicating that sildenafil is useful in patients with poor endothelial function and in those with myocardial ischaemia. We found among 6 volunteer patients with nonST-elevation myocardial infarction that treatment with sildenafil was protective in limiting infarct size. We also observed that sildenafil can decrease blood pressure among hypertensives and provide benefits against heart failure in patients with acute left ventricular failure.

Experimental and clinical experiences support the usefulness of sildenafil in patients with acute myocardial infarction, heart failure and hypertension. Randomized, controlled trials and long-term follow-up are necessary to confirm these observations.

Keywords: Sildenafil, cardioprotective, hypertension, heart failure, nitric oxide

INTRODUCTION

There is consistent evidence that sildenafil can protect against endothelial damage and myocardial injury by enhancing preconditioning [1, 2]. One study showed [2], that opening of mitochondrial ATP sensitive K channels by ischemic preconditioning or Diazoxide protected

* Correspondence: Dr R B Singh, Halberg Hospital and Research Institute, Civil Lines,Moradabad-10(UP)244001, India. Fax 0091 591 2411003,tel 0091 591 2417437; Email: icn2005@mickynline.com.

the endothelium by reducing the bursts of free radicals that occurred at reperfusion. Mitochonchria is rich in the coenzyme Q10 and carnitine, which are cytoprotective antioxidants and bioenergetic agents [3-5]. Both these agents are known to maintain ATP, which poses the possibility that endogenous levels of the agents or their supplementation may be protective against free radical-induced damage to ATP Sensitive K channels. It is also possible that these agents might enhance the capability of the myocardial and endothelial cells in preconditioning which is known to protect the cells against injury responsible for arrhythmias, and can modulate remodeling of the myocardium and endothelium against heart failure and atherogenesis.[4-6]. It has been shown that this widely-used drug for treating erectile dysfunction reduces the apoptosis under heart attack-like conditions in a laboratory model. These findings may help researchers to develop a new treatment for patients with heart failure and acute myocardial infarction (AMI), where the loss of cells is primarily due to cell suicide or ischemic damage respectively [5, 6].

Clinical Observations

In our experience, 3 patients, aged 45-60 years, (1 male and 2 females), presenting with congestive heart failure due to hypertension (systolic >200mmHg and diastolic >110mmHg) and ischemic heart disease, were given furosemide 40mg intravenously daily plus sildenafil 50mg twice daily, plus perindopril 4-8mg daily, there was a marked improvement in New York Heart Association(NYHA) class heart failure and quality of life including improvement in fatigue and dyspnea within 48 hours of treatment. All 3 patients were discharged by the end of one week. All these patients had radiological, electrocardiographic and echocardiographic manifestations of heart failure, including lower ejection fraction between 40-50%. There was a significant reduction in systolic and diastolic blood pressures in all the patients (>150/95mmHg). In another clinical observation, among 6 patients with acute myocardial infarction(AMI),we noted that sildenafil (25mg 2-3 times, daily) can decrease anginal episodes, cause less increase in LDH and reduce electocardiographic QRS score(infarct size) when compared to another 6 age, sex and body mass index matched subjects not given this agent. There was a 20-25% increase in heart rate and decrease in blood pressures initially among patients receiving sildenafil compared to the baseline heart rate, which settled to baseline rates after about 5 days treatment. The patients in both groups also did not receive streptokinase because some of them presented beyond 20-24 hours of onset of chest pain and some had nonST-segment elevation AMI. Their age varied between 45-60 years with 5 males and 1 female in each group. One patient with inferior wall infarction had hypotension, (80/50mmHg) where the dose of sildenafil was decreased to 25mg/day from 25mg thrice daily. There were no adverse effects of sildenafil in both of our observations and all patients gave written informed consent for the administration of sildenafil.

Existing Clinical Evidence

In one study among healthy subjects [7], ischemia/reperfusion on endothelial and neutrophil function was studied, in which the forearm was made ischemic by inflating a blood pressure cuff to 200mmHg for 20 minutes. The dilator response to the endothelial dependent dilator, acetylecholine and the nonendothelial dependent dilator nitroglycerine was determined before and after ischemia/reperfusion. Neutrophil function was studied by determining the upregulation of the CD11b in the circulating blood. Ischemic preconditioning was developed by 3 five minute periods of ischemia/reperfusion prior to the 20 minute ischemic periods. There was a marked decline in radial artery dilation to acetylecholine but not to nitroglycerine and an upregulation of CD11b, due to ischemia/reperfusion in the control subjects. Ischemic preconditioning blunted these responses to ischemia/reperfusion. This study suggests possible pathways of pharmacological preconditioning of the vasculature causing better reflow in patients with endothelial injury. In another more recent study [8], the role of ATP sensitive K channels was studied in mediating the influence of ischemic preconditioning among healthy volunteers after ischemia/reperfusion of the forearm. Intraarterial administration of acetylecholine was used to determine vasodilator response, indicating endothelial function, before and at 15 minutes, after 20 minutes of forearm ischemia/reperfusion under the influence of various drugs. Ischemic preconditioning protected against induced endothelial dysfunction by ischemia/reperfusion and this protection was blunted by cotherapy with glibenclamide. However, pretreatment with diazoxide simulated the effects of preconditioning to protect against endothelial dysfunction, which was blocked by glibenclamide. Interestingly, in the absence of ischemia/reperfusion, diazoxide had no influence on vasodilator responses to acetylecholine. It is possible that ATP sensitive K channels have an important role in ischemia/reperfusion-induced endothelial damage in humans. It is also likely that modulation of channel pathways using certain agents by activation of K channels may have a therapeutic use in patients with AMI. Tomai et al [9], in one early study, reported that repeated episodes of angioplasty induced ischemia blocked by glibenclamide, had no beneficial influence on cardiomyocytes that was to be provided by preconditioning. These clinical studies and our observations in AMI indicate that activation of myocardial and and/or endothelial localized ATP sensitive K channels are useful in patients with coronary artery disease, which might decrease injury to endothelial cells as well as to cardiomyocytes. In a most recent observation, Gori et al [10] studied the effects of treatment with sildenafil (50mg/day) among 10 healthy male volunteers, 2 hours prior to 15 minutes of cuff-induced radial artery ischemia, followed by 15 minutes of reperfusion. In a double blind, randomized, crossover study, flow mediated vasodilation was determined prior to drug or placebo treatment as an indicator of endothelial function. Glibenclamide (5mg) was administered one hour prior to sildenafil administration in a randomized, double blind fashion, in a separate group of 7 healthy volunteers. There was a significant reduction in the endothelial function in placebo-treated controls and this decline was prevented by prior treatment with sildenafil. However, the beneficial effect of sildenafil was blunted by glibenclamide at a dose, which had no influence on endothelial function in the absence of sildenafil. This study has provided proof for the first time that sildenafil provides protection to the endothelium against ischemia/reperfusion in humans and this effect involves activation of vascular ATP sensitive K channels. One earlier study [11] also showed that treatment with sildenafil, acutely in patients with chronic heart failure enhances endothelium-dependent, flow mediated vasodilation in the brachial artery, one hour after sildenafil therapy compared to control subjects. In another study [12], 100mg/day of sildenafil was administered causing dilation of epicardial coronary arteries, and improvement in endothelial function in the brachial artery and it also inhibited platelet function in patients with coronary artery disease.

There was a significant reduction in exercise-induced ischemia upon treatment with sildenafil, which showed moderate effects when compared to placebo and isosorbide dinitrate. It is clear that sildenafil was effective, both in healthy volunteers as well as in patients with chronic heart failure and coronary artery disease [11-13]. Our observations do not provide proof that sildenafil should be administered in the treatment of AMI. However, in view of the above studies, it indicates a need for randomized, controlled trials to determine its exact role in the prevention of complications in these patients, especially in those who have myocardial ischemia in the presence of coronary atherothrombosis and left ventricular dysfunction. There are no serious adverse effects of sildanafil, except hypotension, especially in those patients receiving nitrates and other nitric oxide donors [14, 15].

In one study [16] data were pooled regarding myocardial infarction (MI) and cardiovascular death from more than 120 clinical trials of sildenafil citrate (Viagra) conducted from 1993 to 2001. During placebo-controlled trials, the rate of MI or cardiovascular death was 0.91 (95% CI: 0.52-1.48) per 100 person-years (PY) of follow-up among sildenafil-treated patients compared with 0.84 (95% CI: 0.39-1.60) per 100 PY of follow-up among placebo-treated patients. The relative risk of MI or cardiovascular death was 1.08 (95% CI: 0.45-2.77) for sildenafil compared with placebo ($p = 0.88$). During open-label studies, the rate of MI or cardiovascular death was 0.56 (95% CI: 0.44-0.72) per 100 PY of follow-up. This analysis showed that the rates of MI and cardiovascular death were low and comparable between men treated with sildenafil and those treated with placebo. The use of sildenafil was not associated with an increase in the risk of MI or cardiovascular death.

Experimental Evidence

Several studies [17-21] have examined the cardioprotective effects of sildenafil on myocardial infarct size and arrhythmias. All the studies reported a beneficial influence except one [17] showing that slidenafil-nitric oxide donor combination promotes ventricular tachyarrhythmias in a swine right ventricle. In one study [18], both acute treatment with sildenafil given 30 minutes prior to ischemia, and chronic administration, given 24 hours prior to the index ischemic period produced a marked preconditioning like effect in intact rabbits. After administration of the drug or the vehicle, rabbits were subjected to 30minutes of ischemia and 3 hours of reperfusion. The triphenyletetraz -olium histochemical staining technique was used to determine the infarct size and showed that delayed treatment with sildenafil decreased the infarct size by 41% and acute treatment by 68%, respectively. Treatment with 5-HD, a mitochondrial selective, ATP sensitive K channel antagonist, 10minutes prior to the index ischemic period, blocked these beneficial influences. Oral administration of sildenafil was associated with both acute and delayed cardiac protection.

Further studies [19, 20] showed that reduction of infarct size by sildenafil in acute administration was due to PKC and that an upregulation of both endothelial nitric oxide synthetase (eNOS) and iNOS occurred in a delayed preconditioning model in mouse hearts.

After 24 hours of sildenafil administration, treatment with a selective iNOS inhibitor, 1400W, antagonized the sildenafil-induced cardioprotection, if given 30 minutes prior to index ischemia. It is clear that PKC, nitric oxide and mitochondrial ATP sensitive K channels are involved in providing cardioprotective effects to reduce infarct size in experimental models.

Increased availability of coenzyme Q10 and carnitine may repair or strengthen these mechanisms, resulting in better protective effects.

Nagy et al [20] also showed that sildenafil decreased the severity of ventricular rhythm disturbances in experiments with dogs, 24 hours after oral treatment with this agent. However, when sildenafil was given in combination with nitric oxide donor nitroprusside or nitroglycerine, it became arrhythmogenic in nonischemic, buffer-perfused, isolated right ventricular walls of swine hearts. Myocardial tissue deficiency of coenzyme Q10 and carnitine, which were not available in this experiment, may be the cause of these adverse effects. We also observed a 20-25% increase in baseline heart rate among patients with AMI receiving sildenafil. Other factors responsible for this discrepancy, may be due to protocol differences, a drug interaction or due to species differences between dogs and pigs.

Mechanisms

Recently, it has been reported [2, 6] that treatment with sildenafil citrate at clinically relevant concentrations produced therapeutic levels of nitric oxide (NO) in the heart cells by increasing protein levels of two enzymes responsible for the synthesis of NO. Employing a cellular model where heart attack-like conditions are simulated in a Petri dish, it has been demonstrated that NO produced from sildenafil inhibits cell death by stabilizing mitochondria, thereby increasing the level of the anti-death protein, Bcl-2, and inhibiting caspase 3, the protein considered to be the ultimate weapon in cell suicide. This research has established a strong basis for the design of future studies targeted toward investigating the clinical effects of sildenafil on survival of the heart muscle following a major heart attack. In addition, these findings suggest that this drug may slow or possibly reverse the progressive loss of heart cells during chronic heart failure in patients with acute or chronic coronary artery disease. Researchers used heart cells prepared from genetically engineered mice that lack nitric oxide synthesizing enzymes. The model was particularly useful in studying the protective effect of sildenafil in heart muscle cells independent of any vascular effects or other types of cells. Sildenafil not only protected against necrosis, accidental cell death occurring due to oxygen deprivation, but also against apoptosis, cell death following DNA fragmentation. Furthermore, the researchers found the presence of phosphodiesterase-5 (PDE-5), an enzyme responsible for the destruction of the cGMP molecule, in the heart cells. The cGMP is an intracellular messenger molecule that plays an important role in the dilation of arteries in the body. Sildenafil is able to preserve cGMP, and therefore dilation of the arteries by inhibiting PDE-5.

Conclusion

These observations have far-reaching implications for the treatment of patients with heart failure where loss of cells is primarily due to apoptosis, and in patients with AMI and angina pectoris where the cell loss may be due to ischemic injury. In several other studies [6-21] and due to our observations, it is proposed that sildenafil has a powerful, protective effect in the heart during experimental and clinical heart attack in animal models, and in humans, respectively, indicting that it could be protective against AMI and hypertensive heart failure and also possibly in patients with hypertension for decreasing blood pressure. Randomized, controlled, clinical trials are necessary to demonstrate the role of sidenafil in cardiovascular disease.

ACKNOWLEDGMENTS

We are grateful to Raj Chopra, President of the Tishcon Corporation, Westbury, NY, for support in writing this article.

REFERENCES

[1] Gross GJ.Sildenafil and endothelial dysfunction in humans (Editorial). *Circulation* 2005 (in press).

[2] Beresewicz A, Maczewski M, Duda M. Effect of classical preconditioning and diazoxide on endothelial function and O2 and NO generation in the post-ischemic guinea-pig heart. *Cardiovas Res* 2004,63:118-129.

[3] Chiang CA, Pella D, Singh RB. Coenzyme Q10 and adverse effects of statins. *J Nutr Environ Med* 2004,14:17-28.

[4] Singh RB, Neki NS, Kartikey K, Niaz MA, Thakur AS. Effect of coenzyme Q10 on risk of atherosclerosis in patients with recent myocardial infarction. *Mol Cell Biochem* 2003,246:75-82.

[5] Singh RB, Niaz MA, Agarwal P, Begom R, Rastogi SS, Sachan DS.A randomized, double blind, placebo controlled trial of L-carnitine in suspected acute myocardial infarction. *Postgrad Med* 1996,72:45-50.

[6] Kukreja RC, Ockaili R, Salloum F and Xi, L. Cardioprotection with phosphodiesterase-5 inhibition-a novel preconditioning strategy. *J Mol Cell Cardiol* 2004,36:165-173.

[7] Kharbanda RK, Peters M,* Walton B, Kattenhorn M, Mullen M, Klein N, Vallance P, Deanfield J, MacAllister R.*Ischemic preconditioning prevents endothelial injury and systemic neutrophil activation during ischemia-repurfusion in humans in vivo. *Circulation* 2001, 103:1624-30.

[8] Broadhead MW, Kharbanda RK, Peters M *MacAllister RJ.* K-ATP channels activation induces ischemic preconditioning of the endothelium in humans in vivo. *Circulation* 2004, 110:2077-2082.

[9] Tomai F, Crea F, Gaspardone A, *Gaspardone A, Versaci F, De Paulis R, Penta de Peppo A, Chiariello L, Gioffre PA. *Ischemic preconditioning during coronary angioplasty is prevented by glibenclamide, a selective ATP-sensitive K+ channel blocket. *Circulation* 1994,90:700-705.

[10] Gori T, Sicuro S, Dragoni S, *Donati G, Forconi S, Parker JD.* Sildenafil prevents endothelial disfunction induced by ischemia and reperfusion via opening of ATP sensitive K channels. A human invivo study. *Circulation* 2005, 111:742-6.

[11] Katz SD, Balidamaj K, Homma S *Wu H, Wang J, Maybaum S.*Acute type 5 phosphodiesterase inhibition with sildenafil enhances flow- mediated vasodilation in patients with chronic heart failure. *J Am Coll Cardiol* 2000,36:845-851.

[12] Halcox JPJ, Nour KRA, Seals G *Mincemoyer RA, Waclawiw M, Rivera CE, Willie G, Ellahham S, Quyyumi AA.*The effect of sildenafil on human vascular function, platelet activation and myocardial ischemia. *J Am Coll Cardiol* 2002,40:1232-1240.

[13] Yellon DM, Downey JM. Preconditioning the myocardium: from cellular physiology to clinical cardiology. *Physiol Rev* 2003,83:1113-1151.

[14] Kloner RA. Cardiovascular effects of the 3phosphodiesterase-5 inhibitors approved for the treatment of erectile dysfunction. *Circulation* 2004, 110:3149-3155.

[15] Reffelman T, Kloner RA. Effects of sildenafil on myocardial infarct size, microvascular function and acute ischemic left ventricular dilation. *Cardiovasc Res* 2003,59:441-449.

[16] Mittleman MA, Glasser DB, Orazem J Clinical trials of sildenafil citrate (Viagra) demonstrate no increase in risk of myocardial infarction and cardiovascular death compared with placebo. *Int J Clin Pract.* 2003 Sep;57 (7):597-600.

[17] Ockaili R, Salloum F, Hawkins J and Kukreja RC. Sildenafil(viagra) induces powerful cardioprotective effect via opening of mitochondrial K ATP channels in rabbits. *Am J Physiol* 2002, 283:H1263-H1269.

[18] Das A, Ockaili R, Salloum and Kukreja, R.C. Protein kinase C plays an essential role in sildenafil-induced cardioprotection in rabbits. *Am J Physiol* 2003, 286:H1455-H1460.

[19] Salloum F, Yin C, Xi L and Kukreja RC. Sildenafil induces delayed preconditioning through inducible nitric oxide synthase dependent pathway in mouse heart. *Circ Res* 2003,92:595-597.

[20] Nagi O, Hajnal A, Parratt JR and Vegh A. Sildenafil(viagra)reduces arrhythmias severity during ischemia 24h after oral administration. *Brit J Pharmacol* 2004,141:549-551.

[21] Swissa M, Ohara T, Lee MH, Kaul S, Shah PK, Hayashi H, Chen PS, Karagueuzian HS. Sildenafil-nitric oxide donor combination promotes ventricular tachyarrhythmias in the swine right ventricle. *Am J Physiol* 2001, 282:H1787-H1792.

In: World Heart Research Yearbook. Volume 1
Editors: Franz Halberg and R. B. Singh
ISBN: 978-1-60741-881-8

ASPIRIN RESISTANCE: NEED FOR A SPECIFIC, RAPID, POINT-OF-CARE ASSAY

*Gundu H. R. Rao**
Laboratory Medicine and Pathology; Lillehei Heart Institute, US

ABSTRACT

Background: Aspirin as a therapeutic drug has been in use for over hundred years. Its use as an anti-platelet drug was recognized in the early 70s. For secondary prophylaxis of vascular disease, it is the most useful and cost-effective drug. Large numbers of clinical trials using aspirin have concluded that at any given vascular risk, a low to medium dose of aspirin (80-160mg), is as effective as any other drug of choice. However, in recent years, there are several studies, in which aspirin resistance in patients with various vascular diseases have been demonstrated. Furthermore, some studies have suggested worst outcome in aspirin non-responders.

Methods: A variety of methods have been used in these studies, to determine "non-responders" to the action of aspirin .The definition of "aspirin resistant" individuals is those whose platelet cyclooxygenase are not inhibitable by aspirin. Methods used for monitoring aspirin resistance in these studies are non-specific platelet function tests.

Results: Differences in the definition of aspirin resistance, variations in the methods used to detect "non-responders", inter-individual variations in the response of platelets to the action of different agonists, and lack of data from large clinical trials have hampered the advancement of knowledge in this area.

Conclusion: Therefore, there is a great need to develop specific and rapid Point-of-Care assays that could detect the prevalence of aspirin resistance in patient populations, so that those found to be non-responders to the action of aspirin might be provided alternate treatment regimen.

Keywords: Aspirin resistance, non-responders, thrombosis, stroke

INTRODUCTION

Role of platelets in the pathogenesis of atherosclerosis, thrombosis and stroke is well documented [1]. Therefore, there is a great need for developing specific and effective drugs for modulating platelet function. A thorough understanding of the signaling mechanisms

* MMC 609, University of Minnesota, Minneapolis, MN 55455; E mail: raoxx001@umn.edu, Phone: 612 626 2717.

involved in the regulation of platelet function will facilitate the development of better anti-platelet drugs. Agonists interact with the platelet at specific receptor sites on the plasma membrane and initiate a series of signaling events capable of modulating shape change, adhesion, aggregation, secretion of granule contents and expression of activation markers on the membrane [2-10]. Platelet aggregates are formed when the GP11b/111a receptors get activated and bind fibrinogen and recruit other platelets to form clumps. This phenomenon plays a significant role in the formation of effective haemostatic plug as well as growth of thrombus. Weak agonists such as epinephrine, ADP require the production of pro-aggregatory prostaglandin endoperoxides and thromboxane to cause platelet aggregation and secretion. Aspirin is a specific inhibitor of cyclooxygenase and prevents the formation of pro-aggregatory PG endoperoxides.

Data from a large number of clinical studies have demonstrated that at any given risk, irrespective of the disease state, aspirin at low to medium concentration is as effective as any other drug [2-5]. Although the ability of a plant bark (bark of willow, *Salix alba*) product to reduce fever was discovered two hundred years ago, the mechanism of action of aspirin remained elusive till late 1900 [6]. Nobel laureate Sir John R. Vane and his associates at the Royal College of Surgeons, in London, in 1971 proposed the first satisfactory mechanism as to how aspirin works [7, 8]. Within a short period of time extensive work was done by various groups to elucidate the mechanism of action of aspirin like compounds [8-20]. During the same period, another Nobel Laureate Dr. Bengt Samuelsson of the Karolinska Institute, Stockholm, Sweden, discovered that the prostaglandin synthase produces transient bioactive prostanoids like PGG_2 /PGH_2 and thromboxane A_2 from the substrate arachidonic acid [10]. These findings revolutionized the research in platelet physiology and pharmacology [2-21].

PLATELET PHYSIOLOGY

Blood platelets interact with a variety of soluble agonists such as epinephrine (EPI), adenosine diphosphate (ADP), thrombin and thromboxane (TXA_2); many cell matrix components, including collagen, laminin, fibronectin, and vonWillebrand factor and biomaterials are used for construction of invasive medical devices [21-29]. These interactions stimulate specific receptors and glycoprotein-rich domains (integrin and non-integrin receptors) on the plasma membrane and lead to the activation of intracellular effector enzymes. Agonist–mediated activation of platelets stimulates phospholipase C (PLC) and it then triggers the hydrolysis of Phosphatidyl inositol 4, 5-bisphosphate, the formation of second messengers such as 1, 2-diacyl glycerol and inositol 1, 4, 5 trisphosphate. Diacylglycerol activates protein kinase and inositol trisphosphate facilitates the mobilization of free calcium from the storage sites. The majority of regulatory events appear to require free calcium. Ionized calcium is the primary bioregulator, and a variety of biochemical mechanisms modulate the availability of free calcium [27]. Elevation of cytosolic calcium stimulates phospholipase A_2 and liberates arachidonic acid (AA). Free AA is transformed to a novel metabolite thromboxane, a potent platelet agonist. This is the major metabolite of AA metabolism and plays an important role in platelet recruitment, granule mobilization, secretion of granule contents, and expression of activated GP11b/111a ($\acute{\alpha}_{11b}\,\beta_3$) receptors [22-

30]. Up regulation of activation signaling pathways, will increase the risk for clinical complications associated with thromboembolic episodes.

Arachidonic Acid Metabolism

Arachidonic acid is a 20 carbon polyunsaturated fatty acid (20:4w6) found in membrane phospholipids. Cell activation stimulates Phospholipase A_2, which facilitates the release of this fatty acid from phospholipids. AA is converted to prostaglandin (PG) endoperoxides (PGG_2/PGH_2) by cyclooxygenase (Prostaglandin G/H synthase; COX1)). These transient metabolites are converted by thromboxane synthetase to thromboxane A_2, which is the major metabolite of this pathway in platelets [10]. Whereas, in vascular tissues, the endoperoxides generated by COX1 are transformed by prostacyclin synthetase to prostacyclin (PGI_2). Thromboxane is a potent platelet agonist and a vasoconstrictor. Prostacyclin is an antiplatelet compound and exerts vasodilatory effects on vascular tissues. Thus from a single substrate (AA), two pharmacologically opposing vasoactive prostanoids are generated by platelets and vascular tissues [3]. Aspirin selectively acetylates the hydroxyl groups of a single serine residue (position 529) in the prostaglandin G/H synthase and causes irreversible inhibition of the activity of this enzyme [12, 13]. Inhibition of PG synthase results in the decreased conversion of AA to PG endoperoxides, PGG_2/PGH_2. Molecular mechanisms involved in aspirin-mediated inhibition of prostaglandin G/H synthase are well documented [4-16].

However, little is known about how other non-steroidal anti-inflammatory drugs inhibit this enzyme [14]. To elucidate the mechanism by which this enzyme oxidizes AA, we developed a cell free assay system. This system used ferrous iron induced oxidation of AA. Oxidation of the fatty acids by iron was followed by nitrobluetetrazolium [31]. Several drugs known to be inhibitors of this enzyme were used in this system to evaluate the affinity of these compounds to ferrous iron. Results demonstrated these compounds could form a complex with ferrous iron and inhibit AA metabolism [32, 33]. Using a ferrous iron chelator, bypirydil, we demonstrated the ability of this compound to inhibit platelet prostaglandin synthesis and function [34]. In a separate study, we showed ibuprofen, a short acting drug, interacted with the active site of PG synthase and blocked the ability of aspirin to acetylate COX1 enzyme [35]. Based on these results and other studies, we concluded aspirin like compounds devoid of acetyl group interact with the heme part of the PG synthase and block AA oxidation [31-33]. In platelets AA is converted by lipoxygenase to 12-hydroxyeicosatetraenoic acid. This pathway is not inhibited by aspirin.

Studies on the Use of Aspirin as an Inhibitor of Cox-1 Enzymes

Single oral doses of 10-100 mgs of aspirin can significantly inhibit the platelet PG synthase activity [36]. The inhibitory effect of aspirin on circulating platelets in the blood is fast and probably occurs in the portal circulation. The half-life of aspirin is very short (15-20 minutes) but sufficient to inhibit PG synthase of circulating platelets. Since these cells lack DNA and the ability to resynthesize the enzyme, the dysfunction caused by aspirin cannot be overcome. Therefore, platelets exposed to aspirin lose the ability to make the prostanoids completely. However, one should keep in mind that once the aspirin is hydrolyzed to salicylic acid, ability to inhibit prostaglandin synthase is lost. Hence the platelets produced from the marrow after the aspirin is hydrolyzed, will have active prostaglandin synthase. Approximately 10% of fresh platelets are added on to the circulating blood every day. Although aspirin treated blood platelets do not make prostaglandins, they respond with aggregation to the stimulation by prostaglandin endoperoxides and thromboxane. Fresh platelets formed after the hydrolysis of aspirin, can synthesize prostanoids and these newly formed metabolites of AA can cause aggregation of aspirin exposed platelets. In view of the fact that aspirin irreversibly inhibits prostaglandin synthase, it is possible to take advantage of repeated low-dose aspirin to achieve a cumulative effect [42-55]. Even doses as low as 30-50 mg aspirin taken daily will suppress platelet thromboxane synthesis significantly in 5 to 10 days.

Vascular tissues on the other hand have the ability to resynthesize prostaglandin G/H synthase [36]. Therefore, these cells can recover the enzyme activity following aspirin exposure. It is therefore, possible to develop a strategy to promote the biochemical selectivity of aspirin in terms of inhibition of platelet prostaglandin synthase. This is done by modification of the drug delivery, so the amount of drug delivered is just enough to inhibit platelet enzymes in the peripheral circulation and spare the systemic effect on vascular endothelium [37, 38]. Several studies have demonstrated the feasibility of this approach and various control release or timed release formulations have been developed for this novel therapy [37-39].

As mentioned earlier, aspirin is metabolized rapidly and the major metabolite, salicylic acid is a poor inhibitor of platelet prostaglandin synthase. Therefore, it is essential to develop appropriate strategies to maximize the beneficial effect of this novel drug. As low dose as 20 mg taken daily, reduces the platelet thromboxane formation by more than 90 percent. However, it is generally believed that higher doses are essential for preventing thromboxane dependent platelet activation. Studies by Wilson et al demonstrated that maximal plasma concentration of 12umol/L could be achieved by a single oral 50 mg dose of enteric-coated aspirin [17]. This dose was found sufficient to cause significant inhibition of platelet function and daily ingestion of low-dose aspirin demonstrated a cumulative effect. In a separate study, McLeod et al used doses ranging from 50-3900 mg of aspirin and monitored platelet function, bleeding time, and concluded that maximum dysfunction was obtained with daily doses of about 100 mg and no further changes were observed in these studies with higher doses [18]. Several workers have demonstrated the efficacy of low-dose oral aspirin in preventing platelet thromboxane production [2-4, 18, 44]. Indeed one of these studies has demonstrated beneficial effect of a dermal aspirin preparation on selective inhibition of platelet prostaglandin synthase, sparing the prostacyclin biosynthesis (38). It is very well established that 100 mg of aspirin per day is sufficient to significantly reduce the platelet thromboxane production [2-4, 20, 21, 40-42]. Furthermore, studies by McLeod et al have shown that dosages higher than 100 mg per day do not produce any greater inhibition of platelet function or enhance bleeding times [18]. Therefore, it is reasonable to conclude that 80-160 mgs aspirin per day should be the choice for an ideal preventive protocol [41]. However, there is considerable room for improvement to maximize the benefits by better understanding the pharmacology of aspirin and platelet physiology [2-4]. It is possible to customize the aspirin treatment based on the individual patient needs. One can monitor the platelet prostaglandin synthase activity following aspirin ingestion and recommend a dose that is appropriate [34, 41]. It is possible to monitor the platelet response to agonists such as ADP or arachidonate and determine the degree of inhibition by aspirin like compounds [18]. In order to get maximum inhibition of platelet COX1 enzymes, continuous release aspirin formulations can be developed and tested against currently available aspirin formulations. Platelets are produced and released constantly to the circulation. Therefore, a time release aspirin which would make available small amounts of aspirin into the circulation may be effective. For instance, a 100 mg formulation capable of releasing 10 mg acetyl salicylic acid per hour may be better than a preparation which releases all of its active principle in a short span of time. Using the strategy of slowing down the release of active principle, newer formulations could be used effectively, to provide needed amounts of the drug into circulating blood at regular intervals. These novel formulations may also provide selectivity of aspirin action by preventing platelet thromboxane production and sparing the endothelial prostacylcin synthesis. McLeod et al studied the effect of various doses of aspirin (50, 100, 325, 1000 mg) on platelet and vascular tissues [43]. They did not observe inhibition of urinary 6-keto-PGF1 alpha production at low doses of 50 and 100 mg. They attributed these findings to the differential and selective inhibition of platelet function and the sparring effect of vascular COX1 enzymes. Sullivan and associates studied the effect of two different doses of aspirin on platelet function and TXA_2 production [45]. Platelet function in healthy volunteers was inhibited by both the doses (75 and 300 mg). Low dose failed to inhibit completely TXB_2 production 24 hours later, whereas 300 mg aspirin did. Even alternate day regimen of these doses prevented platelet function and significantly inhibited the urinary levels of the 11-keto-TXB_2. In a separate study, in healthy volunteers, formation of thrombin (Fibrinopeptide A; FPA), alpha granule release (beta-thromboglobulin; beta TG), and thromboxane (TXB_2) were monitored in vivo, in blood emerging from a template bleeding incision [46]. At the site of plug formation significant platelet activation and thrombin generation was observed as indicated by 110 fold, 50 fold, and 30 fold increase in FPA, beta TG, and TXB_2, within the first minute. A low dose regimen (0.42m/kg/day for 7 days) caused greater than 90% inhibition of TXB_2 formation in both bleeding time and clotted blood in these studies, suggesting critical role of platelet activation at the site of haemostatic plug formation. In a study to evaluate the effect of low dose aspirin (0.5and 15 mg/kg/day) on platelet and renal prostanoids, Wilson et al monitored serum TXB_2 and urinary 6-keto PGF1 alpha [47]. Serum TXB_2 level was reduced to 3% of control by low dose and to 0.1% by the higher dose. Urinary TXB_2 was reduced only to 68% by low dose aspirin and to 51% by high dose. Urinary 6-keto-PGF1 alpha was not reduced by either dose. Based on their observation, they concluded low dose aspirin could significantly affect platelet PG production without affecting stimulated release of PGI_2 production.

Clinical Studies on the Use of Aspirin

The two major clinical trials on aspirin concluded that ingestion of 160 mg per day or 325 mg alternative day provided significant benefit in preventing fatal events associated with CAD [20, 21]. Whereas, a 10 year trial involving nearly 40,000 women aged 45 and older with no evidence of cardiovascular disease found that a regular alternate day low-dose

(100mg) aspirin was effective in reducing the incidence of stroke, but it did not have any effect on the incidence of heart attacks [48]. They concluded that the reasons for any sex-based differences in the efficacy of aspirin for primary prevention are unclear. According to Minnesota Heart Survey, about 6% of healthy women under age 65 and 30% of those over 65 take low-dose aspirin to prevent acute vascular events. Data from this primary prevention study dose not apply to women who already have had a heart attack or heart surgery or diagnosed with coronary artery disease. For such women, as found in men, regular daily low dose (80-160mg) of aspirin clearly reduces the risk of developing acute coronary events.

Several earlier studies evaluated the effect of low dose aspirin on normal healthy volunteers as well as patients with various vascular diseases [45-58]. However, earlier studies did not report prevalence of any aspirin resistance. Zucker et al evaluated the effect of low dose aspirin (0.45mg/kg/day) and a high dose (900mg/day) in type 11 hyper-lipoproteinemic subjects [49]. They found that low dose aspirin effectively inhibited platelet function in these patients. Increased platelet thromboxane production has been described in several disorders including type-2 diabetes and type 11a hypercholesterolemia. This increased production of TXB_2 in hyper-cholesterolemic patients is attributed to abnormal cholesterol levels in these patients. It has been shown that even a low dose of aspirin (50 mg/7 days) significantly reduces 11-dehydro-TXB_2, in these patients [50]. The effect of low dose aspirin has been evaluated in patients with diabetes, coronary heart disease, myocardial infarction (MI), cerebrovascular disease, peripheral artery disease and a variety of surgical procedures [45-58]. Diminno et al studied the effect of single doses of 100 and 1000 mg aspirin for 1 month in normal volunteers and patients with diabetic angiopathy [51]. They found a dose schedule of aspirin, which may suffice in normal volunteers, was not effective in patients with diabetic angiopathy. Contrary to this observation, Terres et al found a low dose of aspirin (100mg) caused significant inhibition of platelet function in both healthy subjects and patients with coronary heart disease [52]. Similarly, a low dose (0.45mg/kg/day) was found adequate for selective inhibition of TXA_2-related platelet function, in patients recovering from MI [53]. Looks like the results on the effect of low-dose aspirin vary considerably, depending upon the type and stage of disease, dose of aspirin, and severity of procedure. In a study evaluating the effect of low dose aspirin (100mg) on hematological activity of left ventricular (LV) thrombus in anterior wall acute MI (AMI), Kupper et al found that low-dose had no effect on the incidence of hematologic activity and embolic potential of LV thrombosis in anterior wall AMI [54]. On the other hand, a low dose aspirin (40mg/day) taken daily was found to be as effective as higher doses in preventing platelet functional responses in patients who had recent cerebral ischemia [55]. Uchiyama et al evaluated the effect of low dose aspirin, ticlopidine, and a combination of both these drugs in patients with cerebral ischemia [56]. Aspirin alone markedly inhibited platelet aggregation induced by AA, partially inhibited aggregation induced by ADP and did not inhibit aggregation by platelet activating factor. Combination of these drugs inhibited aggregation by all agonists. Rao et al demonstrated, in healthy volunteers, low doses of aspirin (40-80mg) had no inhibitory effect on the response of platelets to ADP, epinephrine and thrombin, but effectively inhibited the platelet response to threshold concentrations of AA [3, 4]. Epinephrine at concentrations too low to cause aggregation restored the sensitivity of aspirin-treated platelets to AA [59-61]. This phenomenon, in which weak agonists restore the sensitivity of drug-induced refractory platelets to the action of other agonists, was described from our laboratory as "mechanism of membrane modulation" [58-65].

ASPIRIN RESISTANCE

Studies from our laboratory for the first time demonstrated that one could induce drug-mediated resistance in platelets to the action of aspirin [66]. In this study, the subjects were given a short acting inhibitor of COX1, Ibuprofen. This was followed by administration of a full strength (325mg) aspirin. Ibuprofen-mediated inhibition of COX1 enzyme lasts for a short time, whereas, aspirin induced inhibition is irreversible. Ibuprofen treated platelets recovered their sensitivity to the action of AA by 24 hrs. Whereas, aspirin treated platelets failed to respond to the action of AA even after 24 hrs. In those subjects who had ingested aspirin after taking Ibuprofen first, aspirin failed to inhibit irreversibly the COX1; suggesting Ibuprofen molecules effectively prevented the acetylation of COX1enzyme by aspirin. One of the earliest work describing "non-responders" and "responders" evaluated the effect of low dose aspirin and a thromboxane synthetase inhibitor dazoxiben (UK3724B) in healthy subjects [57]. These studies demonstrated that low dose aspirin and ingestion of two dazoxiben tablets prevented the release of granules from platelets in response to AA in some individuals (responders) and not in others (non-responders). These subtle differences in response of platelets to various drugs as well as differences in response to various agonists may be critical when considering the outcome of acute vascular events. For instance, collagen seems to exert its effect by multiple mechanisms. In a study, using aspirin, monoclonal antibodies to 11b-111a receptor and fibrinogen, it was demonstrated that there exists at least three mechanisms by which collagen activates platelets; 1) GP11b-111a associated activation, 2) prostaglandin dependent pathway, 3) alternate pathway responsible for 20-30% platelet aggregation [67].

Although it is well known that there are individual differences in response to drugs as well as agonists, this subject has not been studied thoroughly. Studies from Harvard researchers have demonstrated that the onset of myocardial infarction and sudden death is frequently triggered in early hours of the day. Aspirin and beta adrenergic blocking agents have been shown to prevent morning onset of acute vascular events [68]. In a limited chronobiologic study (n=7) on the efficacy of low-dose aspirin, international womb-to-tomb chronome initiative group demonstrated, that aspirin was more effective in the early hours of the day than late in the afternoon or evening [69, 70] Influence of dietary components and supplements on the efficacy of anti-platelet drugs also is poorly understood. Vitamin E and its quinone are potent inhibitors of platelet function and interfere with the release of arachidonic acid by cell membranes [71, 72]. Studies from our laboratory have demonstrated that heme chelators, non-steroid anti-inflammatory drugs, antioxidants such as butylated hydorxytoulene, butyalted hydroxyanisole and fish lipids compete with arachidonic acid metabolism and prevent the formation of pro-aggregatory PG metabolites [71-74]. Docosahexaenoic acid (DHA) is poorly metabolized by Cox-1 enzymes. However, *in vitro* studies have demonstrated that DHA is a potent inhibitor of AA metabolism and platelet function [74]. Eicosapenaenoic acid, oleic acid, linoleic acid, linolenic acid competitively inhibit COX1 enzymes in in *vitro* studies. We do not know very much about the influence of dietary lipids on AA metabolism by platelets.

Several recent studies have demonstrated drug resistance in patients with a variety of vascular diseases [75-118]. This subject currently is a very hot topic and has made national headlines. Andrew Pollack published an article in July of 2004 in New York Times, on this subject titled, “For Some, Aspirin May Not Help Hearts” [75]. According to this article, 5-40% of aspirin users are “non-responders” or “resistant” to the drug. In the same article, he cites the opinion of Dr. Daniel I. Simon, the associate director of interventional cardiology at Brigham and Women’s Hospital, Boston, which reads as follows: “They are taking it for stroke and heart attack prevention and it’s not going to work”. He also reports the opinion of Dr. Michael J. Domanski; head of clinical trials unit at the NIH, in his opinion, the non-responders may represent a huge number of patients. According to Dr. Deepak L. Bhatt, director of interventional cardiology Cleveland Clinic, aspirin resistance is associated with worst outcome. Professor Eric Topol, Chairman, Cardiovascular Medicine Cleveland Clinic, USA states, “Aspirin resistance carries high risk, with over 20 million Americans taking aspirin to prevent heart attacks or strokes, it is important that further work to be done to confirm our findings and develop a rapid detection method. He also assures that for individuals with aspirin resistance, there are excellent alternatives”. These observances from health care providers and researchers raise a number of issues. Do we know enough about aspirin resistance? What is the prevalence of aspirin resistance in the healthy population? What causes this resistance to develop in patient populations? Are there specific, rapid, cost-effective tests available? What alternative long-term treatments are available, if patients are resistant to common anti-platelet drugs such as aspirin and Clopidogrel? Should the doses of these drugs used for therapy be increased? Should we drop the use of these drugs in non-responders? We need to find answers to these and other emerging questions soon. In the next few paragraphs a brief overview of what is known about the prevalence of aspirin resistance, clinical findings, and methodologies available, will be provided. The first and foremost need at this time is to standardize a definition of aspirin resistance. The mechanism of action of aspirin is very well documented [7-13]. The drug acetylates the platelet COX1 enzyme and irreversibly inhibits its ability to convert AA to PG endoperoxides [12, 13]. In the absence of COX1 enzyme activity, platelets do not respond to AA stimulation with aggregation. Weak agonists such as ADP, Epinephrine depend on the formation of PG endoperoxides to initiate a secondary wave of aggregation and promote release of platelet granule contents [3]. Therefore, weak agonists fail to induce platelet aggregation and release granules from aspirin-treated platelets. Failure of AA, ADP and Epinephrine to cause aggregation of platelets more or less establishes drug-induced platelet dysfunction. If platelets obtained from individuals who have ingested a full strength aspirin, respond with aggregation to the action AA, ADP and EPI, and release their granule contents, then one can safely conclude that these platelets are resistant to aspirin action. Further proof for aspirin resistance of platelets can be provided by studying AA metabolism by such platelets, monitoring serum TXB_2 levels, or urinary levels of TXB_2 or its metabolite, 11-dehydro-TXB_2. Methods are available to monitor all these parameters. According to Cattaneo, “aspirin resistant” should be considered as a description for those individuals whom aspirin fails to inhibit thromboxane A2 production, irrespective of the results of unspecific tests of platelet function [110].

Prevalence of Aspirin Resistance

Aspirin resistance has been poorly defined, variety of non-specific methods have been employed to monitor the “aspirin resistance” and conflicting reports have been published on the rates of prevalence and outcome of continuing this therapeutic modality [75-93]. Aspirin resistance has been reported in patients with cardiovascular, cerebrovascular, and peripheral vascular disease [75-93]. Because of the differences in methodologies used to monitor this phenomenon and lack of a specific assay to determine the true aspirin resistance, there is considerable confusion and the true significance of this observation remains obscure [76- 78]. It also raises the question, as to how we missed this phenomenon of drug resistance all these years? Large numbers of clinical trials have demonstrated the beneficial effects of aspirin therapy irrespective of the disease state [40]. Is it possible that these earlier trials missed aspirin non-responders? On the other hand, it is quite possible that only responders to the action of aspirin received the benefit of this therapy.

Studies in our laboratory over three decades, have failed to show any aspirin resistance in normal healthy subjects. The only subject whose platelets failed to aggregate in response to AA stimulation was found to be deficient in platelet COX1enzyme activity [60]. Platelets obtained from this subject responded with aggregation when stirred with epinephrine and arachidonate, suggesting PG endoperoxides and TAX_2 are not essential to cause irreversible aggregation of platelets. There is not much data on the prevalence of aspirin resistance in general healthy subjects. In patients with various vascular diseases, the rate of non-responders reported varies between less than 2% to over 60%. Since the methods used to monitor aspirin resistance in these reports are not specific, the prevalence rate published is debatable [75-93].

Hurlen et al used the method of Wu and Hoak to determine the platelet aggregation ratio as a marker for assessing platelet function and evaluated the effect of aspirin (160mg/day) in 143 patients who had survived myocardial infarction [80, 81]. Based on their definition of non-responders to the action of aspirin, they could only identify two subjects as primary non-responders. Gum et al from Cleveland Clinic studied 326 stable cardiovascular subjects on aspirin (325mg/day) and tested aspirin sensitivity by platelet response to aggregating agents such as ADP and AA. They found 5.5% as non-responders to aspirin and 24% as semi-responders [82]. Gum and associates used the PFA-100, a method that measures platelet function, to determine aspirin resistance in their patient population [83]. Based on the results of their studies with this methodology, they found 9.5% to be non-responders to aspirin action.

Some studies have reported as high as 30-40% non-responders of stroke or vascular disease patients and predicted >80% increase risk for a repeat event during a 2-year follow up period [84-88]. Eikelboom et al analyzed base line urinary levels of TXB2 metabolites 11-dehydro thromboxane B2 in 5529 patients enrolled in the Heart Outcomes Prevention Evaluation (HOPE) study [88]. Of these subjects 488 were on aspirin regimen. On the basis of their findings they concluded that in aspirin-treated patients, increased levels of urinary metabolite of TXB_2 predict future risk of myocardial infarction or cardiovascular death. The patients with the highest levels of urinary TXB_2 metabolite had 3-5 fold higher risk of cardiovascular death compared to those in the lowest quartile. Another study reporting clinical outcomes of aspirin resistance is from Austria [85, 87, 90]. In this study patients undergoing arterial angioplasty were on 100 mg aspirin per day. Platelet function was assessed by whole blood aggregometry. This study demonstrated that reocculsion at the sites of angioplasty occurred only in men for whom platelet dysfunction was evident by aggregometry [87]. Zimmerman et al identified aspirin non-responders as those who had >90% inhibition of TXB_2 formation in presence of 100umol/L aspirin and 1mmol/L arachidonate [91]. In patients who had undergone coronary bypass surgery (CABG), AA and

Collagen stimulated formation of TXB_2 was the same before and after CABG, indicating oral aspirin did not significantly inhibit platelet COX1. However, the *in vitro* studies with 100umol/L aspirin on blood obtained from these subjects showed decreased TXB_2 (>10%) in most samples studied. They concluded that platelet COX1 inhibition by aspirin is compromised for several days after CABG, probably due to an impaired interaction between aspirin and platelet COX1. This observation indicates how complex the issues are when evaluating the effect of anti-platelet drugs during and after interventional procedures. Sane et al evaluated the effect of aspirin (325 mg/day/month) in patients suffering from congestive heart failure [92]. These researchers used whole blood aggregometry (Chronolog Corp, PA., USA), Platelet receptor expression by flow cytometry and PFA-100. Patients were considered non-responders when 4 of the 5 parameters assayed were observed. Using this complex rating, persistent platelet activation was observed in 50 of the 88 patients (56.8%). These observations remind us of the inadequacy of the existing methods to detect what truly represents "aspirin resistance".

Clopidogrel Resistance

Muller et al have reported the prevalence of Clopidogrel "non-responders" among patients with stable angina scheduled for coronary stent replacement [93]. They evaluated the effect of 100mg/day aspirin with a loading dose of 600mg of Clopidogrel. They defined Clopidogrel non-responders by an inhibition of ADP (5and 30umol/L) induced platelet aggregation to less than 10% of base line values after the ingestion of the drug. They found 5-11% of the patients as non-responders and 9-26% semi-responders. Lau et al studied both normal subjects and patients undergoing stent replacement to determine the prevalence of drug resistance [94]. Since Clopidogrel is activated by hepatic cytochrome P450 (CYP) 3A4, they monitored the activity of this enzyme in both test subjects. They concluded that some patients are resistant to these drugs because of biological variability and drug-drug interactions. They also attributed the difference due to variations in (CYP) 3A4 activity. Angiolillo et al compared the effect of standard dose of 300mg with a high dose of 600mg Clopidogrel after coronary stenting [95]. They concluded that use of higher dose optimizes platelet inhibitory effects. Serebruany et al evaluated the effect of Clopidogrel in a large heterogenous population using ex vivo measurements of platelet aggregation [96], Prevalence of hypo-responsiveness and hyper-responsiveness to Clopidogrel in these patient population was 4.2% and 4.8% respectively. A Polish study with a small sample size (n=31) studied the effect of Clopidogrel (300) in patients with stable angina using a rapid whole blood platelet function assessment [97]. They conclude that the clinical importance of Clopidogrel resistance is still debatable. In view of the fact that data are not available on large number of clinical trials, their conclusion is reasonable.

Methodologies

Researchers have used a variety of methods to assess the aspirin and Clopidogrel resistance [81-98]. In spite of the inherent problems associated with platelet aggregometry, it still is the gold standard to detect aspirin sensitivity of platelets. Studies from our laboratory and that of others have shown even low doses (40-80 mg) of aspirin effectively inhibit arachidonate-mediated platelet aggregation. In the absence of any other specific rapid Point-of-Care assay system for detecting the sensitivity of platelets to aspirin or lack of aspirin sensitivity, it is preferable to use optical whole blood aggregometry to validate the results obtained by other methods. Hurlen et al used platelet aggregate ratio (PAR) to evaluate the effect of aspirin in post-MI patients [80]. Basically the method developed by Wu and Hoak uses a ratio of platelets obtained with EDTA/formalin as anti-coagulants and comparing the counts of platelets obtained with EDTA [80, 81]. In the presence of platelet aggregates the ratio is <1.0. Using this method they found two individuals as primary non-responders and 14 patients as secondary non-responders.

Several researchers have used Platelet Function Analyzer PFA-100 (Dade International Inc, Miami USA), to evaluate aspirin resistance in patients with various vascular diseases [83, 92, 101, 103, 104, 113, 119]. This analyzer measures platelet function as their ability to occlude a membrane coated with collagen and epinephrine (EPI) or collagen and ADP under high sheer stress. Sambola et al evaluated the effect of low dose aspirin (100mg/day/1month, 6month) in 100 patients with acute coronary syndrome [101]. At one-month post-aspirin therapy, they found 49 patients to have sub-optimal response to aspirin (SASAR), whereas only 25 of them showed SASAR by conventional aggregometry. Anderson et al evaluated the effect of 75 mg aspirin in patients (n=202) with MI. In patients on aspirin alone they found 25/71 as non-responders with the epinephrine cartridge. They did not find a significant difference between EPI cartridge and ADP cartridge. Gum et al. evaluated the phenomenon of aspirin resistance in 325 stable cardiac patients [83]. They found 5 per cent were non-responders and 23 per cent semi-responders by optical aggregometry. Whereas, using PFA-100 they found 9.5% as aspirin resistant. This detection system does not seem to detect difference between the effects of low and high-dose aspirin on platelet function. Since it evaluates the synergistic effect of a combination of two agonists on platelet function, the results obtained or similar to that obtained in our aggregation studies [58-66]. In a series of studies we have demonstrated a combination of two agonists overcomes the inhibition by aspirin and other drugs [58-66].

Malinin et al used THE Ultegra RPFA-ASA (VerifyNow; Accumetrics, Inc., San Diego, California, USA) to monitor the effect of a single dose of aspirin (325 mg) in subjects with multiple risk factors [100]. This system uses turbidometric optical detection system. It uses a test cartridge that contains lyophilized preparation of human fibrinogen-coated beads, platelet agonist, and buffer. Fibrinogen-coated beads bind available receptor on platelet membrane. A cationic agonist, propyl gallate, is used to obtain complete activation of platelets. It uses citrated whole blood for assays. The results are expressed in aspirin response units (ARU). Of the 14 subjects studied, only one was found to be non-responsive by aggregometry, whereas they found 10 subjects as non-responders by RPFA-ASA. They concluded this system was a sensitive device for measuring anti-platelet responsiveness. The newly introduced "VerifyNow" kit includes arachidonic acid as an agonist for activating platelets. Inclusion of this agonist instead of propyl gallate has considerably improved the performance of this system. In our hands, this system is as good as whole blood aggregometry (Chronolog Corporation) in identifying aspirin non-responders.

Aspirin resistance could be monitored by a variety of assays, including platelet aggregometry, PAR, PFA100, RPFA-ASA; plasma, serum, urinary TXB_2 and urinary 11-

dehryothromboxane-2 [46, 47, 80-84, 87, 88, 92, 95, 98, 100]. We use majority of these methods to validate data in our efforts to develop a rapid, specific Point-of-Care assay system, for monitoring platelet function. The majority of these methods are labor intensive, time consuming and expensive. Technologies are available to develop a rapid and specific assay system, which can monitor platelet function. Specific fluorescent antibodies can be used to detect platelet bound fibrinogen, P-selectin or released granule products such as beta-thromboglobulin, platelet factor 4 and soluble P-selectin. Furthermore, ATP release or thromboxane generated also could be easily monitored. All the available methods use large quantities of blood and take a considerable amount of time. It is possible to devise methods that use only small quantities of blood obtained from a finger stick. By using state-of-the-art detectors one could detect the luminescence (ATP) or fluorescence (specific antibodies) in minutes and develop needed software to standardize the results. If the assay uses AA as a standard platelet agonist then specificity could be built into this system for monitoring aspirin sensitivity. Similarly by using ADP as an agonist one can build the needed specificity to monitor non-responders to Clopidogrel. The limiting factors for non-availability of such a Point-of-Care assay system are lack of funds and the assumption that currently available methods detect platelet sensitivity or otherwise to anti-platelet drugs effectively.

DISCUSSION

Aspirin is the most-effective, widely used, relatively inexpensive anti-platelet drug currently available. In the developing countries, aspirin is the most cost-effective drug for primary as well as secondary prophylaxis for platelet-mediated vascular complications [3-5]. The mechanism by which it inhibits platelet function is well documented [7-14]. Many large clinical trials have established beyond any doubt that aspirin therapy significantly reduces the incidence of acute events in a variety of vascular diseases [40]. Recent studies have provided evidence to suggest that some sub-populations of patients on aspirin therapy may have developed resistance to the action of aspirin [75-98]. These observations have raised an alarm to the public as to who is getting protection and who is not? Since there is no simple test that can be performed at the doctor's office to detect such a condition there is some panic in the patient population. Furthermore, there is still a lack of awareness of this problem in the medical community at the time of this writing. There are only two major studies, which have described adverse outcome in those patients who are defined as non-responders to the action of aspirin [83, 88].

Based on methods, which still are not very specific, researchers have identified a sub-population of patients who are considered non-responders and another group as semi-responders to the action of aspirin [82-98]. Although the majority of methods used for monitoring this phenomenon lack specificity, it is important to recognize that this problem exists. If these patients for whatever reason are not getting appropriate protection from drug therapy, there is an immediate need to identify them and change their therapeutic regimen. It is equally important to recognize that even those who are considered responders, may need additional protection to prevent adverse out comes, if they have hyper-responsive platelets or hyper-responsive coagulation pathways. Basically, we need to identify aspirin non-responders, individuals with hyperactive platelets/coagulation pathways.

The subject of aspirin resistance has received lot of attention in the press and scientific publications [75-98]. However, the practicing physicians and the pubic are not fully aware of the problem. Therefore, there is an immediate need for the development of awareness programs to educate the health care providers as well as the public who receive health care. Since there is considerable interest in this subject in the research community, a number of reviews have been published on this subject [75-98]. No attempt has been made in this article to extensively review this subject. Focus of this article has been to bring into discussion three specific areas of concern. First and foremost is the molecular mechanism involved in the initiation of thrombosis and stroke. Basically two major pathways (platelet activation dependent and coagulation cascade activation dependent) play a role in the pathophysiology of this process. Therefore, there is a need to identify the hyper-responsiveness of individuals to both these pathways and develop appropriate combination therapy. Secondly, the arachidonic acid pathway blocks only one of the many mechanisms modulating platelet activation. Therefore, there is an immediate need to develop appropriate drugs or drug combinations to prevent the common pathway of platelet activation. Since fibrinogen binding to activated GP 11b/111a receptor promotes thrombus formation and growth, drugs should be designed and developed to modulate these mechanisms. Third, there is a need for better Point-of-Care assays, which can profile the coagulation pathway as well as platelet activation mechanisms. Such an assay system could be effective in identifying non-responders to commonly used anti-platelet drugs, semi responders or hyper responsive individuals and those with hyper coagulable states. Since there is no such detection system a lot of individuals at risk are not getting appropriate treatment or prophylaxis against acute vascular events.

In the early 80s, based on our extensive studies, we concluded that aspirin and other anti-platelet drugs do not prevent platelet activation under a variety of experimental conditions [58-66]. Aspirin only inhibits one of the many platelet activation mechanisms. Furthermore, it does not prevent platelet interaction with vessel wall [63]. However, in a large number of clinical studies, aspirin has been shown to offer significant beneficial effects to patients with various vascular diseases [40]. Several recent studies have demonstrated that there exists some degree of non-responders to the action of aspirin [75-98]. Therefore, it is of great importance to thoroughly examine this issue of drug resistance and determine the prevalence of true "aspirin resistance" among the patients and provide them alternate therapies. Since our studies have clearly demonstrated epinephrine, nor-epinephrine, and ADP can potentiate the action of other agonists on platelets, we may as well screen those who are hyper responsive to various agonists, so that these individuals also could be provided appropriate therapeutic regimen. There are reports suggesting those who are non-responders to the action of aspirin may be more responsive to the action of agonists such as ADP or collagen. Studies should take into consideration that platelets can be stimulated by a variety of soluble agonists as well as cell matrix components and increased shear stress. In spite of the fact that several attempts have been made to explain the mechanisms involved in aspirin resistance, there exists no clear explanation. Studies should be initiated immediately to explore the mechanism by which an individual develops resistance to these drugs. Since platelets lack DNA, it is highly unlikely that these cells re-synthesize COX1 enzyme. Since many of these patients are on long-term aspirin therapy the effect of aspirin on megakaryocytes should be further explored. Platelets are formed from megakaryocytes and these cells do have DNA, hence studies are warranted to explore the effect of aspirin on bone marrow megakaryocytes. The majority of patients with vascular disease also will be taking many other drugs. As such, some amount of drug-drug interaction cannot be ruled out. Whatever may be the mechanism by which individuals with vascular disease develop resistance to aspirin, a better understanding of the molecular mechanisms involved will facilitate the development of the appropriate therapeutic regimen. Now that anti-platelet drug resistance has surfaced out and created concern in the clinical community, there will be renewed interest in the development for improving the available technologies for monitoring platelet and coagulation pathways [75-118] Chronolog corporation, one of the leaders in developing optical aggregometers, has already come up with a less expensive whole-blood aggregometer for monitoring aspirin resistance. The accumetric system has recently introduced arachidonic acid as a stimulant instead of propyl gallate, for monitoring aspirin resistance. Similarly, research and development work is going to improve the PAF-100 system as well, for monitoring aspirin resistance. Currently available data on the use of PFA-100 to monitor aspirin resistance is inconclusive. A large study using 1000 patients is in progress to evaluate the applicability of PFA-100 to monitor drug resistance [119]. Results from this study may shed some light on the useful ness of this detection system. All the currently available methodologies require relatively large quantities of fresh blood. Platelet function assays are labor intensive, non-specific and time consuming. Future direction of research will focus on the development of rapid, specific, Point-of-Care assays using minimal amounts of blood from a finger stick, for monitoring platelet function as well as coagulation profile.

Conclusion

Platelets play a very important role in the pathogenesis of atherosclerosis, thrombosis and stroke. Aspirin, even at a low to medium dose (80-160mg/day) has been shown to offer significant protection to individuals from developing acute vascular events. Aspirin is the most cost-effective drug available for the secondary prophylaxis of cardiovascular diseases. From the available evidence both experimental and clinical, it is reasonable to conclude, that a significant number of patients are not getting full protection from the use of aspirin. Even those who are considered responders to aspirin therapy may need additional protection, if their platelets are hypersensitive or have a hyper-responsive coagulation pathway. Since currently available methods to assess aspirin sensitivity are not specific, labor intensive and time consuming; efforts should be made to develop specific, rapid, detection methods. Serious attempts should be made to develop state-of-the-art Point-of-Care assay systems, which are capable of detecting not only individuals who develop resistance to currently available anti-platelet drugs but also those, who are hyper-responsive to both platelet and coagulation activation mechanisms.

References

[1] Sherry S, Scriabine *A. Platelets and Thrombosis*. University Press, USA 1999. P.309

[2] Suldow C, Baigent C. Randomized Trials of Antiplatelet Therapy. *Handbook of Platelet Physiology and Pharmacology*. Rao GHR, (ed) Kluwer Academic Publishers, USA1999, p526-549.

[3] Rao GHR, Rao AT. Pharmacology of Platelet Inhibitory Drugs. *Ind. J. Physiol.*19994, 38:69-84.

[4] Rao GHR, Rao ASC, White JG. Aspirin in Ischemic Heart Disease-an overview. *Ind. Heart J.*1993, 45: 73-79.

[5] Rao GHR. Aspirin and Coronary Artery Disease: Coronary Artery Disease in South Asians: Epidemiology, Risk Factors and Prevention. Rao GHR, Kakkar VV(eds), *Jaypee Medical Publishers*, India, 2001, p263-278.

[6] Weisman G. Aspirin. *Sci Am.*1991, 264: 84-91.

[7] Vane JR. Inhibition of prostaglandin synthesis as a mechanism of action of aspirin-like drugs. *Nature* 1971, 231: 232-235.

[8] Vane JR, Flower RJ, Botting RM. History of aspirin and its mechanism of action. *Stroke* 1990, 21: IV-12.

[9] Ferreira SH, Vane JR. Newer aspects of the mode of action of non-steroidal anti-inflammatory drugs. *Ann. Rev. Pharmacol.* 1974, 14: 57-73.

[10] Hamberg M, Svensson J Samuelsson B. Thromboxanes: A new group of biologically active compounds derived from prostaglandin endoperoxides. *Proc. Natl. Acad. Sci.* 1975, 72:2994-2998.

[11] Marcus AJ. Aspirin as an anti-thrombotic medication. *N. Engl. J. Med.* 1983, 309: 1515-1517.

[12] Roth JG, Caverley DC. Aspirin, Platelets and Thrombosis: Theory and Practice. *Blood* 1994, 83: 885-898.

[13] Roth JG: Stanford N, Majerus PW. Acetylation of prostaglandin synthetase by aspirin. *Proc. Natl. Acad. Sci.* 1975, 72: 3073-3076.

[14] Meade EA, Smith WL, Dewitt DL: Differential inhibition of prostaglandin endoperoxide syhthase (cyclooxygenase) isoenzymes by aspirin and other non-steroidal anti-inflammatory drugs. *J. Biol. Chem.* 1993, 268: 6610-6614.

[15] Burch JW, Stanford N, Majerus PW. Inhibition of platelets prostaglandin synthetase by oral aspirin. *J. Clin. Invest* 1978: 61: 314-319.

[16] Reilly IA, FitzGerald GA. Aspirin in Cardiovascular Disease. *Drugs* 1988, 35: 154-176.

[17] Wilson KM, Siebert DM, Duncan EM. et al. Effect of aspirin infusions on platelet function in humans. *Clin. Sci.* 1990, 79: 37-42.

[18] McLeod LJ, Roberts MS, Cossum PA. et al. The effects of different doses of some acetyl salicylic acid formulations on platelet function and bleeding times in healthy subjects. *J. Haematol.* 1986, 36: 379-384.

[19] Masptti G, Galanti G, Pogessi L. Differential inhibition of prostacyclin production and platelet aggregation by aspirin. *Lancet* 1972, 2:11213-1216.

[20] Steering Committee of the Physicians Health Study Research Group. Preliminary Report: Findings from the aspirin component of the ongoing physicians' health study. *N. Engl. J. Med.* 1988, 318: 262-264.

[21] Steering Committee of the Physicians Health Study Research Group. Final Report. *N. Engl. J. Med.* 1989, 321: 129-135.

[22] Hallam TJ, Sanchez A, Rink TJ. Stimulus response coupling in Platelets. *Biochem J.* 1984, 218:819-827.

[23] Zucker MB Nachmias VT. Platelet Activation. *Arteriosclerosis*. 1985, 5:2-18.

[24] Edridge MJ. The molecular basis of communication within the cells. *Sci. Am* 1985, 253:142-152.

[25] Holmsen H. Platelet metabolism and activation. *Semin Hematol.* 1985, 22:219-240.

[26] Seiss W. Molecular mechanism of platelet activation. *Physiol. Rev.*1990, 70:115-164.

[27] Rao, GHR. Physiology of blood platelet activation. *Ind J Physiol Pharmacol.* 1993, 37:263-275.

[28] Rao, GHR. Signal transduction, second messengers and platelet function. *J Lab Clin Med.* 1993, 121:18-21.

[29] Rao, GHR. Signal transduction, second messengers and platelet pharmacology. *Pharmacol.* 1994,13:39-44.

[30] Packham MA. Role of platelets in thrombosis and hemostasis. *Can J Physiol. Pharmacol.* 1993, 72:278-284.

[31] Rao GHR, Gerrard JM, Eaton JW, White JG. The role of iron in prostaglandin synthesis: Ferrous iron mediated oxidation of arachidonic acid. *Prost and Med* 1978, 1: 55-70.

[32] Peterson DA, Gerrard JM, Rao GHR, Mills EL, White JG. Interaction of arachidonic acid and heme iron in the synthesis of prostaglandins. *Adv Prost and Thromb Res* 1980, 6; 157-161.

[33] Peterson DA, Gerrard JM, Rao GHR, White JG. Inhibition of ferrous iron induced oxidation of arachidonic acid by indomethacin. *Prost and Med* 1979, 2: 97-108.

[34] Rao GHR, Cox AC, Gerrard JM, White JG. Effects of 2,2' dipyrydil and related compounds on platelet prostaglandin synthesis and platelet function. *Biochem Biphys Acta* 1980, 628: 468-479.

[35] Rao GHR, Johnson GJ, Reddy KR. Ibuprofen protects cyclooxygenase from irreversible inhibition by aspirin. *Arteriosclerosis* 1983, 3: 384-388.

[36] Patrono C. Aspirin as an antiplatelet drug. *N Engl. J Med* 1994, 330: 1287-1294.

[37] Hanley SP, Cockbill SR, Bevan J. et al. Differential inhibition by low-dose aspirin of human venous prostacyclin synthesis and platelet thromboxane synthesis. *Lancet* 1981, 2: 969-971.

[38] Keimowitz RM, Pulvermacher G, Mayo G. et al. Transdermal modification of platelet function: A dermal aspirin preparation selectively inhibits platelet cyclooxygenase and preserves prostacyclin biosynthesis. *Circ* 1993, 88: 556-561.

[39] Clarke RJ, Mayo G, Price P. et al. Suppression of thromboxane A_2 but not systemic prostacyclin by controlled release aspirin. *N Engl. J Med* 1991, 325: 1137-1141.

[40] Antiplatelet Trialists' Collaboration. The Aspirin Papers. Brit. J. Med.1994, 308:71-72, 81-106.

[41] Fuster V. Dyken ML, Vokomas PS. Aspirin as a therapeutic agent in cardiovascular disease. *Circ.* 1993, 87:659-675.

[42] Rao GHR, Reddy KR, White JG. Low-dose aspirin, platelet function and prostaglandin synthesis: influence of epinephrine and alpha-adrenergic receptor blockade. *Prost. and Med.* 1981, 6:485-494.

[43] McLeod LJ, Roberts MS, Seville PR. Selective inhibition of platelet cyclooxygenase with controlled release low dose aspirin. *Aust. N Z J Med.*1990, 20: 652-656.

[44] Rao GHR, Radha E Johnson GJ. et al. Enteric coated aspirin, platelet cyclooxygenase activity and platelet function. *Prost. Leukot. Med.* 1984,13: 3-12.

[45] Sullivan MH, Zosmer A, Gleeson RP. et al. Equivalent inhibition of *in vivo* platelet function by low dose and high dose aspirin. *Prost. Leukot. Fatty Acids.* 1990,39:319-321.

[46] Kyrle PA, Eichler HG, Jager U. et al. Inhibition of prostacyclin and thromboxane A2 generation by low dose aspirin at the site of plug formation in man *in vivo*. *Circ.*1987, 75:1025-1029.

[47] Wilson TW, McCauley FA, Wells HD. Effects of low dose aspirin on responses to Furosamide. *J. Clin. Pharmacol.* 1986, 26:100-105.

[48] Ridker PM, Cook NR, Lee IM, et al. A randomized trial of low-dose aspirin in the primary prevention of cardiovascular disease in women. *N. Engl.J. Med.* 2005, 352, 1293-304.

[49] Zucker Ml, Trowbridge C, Woodroof J. et al. Low- vs high-dose aspirin. Effects on platelet function in hyper-lipoproteinemic and normal subjects. *Arch. Intern. Med.* 1986, 146: 921-925.

[50] Davi G, Averna M, Catalano I. et al. Increased thromboxane biosynthesis in type 11a hypercholesterolemia. *Circ.* 1992, 85: 1792-1798.

[51] Diminno G, Silver MJ, Cerbone AM et al. Trial of repeated low-dose aspirin in diabetic angiopathy. *Blood.*1986, 68: 886-891.

[52] Terres W, Schuster O, Kupper W. et al. Effects of low-dose acetylsalicylic acid on thrombocytes in healthy subjects and in patients with coronary heart disease. *Dtsh Med. Wochenschr* 1989, 18: 1231-1236.

[53] De Caterina R, Giannessi D Bernini W. et al. Low-dose aspirin in patients recovering from myocardial infarction. Evidence for a selective inhibition of thromboxane-related platelet function. *Eur. Heart J.* 1985, 6:409-417.

[54] Kupper AJ, Verheugt FW, Peels CH. et al. Effect of low dose acetylsalicylic acid on the frequency and hematologic activity of left ventricular thrombus in anterior wall acute myocardial infarction. *Am. J. Cardiol.* 1989, 63:917-920.

[55] Weksler BB, Kent JL, Rudolph D. et al. Effects of low dose aspirin on platelet function in patients with recent cerebral ischemia. *Stroke.* 1985, 16: 5-9.

[56] Uchiyama S, Sone R, Nagayama T et al. Combination therapy with low-dose aspirin and ticlopidine in cerebral ischemia. *Stroke.* 1989, 20: 1643-1647.

[57] Jones EW, Cockbill SR, Cowley AJ. et al. Effects of dazoxiben and low-dose aspirin on platelet behavior in man. *Brit. J. Pharmacol.* 1983, 15: 395-445.

[58] Rao GHR, White JG. Epinephrine-induced Platelet Membrane Modulation. The Platelet Amine Storage. Myers KM, Barnes CD (eds) *CRC Press*, Roca Baton, USA.1992, p117-149.

[59] Rao GHR, Johnson GJ, White JG. Influence of epinephrine on the aggregation response of aspirin-treated platelets. *Prost. Med.* 1980, 5:45-58.

[60] Rao GHR, White JG. Epinephrine potentiation of arachidonate-induced aggregation of cyclooxygenase deficient platelets. *Am. J. Hematol.* 1981, 11: 355-366.

[61] Rao GHR, White JG. Role of arachidonic acid in human platelet activation and irreversible aggregation. *Am. J. Hematol.* 1985, 19: 339-347.

[62] Rao GHR, White JG. Aspirin, PGE1 and Quin-2 AM induced platelet dysfunction. Restoration of function by nor-epinephrine. *Prost. Leukot. Essen. Fatty A*cids 1990, 39: 141-146.

[63] Rao GHR, Escolar G, White JG. Epinephrine reverses the inhibitory influence of aspirin on platelet vessel wall interaction. *Thromb. Res.* 1986, 44: 65-74.

[64] Rao GHR, Escolar G, Zavrol J. Influence of adrenergic receptor blockade on aspirin-induced inhibition of platelet function. *Platelets* 1990,1:145-150.

[65] Rao GHR, Reddy KR, White JG. Modification of human platelet response to sodium arachidonate by membrane modulation. *Prost. Med* 1981, 6: 75-90.

[66] Rao GHR, Johnson GJ, Reddy KR. Ibuprofen Protects Platelet Cyclooxygenase from Irreversible Inhibition by Aspirin. *Arteriosclerosis*. 1983, 3: 383-388.

[67] Connelan JM, Thurlow PJ, Barlow B. et al. Investigation of alternative mechanisms of collagen-induced platelet activation using monoclonal antibodies to glycoprotein 11b-111a and fibrinogen. *Thromb. Haemost.*1986, 55: 153-157.

[68] Muller JE, Tolfer GH. Triggering and hourly variation of onset of arterial thrombosis. *Ann Epideniol*. 1992, 2: 393-405.

[69] Rao GHR. Circadian Variations and coronary artery disease. *Chronobiol* 1994, 21: 63-64.

[70] Prikryl P, Siegelova J, Cornelissen G et al. Chronotherapeutic treatment daily low-dose aspirin. University of Minnesota *Medtronic Chronobiology Series* 1991.

[71] White JG, Rao GHR, Gerrard JM. Effects of nitroblue tetrazolium and Vitamin E on platelet ultrastructure, aggregation and secretion. *Am J. Pathol* 1978, 92:745-53.

[72] Rao GHR, Cox CA, Gerrard JM. Et al. Alpha tocopherol quinone: a potent inhibitor of platelet function. *Prog. Lipid Res*. 1981, 6: 51-64.

[73] Rao GHR, Tate MR, Murthy M. et al. Influence of antioxidants on arachidonic acid metabolism and platelet function. *Biocehm Med. and Met Biol*. 1994, 51:74-79.

[74] Rao GHR, Radha E, White JG. Effect of docosahexaenoic acid (DHA) on arachidonic acid metabolism and platelet function. *Biochem Biophs Res Comm.* 1983, 117: 549-556.

[75] Pollack A. For Some, Aspirin May Not Help Hearts. *New York Times*. 2004, July.

[76] Weber AA, Przytuski B, Schanz A. et al. Towards a definition of aspirin resistance: a typological approach. *Platelets*. 2002, 13: 37-40.

[77] Yilmaz MB, Balbay Y, Korkmaz S. Aspirin resistance. *Anadolu. Kardiyol. Derg* 2004, 4: 59-62.

[78] Patrono C, Coller B, FitzGerald GA. et al. Platelet-Active Drugs: The Relationships Among Dose, Effectiveness, and Side Effects. *CHEST* 2004, 126: 234S-264S.

[79] Howard PA. Aspirin resistance. *Ann Pharmacother*. 2002, 36: 1620-1624.

[80] Hurlen M, Seijeflot I, Arnesen. The Effect of Different Regimens on Platelet Aggregation After Myocardial Infarction. *Scand. Cardiovasc*. J. 1998, 32: 233-237.

[81] Wu KK, Hoak JC. A new method for the quantitative detection of platelet aggregation in patients with arterial insufficiency. *Lancet* 1974,11: 924-926.

[82] Gum PA, Kottke-Marchant K, Poggio ED. et al. Profile and prevalence of aspirin resistance in patients with cardiovascular disease. *Am. J. Cardiol*. 2001, 88: 230-235.

[83] Gum PA, Kottke-Marchant K, Welsh PA. et al. A prospective, blinded determination of the natural history of aspirin resistance among stable patients with cardiovascular disease. *J. Am. Coll. Cardiol*. 2003, 41: 961-967.

[84] Deliargyris E, Boudoulas H. Aspirin Resistance. *Hellenic J. Cardiol*. 2004, 45: 1-5.

[85] Grotemeyer KH. Effects of acetylsalicyclic acid in stroke patients; evidence of non-responders in a subpopulation of treated patients. *Thromb. Res*. 1991, 63: 587-593.

[86] Grotemeyer KH. Two-year follow-up of aspirin responder and aspirin non-responder. A pilot-study including 180 post-stroke patients. *Thromb. Res*. 1993, 71:397-403.

[87] Mueller MR, Salat A, Stangi P. et al. Variable platelet response to low-dose ASA and the risk of limb deterioration in patients submitted to peripheral arterial angioplasty. *Thromb. Haemost*. 1997, 78: 1003-1007.

[88] Eikelboom JW, Hirsh J, Weitz JI. et al. Aspirin-resistant thromboxane biosynthesis and the risk of myocardial infarction, stroke, or cardiovascular death in patients at high risk for cardiovascular events. *Circ* 2002, 105: 1650-1655.
[89] Smout J, Stansby G. Aspirin resistance. *Brit. J. Surgery* 2002, 89: 4-5.
[90] Helgason CM, Bolin KM, Hoff JA. et al. Development of aspirin resistance in persons with previous ischemic stroke. *Stroke* 1994, 25: 2331-2336.
[91] Zimmerman N, Wenk A, Kim U. et al. Functional and biochemical evaluation of platelet aspirin resistance after coronary artery bypass surgery. *Circ.* 2003, 108: 542-547.
[92] Sane DC, McKee SA, Malinin AI. Frequency of aspirin resistance in patients with congestive heart failure treated with antecedent aspirin. *Am. J. Cardiol.* 2002, 90: 893-895.
[93] Muller I, Besta F, Schulz C. et al. Prevalence of Clopidogrel non-responders among patients with stable angina pectoris scheduled for elective coronary stenting. *Thromb. Heamost.* 2003, 89: 783-787.
[94] Lau WC, Gubrel PA, Watkins PB. et al. Contribution of hepatic cytochrome P450 3A4 metabolic activity to the phenomenon of Clopidogrel resistance. *Circ.* 2004, 109: 166-171.
[95] Angiolilo DJ, Fernandez-Ortiz A, Bernardo E. et al. High Clopidogrel loading dose during coronary stenting: effect on drug response and inter-individual variability. *Eur. Heart J.* 2004, 25: 1903-1910.
[96] Serebruany VL, Steinhubl SR, Berger PB. et al. Variability in platelet responsiveness to Clopidogrel among 544 individuals. *J. Am Coll. Cardiol.* 2005, 45: 246-251.
[97] Dziewierz A, Dubek D, Heba G. et al. Inter-individual variability in responses to Clopidogrel with cardiac diseases. *Polis Heart J.* 2005, 62: 1-6.
[98] Altman R, Luciardi HL Muntaner J. et al. The anti-thrombotic profile of aspirin, aspirin resistance or simply failure? *Thromb. J.* 2004, 2: 1-8.
[99] De Gaetano G, Cerletti C. Aspirin resistance: a revival of platelet aggregation tests? *J. Thromb. Haemost.* 2004, 1: 2048-2061.
[100] Malinin A, Spergling M, Muhlestein B. et al. Assessing aspirin responsiveness in subjects with multiple risk factors for vascular disease with a rapid platelet function analyzer. *Blood Coag. Fibrinol.* 2004, 1%: 295-301.
[101] Sambola A. Heras M, Escolar G. et al. The PFA-100 detects sub-optimal antiplatelet responses in patients on aspirin. *Platelets.* 2004, 1-8.
[102] Coleman JL, Wang JC, Simon DI. Determination of individual responses to Aspirin therapy using the Accumetric Ultegra. *The J. Near-Patient Testing and Technol.* 2004, 3: 77-82.
[103] Feuring M, Hasseroth K, Janson CP. et al. Inhibition of platelet aggregation after intake of acetylsalicylic acid detected by a platelet function analyzer (PFA-100). *Int. J. Clin Pharmacol Ther.* 1999, 37: 584-548.
[104] Andersen K, Hurlen M, Arnesen H. et al. Aspirin-responsiveness as measured by a PFA-100 in patients with coronary artery disease. *Thromb. Res.* 2002, 108: 37-42.
[105] Singh S, Kothari SS, Bahl VK. Aspirin Resistance: Myth or Reality? *Ind. Heart J.* 2003, 55: 1-8

[106] McKee SA, Sane DC, Deliagyris. Aspirin resistance in cardiovascular disease: A review of prevalence, mechanisms, and clinical significance. *Thromb. Haemost.* 2002, 88: 711-715.

[107] Eikelboom JW, Hankey GJ. Aspirin resistance: a new independent predictor of vascular events? *J. Am. Coll.Cardiol.* 2003, 41: 966-968.

[108] Berger PB. Resistance to antiplatelet drugs: Is it real or relevant? *Cath. And Cardiovasc Interven.* 2004, 62: 43-45.

[109] Shemesh CG, zehavi M, Dinur I et al. Lack of aspirin effect: aspirin resistance or resistance to taking aspirin? *Am. Heart J.* 2004, 147: 293-300.

[110] Cattaneo M. Aspirin and Clopidogrel: efficacy, safety, and the issue of drug resistance. *Arterscler. Vasc. Biol.* 2004, 24: 1980-87.

[111] Nguyen TA, Diodati JG, Pharand C. Resistance Clopidogrel: a review of the evidence. *J. Am Coll Cardiol* 2005, 45: 1157-64.

[112] Sztritha LK Sas K, Vecsei L. *Aspirin resistance in stroke:* 2004. 2005, 230:163-69.

[113] Coma-Canella I, Velasco A, Castano S. Prevalence of aspirin resistance measured by PFA-100. *Int. J. Cardiol.* 2005, 101:71-76.

[114] Kuliczkowski W, Halawa B, Korolko B. Aspirin resistance in ischemic heart disease. *Kardiol Pol.* 2005, 62: 14-25.

[115] Schwartz KA, Schwartz DE, Ghosheh K et al. Compliance as a critical consideration in patients who appear to be resistant to aspirin after healing of myocardial infarction. *Am. J. Cardiol* 2005, 95: 973-75.

[116] Driewierz A, Dudek D, Heba G, Inter-individual variability in response to Clopidogrel in patients with coronary artery disease. *Kardiol Pol.* 2005, 62: 108-118.

[117] Serebruaany VL, Steinhubl SR, Berger PB. et al. Variability in platelet responsiveness to Clopidogrel among 544 individuals. *J Am Coll Cardiol.* 2005 45: 246-51.

[118] Rao GHR. Aspirin resistance: A fact or a myth? *Expt. and Clin. Cardiol.* 2005, 10: 17-20.

[119] Pettersen AA, Seljeflot I, Abdelnoor M et al. Unstable angina, stroke, myocardial infarction and death in aspirin non-responders. A Prospective, randomized trial. The ASCET (Aspirin non-responsiveness and Clopidogrel Endpoint Trial) design. *Scand Cardiovasc. J.* 2004, 38:353-56.

In: World Heart Research Yearbook. Volume 1
Editors: Franz Halberg and R. B. Singh
ISBN: 978-1-60741-881-8

CIRCADIAN CARDIOLOGY

B. Singh,[*] Ashwaria Gupta, Daniel Pella and Adarsh Kumar
Halberg Hospital and Research Institute, Moradabad, Glenmark Pharmaceuticals Limited, Mumbai, India
Safaric University, Kosice Slovakia
Government Medical College, Amritsar, India

ABSTRACT

A circadian cell cycle resides in every cell, and peripheral timing mechanisms are documented in molecular biologic terms at about 24-hour (circadian) and higher (ultradian) frequencies with coordination in mammals by the adrenal and the pineal-hypothalamic-pituitary network. The suprachiasmatic nuclei (SCN) and clock gene contribute to the coordination of the circadian rhythms' phase and amplitude in everyday life. The SCN are influenced by the daily alternation between light and darkness directly via the eyes and by plasma melatonin concentrations secreted by the pineal gland, which is a window to both light and geomagnetics. A clinical event occurs when the neuroendocrine time structures (chronomes) are not able to cope with the adverse effects of stimuli acting from within or from without, e. g., via the sympathetic nervous system. Triggering of the neuroendocrines by environmental factors may activate the pineal gland, pituitary functions and adrenal secretions, resulting in adverse effects on circadian variations, heart rate variability (HRV) and blood pressure variability (BPV). Circadian rhythm has been known to ancient man from the time of Homoerectus and Homosapiens who used to have intercourse in the early morning hours, prior to going hunting in the forests, causing increased secretion of testosterone in the morning. The role of time-adjusted drug intake, especially in the early morning, was also known to ancient Indian physicians. In the Ayurveda, drinking of large amounts of water in the early morning is advised, which appears to be in an attempt to increase vagal tone due to gastric distention. Frey considered the mean distribution of deaths along the scales of the day and the year. In one industrial population, Pell and D'Allonzo, discussed time-macroscopically the occurrence of a peak in the morning hours in a study of acute myocardial infarction (AMI), a proposition also ascertained and extended to the yearly pattern time-microscopically.

The subsequent reports from other countries, the Soviet Union and the extensive data by WHO in the report of myocardial infarction Community Registers from 19 European centers demonstrated a peak incidence of onset of chest pain due to AMI from 8.00 to 11.00 AM with a ratio of approximately 2 In one study from India, in 605 AMI patients, 39% of those who had Q wave infarction (n=174) had the onset between 6. 00 AM to 12.

[*] Correspondence: Dr R B Singh, MD Professor of Medicine, Halberg Hospital and Research Institute Civil Lines, Moradabad-10(UP)244001, Indiaicn2005@mickyonline.com.

00 noon. In a more recent Mechanism of Acute Myocardial Infarction (MAMI) study by Singh et al, among 202 AMI patients, the incidence of onset of chest pain was highest in the second quarter of the day (41. 0%), mainly between 4-8 AM, followed by the 4th quarter, usually after large meals (28. 2%).

Emotion was the second most common trigger (43. 5%), which was the most common in the patients with onset of chest pain in the second quarter of the day (51. 8%). Cold weather was a predisposing factor in 29. 2% and hot temperatures (40°C) was common in 24. 7% of the patients. A large meal, especially a large breakfast in the morning was an important trigger of AMI in this study, which poses the intriguing possibility that some heart attacks could be prevented by not eating breakfast or by eating a small superfood breakfast containing walnuts, almonds, raisins and yogurt which are known to be protective against cardiovascular disease.

Blood pressure is usually lower during the night, starts increasing before awakening, and remains high during the day-time, mostly in the second quarter of the day. Circadian rhythms of triggers and cardiac events and their mechanisms have been described by various workers. It is possible that circadian rhythm could be a new target for treatment with lifestyle changes, nutrient, nutraceuiticals such as w-3 fatty acids and coenzyme Q10, prayer and drug therapy in the management of cardiovascular disease.

INTRODUCTION

Many scientists believe that our universe came into existence about 20 billion years ago after an explosion of a primordial fireball of matter. Within 3 minutes of the explosion, the elementary matter particles coalesced to form the lightest elements, which were responsible for the formation of galaxies. Most of the galaxies appear to be receding from us at high velocities, which has been explained by the expansion model of the universe. Rhythm is a fundamental characteristic of the galaxies in our universe. The sun revolves around the core of the Milky Way Galaxy, rotating on its axis.

The planets revolve around the sun and moon revolves around the planets. One season follows the other season, day follows night, tide-in follows tide-out. Most of the rhythms are linked to the movements of the heavenly bodies.

The rotation of the earth is responsible for the day and night cycle, and the moon orbiting around the earth for the monthly cycle. The procession of the earth on its axis is responsible for the four seasons and the earth orbiting the sun for the annual cycle. Many physiological functions must adapt to these external rhythms, causing dysfunctions resulting in the development of diseases. [1-3].

The universe of living creatures appears to have similar characteristics. All living cells have life cycles and periodicity in their life function [3]. The migration of birds, the hibernation of bears, dogs and several other animals, ripening of fruits and flowering of plants, are driven by the changing seasons.

Similarly, other rhythms, such as sleep and wakefulness, the opening and closing of flowers, feeding and nesting are also driven by the circadian cycle. There is substantial evidence that cardiovascular events occur in the second quarter of the day. [1-3]. The exact pathogenesis and risk factors of circadian rhythms are not known [4-9].

THE INTERACTION OF GENES AND MEANS AND ADAPTATION

Diet and lifestyle, tobacco, pollutants, stress, and alcohol are the most important environmental means, which interact with genes in the pathogenesis of cardiovascular disease, diabetes and cancer. The interaction of genes and environment, nature and nurture, is the foundation for the development of disease and health. It has been shown through molecular biological techniques that genetic factors determine susceptibility to disease and environmental factors determine which genetically susceptible individual will develop a disease [9]. Despite major changes in our diet and lifestyle in the last 10,000 years, our genes have not changed and hence our biological responses are unable to adapt, resulting in greater adverse effects of these factors on our circadian rhythms. The spontaneous mutation rate for nuclear DNA is estimated at 0.5% per million years. The period of 10,000 years of the agricultural revolution appears to be too short to modulate our genes, causing an approximate 0.005% alteration. It seems our genes are much similar today to our ancestors of the Paleolethic period 40,000 years ago, when our genetic profile was established [9]. It is possible to presume that humans today live in an environment that differs completely from that when our genetic constitution was selected and therefore our clock gene remains as potent as several million years ago to initiate the biorhythms of our bodies. Our clock gene does not allow us to adapt to modulate rapid changes in diet and lifestyle, which influence circadian rhythms.

EVOLUTIONARY ASPECTS OF BIOLOGICAL FUNCTION RHYTHMICITY

Homosapiens, along with their predecessors Homo-habilis, were primarily vegetarians, although for more than a million years, they have been hunting. They became omnivorous as they moved away from other primates. Environmental influences, development of social groups and increasing demands for survival made them skillful and caused significant changes in their lifestyle. They went to the forest in the early morning for hunting animals. They were killed early in life due to accidents. It has been proposed that, in order to preserve their progeny, the Homosapiens had intercourse early in the morning resulting in one of the most important physiological adaptations of an increased release of testosterone in the morning, as a circadian rhythm.

The increased release of testosterone occurred to coordinate sexual activity with the aim of conceiving the women. We suggest that since hunting used to start at about sunrise, causing enormous excitement, physical and mental exertion and increased sympathetic activity (associated with marked secretion of cortisol, catecholamines, aldosterone, angiotensin and renin in a state of low melatonin), it also became a circadian rhythm in modern men. Ancient man was able to adapt and fight the adverse effects of testosterone, cortisol and catecholamines, due to their enormous physical activity and lack of time for breakfast. Modern men is not, however, resulting in increased rhythmicity of cardiac events in the second quarter of the day. Late night falling asleep, late awakening, heavy breakfasts, no physical activity and meditation in the morning, and excitement related to rushing to the workplace, trigger a biochemical and biological atmosphere in our body that contributes to the greater cardiovascular events and deaths between 8.00-11.00 hours. [1-3].

We are comparing the diet and lifestyle as well as heart rate and blood pressures around the clock for 7 days in people in tribes living in the adverse conditions of Laddakh, with those living in Moradabad and Tokyo City to determine the pattern of circadian changes, and to provide further insight into the pathogenesis of circadian rhythms.

Evolutionary Aspects of Diet and Lifestyle

Recently, several scholars became interested in health and disease from an evolutionary perspective and consider whether our departure from the hunter-gatherer lifestyle may contribute to contemporary health problems [1, 2].

Foods are probably appropriate for any given species if they were regularly consumed during most of the prior evolution, as in the case of hunter gatherers. Prehistoric human hunter gatherers may have protected themselves by choosing plants that have low concentrations of xenobiotics and by avoiding dangerous plant species. The available food staples during the Palaeolithic period may have been meat, fish, shellfish, leafy vegetables, fruits, nuts, insects and larvae in varying proportions. Since tubers often require cooking for their starch to be digestible their routine consumption may have started in the later period. [6-8].

Prior to the agricultural revolution, about 10,000 years ago, humans ate an enormous variety of wild plants. Meat, fish, green leafy vegetables, fruits, nuts, berries and honey were the food items available to pre-agricultural humans which shaped modern humans' genetic nutritional requirements. Early man also managed to survive in a wide range of environments, from the tropical rainforest to near the Arctic, each of these environments offering a different and limited set of foods. However, all diets of ancient men lacked breakfast foods; milk, cheese, butter, syrups, cereals, and of course, refined carbohydrates and sugar that is sprinkled on them, which are known to have adverse effects on our metabolisms causing insulin resistance. These foods supply approximately 70% of the energy in the diets of the Western world today. Irrespective of the specific proportions of meat and vegetables, prehistoric hunter-gatherers' diets would have been very different from those of contemporary humans with regard to their nutritional value.

Hunting was the major part of the occupational physical activity of prehistoric men, which might have continued throughout the entire day. After they returned from the forest in midday or evening, they may have had a late heavy lunch, followed by dancing and eating again in the late evening.

Many experts suggest that reversion to the original Palaeolithic human lifestyle (1. 5 million-10, 000 years BP) might be useful in the prevention of chronic diseases of Western populations [6-8]. The main symbols of Gods of early men were the sun, fire, sea and hills, which they worshiped to decrease their mental stress.

Several biological functions, such as temperature regulation, blood circulation in the nasal mucosa, the caliber of the tracheobronchial airway, blood pressure, heart rate, cortisol and growth hormone release exhibit an intrinsic circadian rhythm [1-5].

Most physiological rhythms may be ultradian having a duration of seconds, minutes, or at most a few hours. Circadian means 24 hours, circamensual, 30 days and circaannual, one year. The sleep phases, heart rate, respiratory rate and the functional peaks of many enzymes, receptors and endothelial nitric oxide releases show ultradian variations, depending upon triggers and clocks. (Table 1).

Table 1. Neuropsychiatric risk factors of acute myocardial infarction

Precursors	Healthy Subjects (n-595)	AMI (n=202)
Anxiety	88 (14. 8)	122 (60. 4)*
Depression	42 (7. 0)	45 (22. 3)*
Type A behaviour	103 (17. 3)	95 (47. 2)*
Emotional stress	147 (24. 2)	92 (45. 5)*
Sleep deprivation	42 (7. 0)	56 (27. 7)*
Cold Climate	-	59 (29. 2)*
Hot climate (>40 degree celsius)	-	50 (24. 7)*
Large Meals	147 (24. 7)	96 (47. 5)*
Physical Exertion	173 (29. 1)	63 (31. 2)*
Diabetes mellitus	70 (11. 7)	53 (26. 2)*
*=P<0. 05 by Chi square test		

CIRCADIAN

The words circadian and chronobiology were used for the first time by Franz Halberg in 1950 and officially introduced to a nomenclature committee in Stockholm for the first time in 1955 [4, 5]. Chonobiology developed globally after 1969 when an article entitled "Chronobiology" was published in the *Annual Review of Physiology* and became a Current Contents citation classic. Body temperature shows circadian variation; it is lowest in the morning, peaks in the afternoon and falls again during the night. In contrast, cortisol release peaks in the morning. Blood pressure varies by up to 40mm Hg over the time structure of the day with a clear-cut peak in the morning.

Cholesterol is synthesized mainly in the nighttime. An annual variation has also been reported in aldosterone secretion showing a peak during the winter. The cycle of the reproductive organs is the best-known circamensual rhythm. Ultradian sleep phases (up to a few hours), heart rate, respiratory rate, circadian temperature changes in the interior of the body, all have a circadian rhythm.

A circaannual rhythmicity has been observed for serum cholesterol levels with the winter values being much higher. Halberg feels that apart from circadian, circaseptan (weekly), monthly, yearly or even longer term physiological variations occur.

Otsuka proposed that the physiological chronomes such as heart rate variability have counterparts in our environment and our genetic makeup over time may have evolved from our adaptation to and integration with the cosmos. There is a need to examine how these phenomena including heliomagnetics and geomagnetics, can influence physiological chronomes, especially for heart rate and blood pressure variability [10].

CLOCKS

The circadian rhythms enable the body to adapt in an optimum manner to changes in its environments including geomagnetic forces. These rhythms are set up endogenously in the body and the entire system of hormonised rhythms, the biological time structure can be influenced by external and internal factors, which are called clocks. It is very difficult to assess the internal factors that govern the circadian rhythms. Hence, we know very little about internal clocks.

It is indeed very difficult to assess the internal factors that govern biological rhythms, however. Halberg has proposed that a circadian cycle resides in every living cell and peripheral timing mechanisms are being documented in molecular biological terms at about 24 hour (circadian) and utradian frequencies, with coordination in mammals by the Adrenal, pineal-hypothalamic-pituitary network (Figure 1). Suprachiasmatic nuclei (SCN) is one known specific area of the brain that works as an internal clock and is responsible for the regulation of central nervous functions, phase and amplitude, as it receives information from the eyes. The information from the brain is transferred to the pineal gland. Melatonin released from the pituitary gland during the dark hours of the days in a circadian cycle regulates sleep and awake periods. The SCN are influenced by the daily alternation between light and darkness direcly via the eyes and melatonin levels. A cardiovascular event occurs when our neuroendocrine time structures (chronomes) are not able to cope with the adverse effects of stimuli from within or without acting eg via the sympathetic nervous system [10-13]. It appears that the two most powerful external clocks for humans are light at high intensity and social contacts. The results of initial attempts to use bright light to adapt shift workers were encouraging [14]. Most organisms from cyanobacteria to mammals are known to use circadian clocks to coordinate their metabolisms with the natural circadian light/dark cycle. The human clock gene was discovered and mapped to chromosome17p12-13. 1 in 1997 [15]. It is surprising that the clock gene is similar in all life forms on earth. In plants, several molecular components have been described for the circadian system.

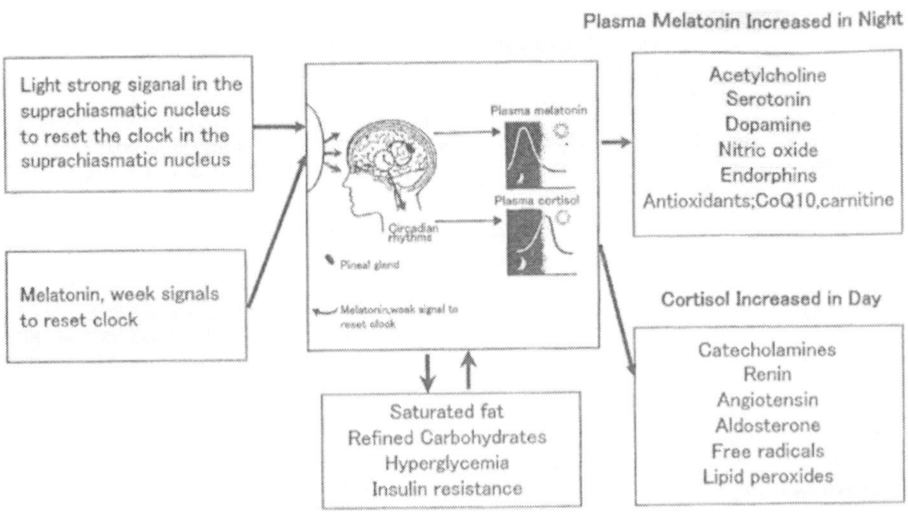

Figure 1. Control of Daily Rhythms By Molecular Clock.

STIMULUS TIMING CONTRIBUTES TO CHANCE OF DEATH VS SURVIVAL

CIRCADIAN AMPLITUDE (AND PHASE ?) DIFFERENCE IN SUSCEPTIBILITY TO A CARDIAC DRUG, OUBAIN, OF TWO INBRED MOUSE STRAINS*

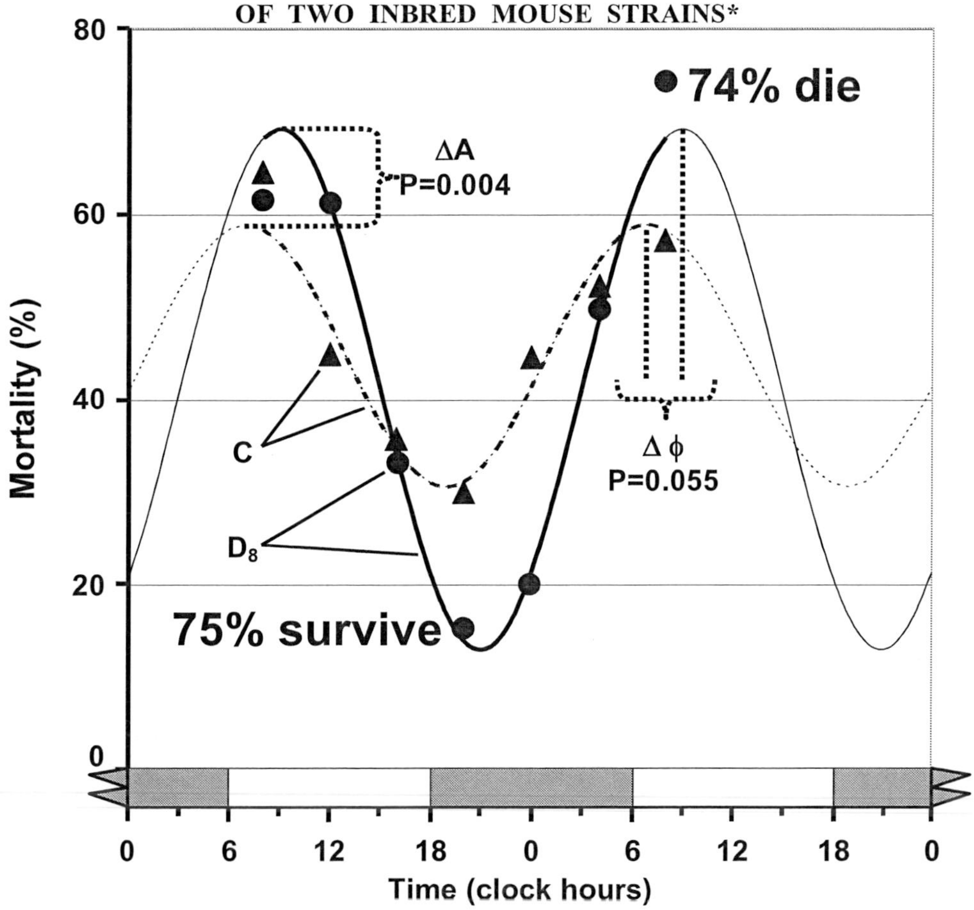

Strain	P	M	Amplitude (A)	Acrophase (ϕ**)
D_8	P < 0.001	40.0	28.1 (21.5; 34.8)	-135 (-119; -150)
C	P = 0.011	45.2	14.2 (7.3; 21.0)	-104 (- 73; -136)

*** C = Bagg albino, D_8 = subline 8 of Dilute Brown strain; oubain 0.15 or 0.5 mg/20 g of body weight, respectively. Thin lines in the graph are extrapolations of fitted cosine curves. ** In the table: 95% confidence limits in parentheses, ϕ in degrees (360° = 24 hours). M = MESOR; P from zero-A (no-rhythm) test.**
Data from F.Halberg et al., Minnesota Acad Sci Proc 1959; 27: 139-143.

Figure 2. First demonstration of the importamnce of timing with a drug, in this case > a cardiac drug and also a demonstration more generally of the importance> of statistics along the circadian scale. Feel free to use it.

TRIGGERS

Triggering of the chronomes by environmental factors may activate the pineal gland, pituitary functions and adrenal secretions, causing adverse effects on circadian rhythms, heart rate variability and blood pressure variability [10-14], resulting in cardiovascular events [11-15]. The various clinical manifestations of cardiovascular events do not occur at random times, but according to a time structure. It is possible that certain external activities known as triggers may play a major role in causing myocardial ischaemia, myocardial infarction, sudden cardiac death and stroke [11-15]. The MILIS (Multicentre Investigation of Limitation of Infarct Size) study showed that half of all myocardial infarction patients reported a temporal relationship between characteristic activities and occurrence of infarction. Emotional stress, mild and heavy physical exersion, sleep deprivation and large meals were the most frequently reported triggering activities [16].

The TRIMM (Triggers and Mechanisms of Myocardial Infarction) study showed that 76% of all infarction patients reported an unusual event shortly before the onset of infarction [17]. Emotional upset or stress was reported by 52% of the subjects and 10% reported multiple trigger activities coinciding just before the event. A morning increase in platelet aggregation appears to be one of the most important triggers for cardiovascular events in the second quarter of the day [18]. It seems that there is powerful evidence of a link between these triggers and the sequences of cellular and pathophysiological events that are proposed to be responsible for coronary artery ischaemia. In one study among 58 patents with AMI, large meals including a large breakfast, emotional stress, cold climate and hot climate (>40°C) were important triggers. A large breakfast in the morning was associated with increased concentration of proinflammatory cytokines; tumour necrosis factor-alpha and interleukin-6 as well as insulin and glucose in the blood [11] (Table 2). In the MAMI study [2], large meals, sleep deprivation, emotional stress, cold climate and hot climate were quite commonly observed (Table 3). Circadian rhythms of myocardial ischaemia, angina pectoris, myocardial infarction, sudden cardiac death and stroke have been described by several experts which are triggered by environmental factors as well as biochemical and biological triggers present in every living cell.

Table 2. Clinical Characteristics of subjects in various subgroups in relation to circadian pattern

Sub Group Total n=202	1-6 hours 34 (16. 8)	6-12 hours 83 (41. 0)	12-18 hours 28 (13. 8)	18-24 hours 57 (28. 2)
Male (n=160)	24 (15. 0)	60 (37. 5)	25 (15. 6)	51 (31. 8)
Female (n-132)	10 (23. 8)	23 (54. 7)	3 (7. 1)	6 (14. 2)
Age>60 (n=70)	12 (17. 1)	32 (45. 7)	8 (11. 4)	18 (25. 7)
60 and less (n=132)	12 (16. 6)	51 (38. 6)	20 (15. 1)	39 (29. 5)
History of CAD	16 (30. 7)	24 (46. 1)	7 (13. 4)	5 (9. 6)
Known Diabetes (n=53)	10 (18. 8)	22 (41. 5)	8 (15. 0)	13 (24. 5)
Known Hypertension (n-75) (>140/90)	13 (17. 3)	30 (40. 0)	11 (14. 6)	21 (28. 0)

Values are number (%). P value was obtained by comparison of subgroups by chi square test. *P>0. 05m *=P<0. 02, CAD= Coronary artery disease.

Circadian Rhythms in Ischemic Heart Disease

In the decade since the 1985 observation by Muller et al. that the frequency of onset of myocardial infarction peaks at 9 a. m., numerous publications have supported this observation not only for myocardial infarction, but also for sudden cardiac death, transient myocardial ischemia, and stroke. Refinement of these epidemiological observations has led to the conclusion that the morning peak in disease onset is due in part to the physical and mental stressors associated with morning awakening and activity. The observations also showed that stressors such as heavy physical activity and anger can trigger acute cardiovascular events [19].

Why Morning Is so Risky?

Circadian rhythm peaking in the morning is also found for so-called silent myocardial ischaemia, which occurs in more than 20% of patients with arterial hypertension, and can be regularly detected in combined 24-h-ABPM/EKG examinations. Comparative studies have shown that hypertensives with SMI suffer more cardiac events than those with no SMI. It has further been demonstrated that an elevated blood pressure amplitude, which is considered an independent risk factor for cardiac events, is associated with an increased incidence of SMI in patients with micro- or macro-angiopathy [20].

The Possible Mechanisms Involved

Transient myocardial ischemia, detected by ambulatory ST segment monitoring, is also unevenly distributed during the day. The pathophysiology and the mechanisms underlying these variations are the focus of much investigation. Heart rate, blood pressure, neural and humoral vasoactive factors such as plasma norepinephrine levels and renin activity, and probably also contractility, are increased in the morning hours, indicating that an increase in myocardial oxygen demands contribute importantly to the increased prevalence of ischemia in the morning. A study by Li JJ found that the circadian rhythm of the ischemic threshold detected by repetitive exercise treadmill tests in patients with chronic coronary artery disease is also apparently associated with levels of plasma ET-1 [21].

Relation to Plasma Endothelin-1

Li JJ et al. demonstrated that ET-1 values were higher in the morning hours as compared to afternoon hours. Circadian variations of plasma levels of ET-1 are likely to be one of the most likely mechanisms involved of reduction of the ischemic threshold in the morning hours [22].

Table 3. Triggers observed in 202 patients of acute myocardial infarction in relation to circadian periods

Quarter of 24 hrs	1-6 hours	6-12 hours	12-18 hours	18-24hours	Total
Subjects	34	83	28	57	202
Trigger total	25 (73. 5)	70 (84. 3)	15 (53. 5)	42 (73. 7)	162 (82. 2)
Large meals	18 (52. 9)	41 (49. 4)	12 (42. 8)	26 (45. 6)	96 (47. 5)
Emotional stress	15 (44. 1)	43 (51. 8)	14 (50. 0)	20 (35. 0)	92 (45. 5)
Physical Exertion	12 (35. 3)	25 (30. 1)	8 (28. 5)	18 (31. 6)	63 (31. 2)
Sleep deprivation	8 (23. 5)	32 (38. 5)	6 (21. 4)	10 (17. 5)	56 (27. 7)
Cold climate	10 (29. 4)	35 (42. 1)	5 (17. 8)	9 (15. 5)	59 (29. 2)
Hot climate (>40 celsius)	8 (23. 5)	30 (36. 1)	5 (17. 8)	7 (12. 3)	50 (24. 7)

Values are number (%) *=P<0. 05, Pvalues were obtained by comparison of subgroups by chi square test.

Fluctuation in Endothelial Function

Coronary spasms are induced by acetylcholine (ACh), which causes vasodilation when the endothelium is functioning normally. The spasms are promptly relieved by nitroglycerin (NTG), which causes vasodilation through its direct action on the smooth muscle. The frequency of ischemic attacks displays diurnal variations in patients with VA (i. e., coronary spastic angina). The number of attacks increases in the early morning and decreases in the afternoon.

Mechanism of Coronary Spasms

In patients with coronary spasms, coronary dilation caused by endothelium-dependent vasodilators is reported to be impaired. In addition, antioxidants such as vitamin C and glutathione, attenuate the constrictor response to ACh. The plasma levels of vitamin E, a natural antioxidant, are decreased. The coronary arteries of patients with VA exhibit a circadian variation in tone. As the endothelial function of the brachial artery and that of the coronary artery are closely related [22], the fluctuation of endothelium-dependent dilation in the brachial artery most likely takes place in the coronary arteries as well.

Mechanism of Diurnal Variation in Flow-Mediated Vasodilation

It is known that the day/night pattern in the intensity of physical activity causes diurnal variation of hemodynamics. In the evening and afternoon, peripheral blood flow to the skeletal muscle is increased through local regulation in proportion to its need for oxygen and nutrients. Endothelial nitric oxide synthase is known to be upregulated by increased blood flow or shear stress.

Therefore, it is possible that the variation in baseline blood flow may upregulate nitric oxide synthase and contribute to the fluctuation of the flow-mediated, endothelium dependent vasodilation in patients with VA. Diurnal fluctuations of the endothelial function may play an important role in the occurrence of ischemic episodes in patients with VA [23].

Heart Rate Variability and the Rate of Autonomic Change

The incidence of sudden cardiac death peaks during the early morning hours when there is a rapid withdrawal of vagal and an increase of sympathetic tone. The rate of autonomic change could be of prognostic importance. B. Wennerblom showed that during the night/morning hours, healthy controls demonstrated faster HF max. velocity and higher HF gradient than angina patients. The authors concluded that rapid vagal withdrawal seemed to be a sign of a healthy autonomic nervous system in the control group but was significantly slower in angina patients. IS-5-MN and metoprolol tended to normalise vagal withdrawal and metoprolol slowed down the rapid increase in sympathetic predominance in the morning in these patients [24].

Circadian Rhythm in Myocardial Infarction

Despite impressive strides in diagnosis and management over the past three decades, acute myocardial infarction (AMI) continues to be a major public health problem in the industrialized world and is becoming an increasingly important problem in developing countries. About 50 percent of the deaths associated with AMI occur within 1 hour of the event and are attributable to arrhythmias, most often ventricular fibrillation. Because AMI may strike an individual during the most productive years, it can have profoundly deleterious psychosocial and economic ramifications [25].

Circadian Periodicity

An analysis of a large number of patients hospitalized with MI, studied as a part of the Multicenter Investigation of Limitation of Infarct Size (MILIS), revealed a pronounced circadian periodicity for the time of onset of AMI, with peak incidence of events between 6 a. m. and 12 p. m. About 20% of myocardial infarctions occur between midnight and 6 AM. The circadian distribution of acute myocardial infarction has a morning peak, especially during the first few hours after awakening [26].

Pathogenesis

Circadian rhythms affect many physiological and biochemical parameters; the early morning hours are associated with rises in plasma catecholamines and cortisol as well as increases in platelet aggregability. At this time, sympathetic activation is thought to disrupt atherosclerotic plaque through vasoconstriction and an increase in blood pressure. In addition, early morning changes in hemostatic activity may lead to thrombosis. In contrast, sleep may be protective, both because of the absence of external triggers and the decline in sympathetic activity during non–rapid eye movement (REM) sleep, which accounts for about 80% of total sleep time. However, about 20% of myocardial infarctions occur between midnight and 6 AM. REM sleep, which is characterized by sympathetic surges, might be involved—as it is in vasospastic angina - but REM sleep constitutes less than 20% of total sleep time in adults [27].

Hence, the pathogenesis of nocturnal myocardial infarctions may differ from those that occur during the daytime, since they may not be related to sympathetic activation or triggering events. Other sleep-induced cardiovascular changes that affect the coronary circulation or cardiac function may be involved. For example, sleep-induced variations of flow patterns in coronary arteries might be involved, or shifts in blood volume might affect the dimensions and hemodynamic function of the right ventricle [28, 29].

Circadian Variation in Plaque Rupture

Pathologic studies have revealed that plaque rupture is one of the major causes of AMI. One large-scale multicenter study has demonstrated that AMI is 1.28 times more likely to begin between 6:00 A. M. and 12:00 P. M. than during the other three 6-hour intervals of the day[2]. Pathologic studies have revealed that plaque rupture and subsequent thrombosis is one of the major causes of AMI. Therefore, the hypothesis that increased physiologic activities in morning hours may trigger plaque disruption has been proposed [30].

A. Tanaqa et al. demonstrated that in the plaque rupture group, a morning increase (from 6:00 A. M. to 12:00 P. M) was observed, whereas in the nonrupture group there was a nocturnal nadir (from 12 to 6:00 A. M) and no significant morning increase was detected. 53% of the patients in the nonrupture group had preinfarction angina and only 31% of patients had an AMI at rest. This circadian pattern was not detectable in the nonrupture group. This morning increase in the incidence of plaque rupture accounts for the characteristic circadian rhythm of AMI [31]. Various physiologic studies have highlighted the fact that systemic physiologic processes increase in intensity in the morning, such as an arterial pressure surge accompanied by an increase in heart rate [32] and increased vascular tone [33]. Serum cortisol levels also decrease during the period of increased plaque disruption. Because the Japanese population of patients with AMI compared with whites shows a higher incidence of spasm and greater vasoconstriction of nonspastic segments after acetylcholine [34], this decrease in serum cortisol levels could enhance the sensitivity of the coronary arteries to the vasoconstrictive effects of catecholamines. Such physiologic alterations may, alone or in combination, account for the morning increase in plaque rupture. When plaque rupture occurs, the contents of the lipid core that form the most thrombogenic components of the plaque may be released into the lumen and precipitate a cascade that produces thrombosis. Increased platelet activity, increased blood viscosity, and the minimal level of fibrinolytic activity may further contribute to thrombosis in this setting during the morning hours. The efficacy of β blockers and aspirin in preventing AMI indirectly lends support to the idea that these physiological variations may play an etiologic role in plaque disruption and resultant thrombosis [31].

Several studies have shown that in many instances, MI may occur without any obvious precipitating events and may occur at rest. Grines et al [35] reported that one independent predictor of a higher frequency of onset during the morning hours was the absence of a history of angina.

Q-WAVE VERSUS NON-Q WAVE MI

V. Culic et al. [36] demonstrated that both AMI types showed a nonuniform daily distribution of onset with a night nadir (0 to 4 A. M.), and Q-wave AMI also showed a late morning peak (8 A. M. to noon). The study demonstrated that wakeful patients with Q-wave infarction were more likely to have AMI onset in the presence of a possible external trigger than those with non–Q-wave AMI. This is consistent with the hypothesis that powerful hemodynamic stresses may produce more extensive plaque rupture, often leading to complete occlusion of the coronary lumen and Q-wave infarction. Non–Q-wave infarction is more likely to result from a shorter occlusion of a major coronary artery, with earlier and more frequent reopening than from firm occlusion of a small branch.

Table 4. Circadian pattern of acute myocardial infection in relation to drug therapy

Subgroups	1-6 hours 34	6-12 hours 83	12-18 hours 28	18-24 hours 57	Total 202
Beta-blockers Calcium	10	8	6	6	30
Blockers	2	2	2	6	12
ACE-inhibitor	4	4	-	6	14
Fish Oil Coenzyme	5	2	-	2	9
Q10	8	2	12	4	26
No Drug Therapy	(4. 3)	64(54. 7)**	10(8. 5)	37(31. 6)**	117
Drug Therapy Total	29(34. 1)	19(22. 3)	18(21. 2)	20(23. 5)	85

Values are number (%) out of totals = P<0. 05, **P=P<0. 01m O value were obtained by comparison of sub-groups by Chi square test.

Table 5. Clinical characteristics of subjects

	Acute myocardial infarction (n=54)	Controls (n=85)
Sex- males	45 (83. 3)	76(89. 4)
Mean age (years)	49. 5± 4. 2	52. 1± 5. 2
Body mass index (kg/m2)	23. 7± 3. 2	22. 4±3. 4
Hypertension (>140/90 mmhg)	25(46. 3)*	25(29. 4)
Glucose intolerance	12(22. 2)*	10(11. 8)
Diabetes mellitus	14(25. 9)	--
Smoking	24(44. 4)*	28(32. 9)
Higher transfattyacids (>5g/day) Large meals(>1000 Kcal) Large breakfast(>1000 Kcal)	27(50. 0)** 27(50. 0)** 22(40. 7)**	-- 25(29. 4) 10(11. 8)

*=P <0. 05 P value was obtained by z score test for proportions by comparison of two groups. Values are number (%) and mean(Standard deviation).

An acceptable explanation for a diverse circadian pattern in 2 AMI types, with late morning peak only in the Q-wave AMI, is that hemodynamic, prothrombotic, and vasoconstrictive forces resulting from a morning rise in sympathetic activity and cortisol levels contribute to the formation of sustained coronary occlusion and Q-wave infarction. A lower incidence of both infarction types during the early morning hours corresponds to the time when most patients would be expected to be asleep, so hemodynamic and other triggering forces may be reduced in patients with both types of AMI.

Table 6. Circadian rhythm of cardiac events in patients with acute myocardial infarction

Quarters of the day	Number of subjects (%)
1-6 Hours	10(18. 5)
6-12 Hours	20(40. 7)**
12-18 Hours	7(12. 9)
18-24 Hours	15(27. 7)*

=P <0. 05, **=P>0. 02 , P value was obtained by Z score test for proportions.

Table 7. Laboratory data in patients of acute myocardial infarction at baseline and after 4 weeks in relation to meal size

Data	Large breakfast, (n=22)		Small breakfast, (n=32	
	Baseline	After4	Baseline	After4
Lipoprotein(a)mg/dl	23.1+5.4	20.1+4.2*	22.5+4.6	19.7+4.1*
Triglycerides (mmol/L)	1.88+0.61	1.70+0.38*	1.81+0.60	1.64+0.32*
Blood glucose(mmol/l)	7.7+1.6	6.0+1.2*	6.6+1.4*	5.5+0.30*
Plasma insulin(mg/dl)	47.5+11.3	36.3+5.6**	43.2+8.8*	27.6+3.5*
TBARS(pmol/l)	1.87+0.46	1.32+0.33*	1.77+0.42	1.30+0.31*
MDA(pmol/l)	2.68+0.34	2.02+0.21*	2.66+0.33	2.01+0.21*
Diene conjugate(OD)	27.5+4.2	24.6+4.0*	26.2+4.1	24.2+3.5*
CoenzymeQ10(ug/ml)	0.21+0.02	0.32+0.23*	0.23+0.03	0.45+0.24*
Interleukin-6(pg/ml)	32.6+6.2	22.5+4.3*	27.5+5.2*	20.6+0.22*
TNF-alpha(ug/dl)	42.5+12.8	23.6+4.1*	38.2+10.6*	19.6+0.18*
	32.6+6.2	22.5+4.3*	27.5+5.2*	20.6+0.22*
	42.5+12.8	23.6+4.1*	38.2+10.6*	19.6+0.18*

* = P < 0.05,**=P<0.002, TNF=Tumour necrosis factor,MDA=malonaldehyde.

Table 8. Circadian distribution of cases in relation to 4 hourly period

Periods	Men	Women	Total
0-4 hours	6(3.7)	2(4.7)	8(3.9)
4-8 hours	58(36.2)*	22(51.7)*	80(39.6)*
8-12 hours	25(15.6)	4(9.4)	29(14.3)
12-16 hours	8(5.0)	---------	8(3.9)
16-20 hours	40(25.2)*	10(23.5)*	50(24.7)*
20-24 hours	23(14.3)	4(9.4)	27(13.3)

Values are numbers (%) *=P<0.05 P values are abtained by comparison of subjects in various sub groups of periods.

Table 9. Biochemical data in patient with acute myocardial infarction compared to healthy subject

Data	Healthy subjects (n=595)	Acute myocardial infarction (n-202)
Serum magnesium (m EQ/L)	1.64(0.25)	1.51(0.23)*
Serum potassium (m EQ/L)	4.3(0.96)	3.7(0.82)*
Vitamin C (mmol/l)	37.5(6.8)	18.6(4.3)*
Vitamin E(mmol/l)	20.1(3.7)	14.5(2.5)*
Vitamin A(mmol/l)	2.25(0.19)	1.86(0.15)*
Interleukin-6 (pg/ml)	15.6(3.2)	30.5(5.7)*
Tumour necrosis factor-alpha (pg/dl)	18.8(4.5)	41.6(8.4)*
Insulin (mg/dl)	17.6(4.2)	48.8(12.8)*

Results of a study by V. Culic suggest that pain at different body areas and other relevant symptoms more frequently follow Q-wave infarction. Both sympathetic and vagal afferent fibers can transmit cardiac pain to remote body areas due to convergence of visceral and somatic fibers on the same neurons within the central nervous system. Accordingly, a greater area of myocardial damage and more extensive stimulation of afferent fibers could induce pain sensation in a greater number of somatic regions and cause a higher frequency of other symptoms in patients with Q-wave AMI. The study also demonstrated that dyspnea was more associated with non–Q-wave infarction. A similar frequency of pulmonary congestion in 2 AMI type subsets, even in the presence of lower left ventricular ejection fraction among patients with Q-wave infarction, has been attributed to acute transient myocardial ishemia associated with non–Q-wave infarction, whereas irreversible ishemia could be the dominant mechanism of ventricular dysfunction in patients with Q-wave AMI [37].

Circadian Differences in the Site of Myocardial Infarction and in the Involved Coronary Arteries

P. Moruzzi and colleagues [27] demonstrated that 55% of the infarctions were anterior or anterolateral and 45% were inferior, including posterior or involving the right ventricle. They found that there was a slight peak in the incidence of myocardial infarction between 6 AM and noon. Anterior infarctions were more common from 6 AM to midnight, whereas inferior infarctions were more common between midnight and 6 AM.

Coronary involvement varied by the time of symptom onset among patients with inferior infarctions: right coronary artery involvement was much more common than left circumflex artery involvement among those with symptom onset from midnight to 6 AM. Among those with right coronary artery involvement, the proximal segment was more common as the site of the culprit lesion between midnight and 6 AM than between 6 AM and midnight.

The right coronary artery, which maintains its large caliber down to the crux, is characterized by slow flow velocity [38, 39]. It is possible that by decreasing the pressure gradient across a coronary artery stenosis, sleep-induced reduction in aortic pressure increases distal stasis, thereby facilitating thrombosis. This may be more of a problem in the right coronary artery than in the left coronary artery because the pressure gradient is inversely related to the fourth power of the minimum lumen diameter [27].

If the rhythmic processes that drive the circadian rhythm of myocardial-infarction onset can be identified their modification may delay or prevent the occurrence of infarction.

Circadian Rhythm and Sudden Cardiac Death

Sudden cardiac death (SCD) is natural death due to cardiac causes, heralded by abrupt loss of consciousness within 1 hour of the onset of acute symptoms in a person with or without known preexisting heart disease, but in whom the time and mode of death are unexpected. The worldwide incidence of SCD is difficult to estimate but estimates for the United States range from 300, 000 to nearly 400, 000 SCDs annually [40].

Circadian Rhythm and SCD

The biologic functions of mammals vary according to a circadian rhythm of about 24 hours, which is governed by the hypothalamus. These rhythms can be altered by disease and the actions of drugs can be affected by the time of day at which they are administered. A number of important physiological parameters such as heart rate, blood pressure, vascular reactivity, cardiac contractility, and various hemostatic factors all demonstrate a circadian pattern similar to that described for cardiovascular disorders. Circadian patterns have been observed for several supraventricular arrhythmias, premature ventricular beats, ventricular tachycardias including sudden cardiac death [41].

Sudden cardiac death has a circadian pattern, with the peak incidence occurring from 7 to 11 A. M. [42], from 7 to 9 A. M., with more sudden cardiac deaths occurring between 6 A. M. and 12 P. M. than during the other quarters of the day [43]: from 9 A. M. to 12 P. M. [44], and from 6 A. M. to 12 P. M. [45]. A study by Aronow and colleagues [46] showed that there was a circadian pattern in the number of deaths per hour in patients with CHF after prior myocardial infarction. The primary peak occurred between 6 A. M. and 12 P. M., with 39% of deaths occurring in that 6-hour period.

Flack and Yunis [47] indicate that the morning peak from 6 am to 12 noon of such occurrences as MI, thrombotic stroke, transient myocardial ischemia, and SCD is due to the high levels of coronary vasomotor tone, plasma catecholamines, and platelet aggregability, and the low levels of coronary blood flow and plasma fibrinolytic activity. At this same time, there is a rapid increase in blood pressure during the early morning hours. They also feel that it is important to maintain control of blood pressure throughout the early morning to try to avoid adverse events. A study in Auckland, New Zealand, by Van der Palen et al [48] had some slightly different findings on circadian rhythm. They report an afternoon peak in SCD (32. 5%) and a secondary morning peak (27. 6%). Also, they found a Saturday high (18. 6%) for SCD. Peckova and colleagues [49] showed a similar pattern of cardiac arrest: a low incidence at night, a sharp increase between 8 AM and noon with peaking at 10 AM, a relatively high incidence during the day, and another peak between 5 and 8 PM. Both morning and evening peaks were of a similar magnitude. Young patients had a relatively higher incidence at night than older patients and also exhibited a higher incidence in the morning than in the evening. Patients in the age category 41 to 65 years had a higher evening peak. Elderly patients maintained a rather high incidence during the daytime hours, with less pronounced peaks.

Mechanisms Underlying Sudden Cardiac Death

Cardiac arrest may have either a cardiac or a non-cardiac aetiology and may present with a variety of arrhythmias, including ventricular tachycardia, ventricular fibrillation, asystole, and electromechanical dissociation. The likelihood of a "sudden death" episode occurring and being witnessed is not constant throughout the day. Soo and colleagues [50] observed that there were three major time periods when a cardiac arrest was most likely to occur—an *early* peak in the morning around 1100 hours, a *late* peak in the evening around 2200 hours, and, for those whose arrest was from a cardiac disease, a third time period—around 1600 hours—also seemed to be critical In Seattle [51] and Berlin [52], the most important times for a cardiac arrest seemed to be around 1000 and 1800 hours. Ventricular fibrillation was most frequent around 2000 hours in the series by Peckova and colleagues[49], while Arntz and associates found that ventricular fibrillation occurred most often around 1000 hours, with the exception of ventricular fibrillation, the circadian variation of the arrest rhythm in both cardiac and non-cardiac groups appeared to be identical. The triggers for a cardiac arrest in both groups are likely to be similar when the arrhythmia is something other than ventricular fibrillation, irrespective of the aetiology of arrest [51].

Electrical Factors and Sudden Cardiac Death

The mechanisms underlying sudden cardiac death are probably multifactorial, and in some patients, primarily electrical factors or an interaction between electrical abnormalities and myocardial ischemia may be responsible for sudden cardiac death. Ambulatory recordings at the moment of sudden death have shown that ventricular tachycardia degenerating into ventricular fibrillation is a common terminal rhythm and often occurs in the absence of antecedent ischemic ST segment shifts [52]. In addition, the frequency of complex ventricular ectopy and the occurrence of sustained monomorphic ventricular tachycardia also are greatest in the early morning hours when the incidence of sudden death is greatest. Thus, a circadian variation in cardiac electrophysiological parameters may be an alternate mechanism contributing to the circadian variation in sudden death [53].

The distribution of ventricular fibrillation events followed the general pattern except that the evening peak is substantially higher than the morning peak. Peckova and colleagues [49] suggest the evening peak to be of approximately the same magnitude as the morning peak of incidence. They found that the bimodal pattern is mainly an attribute of ventricular fibrillation and that patients with asystole or pulseless electrical activity had a less pronounced evening peak. There was no difference in circadian variation between sexes, races, or days of the week. The analysis suggested that differences between the age categories are probably explicable by different rhythm distributions and thus are more likely due to sociodemographic factors than to biological differences.

Circadian Variation and Refractoriness

The circadian variation in the incidence of sudden cardiac death mainly appears to be due to variability in the time of onset of ventricular fibrillation [53]. Evidence has provided confirmation of the traditional hypothesis that ventricular fibrillation is due to multiple functional reentrant circuits, which change over time [54, 55]. Shorter refractory periods promote reentry by allowing reentrant circuits to be maintained in a smaller mass of tissue and by decreasing the length of lines of the block, leading to the variability in reentry observed during ventricular fibrillation.

Experimental studies also have demonstrated that shortening of refractory periods under a variety of conditions may be proarrhythmic [56]. In the present study, maximal shortening between hourly refractory periods as well as the shortest absolute refractory periods were observed around the hour of waking, raising the possibility of a close relation between these findings and the increased morning incidence of arrhythmic sudden death. Although not measured in this study, an increased dispersion of refractoriness, which has been shown to promote ventricular arrhythmias [57], might be expected when overall ventricular refractoriness is rapidly changing. The circadian variation in refractory periods may be associated with a circadian variation in other electrophysiological properties, such as conduction velocity, which also may promote the emergence of reentrant circuits and arrhythmias. Fluctuations in sympathetic tone are mainly responsible for temporal changes in ventricular refractoriness [53].

Studies also have shown that acute cardiac events are temporally linked to waking [58]. In the Physicians' Health Study [59], 25% of myocardial infarctions occurred within 3 hours of waking, and the relative risk of infarction during this time interval was almost twice that during any other 3-hour period during the day. In the study by Kong QT et al [53], the most pronounced changes in ventricular refractoriness were also more closely linked to the hour of waking than to the absolute time of day.

Results of the study therefore suggest that the time around waking is characterized by marked electrophysiological changes and possibly an increased vulnerability to arrhythmias.

Circadian Variation and Repolarization

The QT interval as measured on a surface ECG reflects global ventricular myocardial repolarization. A circadian variation in the QT interval has been described previously [61] and has been attributed to a circadian variation in ventricular repolarization. The QT interval has been found to be longest during sleep and shortest during the waking hours.

However, the relevance of these observations to a potential circadian variation in ventricular refractoriness is not completely clear because the refractory period and action potential duration (as reflected globally by the QT interval) may be dissociated in some situations [62].

In addition, evaluation of the QT interval at different times of the day requires a correction for heart rate, which could limit the accuracy of the analysis of circadian changes in the QT interval. Finally, unlike refractory periods that were generally reproducible to within 4 ms with the methodology used in the study by Kong QT and colleagues [53], estimation of the QT interval may be somewhat less reproducible.

Despite these potential differences, the results of the study suggest that the circadian variation in ventricular refractoriness qualitatively parallels the previously described circadian variation in the QT interval.

Yi et al [62] examined circadian variation of the QT interval in post MI patients and normal controls and its relation to SCD. They found the SCD victims did not show a significantly longer QT interval at night when compared to day as the normal subjects and MI survivors did, and the SCD victims did show a significantly longer QTc averaged over 24 hours. So, the circadian variation of the QT interval did vary when compared to normal subjects and those who survived the year following a MI.

Circadian Variation in Serum Potassium and Plasma Catecholamine Levels

Kong QT and colleagues [53] demonstrated a significant circadian variation in mean serum potassium levels, with the highest levels observed during the waking hours and the lowest levels during sleep. In eight of nine subjects, the minimum potassium levels were observed between the hours of 1:00 AM and 4:00 AM; the ninth subject had a minimum level at 2:00 PM.

A significant circadian variation was also observed in mean levels of plasma epinephrine and norepinephrine. Mean levels of each were highest during the day and lowest during sleep. A single harmonic model with a peak at 3:00 PM provided the best fit for epinephrine levels, and a double harmonic model with peaks at 9:00 AM and 9:00 PM provided the best fit for norepinephrine levels.

We also observed low levels of magnesium and potassium as well as vitamine E and C and higher levels of TBARS and MDA, which are indicators of oxidative damage, in the second quarter of the day compared to evening values.

Circadian Variation in Cardiac Events

Some of the circadian variability in the incidence of sudden death may be due to a morning increase in myocardial ischemia [63, 64, 65, 66]. However, ischemic events do not account for all instances of sudden cardiac death, as autopsy studies of sudden death victims have failed to demonstrate acute coronary lesions in up to 42% of cases [67]. Furthermore, the occurrence of sustained monomorphic ventricular tachycardia, which is not generally a consequence of acute ischemia [68], also demonstrates a substantial variation [69]. Therefore, a circadian variation in cardiac electrophysiological parameters could potentially contribute to the increased morning incidence of sudden cardiac death.

Circadian Rhythm and Stroke

Monday Preference in Onset of Ischemic Stroke

The onset of stroke has a specific temporal pattern [70], characterized by a higher frequency in winter and in the mornings. According to a meta-analysis of more than 11, 000 patients, an estimated 37% of strokes occurred during morning hours [71].

A circaseptan rhythm, with a significant peak on Mondays was observed for all strokes and for ischemic strokes.

Data from a Norwegian study [72] suggested that biochemical factors associated with cardiovascular risk—such as measures of hematosis and carbohydrate and lipid metabolism—were less favorable on Mondays compared with other days of the week. Thus, similar to the association between increased thrombophilia in the mornings [73] and the circadian pattern of other thrombotic disease such as myocardial infarction [74] and limb ischemia [75], the Monday risk of ischemic stroke may reflect an increased thrombogenic condition [76].

Circadian Variation in Acute Ischemic Stroke

The existence of a circadian rhythm in ischemic stroke has been established, with a higher frequency in the early hours of the morning. The cause of this diurnal variation is uncertain. It has been related to the circadian rhythm of fibrinolysis, platelet aggregability [77] and mainly, arterial blood pressure, with its minimum value during sleep and maximum value in the early hours in the morning, in both normotensive and hypertensive patients [78]. However, it has been suggested that an increase in morning stroke onset could be due to patients awakening with neurological deficits as a result of a stroke that could have occurred during the night [79].

A. Lago et al. [79] found a higher frequency of stroke during the day and a lower frequency between 6:01 PM and 12:00 AM, obvious in all the different types of ischemic stroke viz. lacunar, thrombotic, embolic stroke.

In acute myocardial ischemia, the time of onset is easily determined [80, 81] corresponding with the onset of thoracic pain. This does not occur when the patient with ischemic stroke is discovered upon awakening; the onset may have occurred at any time during sleep. Unfortunately, at present there is no marker that indicates the time of stroke onset.

Stroke is classified within a heterogeneous group of vascular diseases, unlike myocardial ischemia, with different ethiopathogenic mechanisms. Arterial pressure, as other factors, may play an important role, favoring an increase in morning stroke onset. But these same factors, such as lower arterial pressure and heart rate during the night may contribute, through a hemodynamic mechanism, to a stroke onset during the sleeping hours, particularly in the case of thrombotic stroke. Results of study by A. Lago et al. [79] show that thrombotic and lacunar strokes have a higher onset during sleeping hours when compared with embolic stroke. The circadian rhythm of arterial blood pressure may be disturbed in patients who have suffered from stroke.

Loss of Circadian Rhythm of Blood Pressure Following Acute Stroke

Hypertension remains a dominant risk factor and prognostic indicator in patients with stroke in all communities. The risk of stroke is directly related to elevations of blood pressure.

S. Jain et al [82] showed a pathologically reduced or abolished circadian BP variation after stroke. The absence of normal dipping results in a higher 24 hour blood pressure load and may have more target organ damage than those with normal diurnal variations of blood pressure. The epidemiology of acute stroke is different in developing countries than that in the developed world. The age at stroke, risk factors, subtypes of stroke and prognosis are different in developing countries. In India, ischemic strokes constitute 70–75% while hemorrhagic strokes account for 20-25% of total cases [82]. However, hypertension remains a dominant risk factor and prognostic indicator in patients with stroke in all communities. The risk of stroke is directly related to elevations of blood pressure.

The accurate measurement of blood pressure after an acute stroke is important because antihypertensive therapy may be considered in some patients. However, blood pressure may be falsely elevated or depressed immediately after a stroke depending on the level of consciousness, severity of neurological deficit and physical activity.

The normal diurnal variation in blood pressure i. e., nighttime dipping was abolished in 88% patients in study by Jain and colleagues [82]. This nondipping was seen equally in both hemorrhagic and ischemic subgroups without any statistically significant difference.

In studies of patients with stroke, abnormal pattern of circadian rhythm of blood pressure using ambulatory blood pressure monitoring (ABPM) has been reported [83-85]. In a different study, Dawson et al[86] found a significant reduction in diurnal variation in systolic blood pressure in cortical infarct and intracerebral hemorrhage subgroups, compared with control subjects. The subcortical infarct subgroup demonstrated only minimal reduction in normal circadian variation. Fujishima et al [87] reported that blood pressure was elevated in the acute phase of a single lacunar infarction and it declined with time. No night time fall was noted in acute phase, but the circadian variation in blood pressure normalized in the subacute and chronic phase.

Circadian Variation in the Timing of Stroke Onset

Early studies of the timing of acute stroke, however, indicated that many afflicted patients reported awakening with new neurologic deficits, and several reports indicated that acute strokes tended to occur either during the evening hours or during sleep [88]. This led to the conclusion that especially because acute therapies for stroke-in-evolution were not particularly effective, there was little reason to consider acute stroke as a medical emergency because the onset of symptoms was thought to occur during sleep, when most patients would not recognize them [89].

The highest risk is found between 8:01 AM and noon; the lowest is found between midnight and 4 AM. Because there are some reports from Japan [90], especially regarding hemorrhagic stroke [91], which suggest that there may be differences in circadian variation of stroke timing according to the subtype of stroke of interest, meta-analyses of ischemic and hemorrhagic stroke (including subarachnoid and intracerebral bleeds), and transient ischemic attack were also carried out. Results of the study by WJ Elliott and colleagues [89] suggest that for each subtype of stroke studied, there is an increase in risk during the early morning hours. The data are remarkably consistent across the various subtypes of stroke, and indicate, for ischemic stroke, hemorrhagic stroke, and even transient ischemic attacks, that the excess risk during the 6 AM to noon time period is significantly higher than would be expected by chance: 89%, 52%, and 80%. Similarly, there was a significantly lower risk of stroke during the nighttime hours (midnight to 6 AM) for each stroke subtype: 30%, 54%, and 81%.

The finding that the early morning hours (and not the nighttime hours) have the highest risk for the onset of stroke symptoms has two broad implications. The first is that patients should no longer be told that stroke symptoms are not a medical emergency. Although this may have been sound public policy when acute treatments for stroke were not available, there is now some evidence that acute emergent treatments for cerebral ischemia can be delivered in a timely fashion and result in improved long-term outcomes. The results of meta-analysis contradict older conclusions that "strokes are more likely to occur during sleep". Meta-analysis indicates that irrespective of the type of stroke, most patients will be awake when the onset of stroke symptoms occurs. The recognition of new neurologic deficits should prompt afflicted patients and their families to consider these as a medical emergency (or "brain attack"). The second implication has to do with some modalities useful in stroke prevention. Blood pressure is often considered one of the most powerful risk factors for stroke and has a circadian variation that essentially parallels the circadian variation in stroke onset. Antihypertensive agents administered in the morning ought to have a long duration of action to still have an effect on the early morning rise in blood pressure. It is tempting to speculate that antihypertensive agents that specifically target the early morning rise in blood pressure and heart rate, without reducing blood pressure severely during the night, might be more advantageous in controlling the 20% rise in blood pressure during the hours around awakening. This appears also to be the time of day associated with an increased risk of stroke, myocardial infarction, and sudden cardiac death [89].

Circadian and Seasonal Occurrence of Subarachnoid and Intracerebral Hemorrhage

Subarachnoid hemorrhage (SAH) and intracerebral hemorrhage (ICH) are associated with high morbidity and mortality, and they represent about 20% of all strokes [92].

The occurrence of cerebral infarction has been reported to vary with the time of day; cerebrovascular ischemic events predominantly occur in the early morning and late afternoon [88, 93-95]. Recently, seasonal variations in the incidence of this disorder have also been detected, the peak occurrence being in the winter and autumn [96].

In some studies, the occurrence of SAH in individuals with a history of hypertension has been reported to vary with time of day [97-99].

P.A. Nyquist et al. [96] reported that the occurrence of ICH and SAH combined was increased during the winter. However, when the hemorrhage subtypes were evaluated, the main trend for seasonal differences was noted in SAH but not in ICH.

The circadian variation of blood pressure seems to mirror the time for onset of hemorrhagic stroke in that daily increases in blood pressure occur in the morning and early afternoon and lower levels occur at night [88, 98, 100]. Some investigators have hypothesized that this increase in blood pressure may be responsible for the increase in hemorrhagic stroke frequency in the early morning and afternoon. In addition, others have noted that normotensive individuals who experience SAH or ICH may have a late-afternoon locus of onset instead of an early morning locus of onset [98]. Other authors have suggested that the occurrence of SAH and ICH during the working hours may suggest an activity precipitant for SAH or ICH [101]. Factors that might contribute to an increased risk during the winter are uncertain. However, cardiovascular stresses occur during the winter, particularly in areas with extremes of seasonal climates, which may result in fluctuations in blood pressure, blood coagulability, and cardiovascular performance. These stresses include deconditioning, stress of physical activity in temperature extremes, types of activity required in a cold climate, and more specific effects of abrupt temperature changes and temperature extremes on the blood pressure and vascular system. Inflammatory factors such as cytokine levels and cortisol levels fluctuate with a circadian and circannual rhythmicity. These factors may play a role in priming the vasculature to respond in a manner predisposing the endothelium to rupture [96].

Circadian Variation in Transient Ischaemic Attack

A metaanalysis of 31 publications reporting the circadian timing of 11,816 strokes found a 49% increase in stroke of all types between 0600 and 1200 [89]. Possible explanations for the circadian pattern of cerebrovascular events have focused on circadian or postural changes in platelet aggregation, thrombolysis, blood pressure, heart rate, and catecholamine concentrations that occur after awakening with resumption of physical and mental activities. In a minority of cases, which varies in the literature from less than 10% to as much as 44%, stroke occurs at night [88, 93, 102]. This suggests that sleep, although "protective" for most cerebrovascular events, may represent a vulnerable state for a subset of patients at risk for stroke. Nocturnal blood pressure swings, cardiac arrhythmias, and sleep disordered breathing have been suggested as possible explanations for the nocturnal onset of stroke. Not only acute ischaemic stroke but also transient ischaemic attacks have a circadian pattern with a peak of onset between 0600 and 1200 and about 20% of events occurring at night time [103-105]. Furthermore, it is shown for the first time that patients with daytime and night time onset of transient ischaemic attack/stroke are similar with regard to most cardiovascular risk factors; clinical and polysomnographic sleep characteristics; and stroke parameters.

Findings by C. Bassetti et al. [106] suggest that low diastolic blood pressure values may predispose to nighttime onset of cerebrovascular events enhancing the sleep related fall in blood pressure.

Onset of Transient Ischaemic Attack/Stroke and Sleep Characteristics

Sleep disordered breathing is present in about 50% of patients with acute cerebrovascular diseases [107, 108]. Sleep apnoea—while being a risk factor for stroke [109, 110]—may only rarely represent the immediate cause of transient ischaemic attack or stroke. Rather, respiratory events during sleep may cause haemodynamic and haematological changes which increase the risk of cerebrovascular events at the transition from sleep to wakefulness and during the subsequent few hours.

It is nevertheless conceivable that in a patient with severe sleep apnoea swings in blood pressure, decreased cerebral blood flow, and cardiac arrhythmias produced by respiratory events may trigger cardiovascular and cerebrovascular events during sleep [106].

Onset of Transient Ischaemic Attack/Stroke and Stroke Characteristics

In a study of 1,233 patients, Lago et al [79] also found a higher frequency of all types of stroke during the day and a higher night time onset in macroangiopathy and microangiopathy compared with other stroke subtypes. Macroangiopathic and microangiopathic strokes may be particularly susceptible to nocturnal haemodynamic changes and decreased cerebral perfusion. Although yet to be proved, it is possible that intrathoracic pressure variations related to sleep apnoea may also predispose to cardioembolic strokes secondary to right-left shunt (for example, patent foramen ovale).

C. Bassetti et al. [106] have thus proven that [107] night time and daytime transient ischaemic attack/ stroke are similar in sleep and stroke characteristics, and [70, 71] diastolic hypotension may predispose to night time cerebrovascular events.

Nonpharmacological Treatment

Nonpharmacological management of circadian rhythm with yoga, physical activity, moderate alcohol intake, functional foods such as almonds, walnuts, rape seed oil, and neutraceuticals, eg coenzyme Q10 and w-3 fatty acids appear to be protective against circadian rhythms of cardiovascular events.

Pharmacotherapy

The concept of homeostasis in biology postulates that there is constancy of the intern milieu. Thus, it is assumed the risk and exacerbation of disease are invariable and independent of the time of day, day of month, and month of year as are the responses of patients to diagnostic tests and medications. Findings from the field of chronobiology, the study of biological rhythms, challenge the concept of homeostasis and the many assumptions and procedures of clinical medicine based on it. It is now recognized that human functions have daily, weekly, monthly and yearly biological rhythms. Plants, animals, and insects also have chronobiological rhythms. Circadian patterns have been observed for a variety of cardiovascular disorders, including cardiac arrhythmias, sudden cardiac death, cerebrovascular events, episodes of stable angina, unstable angina and acute myocardial infarction. The morning predominance of these events has been well documented in a number of large population studies. It is now recognized that circadian and other rhythms of the gastrointestinal tract and vital organs are capable of significantly affecting the pharmacokinetics and dynamics of cardiovascular and other medications. This means that the effects of therapeutic interventions administered in identical doses in the morning versus the evening may not be equivalent. The prevention and treatment of cardiovascular disease must take into account chronobiological factors [111].

CHRONOTHERAPEUTICS

Chronotherapeutics is the delivery of drugs at levels that match the body's needs at certain times of day or night. Chronotherapy links the effects of a disease to time, and thus the timing of drug delivery. The main objective of chronotherapy for heart disease would be to deliver needed drugs in higher concentrations during the time they are needed the most (early morning after-waking period) ; and at reduced drug levels when the need is less (during the middle of the sleep cycle) [112].

The goal of chronotherapeutics is to match the timing of treatment with the intrinsic timing of illness. Theoretically, optimum therapy is more likely to result when the right amount of drug is delivered to the correct target organ at the most appropriate time. In contrast, many side effects can be minimized if a drug is not given when it is not needed [113].

TIME-TAILORED DRUGS

Many drugs display normal, reproducible daily variations in pharmacokinetics and pharmacodynamics. Lemmer identified more than 100 drugs that display significant variation in concentrations or effects, or both, over 24 hours. Perhaps the best example is heparin. Even when it is administered at a constant infusion rate, the activated partial thromboplastin time and the risk of bleeding vary significantly according to the hour of the day and are higher at night [114]. The narrower the therapeutic window (i.e., risk-benefit ratio) for a specific drug, the more important the implication of the circadian variation in plasma levels [110].

Selected Medications Exhibiting Circadian Variations in Pharmacokinetic and Pharmacodynamic Action

Cardiovascular agents

- Enalapril
- Diltiazem HCl
- Nifedipine
- Propranolol HCl
- Verapamil

Antiasthmatic agents

- Terbutaline sulfate
- Theophylline

- Gastrointestinal agents:
- Cimetidine
- Omeprazole

Nonsteroidal anti-inflammatory drugs

- Acetylsalicylic acid
- Indomethacin
- Ketoprofen

Anticancer agents

- Cisplatin
- Doxorubicin
- Methotrexate

Other

- Diazepam
- Haloperidol

In selecting the most appropriate treatment for diseases that can be managed with chronotherapy, clinicians should understand that pharmacodynamic profiles of chronotherapeutic formulations are often different from those of traditional homeostatic formulations, even when the active drug itself is the same. Such differences may have important clinical consequences. Unlike homeostatic formulations, which provide relatively constant plasma drug levels over 24 hours, chronotherapeutic formulations may use various release mechanisms (e.g., time-delay coatings, osmotic pump mechanisms, matrix systems) that provide for varying levels throughout the day [115].

Potential Role of Chronotherapy in Cardiovascular Diseases

Angiotensin Converting Enzyme Inhibitors

In one study, an ACE inhibitor was dosed either in the early morning or at bedtime in 18 patients with moderately high blood pressure. Palatini et al showed that nighttime dosing resulted in a greater effect on nighttime pressure than morning dosing. There was no difference in daytime pressure between the 2 groups. Measurement of ACE activity showed that nighttime dosing caused a more even, lasting reduction in blood levels of ACE.

In contrast to the ACE inhibitor study, studies with the beta-blocker atenolol, and the calcium channel blockers nifedipine and amlodipine, showed no different effects on pressure when dosed in the morning versus evening. Like many such studies, too few patients were studied to draw strong conclusions.

It is obvious, though, that drug class, formulation, and size of dose have a large influence on the effect seen [116].

Calcium Channel Blockers

In a study by Yosefy and colleagues from Israel it was found that long acting calcium channel blockers prevent the rise in blood pressure in morning hours and decreased the incidence of stroke by around 50%; thus providing a comprehensive cover during the dangerous hours in the morning [117].

Currently, preparations of verapamil hydrochloride are recommended for dosing at night to provide higher drug levels in the morning, when blood pressure, heart rate, and the risk of cardiovascular events are highest. Studies in hypertension [118] and angina pectoris [119] have demonstrated the benefits of a chronotherapeutic approach to these conditions.

Aspirin

The Physicians' Health Study, a randomized, double-blind, placebo-controlled trial of alternate-day aspirin intake (325 mg) among 22, 071 US male physicians, afforded the opportunity to assess this circadian pattern and examine whether it is altered by aspirin therapy. During a 5-year period of follow-up, 342 cases of nonfatal myocardial infarction were confirmed, of which the time of onset was available in 211 (62%). In the aspirin group, circadian variation was minimal, due primarily to a marked reduction in the morning peak of infarction. Specifically, aspirin was associated with a 59. 3% reduction in the incidence of infarction during the morning waking hours, compared with a 34. 1% reduction for the remaining hours of the day. The greater reduction was observed during the 3-hour interval immediately after awakening, a period with a risk of infarction twice that of any other comparable time interval. Aspirin intake was associated with a mean reduction in the incidence of infarction of 44. 8% over the entire 24-hour cycle. Aspirin reduces the risk of infarction by inhibiting platelet aggregation during the critical periods [118].

Beta Blockers

Drugs may suppress diurnal variation, specifically b-blockers [120, 121], antiarrhythmic drugs, and aspirin. The fact that b-blockers suppress circadian variation of myocardial infarction was already noted in several studies. If b-blockers also suppress circadian variation of cardiac arrests, we would expect that the interval between the times of day of the two arrests would widen, because the expected difference between the arrest times if no circadian variation is present is larger than in the presence of circadian variation [121].

CONCLUSION

The recognition of circadian rhythms in both normal human biologic function and disease has heightened awareness that the timing of drug regimens may have an important impact on effectiveness of treatment. Outcomes in several diseases that have predictable circadian variations have been improved by matching the timing of medication use to the circadian rhythm of the illness.

REFERENCES

[1] Singh, RB;Weydahl, K;Otsuka K et al. Can nutrition influence circadian rhythm and heart rate variability? *Biomed Pharmacother* 2001, 55:(Supple)115-24.

[2] Singh, RB;Kartik, C;Otsuka K;Pella D;Pella J. Brain-heart connection and the risk of heart attack. (Editorial). *Biomed Pharmacother* 2002, 56:(Supple)257-265

[3] Otsuka, K;Cornelissen, G;Halberg, F. Circadian rhythms and clinical chronobiology. *Biomed Pharmacother* 2001, 55:(Supple)7-18.

[4] Halberg, F;Stephens, AN. Susceptibility to quabain and physiologic circadian periodicity. *Proc Minn acad Sci* 1959;27:139-43.

[5] Halberg F;Visscher MB. Regular diurnal physiological variation in eosinophil levels in five stocks of mice. *Proc Soc Exp Biol* (NY)1950, 75:846-47.

[6] Downing D. The history of man in four diets, editorial. *J Nutr Environ Med* 2003, 13:139-41.

[7] Trowell HC, Burkitt DP(eds). *Western Disease:their emergence and prevention.* London, Edward Arnold, 1981.

[8] Eaton SB, Strassman BI, Nesse RM et al. Evolutionary health promotion. *Prev Med* 2002, 34:109-18.

[9] Simopoulos AP. Genetic variation and dietary response:Nutrigenetics/nutrigenomics. *Asia Pac J Clin Nutr* 2002, 11(S6):117-128.

[10] Otsuka K, Shohgo M, Kozo M, Zi-yan Z, Weydahl A, Hansen TL. et al. Chronomes, aging and disease. In Furukawa H, Nishibuchi M, Kono Y, Kaida Y editors;*Ecological Destruction, Health and Development:Advancing Asian Paradigms*, 2004, p 367-94.

[11] Singh RB, Pella D, Rastogi S, Sharma JP, K Kartikey, Goyal VK et al. Increased concentrations of lipoprotein(a), circadian rhythms, and metabolic reactants evoked by acute myocardial infarction in relation to large breakfast. *Biomed Pharmacother* 2004, 58(Supplement):116-122.

[12] Singh RB, Pella D, Neki NS, Chandel JP, Gupta P, Rastogi S et al. Mechanism of acute myocardial infarcion(MAMI) study. *Biomed Pharmacother*, 2004, 58(Supplement): 111-115.

[13] Singh RB, Cornelissen G, Weydahl A, Schwartzkopft O, Katinas G, Otsuka K et al, Circadian heart rate and blood pressure variability considered for research and patient care. *Int J Cardiol* 2003, 87:9-28.

[14] Czeisler CA, Johnson MP, Duffy JF, Brown EN, Rondo JM, Kronauer RE. Exposure to bright light and darkness to treat physiologic maladaptaion to night work. *N Engl J Med* 1990, 18:1253-59.

[15] Tei H, Okamura H, Shigeyoshi Y, Fukuhara C , Ozawa R, Hirose M, Sakaki Y. Circadian oscillation of a mammalian homologue of the Drosophila period gene. *Nature* 1997, 389, pp512-516.

[16] Tofler GH, Stone PH, Maclure M, Edelman E, Davis VG, Robertson T, Antman EM, Muller JE. Analysis of possible triggers of myocardial infarction(The MILIS Study). *Am J Cardiol* 1990, 66:22-27.

[17] Willich SN, Loewel H, Lewis M, Arntz R, Baur R, Winther K, Keil U, Shroeder R, TRIMM study group. Association of wake time and the onset of infarction. *Z Kardiol* 1991, 80(suppl 3):105-10.

[18] Tofler GH, Brezenski D, Schafer AI, Czeisler CA, Rutherford JD, Willich SN, Gleason RE, Williams GH, Mullar JE. Concurrent morning increase in platelet aggregability and the risk of myocardial infarction and sudden cardiac death. *N Engl J Med* 1987, 316:1514-18.

[19] Kozak M. Circadian rhythms in cardiovascular diseases, ischemic heart disease . *Vnitr Lek.* 2003 Apr;49(4):302-7.

[20] Un S, Baulmann J, Weisser B, Dusing R, Vetter H, Mengden T. Circadian rhythm of silent myocardial ischemia. Why morning is so risky for hypertensive patients. *MMW Fortschr Med.* 2003 Nov 20;145(47):34-8.

[21] Li JJ. Circadian variation in myocardial ischemia:the possible mechanisms involving in this phenomenon. *Med Hypotheses*. 2003 Aug;61(2):240-3.

[22] Li JJ; Huang CX; Fang CH; Chen F; Jiang H; Tang QZ; Li GS. Circadian variation in ischemic threshold in patients with stable angina: relation to plasma endothelin-1. *Angiology* - 01-Jul-2002; 53(4): 409-13.

[23] Kawano H; Motoyama T; Yasue H; Hirai N; Waly HM; Kugiyama K; Ogawa H. Endothelial function fluctuates with diurnal variation in the frequency of ischemic episodes in patients with variant angina. *J Am Coll Cardiol* - 17-Jul-2002; 40(2): 266-70

[24] Wennerblom B; Lurje L; Karlsson T; Tygesen H; Vahisalo R; Hjalmarson A. Circadian variation of heart rate variability and the rate of autonomic change in the morning hours in healthy subjects and angina patients. *Int J Cardiol* - 01-Jun-2001; 79(1): 61-9.

[25] Antman ME, Braunwald E. Acute myocardial infarction. In Braunwald (Eds.): *Heart disease: A Textbook of Cardiovascular Medicine 6th ed*; Philadelphia, W. B. Saunders Company, 2001, p. 1114.

[26] MILIS Study Group. Muller JE, Stone PH, Turi ZG, Rutherford JD, Czeisler CA, Parker C, Poole WK, Passamani E, Roberts R, Robertson T. Circadian variation in the frequency of onset of acute myocardial infarction. *N Engl J Med* 1985;313:1315-22.

[27] Moruzzi P, Marenzi G, Callegari S, Contini M. Circadian distribution of acute myocardial infarction by anatomic location and coronary artery involvement. *Am J Med.* 2004 Jan 1;116(1):24-7.

[28] Kirby DA, Verrier RL. Differential effects of sleep stage on coronary hemodynamic function. *Am J Physiol* 1989;256:H1378-83.

[29] Verrier RL, Dickerson LW. Autonomic nervous system and coronary blood flow changes related to emotional activation and sleep. *Circulation* 1991;83 (suppl II):II-81-9.

[30] Muller JE, Tofler GH, Stone PH. Circadian variation and triggers of onset of acute cardiovascular disease. *Circulation* 1989;79:733-43.

[31] Tanaka A, Kawarabayashi T, Fukuda D, Nishibori Y, Sakamoto T, Nishida Y, Shimada K, Yoshikawa J. Circadian variation of plaque rupture in acute myocardial infarction. *Am J Cardiol.* 2004 Jan 1;93(1):1-5.

[32] Millar-Craig MW, Bishop CN, Raftery EB. Circadian variation of blood-pressure. *Lancet* 1978;1:795-7.

[33] Fujita M, Franklin D. Diurnal changes in coronary blood flow in conscious dogs. *Circulation* 1987;76:488-91

[34] Pristipino C, Beltrame JF, Finocchiaro ML, Hattori R, Fujita M, Mongiardo R, Cianflone D, Sanna T, Sasayama S, Maseri A. Major racial differences in coronary constrictor response between Japanese and Caucasians with recent myocardial infarction. *Circulation* 2000;101:1102-8.

[35] Grines CL, Booth DC, Nissen SE, Gurley JC, Bennett KA, O'Connor WN, DeMaria AN. Mechanism of acute myocardial infarction in patients with prior coronary artery bypass grafting and therapeutic implications. *Am J Cardiol* 1990;65:1292-6.

[36] Culic V, Miric D, Eterovic D. Different circumstances, timing, and symptom presentation at onset of Q-wave versus non-Q-wave acute myocardial infarction. *Am J Cardiol.* 2002 Feb 15;89(4):456-60.

[37] Benhorin J., Moss A. J., Oakes D. , Marcus F. , Greenberg H. , Dwyer Jr E. M., Algeo S. , Hahn E.. Multicenter Diltiazem Post-Infarction Group. The prognostic significance of first myocardial infarction type (Q wave versus non-Q wave) and Q wave location. *J Am Coll Cardiol* 1990;15:1201-7.

[38] Ofili EO, Labovitz AJ, Kern MJ. Coronary flow velocity dynamics in normal and diseased arteries. *Am J Cardiol* 1993;71:3D-9D.

[39] Anderson HV, Stokes MJ, Leon M, Abu-Halawa SA, Stuart Y, Kirkeeide RL. Coronary artery flow velocity is related to lumen area and regional left ventricular mass. *Circulation 2000*;102:48-54.

[40] Myerburg JR, Castellanos A. Cardiac arrest and sudden cardiac death. In Braunwald (Eds.): *Heart disease: A Textbook of Cardiovascular Medicine 4th ed*; Philadelphia, W. B. Saunders Company, 2001, p. 756.

[41] Kozak M. Circadian rhythms in cardiovascular diseases—arrhythmias. *Vnitr Lek.* 2003 Apr;49(4):297-301

[42] Muller JE; Ludmer PL; Willich SN; Tofler GH; Aylmer G; Klangos I; Stone PH. Circadian variation in the frequency of sudden cardiac death. *Circulation* - 01-Jan-1987; 75(1): 131-8

[43] Willich SN; Levy D; Rocco MB; Tofler GH; Stone PH; Muller JE. Circadian variation in the incidence of sudden cardiac death in the Framingham Heart Study population. *Am J Cardiol* - 1-Oct-1987; 60(10): 801-6.

[44] Willich SN; Goldberg RJ; Maclure M; Perriello L; Muller JE. Increased onset of sudden cardiac death in the first three hours after awakening. *Am J Cardiol* - 1-Jul-1992; 70(1): 65-8

[45] Levine RL; Pepe PE; Fromm RE Jr; Curka PA; Clark PA. Prospective evidence of a circadian rhythm for out-of-hospital cardiac arrests. *JAMA* - 3-Jun-1992; 267(21):2935-7

[46] Aronow WS, Ahn C. Circadian variation of death from congestive heart failure after prior myocardial infarction in patients >60 years of age. *Am J Cardiol.* 2003 Dec 1;92 (11):1354-5.

[47] Flack JM, Yunis C. Therapeutic implications of the epidemiology and timing of myocardial infarction and other cardiovascular diseases. *J Hum Hypertens.* 1997 Jan;11(1):23-8.

[48] Van der Palen J, Doggen CJ, Beaglehole R. Variation in the time and day of onset of myocardial infarction and sudden death. *N Z Med J.* 1995 Aug 25;108 (1006):332-4.

[49] Peckova M; Fahrenbruch CE; Cobb LA; Hallstrom AP. Circadian Variations in the Occurrence of Cardiac Arrests: Initial and Repeat Episodes. *Circulation.* 1998;98:31-39.

[50] Soo L H, Gray D, Young T, Hampton JR. Circadian variation in witnessed out of hospital cardiac arrest. *Heart* 2000;84:370–376.

[51] Arntz HR, Willich SN, Oeff M, Bruggemann T, Stern R, Heinzmann A, Matenaer B, Schroder R. Circadian variation of sudden cardiac death reflects age-related variability in ventricular fibrillation. *Circulation.* 1993 Nov;88(5 Pt 1):2284-9.

[52] Leclercq JF, Maisonblanche P, Cauchemez B, Coumel P. Respective role of sympathetic tone and of cardiac pauses in the genesis of 62 cases of ventricular fibrillation recorded during Holter monitoring. *Eur Heart J.* 1988 Dec;9 (12):1276-83.

[53] Thomas Q. Kong, Jr, Jeffrey J. Goldberger, Michele Parker, RN, Ted Wang, Alan H. Kadish. Circadian Variation in Human Ventricular Refractoriness. *Circulation.* 1995;92:1507-1516.

[54] Cha YM, Birgersdotter-Green U, Wolf PL, Peters BB, Chen PS. The mechanism of termination of reentrant activity in ventricular fibrillation. *Circ Res.* 1994 Mar;74(3):495-506.

[55] Frazier DW, Wolf PD, Wharton JM, Tang AS, Smith WM, Ideker RE. Stimulus-induced critical point. Mechanism for electrical initiation of reentry in normal canine myocardium. *J Clin Invest.* 1989 Mar;83(3):1039-52.

[56] Sheridan DJ, Culling W. Electrophysiological effects of alpha-adrenoceptor stimulation in normal and ischemic myocardium. *J Cardiovasc Pharmacol.* 1985;7 Suppl 5:S55-60.

[57] Kuo CS, Atarashi H, Reddy CP, Surawicz B. Dispersion of ventricular repolarization and arrhythmia: study of two consecutive ventricular premature complexes. *Circulation.* 1985 Aug;72(2):370-6.

[58] Goldberg RJ, Brady P, Muller JE, Chen ZY, de Groot M, Zonneveld P, Dalen JE. Time of onset of symptoms of acute myocardial infarction. *Am J Cardiol.* 1990 Jul 15;66(2):140-4.

[59] Ridker PM, Manson JE, Buring JE, Muller JE, Hennekens CH. Circadian variation of acute myocardial infarction and the effect of low-dose aspirin in a randomized trial of physicians. *Circulation.* 1990 Sep;82(3):897-902.

[60] Bexton RS, Vallin HO, Camm AJ. Diurnal variation of the QT interval--influence of the autonomic nervous system. *Br Heart J.* 1986 Mar;55(3):253-8.

[61] Rozanski GJ, Jalife J, Moe GK. Determinants of postrepolarization refractoriness in depressed mammalian ventricular muscle. *Circ Res.* 1984 Oct;55(4):486-96.

[62] Yi G, Guo XH, Reardon M, Gallagher MM, Hnatkova K, Camm AJ, Malik M. Circadian variation of the QT interval in patients with sudden cardiac death after myocardial infarction. *Am J Cardiol.* 1998 Apr 15;81(8):950-6.

[63] Tofler GH, Brezinski D, Schafer AI, Czeisler CA, Rutherford JD, Willich SN, Gleason RE, Williams GH, Muller JE. Concurrent morning increase in platelet aggregability and the risk of myocardial infarction and sudden cardiac death. *N Engl J Med.* 1987 Jun 11;316(24):1514-8.

[64] Muller JE, Stone PH, Turi ZG, Rutherford JD, Czeisler CA, Parker C, Poole WK, Passamani E, Roberts R, Robertson T, et al. Circadian variation in the frequency of onset of acute myocardial infarction. *N Engl J Med*. 1985 Nov 21;313(21):1315-22.

[65] Willich SN, Linderer T, Wegscheider K, Leizorovicz A, Alamercery I, Schroder R. Increased morning incidence of myocardial infarction in the ISAM Study: absence with prior beta-adrenergic blockade. ISAM Study Group. *Circulation*. 1989 Oct;80(4):853-8.

[66] Fujita M, Franklin D. Diurnal changes in coronary blood flow in conscious dogs. *Circulation*. 1987 Aug;76(2):488-91.

[67] Roberts WC. Qualitative and quantitative comparison of amounts of narrowing by atherosclerotic plaques in the major epicardial coronary arteries at necropsy in sudden coronary death, transmural acute myocardial infarction, transmural healed myocardial infarction and unstable angina pectoris. *Am J Cardiol*. 1989 Aug 1;64(5):324-8.

[68] Davies MJ, Bland JM, Hangartner JR, Angelini A, Thomas AC. Factors influencing the presence or absence of acute coronary artery thrombi in sudden ischaemic death. *Eur Heart J*. 1989 Mar;10(3):203-8.

[69] Lampert R, Rosenfeld L, Batsford W, Lee F, McPherson C. Circadian variation of sustained ventricular tachycardia in patients with coronary artery disease and implantable cardioverter-defibrillators. *Circulation*. 1994 Jul;90(1):241-7.

[70] Manfredini R, Gallerani M, Portaluppi F, Salmi R, Fersini C. Chronobiological patterns of onset of acute cerebrovascular diseases. *Thromb Res*. 1997 Dec 15;88(6):451-63.

[71] Elliott WJ. Circadian variation in the timing of stroke onset: a meta-analysis. *Stroke*. 1998 May;29(5):992-6.

[72] Urdal P, Anderssen SA, Holme I, Hjermann I, Mundal HH, Haaland A, Torjesen P. Monday and non-Monday concentrations of lifestyle-related blood components in the Oslo Diet and Exercise Study. *J Intern Med*. 1998 Dec;244(6):507-13.

[73] Brezinski DA, Tofler GH, Muller JE, Pohjola-Sintonen S, Willich SN, Schafer AI, Czeisler CA, Williams GH. Morning increase in platelet aggregability. Association with assumption of the upright posture. *Circulation*. 1988 Jul;78(1):35-40.

[74] Cohen MC, Rohtla KM, Lavery CE, Muller JE, Mittleman MA. Meta-analysis of the morning excess of acute myocardial infarction and sudden cardiac death. *Am J Cardiol*. 1997 Jun 1;79(11):1512-6.

[75] Manfredini R, Gallerani M, Portaluppi F, Salmi R, Zamboni P, Fersini C. Circadian variation in the onset of acute critical limb ischemia. *Thromb Res*. 1998 Nov 15;92(4):163-9.

[76] Manfredini R, Casetta I, Paolino E, la Cecilia O, Boari B, Fallica E, Granieri E. Monday preference in onset of ischemic stroke. *Am J Med*. 2001 Oct 1;111(5):401-3.

[77] Kelly-Hayes M, Wolf PA, Kase CS, Brand FN, McGuirk JM, D'Agostino RB. Temporal patterns of stroke onset. The Framingham Study. *Stroke*. 1995 Aug;26(8):1343-7.

[78] Millar-Craig MW, Bishop CN, Raftery EB. Circadian variation of blood-pressure. *Lancet*. 1978 Apr 15;1(8068):795-7.

[79] Lago A, Geffner D, Tembl J, Landete L, Valero C, Baquero M. Circadian variation in acute ischemic *stroke*: a hospital-based study. *Stroke*. 1998 Sep;29(9):1873-5.

[80] Quyyumi AA. Circadian rhythms in cardiovascular disease. *Am Heart J*. 1990 Sep;120(3):726-33.

[81] Muller JE, Tofler GH, Stone PH. Circadian variation and triggers of onset of acute cardiovascular disease. *Circulation*. 1989 Apr;79(4):733-43.
[82] Jain S, Namboodri KK, Kumari S, Prabhakar S. Loss of circadian rhythm of blood pressure following acute stroke. *BMC Neurol*. 2004 Jan 6;4(1):1.
[83] Collins R, MacMahon S. Blood pressure, antihypertensive drug treatment and the risks of stroke and of coronary heart disease. *Br Med Bull*. 1994 Apr;50(2):272-98.
[84] Sander D, Klingelhofer J. Changes of circadian blood pressure patterns after hemodynamic and thromboembolic brain infarction. *Stroke*. 1994 Sep;25(9):1730-7.
[85] Yamamoto Y, Akiguchi I, Oiwa K, Satoi H, Kimura J. Diminished nocturnal blood pressure decline and lesion site in cerebrovascular disease. *Stroke*. 1995 May; 26 (5):829-33.
[86] Dawson SL, Evans SN, Manktelow BN, Fotherby MD, Robinson TG, Potter JF. Diurnal blood pressure change varies with stroke subtype in the acute phase. *Stroke*. 1998 Aug;29(8):1519-24.
[87] Fujishima S, Abe I, Okada Y, Saku Y, Sadoshima S, Fujishima M. Serial changes in blood pressure and neurohormone levels after the onset of lacunar stroke. *Angiology*. 1996 Jun;47(6):579-87.
[88] Marshall J. Diurnal variation in occurrence of strokes. *Stroke*. 1977 Mar-Apr;8(2):230-1.
[89] Elliott WJ. Circadian variation in the timing of stroke onset: a meta-analysis. *Stroke*. 1998 May;29(5):992-6.
[90] Hayashi S, Toyoshima H, Tanabe N, Miyanishi K. Daily peaks in the incidence of sudden cardiac death and fatal stroke in Niigata Prefecture. *Jpn Circ J*. 1996 Apr;60(4):193-200.
[91] Vermeer SE, Rinkel GJ, Algra A. Circadian fluctuations in onset of subarachnoid hemorrhage. New data on aneurysmal and perimesencephalic hemorrhage and a systematic review. *Stroke*. 1997 Apr;28(4):805-8.
[92] Brown RD, Whisnant JP, Sicks JD, O'Fallon WM, Wiebers DO. Stroke incidence, prevalence, and survival: secular trends in Rochester, Minnesota, through 1989. *Stroke*. 1996 Mar;27(3):373-80.
[93] Van der Windt C; Van Gijn J. Cerebral infarction does not occur typically at night. *J Neurol Neurosurg Psychiatry* - 01-Jan-1988; 51(1): 109-11.
[94] Wolf PA, Caplan LR, Foulkes MA. Morning increase in onset of ischemic stroke. *Stroke*. 1989 Apr;20(4):473-6.
[95] Argentino C, Toni D, Rasura M, Violi F, Sacchetti ML, Allegretta A, Balsano F, Fieschi C. Circadian variation in the frequency of ischemic stroke. *Stroke*. 1990 Mar;21(3):387-9.
[96] Nyquist PA, Brown RD Jr, Wiebers DO, Crowson CS, O'Fallon WM. Circadian and seasonal occurrence of subarachnoid and intracerebral hemorrhage. *Neurology*. 2001 Jan 23;56(2):190-3.
[97] Sloan MA, Price TR, Foulkes MA, Marler JR, Mohr JP, Hier DB, Wolf PA, Caplan LR. Circadian rhythmicity of stroke onset. Intracerebral and subarachnoid hemorrhage. *Stroke*. 1992 Oct;23(10):1420-6.
[98] Kleinpeter G, Schatzer R, Bock F. Is blood pressure really a trigger for the circadian rhythm of subarachnoid hemorrhage? *Stroke*. 1995 Oct;26(10):1805-10.

[99] Gallerani M, Manfredini R, Ricci L, Cocurullo A, Goldoni C, Bigoni M, Fersini C. Chronobiological aspects of acute cerebrovascular diseases. *Acta Neurol Scand.* 1993 Jun;87(6):482-7.

[100] Rautaharju PM, Manolio TA, Furberg CD, Siscovick D, Newman AB, Borhani NO, Gardin JM. Ischemic episodes in 24-h ambulatory electrocardiograms of elderly persons: the Cardiovascular Health Study. *Int J Cardiol.* 1995 Sep;51(2):165-75.

[101] Vermeer SE, Rinkel GJ, Algra A. Circadian fluctuations in onset of subarachnoid hemorrhage. New data on aneurysmal and perimesencephalic hemorrhage and a systematic review. *Stroke.* 1997 Apr;28(4):805-8.

[102] Chamorro A, Vila N, Ascaso C, Elices E, Schonewille W, Blanc R. Blood pressure and functional recovery in acute ischemic stroke. *Stroke.* 1998 Sep;29(9):1850-3.

[103] Marsh EE 3rd, Biller J, Adams HP Jr, Marler JR, Hulbert JR, Love BB, Gordon DL. Circadian variation in onset of acute ischemic stroke. *Arch Neurol.* 1990 Nov;47(11):1178-80.

[104] Wroe SJ, Sandercock P, Bamford J, Dennis M, Slattery J, Warlow C. Diurnal variation in incidence of stroke: Oxfordshire community stroke project. *BMJ.* 1992 Jan 18;304(6820):155-7.

[105] Haapaniemi H, Hillbom M, Juvela S. Weekend and holiday increase in the onset of ischemic stroke in young women. *Stroke.* 1996 Jun;27(6):1023-7.

[106] Bassetti C, Aldrich M. Night time versus daytime transient ischaemic attack and ischaemic stroke: a prospective study of 110 patients. *J Neurol Neurosurg Psychiatry.* 1999 Oct;67(4):463-7.

[107] Bassetti C, Aldrich MS, Chervin RD, Quint D. Sleep apnea in patients with transient ischemic attack and stroke: a prospective study of 59 patients. *Neurology.* 1996 Nov;47(5):1167-73.

[108] Dyken ME, Somers VK, Yamada T, Ren ZY, Zimmerman MB. Investigating the relationship between stroke and obstructive sleep apnea. *Stroke.* 1996 Mar;27(3):401-7.

[109] Palomaki H, Partinen M, Erkinjuntti T, Kaste M. Snoring, sleep apnea syndrome, and stroke. *Neurology.* 1992 Jul;42(7 Suppl 6):75-81; discussion 82.

[110] Partinen M. Ischaemic stroke, snoring and obstructive sleep apnoea. *J Sleep Res.* 1995 Jun;4(S1):156-159.

[111] Kozák M. Use of chronobiology findings in therapy of cardiovascular diseases. *Vnitr Lek.* 2003 Apr;49(4): 308-13.

[112] Sica DA, White W. Chronotherapeutics and Its Role in the Treatment of Hypertension and Cardiovascular Disease. *J Clin Hypertens* 2000; 2(4):279-286.

[113] Elliott WJ. Timing treatment to the rhythm of disease: a short course in chronotherapeutics. *Postgrad Med* 2001;110(2):119-29.

[114] Reinberg AE. Concepts of circadian chronopharmacology. *Ann N Y Acad Sci* 1991;618:102-15.

[115] Bhalla A, Singh R, Sachdev A, D'Cruz S, Duseja A. Circadian pattern in cerebro vascular disorders. *Neurol India* 2002;50:526-7.

[116] White WB, Black HR, Weber MA, et al. Comparison of effects of controlled onset extended release verapamil at bedtime and nifedipine gastrointestinal therapeutic system on arising on early morning blood pressure, heart rate, and the heart rate-blood pressure product. *Am J Cardiol* 1998;81:421-31

[117] Frishman WH, Glasser S, Stone P, et al. Comparison of controlled-onset extended-release verapamil with amlodipine and amlodipine plus atenolol on exercise performance and ambulatory ischemia in patients with chronic stable angina pectoris. *Am J Cardiol* 1999;83:507-14.

[118] Ridker PM, Manson JE, Buring JE, Muller JE and Hennekens CH. Circadian variation of acute myocardial infarction and the effect of low-dose aspirin in a randomized trial of physicians. *Circulation.* 1990 Sep;82(3):897-902.

[119] Willich SN, Linderer T, Wegscheider K, Leizorovicz A, Alamercery I and Schroder R. Increased morning incidence of myocardial infarction in the ISAM Study: absence with prior beta-adrenergic blockade. ISAM Study Group. *Circulation* 1989;80:853– 858.

[120] Kupari M, Koskinen P, Leinonen H. Double-peaking circadian variation in the occurrence of sustained supraventricular tachyarrhythmias. *Am Heart J.* 1990 Dec;120(6 Pt 1):1364-9.

[121] Peckova M; Fahrenbruch CE; Cobb LA; Hallstrom AP. Circadian Variations in the Occurrence of Cardiac Arrests: Initial and Repeat Episodes. *Circulation.* 1998; 98:31-39.

[122] Singh RB, Niaz MA, Cornelissen G, Otsuka K, Siegelova J, Fiser B, Halberg F. Circadian rhythmicity of circulating vitamin concentrations. *Scripta Medica (BRONO)*, 2001, 74:93-96.

In: World Heart Research Yearbook. Volume 1
Editors: Franz Halberg and R. B. Singh
ISBN: 978-1-60741-881-8

Decreased Potential of Mitochondria May Increase Risk of Cardiovascular Disease

***Dasa Dudova*[1], *Daniel Pella*[1,*], *Rajeev Kumar*[2] and *Anant Madaan*[2]**
[1]Faculty of Medicine, Safaric University, Kosice, Slovakia
[2]Madan Hospital, Panipat, India; Raj Chopra, Tishcon Corporation, Westbury, NY, US

The ability of people to perform aerobic exercise varies. Recent experimental studies with rats indicate that those individuals with a low tolerance for aerobic exercise may have a lot more to worry about than just their inability to run fast and for long distances. The same underlying defect that reduces aerobic capacity may also predispose a person and could increase the possibility of coronary artery disease and strokes.

A research team including Ulrik Wisloff of the Norwegian University of Science and Technology in Trondheim, Sonia Najjar of the Medical College of Ohio in Toledo, and Steven Britton of the University of Michigan, Ann Arbor, reports that rats that have been selectively bred to have reduced capacity for aerobic exercise show obesity, insulin resistance and high blood pressure, all symptoms of the so-called metabolic syndrome that increases the risk of cardiovascular disease. The researchers also provide evidence that impaired function of the mitochondria, small structures that produce most of a cell's energy, underline the metabolic problems of the rats with low aerobic capacity. (*Science*,Jan 21,2005,307:418).

Previous work had implicated poor mitochondrial function with individual components of the metabolic syndrome, but this is the first time researchers have linked it to all of them at once, " This is an incredibly provocative study, according to Vamsi Mootha of Massachusetts General Hospital in Boston, whose own work has linked mitochondrial malfunction to type II diabetes. "They linked metabolic syndrome to mitochondria in a way that hasn't been done before." The rat-breeding experiments began in 1996,motivated mainly, by dissatisfaction with existing animal models for diabetes and cardiovascular disease. Most of those models were created by very nonphysiological means, such as tying off the coronary artery or administering a drug destroying the beta cells of the pancreas, far removed from the way the conditions develop naturally.

To produce animals whose diseases more closely mimic those in humans, the researchers selectively bred rats to have either high or low capacity for aerobic exercise. They identified

* Email: pellad@hotmail.com.

rats with a high capacity to run on a treadmill and mated them with one another, and they did the same for animals with a low running capacity. Since oxygen metabolism is such a large part of biology, defects in it should manifest. The animals described in the current report, the products of 11 generations of selective breeding, have a 350% difference in their running abilities. And by every measure tested, the couch potato rats rank high on the cardiovascular risk factor scale; Compared to high-capacity runners, they are more obese, have higher blood pressures and higher levels of blood fats and have increased insulin resistance.

It is known that obesity itself can decrease aerobic running capacity, a statistical analysis showed that it accounts for no more than 20% of the decreased aerobic capacity. . Indeed, studies of very young rats who were poor exercisers showed that metabolic changes, hyperlipidemia and hyperglycemia occurred before any weight differences became apparent. Rural and urban differences in India also indicated higher

Prevalence of metabolic syndrome in urbans compared to rurals who have enormous physical activity. Because mitochondria provide the energy for exercise, Britton and his colleagues examined whether these organelles exhibited signs of reduced function in the low-aerobic-capacity rats .The researchers found that muscle from those rats had much lower concentrations of a number of key mitochondrial proteins than did muscle from the high-capacity animals. This indicates that they had either fewer mitochondria or less effective ones. This may be similar to subjects with high arerobic capacity compared to obese people with low capacity. The work provides "a strong link among people who suspect that their own aerobic capacity may be on the low side." Wisloff's team is testing whether regular exercise can reduce the various risk factors in the low-aerobic –capacity rats, and early results look promising that aerobic capability depends on mitochondria.

What is most interesting is that RB Singh, Rajeev Kumar from Moradabad, S.S. Rastogi from Delhi and Reema Singh Rao from Mumbai; all from India have demonstrated that treatment with Coenzyme Q10 can decrease the various components of the metabolic syndrome within a period of 12 weeks. Coenzyme Q10 is very rich in mitochondrial cell membrane and responsible for ATP sparing and energy generation. Abstract presented in the 4th World Conference of the International Coenzyme Q10 Association, LA, USA, April 14-17,2005, Abstract book, p155).

In: World Heart Research Yearbook. Volume 1
Editors: Franz Halberg and R. B. Singh
ISBN: 978-1-60741-881-8

NOT ONLY A COLD CLIMATE BUT ALSO A HOT CLIMATE CAN TRIGGER CARDIAC EVENTS

***Daniel Pella*[1], *Dasa Dudova*[1], *Rajiv Kumar*[2] *and S. B. Gupta*[2]**
[1]Faculty of Medicine, Safaric University, Kosice, Slovakia
[2]Halberg Hospital and Research Institute, Moradabad, India

Acute myocardial infarction (AMI) is a highly dynamic event, which is associated with marked neuroendoorinological dysfunction in addition to cardiac damage. The immediate trigger for AMI is not precisely known. Studies conducted by Lown, Braunwald, Halberg, Otsuka, and our group have demonstrated a marked increase in sympathetic activity, oxidative stress, and magnesium and potassium deficiency during AMI. Clinical studies have reported an increased incidence of AMI sudden death and ischemia during the first quarter of the day when there is a rapid withdrawal of vagal activity and an increase in sympathetic tone. In one case-control study of 202 patients with AMI, there was a significant ($P>0.02$) increase in cardiac events in the second quarter of the day compared to other quarters, respectively (16.8%, 41.0%,13.8%,28.2% per quarter). This characteristic remained prevalent in both men and women and among patients with and without known AMI (n=52), diabetes (n=53) or hypertension (n=75).Triggers of AMI were noted among 162(82.2%) of the patients, Neuropsychological mechanisms were observed as follows: emotional stress (45.5%), sleep deprivation (27.7%), cold climate (29.2%) , hot climate (24.7%), large meals(47.5%) and physical exertion (31.2%).These triggering factors are known to enhance sympathetic activity and decrease vagel tone, resulting in an increased secretion of plasma cortisol, noradrenaline aldosterone, angiotension-converting enzyme (ACE), interleuking (II.)-1,-2,-6,-18, and timor necrosis factor-alpha (TNF-alpha), all of which are proinflammatory agents . There is also a deficiency in the serum levels of vitamin A, E and C and magnesium, potassium, melatonin, and IL-10 (an anti-inflammatory agent). In the above study, a decrease in magnesium, potassium, vitamin A, E, C and beta carotene combined with an increase in thiobarbituric acid-reactive substances (TBARS), MDA and diene conjugates, TNF-alpha and IL-6,were observed, all of which are indicators of oxidative damage and proinflammatory activity, respectively. Hot climate as a trigger of AMI has not been reported in the earlier studies. *(Singh et al, Biomed Pharmacother 2004,58:(Supple)111-115).*

In: World Heart Research Yearbook. Volume 1
Editors: Franz Halberg and R. B. Singh
ISBN: 978-1-60741-881-8

Scientific Session News from the American College of Cardiology, 54th Annual Scientific Session, Orlando, March 6-9, 2005. Trials Cover Stem Cells, Low LDL, Medication Effectiveness

Dasa Dudova, Daniel Pella* and Rafae Ryber
Faculty of Medicine,Safaric University,
Kosice, Slovakia

Participants and attendees of ACC" 05 took in emerging procedures and technology during four days of late-breaking clinical trials. The following represent just a few trials presented during this year's Scientific Sessions.

The ACC Scientific Session presented a late-breaking clinical trial session on small, provocative or experimental trials that delved into the following promising areas of clinical research for the first time this year.

Stem Cells in Acute Myocardial Infarction

Four-month results from the first double-blind placebo-controlled, randomized trial to evaluate the safety and effectiveness of intracoronary transplantation of autologous bone-marrow-derived mononuclear stem cells into patients with acute myocardial infarction (MI) found that the procedure is safe and capable of reducing infarct size. Sixty-seven patients who had suffered an acute MI and presented for treatment two hours after onset of pain were randomized to receive a stem-cell infusion or a placebo within 24 hours after successful mechanical reperfusion of the infarcted artery.

"Bone-marrow cell infused after myocardial infarction can significantly alter the structural adaptation of the heart to transient coronary occlusion –infarct healing", said the study's presenter Stefan Janssens, M.D., University of Leuven, Belgium. The reduction in the compensatory hypertrophy of the remote myocardium in association with the finding suggests a benefit in diastolic function indicating a preventive role of stem cells in heart failure.

* Email, pellad@mickyonline.com

Autologous Myoblasts in Ischemic Cardiomyopathy

Three-year follow-up results from a study evaluating the safety and feasibility of transplanting the autologous myoblasts into 22 patients with ischemic cardiomyopathy undergoing coronary artery bypass grafting showed the procedure to be both safe and feasible for these patients and that efficacy trials are warranted. Patients with a previous MI and left-ventricular ejection fraction of less that 40 percent were enrolled in the trial and injected with skeletal muscle myoblasts in the area of infarction, said Nabil Dib, M.D., director of cardiovascular research, Arizona Heart Institute, Phoenix. Positron-emission tomography and magnetic resonance imaging scans showed evidence of myoblast viability in the area of graft scar tissue, and the patients' ejection fraction improved almost one New York Heart Association (NYHA) functional class.

The results of a small phase I study of the effect of percutaneous transendocardial injection of autologous skeletal myoblast cells on left-ventricular (LV) function in 15 post-MI patients with chronic heart failure indicates that the procedure improves ejection fraction and LV wall motion but is also associated with an increased risk of ventricular arrhythmias. "Randomized, properly powered and closely monitored trials are needed to assess the true safety and efficacy of this treatment in these high-risk patients," said Patrick Serruys, M.D. Chief of Interventional Cardiology, Thorax center, Erasmus University, the Netherlands.

Metalloproteinase Inhibitor (PG116800) in AMI

A randomized experimental study of the effectiveness of a matrix metalloproteinase inhibitor (PG-116800) in preventing LV remodeling in 253 patients with acute MI concluded that at 90 days post-MI, there was no difference in LV remodeling among patients who received a placebo. In addition, 60 percent of the patients had an increase in LV end-diastolic volumes that could potentially lead to heart failure, according to W. Douglas Weaver, M.D., Henry Ford Heart and Vascular Institute, Detroit.

Gene Therapy in Coronary Artery Disease

The final results of the largest gene-therapy trial to promote myocardial angiogenesis (AGENT-3) using Ad5FGF-4, a replication-deficient, serotype-5-adenovirus-encoding fibroblast growth factor, found that this therapy failed to accomplish the trial's primary endpoint of increasing exercise duration for the 416 patients with class II to IV angina enrolled in the trial.

However, researchers from the 65 U.S. centers where the trial was conducted did see some improvement in exercise time in a subset of very high-risk patients, including those with severe class III and IV angina, said Timothy Henry, M.D., director of clinical research, Minneapolis Heart Institute Abbott Northwestern Hospital.

BRAVE-2 Trial with Abciximab

The BRAVE-2 trial, a randomized European multi center trial to assess the value of mechanical reperfusion (percutaneous coronary intervention plus glycoprotein IIb/IIIa inhibition with abciximab) in 365 patients with ST-segment elevation acute MI presenting more than 12 hours after onset of symptoms, demonstrated that this therapy reduces infarct size. The results of the trial support the use of mechanical reperfusion in patients with acute MI who present late, said Adnan Kastrati, M.D., Deutches Herzzentrum (German Heart Centre), Munich, Germany.

The CACAF Study

This prospective, randomized, controlled study of the effect of catheter ablation on atrial fibrillation (AF), showed that catheter-ablation therapy combined with antiarrhythmic drug therapy alone in preventing recurrences of atrial arrhythmias in 137 patients with paroxysmal or persistent AF who had already failed antiarrhythmics. The patients in the ablation group underwent cavatricuspid and left-inferior pulmonary vein mitral isthmus ablation plus circumferential pulmonary vein ablation, said Emanuele Bertaglia, M.D., chief of the electrophysiology lab, Civic Hospital of Mirano, Venice, Italy. Ninety-four percent of the patients in the control group had at least one AF recurrence versus 40.6 percents in the ablation group.

CPAP for Heart Failure

A trial of the use of continuous positive airway pressure (CPAP) for 258 heart-failure patients with central sleep apnea failed to show that CPAP reduces mortality in these patients , according to T. Douglas Bradley , M.D ., Professor of Medicine, University of Toronto. Mortality rates were the same among patients who received CPAP versus those in the control group. However the CPAP-treated patients did have improvements in LV function and exercise tolerance. In addition, their sleep apnea was alodrepinephrine at 12 weeks follow-up.

The PEECH Trial for Heart Failure

Finally, in the PEECH trial a prospective evaluation of the use of enhanced external counterpulsation (EECP) in combination with optimal care for 186 heart-failure patients, demonstrated that EECP improves exercise time but not peak VO2, said Arthur Feldman, M.D., Ph.D., Chairman, Department of Medicine, Jefferson Medical college, Philadelphia. In addition, patients who received EECP had significant improvements in quality of life and NYHA function class versus patients who received optimal therapy alone.

In: World Heart Research Yearbook. Volume 1
Editors: Franz Halberg and R. B. Singh
ISBN: 978-1-60741-881-8

CORONARY ARTERY DISEASE: RISK PROMOTERS, PATHOPHYSIOLOGY AND PREVENTION

Reviewed by R. B. Singh
Professor of Medicine, Subharti Medical College
Founder President, International College of Cardiology
Hon Fellow, Halberg Chronobiology Centre,
University of Minnesota, Minneapolis, Minnesota, US

Editors; Gundu HR Rao, S Thanikachalam, Publishers, Jaypee Brothers, New Delhi, India.2005, email: jaypee@jaypeebrothers.com

The editors of this book, which assembles world-renowned authorities to discuss most of the areas of cardiology, are among the best in their field. The contents of the book are valuable and its form compares favorably with other books published in India (despite a few typographical lapses such as instructions to the typesetter appearing in print). The book was published in 2005 but references quoted are hardly up to 2002; only some authors publishing in 2003 are being considered. The chapters by Drs U.N. Das, Enas A. Enas, P.C. Manoria, V.S. Narain, Gundu H.R. Rao, Y.K. Seedat and Bela Shah are outstanding. Considerations revolving around diet, sedentary behaviour, tobacco and other loads, associated with coronary artery disease (CAD) are discussed by most of the authors, although more emphasis may be welcome in the future. In any future editions of this book, each author should be persuaded to revise his chapter to quote studies published in the intervening years. There is no chapter on physical activity, dietary prevention and stress management indicating their role in the pathophysiology and prevention of CAD. In recent years there has been a flurry of activity in developing new pharmaceutical agents that target both conventional and newly discovered pathways in the development of vascular disease. This book has quite authentically discussed the role of low molecular weight heparin, direct thrombin inhibitors, tissue factor pathway inhibitors and of an oral form of unfractionated heparin but some of the authors have not been able to take the task as seriously as desirable for the readers.

Many authors on classical epidemiology and prevention have merely repeated the same studies multiple times. In the future, all experts interested in epidemiology should join hands to write one large chapter on CAD in south Asians and another chapter on CAD among south Asian immigrants to developed countries. The challenge and opportunity of blood pressure chronomics in India by the BIOCOS group is unique in the sense that its implementation avoids the need for fixed limits to the fiction of a "true" blood pressure. The role of alterations in the variability of pressures is important and is an early warning as a desideratum and is probably contributory, if not responsible for CAD and stroke. It can be treated for stroke and other serious CAD and stroke prevention!

With this rare but important emphasis of chronomic (time-structural) studies now under way in Amritsar, Lucknow and Moradabad, the book can be warmly and unreservedly recommended to cardiologists, other physicians, community medicine experts, still other health professionals, cardiac surgeons, nutritionists, biochemists and dietitians and appears to be the best among all the books published on this subject during the last five years from India.

In: World Heart Research Yearbook. Volume 1
Editors: Franz Halberg and R. B. Singh
ISBN: 978-1-60741-881-8

TRENDS IN ATHEROSCLEROSIS RESEARCH

Reviewed Dr. Chi-Woon Kong*
President, International College of Cardiology, Taiwan

Edited by Leon V.Clark, Nova Biomedical Books, 2004, NY, USA; email, Novascience@earthlink.net, www.novapublishers.com

The editor Dr Clark appears to be extremely good in selecting the authors for various chapters included in this book. The book posses the material which is of international standard. Each chapter has been written by a well known expert in the concerned field.

Mechanistic Approaches to Therapy for Vascular Injury, Surgical Myocardial Revascularization: Off Pump or on a Better Pump?. Targeting the CD40-CD40 Ligand (CD154) System as Therapeutic Intervention for the Treatment of Atherosclerosis.

The role of Matrix Metalloproteinases in Atherosclerotic Plaque Instability.

Investigation of the Role of Endogenous Nitric Oxide Synthesis in Determining Patterns of Arterial Wall Permeability and Diet-Induced Lipid Deposition in the Rabbit.

Large Artery Stiffness: Structural and Genetic Aspects. Small Vessel Ischemic Disease and Atherosclerosis: From Pathophysiology to Risk Factors. Pathophysiology and Pathogenesis of Vascular Cognitive Impairment: A Critical Update. Assessment of Reverse Cholesterol Transport. The Therapeutic Possibilities for the Regression of Vascular Changes in Hypertension. Analytical Methods of Atherosclerosis Research are various chapters available in this book. This may be quite interesting to internists, physicians, cardiologist, basic scientist, health workers, pharmacologists and nutritionists. However, role of nutrition in the atherosclerosis has not been dealt adequately.

* Email: cwkong@vghtpe.gov.tw.

In: World Heart Research Yearbook. Volume 1
Editors: Franz Halberg and R. B. Singh

ISBN: 978-1-60741-881-8

FOCUS ON ATHEROSCLEROSIS RESEARCH

Reviewed Dr. Chi-Woon Kong *

President, International College of Cardiology, Taiwan

Edited by Leon V.Clark, Nova Biomedical Books, 2004, NY, USA; email, Novascience@earthlink.net, www.novapublishers.com

The authors appear to be the great servants of cardiovascular sciences. The book has provided most interesting material to the basic scientist as well as to clical cardiologist and health scientists.The Role of Infection in Atherosclerosis . Cardiorespiratory Fitness and Atherosclerotic Cardiovascular Diseases. Childhood Risk Factors Predict Adult Risk Associated with Subclinical Cardiovascular Disease and Strategies for Prevention: The Bogalusa Heart Study.A Role for Chlamydia pneumoniae in Atherosclerosis: Fact or Fictions? Oxidized Low-Density Lipoprotein Complexed with в2-Glycoprotein I as a Common Metabolic From in Atherogenesis and Autoimmune-Medical Athero-sclerisis.

Impact of Lipoprotein Metabolism on Extreme Longevity. Fatty Acids: Determinants of Endothelial Function, Inflammation, Insulin Resistance and Atherosclerosis. Involvement of Endothelial Dysfunction in Atherogenesis. Oxidative Stress Hypothesis of Atherosclerosis. Vascular Oxidant Stress and Endothelial Dysfunction in Hyperhomocysteinemia.

* Email: cwkong@vghtpe.gov.tw.

In: World Heart Research Yearbook. Volume 1
Editors: Franz Halberg and R. B. Singh
ISBN: 978-1-60741-881-8

CAN WILD WHOLE SEEDS PROTECT AGAINST CARDIOVASCULAR DISEASE?

***Viola Mechirova*[1], *Ram B. Singh**[*,2], *Fabien DeMeester*[3], *Ronald R. Watson*[4], *Lekh Juneja*[5], *Jan Fedacko*[1] *and Daniel Pella*[1]**

[1] Faculty of Medicine, Safaric University, Kosice, Slovakia
[2] Halberg Hospital and Research Institute, Moradabad, India
[3] Columbus Paradigm Institute, Waterloo, Belgium
[4] College of Public Health, University of Arizona, Tuscon, AZ, US
[5] Taiyo Kagaku, Yokkaichi, Japan

Katcher and co-workers' study on whole grains appears to be of great interest [1].

Whole-grain foods appear to be protective against cardiovascular disease (CVD) including acute coronary syndromes (ACS)[2]. However, no guidelines exist for administration of such foods in ACS patients. Katcher and co-workers have very nicely demonstrated that a whole grain-enriched hypocaloric diet may be superior to refined grain foods in decreasing risk of CVD in patients with metabolic syndrome [1]. However, no consideration has been given to w-6/w-3 fatty acid ratio of the two diets, which could have been the important factor in decreasing inflammation [2-5]. Wild whole seeds rich in w-3 fatty acids, antioxidants and magnesium may provide even better results compared to whole grain grown by modern farming.

Prior to the Agricultural Revolution, our diet was based on wild seeds, plants, eggs, fish and meat from wild animals, whereas today, the greatest percentage of food supply is contributed by refined cereal grains, refined carbohydrates and meat from supplemented farm sources. These foods are rich in w-6 fatty acids and low in w-3 fatty acids, fiber, phytoestrogens, minerals and antioxidants. CVD, diabetes mellitus, obesity, cancer, autoimmune diseases, rheumatoid arthritis, asthma and depression are associated with increased production of thromboxane A2(TXA2), leucotrienes, protacyclin, interleukins-1 and 6, tumor necrosis factor-alpha and C-reactive proteins. Increased dietary intake of w-6 fatty acids is known to enhance all these risk factors as well as atherogenicity of cholesterol which have adverse proinflammatry effects resulting into thrombosis and ACS [2-7].

ACS may be due to thrombosis in the unstable plaque, and may be associated with activation of neurohormones and proinflammatory cytokines, resulting into neuroendocrine

* E-mail: drkk@dataone.in

dysfunction, which worsens the prognosis in these patients [8-10]. There also may be oxidative stress, hyperglycemia, hyperinsulinemia, hypertriglyceri-demia, increased levels of catecholamines, free fatty acids and cortisol.

Recent studies [2-5, 8-10), indicate that eating high fat, refined carbohydrate rich fast foods (Western diet), can produce a similar proinflammatory state in our body. It increases oxidative stress, free fatty acids and triglycerides, resulting into endothelial dysfunction, which may have adverse effects in patients with ACS. It is therefore, logical to avoid Western diet in patients with ACS, and to administer Indo-Mediterranean foods, beneficial to vascular endothelium and myocardium [2-5,8-10]. There is no precise and proven guideline for dietary advice for patients with ACS to protect against recurrent cardiac events. A Columbus soup (tomatoes, grapes, vegetables, walnuts, almonds + lin/chia seeds and olive oil) or yogurt containing, walnuts, almonds, raisins, could be prepared for nonpharmacological intervention among patients of ACS. These foods appear to be protective against metabolic syndrome [2]. Recipes have been commonly used in our studies and clinical practice [2-5,8-10]. For prevention of metabolic syndrome, or ACS, we recommend eating 400g/day of fruits and vegetable and another 400g/day of legumes and other whole grains, and 50g/day of almonds and walnuts, in conjunction with 25-50g/day of Columbus oil(olive oil 88 %+ flax seed oil 12.0%) P:S = w-6:w-3 = 1:1 (Patent Application WO2005020698). Increased physical activity to control sedentary behavior is important in urban and affluent populations for prevention of metabolic syndrome and ACS as part of Columbus lifestyle [2]. Apart from designer foods and lifestyle changes, drug therapy with fibrates, statins, coenzyme Q10, w-3 fatty acids, ACE-inhibitors, beta blockers, metformin and glitozones may be useful for prevention and treatment of metabolic syndrome in w-6 fatty acid rich dietary environment.

In one study [11], among 54 patients with ACS, the control subjects (n=85) were randomly selected from the population. Increased consumption of trans fatty acids (TFA) (>5g/day) was significantly greater among ACS patients compared to controls (50.0 vs. 0.0%, n=27 vs. 0). Large meals (>1000 Kcal) (50.0 vs. 29.4%, n=27 vs. 25) and large breakfast (40.7% vs. 11.8%, n=22 vs. 10), rich in TFA, linoleic acid, saturated fat and refined carbohydrates and poor in whole grains intakes were also significantly ($p<0.02$) greater among patients, compared to control subjects. Metabolic syndrome was noted among half of the ACS patients.

Serum levels of nitrite (an indicator of nitric oxide, NO) were significantly lower in patients with ACS, compared to controls (mean+SD:0.36+1.42 vs. 0.96+1.48uM, CI difference 0.60,0.34-1.02,$p<0.03$).Serum levels of vitamins E, C and beta-carotene, coenzyme Q10,magnesium and potassium were significantly lower and insulin, glucose, triglycerides, and lipoprotein(a), TNF-alpha, and IL-6 were significantly higher in ACS, compared to their levels after 4 weeks of follow up. Nitrite deficiency as a risk factor for heart attack has been emphasized in recently [12].

In India ACS, diabetes and hypertension are more common among higher social classes compared to lower social classes, possibly due to lower fat intake and enormous occupational physical activity in lower social classes. What are the social class differences in the western subjects?(delete)

However, it would be very interesting to know the role of refined starches and sugar, large meals, decreased intake of fruits, vegetables, whole grains and nuts and serum nitrite levels as risk predictors of ACS. Fruits, vegetables, nuts, whole grains, animal foods rich in w-3 fatty acids are slowly absorbed and may prevent the increase in free fatty acids, and inflammation, which is a characteristic of Columbus foods (www.columbus-concept.com). Therefore such foods may decrease the risk in ACS as well as metabolic syndrome [2,5,8].Omega-3 fatty acids can regulate leptin gene expression and the concentrations of anandamides in the brain, which in turn binds to endogenous cannabinoid receptors and regulate food intake and satiety and weight gain. International College of Cardiology is developing guidelines to include wild foods in the prevention of ACS.

REFERENCES

[1] Katcher HI, Legro RS, Kunselman AR et al. The effects of whole grain- enriched hypocaloric diet on cardiovascular disease risk factors in men and women with metabolic syndrome. *Am. J. Clin. Nutr.* 2008, 87:79-90.

[2] Singh RB, DeMeester F, Mechirova V, Pella D, Otsuka K. Fatty acids in the causation and therapy of metabolic syndrome. In *Wild Type Foods in Health Promotion and Disease Prevention*, editors Fabien DeMeester and RR Watson, Humana Press, NJ 2008,p 263-284.

[3] Harris WS, Reid KJ, Sands SA, et al. Blood omega-3 and trans fatty acids in middle aged acute coronary syndrome patients. *Am. J. Cardiol.* 2007;99:154–158.

[4] Singh RB,Dubnov G,Niaz MA,Ghosh S,Singh R,Rastogi SS,Manor O,Pella D,Berry EM. Effect of an Indo-Mediterranean diet on progression of coronary disease in high risk patients: a randomized single blind trial. *Lancet* 2002,360:1455-1461.

[5] Harper CR,Jacobson TA. Usefulness of omega-3 fatty acids and the prevention of coronary heart disease. *Amer. J. Cardiol.* 2005,96:1521-29.

[6] Ailhaud G, Massiéra F, Weill P, Legrand P, Alessandri JM, Guesnet P. Temporal changes in dietary fats: role of n-6 polyunsaturated fatty acids in excessive adipose tissue development and relationship to obesity. *Prog Lip Res* 2006;45:203-236.

[7] Rolland-Cachera MF, Maillot M, Deheeger M, Bellisle F. Prediction of adult adiposity using two indicators: a 20 year follow-up study. *Int J Obes* 2006;30:S12.

[8] Singh RB, Rastogi SS, Verma R et al. An Indian experiment with nutritional modulation in acute myocardial infarction. *Am. J. Cardiol. 1992, 69: 879-885.*

[9] Singh RB, Niaz MA, Kartik C.Can n-3 fatty acids provide myocardial protection be decreasing infarct size and inhibiting atherothrombosis? *Eur. Heart J.* 2001;3(Suppl. D)62-69.

[10] Singh RB,Pella D,DeMeester F..What to eat and chew in acute myocardial infarction. *Eur. Heart J.* 2006, 27:1628-29.

[11] Singh RB, Pella D, Sharma JP et al. Increased concentrations of lipoprotein(a), circadian rhythms and metabolic reactions, evoked by acute myocardial infarction in relation to large breakfast. *Biomed. Pharmacother.* 2004;58(Suppl.): 116-21.

[12] Maher AR, Milsom AB, Gunaruwan P, Abozguia K, Ahmad I,Weaver RA, Thomas P, Ashrafian H, Born GVR, James PE, Frenneaux MP. Hypoxic-modulation of exogenous nitrite-induced vasodilation in humans. *Circulation* 2008: 117: 670-677.

In: World Heart Research Yearbook. Volume 1
Editors: Franz Halberg and R. B. Singh

ISBN: 978-1-60741-881-8

FRONTIERS IN WOMEN'S CARDIOVASCULAR HEALTH PREVENTION: WHAT HAVE WE LEARNED SO FAR?

***Rebecca M. Scandrett*[1] *and Sandip K. Mukherjee*[2]**
[1] Cardiovascular Fellow, Yale School of Medicine, US
[2] Associate Clinical Professor of Medicine, Yale School of Medicine, US

INTRODUCTION

Cardiovascular disease affects over 200 million people worldwide and accounts for nearly 30% of global mortality. Approximately 80% of these cardiovascular deaths occur in low and middle-income countries. By the year 2020, ischemic heart disease mortality in developing countries is predicted to increase by 120% for women and 137% for men [1]. In the United States alone, cardiovascular disease (CVD) affects over 37 million American women, representing over one third of the American female population, with coronary heart disease (CHD) affecting 5.9 million women. By age 55, the prevalence of cardiovascular disease in women exceeds that in men. Cardiovascular disease accounts for 1 in 2.5 female deaths compared to 1 in 30 deaths attributable to breast cancer. Despite the high prevalence and mortality rate of cardiovascular disease, only 13% of women consider it to be their greatest health risk [2]. While a recent survey of 1008 women found that the level of awareness regarding CVD mortality in women has nearly doubled since 1997, still only 55% of women recognize CVD as the leading cause of mortality in women. In addition, the survey found that the level of awareness in minorities continues to significantly lag behind the white population with only 38% of blacks and 34% of Hispanics recognizing the magnitude of the problem [3]. Although the past two to three decades has seen a decline in the overall mortality rate from CHD in men, the mortality rates for women have remained stable. The overall incidence of CHD in women has actually increased, as evidenced by a 47% increase in hospital discharges related to CHD [2,4] A prospective registry study of men and women who presented with an acute myocardial infarction found that women were at increased risk for 28-day case fatality (18.5% vs. 8.3%), 6-month mortality (28.5% vs. 10.8%) and readmission rates (23.3% vs. 12.2%) after a first myocardial infarction compared with men, independent of co-morbidities, coronary risk factors and the use of thrombolytics [5]. Not only did women in this study have a higher mortality from their first MI compared to men, it was also found that the median time between symptom onset and initial presentation to the hospital was on average one hour longer in women compared to men. Furthermore, the delay between the emergency room and admission to the coronary care unit was also on average over two hours longer in women than in men. The results from this registry were recently mirrored in the Euro Heart Survey of Stable Angina. This prospective observational trial found that women who presented with a new diagnosis of stable angina were less often referred for noninvasive or invasive studies and were less likely to undergo revascularization or given optimal secondary prevention medication even in the presence of confirmed obstructive coronary artery disease compared to men [6]. These studies highlight the discrepancies in the recognition and appropriate treatment of CHD in women as compared to men and underscore the importance of appropriately identifying women who are at risk for CHD. The aim of this report is to review the primary and secondary prevention measures that are unique to women and to examine the sensitivity and specificity of the current diagnostic modalities in detecting CHD in women.

Hormone Replacement Therapy

Chapter 1: Proposed Mechanism for Estrogen's Cardiovascular Protection

The role of estrogen replacement therapy (ERT) and combined estrogen/progestin hormone replacement therapy (HRT) in the primary and secondary prevention of CHD has been an issue of debate for the past several decades. Given that estrogen is believed to be a cardioprotective agent, it is no surprise that the rates of coronary heart disease in postmenopausal women are two to three times greater than in premenopausal women of the same age [2]. In the basic science arena researchers have demonstrated that estrogen has systemic effects as well as direct effects on the vasculature. These systemic effects of estrogen include alteration in lipoprotein profiles, changes in the coagulation, fibrinolytic and antioxidant systems, as well as production of other vasoactive substances [7]. Activation of estrogen receptors located in hepatic tissue results in alteration of expression of apoprotein genes which in turn results in a decrease in total cholesterol and low-density lipoprotein (LDL) cholesterol, an increase in high density lipoprotein (HDL) cholesterol and triglyceride levels, and a decrease in serum Lp(a) lipoprotein. These effects of estrogen on lipid concentrations have been demonstrated in several large-scale clinical trials. In the Postmenopausal Estrogen/Progesterone Interventions (PEPI) trial [8,9], orally administered estrogen was shown to decrease LDL by about 15%, increase HDL level by about 15% and increase triglyceride level by about 20-25% in postmenopausal women. In addition to its effects on lipids, estrogen has been shown to regulate the hepatic expression of fibrinogen and the anticoagulant proteins antithrombin III and protein S, and to have direct effects on vascular cells and tissues [7]. Estrogen has both rapid effects on the vasculature, resulting in vasodilatation and increase in nitric oxide production, as well as long term effects mediated through its receptors, α and β, resulting in alterations in gene expressions that decrease atherosclerosis, decrease vascular injury, decrease smooth muscle cell growth and increase endothelial cell growth. In addition to the above beneficial effects in preventing atherosclerosis, estrogen has also been shown to have a proinflammatory effect as reflected in the increase in C-reactive protein (CRP) levels that is observed in subjects treated with HRT [10, 11]. Based on these effects of estrogen on the vasculature, coagulation milieu, and cholesterol profile, it is not surprising that the initial observational studies found a protective effect of ERT/HRT in postmenopausal women.

Chapter 2: Data from Randomized Control Trials: Why Placebo Matters

The role for ERT and HRT was initially supported by numerous observational epidemiological studies. A meta-analysis of these initial studies published from 1970 through the 1990s showed a significant reduction (35-40%) in risk of CHD in women taking HRT [12]. Based on these observational data, the use of HRT/ERT in the primary and secondary prevention of CHD in women was the standard of care until 1998 when results from large, randomized control trials contradicted the findings from observational studies. The largest of the secondary prevention trials was the Heart and Estrogen/Progestin Replacement Study (HERS) [13]. This study evaluated the hypothesis that treatment with HRT (conjugated equine estrogen [CEE] and medroxyprogesterone [MPA]) would reduce future CHD events in postmenopausal women with documented CHD. In contrast to findings from observational studies, the authors found that after a mean follow-up of 4.1 years, there was no difference in recurrent CHD events between the treatment group and the control group (relative hazard (RH) 0.99, 95% CI 0.80 to 1.22). The post-hoc time trend analysis showed a 52% increase in CHD events during the first year of HRT use compared to placebo (95% CI 1.01-2.29) and a trend towards a decrease in CHD events in years 3 and 4 (RH 0.87, 95% CI 0.55-1.37; RH 0.67, 95% CI 0.43 – 1.04, respectively) [13]. In order to explore whether the beneficial effects of HRT would be recognized with longer follow-up, the participants in HERS who continued the assigned study drug after completion of the initial trial (93% agreed to continue to be followed) were followed for another 2.7 years. After a total of 6.8 years of follow-up there was still no significant difference in recurrent CHD events between the HRT group and the placebo group [14].

Chapter 3: Does the Type of HRT or the Method of Delivery Matter in Secondary Prevention? No

Once HERS and HERS II proved that combined estrogen plus progestin did not successfully reduce recurrent CHD events, it was hypothesized that perhaps progestin attenuated the beneficial effects of estrogen and that estrogen alone would prove to be beneficial. In a test of this hypothesis, a study of 1,017 postmenopausal women aged 50-69 years who had survived their first myocardial infarction were randomized to receive either estradiol valerate (E_2) or placebo and then followed for two years. The frequency of reinfarction or cardiac death did not differ between the two groups after 24 months of follow-up [15]. Similarly, in a study of transdermal estrogen delivery in 255 postmenopausal women with known CHD, there was no difference in recurrent CHD between the treatment arms and there was a non-significant trend towards increased CHD events in the HRT groups compared to placebo in the first two years of treatment [16].

Chapter 4: Is There a Role of HRT in the Primary Prevention of CHD?

A potential explanation for the lack of benefit of ERT/HRT in the secondary prevention trials was the delay in pharmacotherapy. It has been postulated that estrogen is only effective at preventing the development of atherosclerosis in healthy women. Once atherosclerosis is established, estrogen is ineffective at preventing its progression. This hypothesis, however, did not hold true when tested in a large randomized control clinical trial. The Women's Health Initiative [17, 18] evaluated the role of HRT (CEE plus MPA) and ERT (CEE) on the primary prevention of CHD. Over 16,000 generally healthy postmenopausal women ranging in age from 50 to 79 years old were randomly assigned to HRT or placebo and were followed for a mean of 5.2 years. The authors actually found a trend towards an increase in CHD events with an adjusted hazard ratio for CHD in the HRT group 1.24 (95% CI 1.00-1.54), with the greatest amount of risk occurring in the first year after randomization with a hazard ratio of 1.81 (95% CI 1.09-3.01). A subgroup analysis of women stratified according to years since menopause, however, revealed a non-significant trend towards a reduction in CHD in women with less than 10 years since menopause (HR 0.89, 95% CI 0.5-1.7). Over 10,000 women with a hysterectomy were randomized into the estrogen-alone trial and were followed for an average of 6.8 years [19]. As with the HRT trial, there was no significant difference between the ERT group and the placebo group in CHD event rate (HR 0.91, 95% CI 0.75 – 1.12).

Chapter 5: Why Did ERT/HRT Fail? Unanswered Questions and Future Trials

Regardless of the type of estrogen used, the method of hormone delivery or the combination of hormone replacement with estrogen and progestin, no significant benefit in CHD prevention was found in the aforementioned randomized trials. Many theories have been set forth to explain the significant discrepancy between observational and placebo controlled trials. One possible explanation is that the women in the observational trials who took HRT /ERT were a healthier cohort than those women who did not take HRT/ERT (selection bias). Another theory is that women in the observational studies on HRT/ERT were followed more closely than women not on HRT/ERT (prevention bias) [8]. The pro-inflammatory effect of HRT as reflected in the increase in C-reactive protein seen in women taking HRT [10] has been proffered as an explanation for the early increased risk of CHD events that was observed in both the HERS trial and in the Women's Health Initiative.

Finally, in the randomized trials, the average time between menopause and enrollment in the studies ranged from 16 years to over 20 years. The initiation of hormone or estrogen therapy at this late stage may not truly represent a physiologic replacement and may contribute to lack of benefit in both primary and secondary prevention of CHD. The delay in HRT/ERT may have allowed subclinical atherosclerosis to develop and may have reduced the cardiovascular benefits of estrogen.

The trend toward a reduction in CHD events in the subgroup analysis in the Women's Health Initiative of women who began HRT/ERT within 10 years of menopause [17] as well as a series of experiments in primates which showed a benefit of ERT on atherogenesis progression only when started immediately post oophorectomy [20] lends support to this theory. These observations have kept the door open for a possible role of HRT in primary prevention in women at the inception of menopause and is the basis for the ongoing Kronos Early Estrogen Prevention Study (KEEPS) [21].

For now, however, there is no clear role of HRT or ERT for either primary or secondary prevention of CHD in postmenopausal women. A summary of the aforementioned trials can be found in Table 1.

OBESITY

Over the last 20 years obesity has become a pandemic, affecting over half of women in the United States -- an increase of over 30% in the past three decades [22]. Furthermore the rate of obesity is increasing more rapidly in women than men. In addition to being linked to several CHD risk factors (namely hypertension, diabetes, dyslipidemia, hyperinsulinemia, and increased levels of procoagulant and proinflammatory markers), obesity has also been shown to be an independent risk factor for CHD in women.

In the Nurses Health Study, 115,818 women aged 30 to 55 years who were free of CHD at study entry were followed for 14 years. The investigators found not only a significant increase in the relative risk for CHD events in the group with the highest body mass index (BMI), but also an increase risk in CHD with modest increases in BMI (multivariate RR for BMI 23-24.9: 1.46, BMI 25-28.9: 2.06, BMI >29: 3.56) [23].

In addition, the authors found that women who gained more than 5 kg compared to their weight at age 18 years were at increased risk for CHD events (gain 5-7.9 kg multivariate RR: 1.25, gain 8-10.9 kg multivariate RR: 1.65, gain 11-19 kg multivariate RR: 1.92, gain >20 kg multivariate RR: 2.65).

A recent re-analysis of 20-year follow-up data from the Nurses Health Study reinforces the above findings, showing that both obesity and inactivity are strong independent predictors of CHD events in women [24].

The question of how adipose distribution affects CHD risk has also been raised. It has been shown that abdominal adiposity is independently linked to significant metabolic abnormalities (insulin resistance, elevated triglycerides, hypertension, glucose intolerance and diabetes) and is an independent risk factor for CHD in men and possibly in women.

Using a subset of women from the Nurses Health Study, Rexrode et al examined the impact of abdominal adiposity (as measured by waist hip ratio [WHR] and waist circumference) on the incidence of CHD over 8 years of follow-up.

When controlled for BMI, WHR and waist circumference were independent predictors of CHD events. In women with a WHR of 0.88 or higher, the RR was 3.25 compared with women with a WHR < 0.72. Similarly, a waist circumference of > 96.5 cm had a RR of 3.06 when compared to women with a waist circumference of < 71.1 cm.

This increase in risk remained significant even when adjustment for biological mediators was performed and when results were stratified by BMI (RR for BMI < 25 and WHR > 0.88: 3.54), suggesting that abdominal adiposity is a strong independent predictor of CHD in women regardless of BMI [25].

Table 1. Hormone Replacement Therapy and Cardiovascular Outcomes

Study	Published	# Subjects	Endpoint	Follow-Up Time	Intervention	Results
Observational Studies						
Nurse's Health Study	*NEJM*. 1996; 335: 453-61	59,337 postmenopausal women free of CVD at study entry	CVD = nonfatal MI, fatal coronary disease, CABG/PTCA, fatal or nonfatal CVA	16 years	Estrogen Estrogen + Progestin	RR 0.60 (0.43-0.83) RR 0.39 (0.19-0.78)
	Ann Int Med. 2001; 135: 1-8.	2,489 postmenopausal women with previous MI or documented CAD	Non-fatal MI or coronary death	20 years	Estrogen alone OR estrogen + progestin	RR 0.65 (0.45-0.95)
Effect on Cholesterol and Inflammatory Markers						
PEPI	*JAMA*; 1995; 273: 199-208	875 healthy postmenopausal women	HDL-c SBP Insulin Fibrinogen	3 years	1) placebo 2) CEE 3) CEE + MPA cyclic 4) CEE + consecutive MPA 5) CEE + MP	CEE alone: Inc. HDL 5.6 mg/dL (5.4-6.7), dec. LDL 14.5 mg/dL (12.1-16.8) MPA regimens: Inc. HDL 1.2-1.6 mg/dL, Dec. LDL 16.5-17.7 mg/dL CEE + MP: Inc HDL 4.1 mg/dL, Dec LDL 14.8 mg/dL (12-17) No effect on insulin, sbp or fibrinogen
	Circ. 1999; 100: 717-722	365 healthy postmenopausal women	CRP E-selectin	3 years	As above	All active treatment groups: CRP inc. 85% E-selectin decreased by 18%
Women's Health Study	*Circ*. 1999; 100: 713-716	493 healthy women	CRP		Any HRT regimen	CRP 2x higher among women on HRT compared to no HRT (0.27 vs. 0.14 mg/dL, p = 0.001)
Primary Prevention Randomized Control Clinical Trials						
EPAT	*Ann Int Med*. 2001; 135: 939-953	222 healthy women	Carotid intima-media thickness	2 years	17β-E_2 or placebo	Less progression in E_2 group c/t placebo (-0.0017 vs. 0.0036 mm/yr) Avg. rates of progression did not differ in patient who also took lipid lowering meds

Study	Published	# Subjects	Endpoint	Follow-Up Time	Intervention	Results
WHI	*NEJM*. 2003; 349: 523-534	16,608 healthy postmenopausal women	1) CHD = nonfatal MI and CHD death 2) Invasive breast ca	5.2 years (stopped early 2° risks exceeding benefits)	CEE + MPA vs. placebo	CHD: RR 1.24 (1.00-1.54) 1st year CHD: RR 1.81 (1.09-3.01) Menopause < 10 yrs CHD: RR 0.89 (0.5-1.7)
	JAMA. 2004; 291: 1701-1712	10,739 women with hysterectomy	CHD = nonfatal MI or CHD death	6.8 yrs	CEE vs. placebo	CHD: 0.91 (0.75-1.12) 1st year CHD: 1.16
Secondary Prevention Randomized Clinical Control trials						
HERS	*JAMA*. 1998; 280: 605-613	2,763 postmenopausal women with intact uterus and history of CAD	1° endpoint: nonfatal MI or CHD death 2° endpoint: revascularization, UA, cholesterol, CVA/TIA, PAD, all cause mortality	4.1 years	CEE + MPA or placebo	No difference in 1° or 2° endpoints 1° endpoint: RR 0.99 (0.80-1.22) 1st yr RR: 1.52 (1.01-2.29) Year 3 RR: 0.87 (0.55-1.37) Year 4 RR: 0.67 (0.43-1.04)
HERS–II	*JAMA*. 2002; 288: 49-57.	2,321 of original HERS participants	1° endpoint: nonfatal MI or CHD death	6.8 years	CEE + MPA or placebo (open label)	RR 1.00 (0.77-1.29)
PHASE	*BJOG*. 2002; 109: 1056-1062.	255 postmenopausal women with angiographically proven CAD	CHD death, nonfatal MI, hospitalization for UA	30.8 months	Transdermal 17β E_2 or 17 β E_2 + norethisterone or placebo	HRT/ERT vs. placebo RR 1.29 (0.84-1.95)
ESPRIT	*Lancet*. 2003; 360: 2001-2008	1,017 women who survived first MI	Reinfarction of cardiac death and all-cause mortality	2 years	Oral estradiol vs. placebo	Reinfarction/CHD death RR 0.99 (0.7-1.41) All cause mortality RR 0.79 (0.5-1.27)
ERA	*NEJM*. 2000; 343:522-529	309 women with angiographically confirmed CAD	Mean minimal coronary artery diameter	3.2 ± 0.6 years	CEE or CEE + MPA or Placebo	No difference between treatment groups
WELL-HART	*NEJM*. 2003; 349: 535-545.	226 postmenopausal women with at least 1 coronary lesion	% coronary stenosis (QCA)	3.3 years	Usual care or 17β E_2 or 17β E_2 + MPA (all groups LDL < 130 mg/dL)	No difference in change in % stenosis between groups

Abdominal adiposity is 1 of 5 clinical criteria for metabolic syndrome. It has been suggested that the effect of obesity on CHD risk in women observed in the Nurses Health Study was actually a surrogate for the increased risk associated with the metabolic syndrome. In order to address this theory, Kip et al evaluated the prevalence of CHD and subsequent development of CHD events over 3.5 years in a group of 780 women with suspected myocardial ischemia enrolled in the Women's Ischemia Syndrome Evaluation (WISE) study [26]. Women were classified by their BMI and as being either dysmetabolic or metabolically normal. Although the authors found a strong correlation between the metabolic syndrome and obesity, only the metabolic syndrome was associated with significant underlying CAD, death or major adverse cardiovascular events (HR 2.01 death, HR 1.88 MACE). In fact, normal weight women (BMI < 25) who were dysmetabolic had the highest rate of MACE (25% 3 year event rate) and death (13.4% 3 year event rate). These findings suggest that screening women for metabolic syndrome, even women with normal BMI (< 25), may prove a useful intervention in the primary prevention of CHD events. This study, however, did not assess whether measurements of abdominal adiposity were independent predictors of MACE when metabolic status was also accounted for. See Table 2 for ideal weight and body measurement goals.

Table 2. Weight and Body Measurement Goals

Weight and Body Measurement Goals
1. BMI < 23
2. WHR < 0.72 (waist measured at the level of the umbilicus, hips measured at the largest circumference)
3. Waist circumference < 71.1 cm (measured at the level of the umbilicus)

DIET AND LIFESTYLE

The ideal diet for primary and secondary prevention of CHD in women has been an issue of much debate over the past several decades. The recommendation of the traditional high carbohydrate, low fat diet espoused for the prevention of CHD is now being questioned. It has now been shown that this diet reduces levels of HDL and increases triglyceride levels, both of which independently increase the risk of CHD in women. In addition, the growth in popularity of high fat diets, such as the South Beach Diet and the Atkins diet, has made the question of diet in the prevention of CHD an even more pressing issue for physicians.

Using the Nurse's Health Study database Hu et al examined the role of dietary intake of specific types of fat on risk of CHD. While a higher total fat intake was associated with an increased risk of CHD over 14 years of follow-up, this association almost disappeared when one accounted for confounders such as smoking, alcohol use, vigorous exercise and vitamin E supplementation (relative risk 1.02 for an increase of 5% in energy obtained from total fat as compared with the equivalent energy obtained from carbohydrates). However, a comparison of the different types of fat as percentage of total energy intake revealed that replacing 5% of energy from saturated fat with energy from unsaturated fats was associated with a 42% lower risk of CHD events. This reduction in CHD events was larger than the one observed when carbohydrates replaced saturated fat or trans unsaturated fat in the diet [27]. Further exploring the role of carbohydrates on CHD risk, Liu et al examined the role of glycemic load on CHD risk in women enrolled in the Nurse's Health Study. After accounting for possible confounding clinical and dietary factors, they found that women who had diets with the highest glycemic load had a relative risk for CHD events of 1.98 compared to the women with the lowest glycemic load. The adverse effect of a high glycemic load was observed in women of all body weights; however, the effect was most evident in women with average or above average BMIs [28]. As fruits and vegetables represent examples of foods high in fiber and a low glycemic index, it would follow from these observations that women with diets high in fruits and vegetables would have a lower risk of CHD. Data from the Nurse's Health Study and the Health Professionals' Follow-Up support this observation. Compared to women who ate fewer than three servings of fruit and vegetables a day, women who consumed more than eight servings a day had a 20% lower risk of CHD events over 14 years of follow-up. The lowest risk of CHD events were observed in women who consumed green leafy vegetables, cruciferous vegetables and vitamin C-rich fruits and vegetables [29]. However, the authors estimated that in order for one woman to avoid a coronary heart disease event, 1,443 people would have to increase their consumption of fruits and vegetables by one serving a day for 12 years. To further evaluate the role of fiber in the prevention of CHD in women, Wolk et al looked at 68,782 women aged 37 to 64 years who were free of CHD, diabetes and hyperlipidemia at study entry over 10 years. After accounting for possible confounders, they found that women with the highest intake of total fiber had a nonsignificant trend towards lower CHD events (RR 0.77, 95% CI 0.57-1.04, $p = 0.07$). However, when the sources of fiber were evaluated independently (cereal, fruit, vegetable), women with the highest intake of cereal fiber had a 34% reduction in CHD events over 10 years (RR 0.66, 95% CI 0.49-0.88, $p < .001$). The relationship with cereal fiber was strongest in women who were nonsmokers, BMI < 25, and those in the lowest tertile of saturated and trans unsaturated fat. Interestingly, consumption of vegetable and fruit fiber was not significantly associated with risk of CHD. The beneficial effect of fiber on CHD risk may be explained in part by its role in reducing total and LDL cholesterol via increased bile acid excretion and decreased hepatic synthesis of cholesterol. Fiber may also play a role in delaying absorption of macronutrients, which would lead to decreased insulin sensitivity and lower triglyceride levels [30].

While these studies suggest a role of individual foods and nutrients in the reduction of CHD in women, they do not address how overall eating patterns affect the incidence of CHD. In an effort to answer this question Fung et al evaluated the diet patterns of women in the Nurse's Health Study. Comparing a prudent diet (characterized by high intakes of fruits, vegetables, legumes, fish, poultry and whole grains) to a Western diet (characterized by higher intakes of red and processed meats, sweets and desserts, French fries and refined grains) they found that women in the highest quintile of the prudent diet had a relative risk of 0.76 for CHD events over 10 years compared to those in the lowest quintile. In contrast, those in the highest quintile of the Western diet had a relative risk of 1.46 compared to those in the lowest quintile [31]. This study supports the role of a diet high in polyunsaturated fat, high in fiber, and low in foods with a high glycemic index in the primary prevention of CHD in women.

Although the recently published Women's Health Initiative Dietary Modification Trial which compared a diet low in fat and high in fruit, vegetable and fiber intake to a standard diet on CVD risk in healthy postmenopausal women did not support these observational findings [32], the secondary prevention Lyon Diet Heart Study did find a similar decrease in subsequent cardiac events and mortality in men and women who followed a Mediterranean diet with a high amount of α linolenic acid compared to the standard recommended low fat post-MI diet following a first myocardial infarction (RR 0.28, $p = 0.0001$) [33]. The suboptimal reduction in fat intake in the study group (only a 8% reduction in total fat intake) in the Women's Health Initiative rendered the study with inadequate power to detect a true difference in CVD outcomes between the groups (power estimation of about 40%). Therefore the conclusions from this study regarding the utility of a low fat diet in the primary prevention of CVD must be viewed with caution. Based on the observational data and the date from the Lyon Diet Heart Study, it appears that a Mediterranean type diet that is high in fiber, low in foods with a high glycemic index, low in trans-fatty acids and saturated fats and high in polyunsaturated fat would be beneficial in the primary and secondary prevention of CHD events in women of all weights.

Exercise – How Much and How Often?

The role of exercise and the type of exercise (walking versus vigorous exercise) in the prevention of CHD in women is somewhat controversial. Although there have not been randomized control trials, data from the Nurse's Health Study and the Women's Health Initiative Observational study have shed some light on this topic. Manson et al evaluated the role of walking versus vigorous exercise in the primary prevention of CHD in women over 8 years of follow-up. When adjusting for potential clinical confounders, the authors found a strong positive relationship between increased physical activity and reduced risk of the CHD events. There were significant 34% reduction in CHD events in women who exercised for more than 10.5 MET-hours per week (equivalent of ≥ 3 hours per week of brisk walking or 1.5 hours per week of vigorous exercise). This decrease in risk was found regardless of BMI, smoking status and family history of premature coronary artery disease. A similar reduction in risk was observed in women who only participated in walking (no vigorous activity) with a relative risk of 0.70 in women with a walking score of 3.9 to 9.9 MET-hours per week (equivalent to 1 to 2.9 hours of walking per week at a brisk pace) and a relative risk of 0.60 in women who walked for more than 5 hours per week. Walking pace, in addition to total time walking, also emerged as an independent predictor of CHD events. The magnitude of risk reduction was similar with brisk walking and with vigorous exercise if the total energy expenditures were roughly equivalent [34]. Similar reductions were seen in CHD risk when diabetic women from the Nurse's Health Study were evaluated separately (50% reduction in CHD events in the women who exercise > 7 MET-hours per week compared to < 1 MET-hour per week) [35]. Investigators from the Women's Health Initiative also addressed the role of the walking and vigorous exercise in the prevention of CHD in a more ethnically diverse population of postmenopausal women. Paralleling the results from the Nurse's Health Study, a risk reduction of about 30% was seen in the women with the highest energy expenditure, regardless if the activity was walking or vigorous exercise. In addition, the authors found that longer duration of sitting was associated with a substantially increased risk of cardiovascular events (RR 1.68 for women who sit for 16 hours a day compared to women who sit for less than 4 hours a day). These changes in cardiovascular risk were seen in all women, regardless of race, BMI or age [36]. From these observational studies, it is reasonable to recommend moderate intensity exercise (walking briskly 3 hours per week or vigorous exercise for 1.5 hours per week) to women of all races, body weights and age, in an effort to reduce the risk of CHD. The use of a pedometer to measure the number of steps walked may be a useful objective barometer of exercise and may help facilitate the development of an exercise goals for women.

What Does It All Mean?

When evaluating lifestyle as a whole, Stampfer et al found that women who adhered to a "low risk" lifestyle (defined as not currently smoking, BMI less than 25, consuming at least a half an alcoholic beverage a day, engaging in moderate to vigorous physical activity for at least 30 minutes a day, and being in the highest 40 percent of the cohort in consumption of cereal fiber, marine n-3 fatty acids, folate, ratio of polyunsaturated to saturated fats, lack of consumption of trans fat and low glycemic load) had a significantly reduced risk of CHD events compared to those who did not adhere to such a lifestyle (RR 0.17). This model suggested that 82% of the CHD events in this large cohort of women could have been prevented if all women had followed a low risk lifestyle [37]. See Table 3 for a summary of recommended diet and lifestyle modifications.

Table 3. Diet and Exercise Recommendations

Diet and Exercise Recommendations
1. Diet with a low glycemic load (glycemic load = glycemic index%/100 gm of carbohydrate)
2. Diet low in saturated (≤ 11% of total energy intake)
3. Diet low in trans-unsaturated fats (≤ 2% of total energy intake)
4. Diet high in polyunsaturated fats (≥ 6% of total energy intake)
5. 8 servings of fruits and vegetables a day
6. 5 servings of fish per week
7. Diet high in cereal fiber (> 4 g/day)
8. Brisk walking 3 hr/wk OR vigorous exercise 1.5 hr/wk (at least 30 min of moderate exercise per day, 5 days a week)

DIETARY AND VITAMIN SUPPLEMENTS

Is There a Role for Anti-Oxidant Vitamin Supplements in the Primary or Secondary Prevention of CHD in Women?

As with the debate over hormone replacement therapy in the primary and secondary prevention of CHD in women, the role of antioxidant vitamins has been investigated over the past two decades. The initial data from a large, prospective cohort study suggested a modest benefit of Vitamin E in the reduction of primary cardiovascular events in women. Like estrogen, Vitamin E had a plausible biological basis in which it was postulated it could prevent atherosclerosis. This theory was based on the hypothesis that oxidative modification of low-density lipoprotein initiates atherosclerosis and the idea that anti-oxidant vitamins, such as Vitamin E, could inhibit this lipid peroxidation thereby preventing the development or progression of atherosclerosis and CHD [38]. Observational data from the Nurses Health Study and Iowa Women's Study initially supported this hypothesis [39, 40]. However, the positive benefit of vitamin E supplements noted in observational studies has not been supported by subsequent randomized placebo-controlled clinical trials. Although the Cambridge Heart Antioxidant Study (CHAOS) [41] suggested a beneficial effect on the secondary prevention of CHD, subsequent trials of Vitamin E or combinations of antioxidant vitamins (vitamin E and C) in the secondary prevention of CHD have not shown a similar benefit. The GISSI-Prevenzione trial [42], the Heart Protection Study (HPS) [43] and the WAVE trial [44] found no benefit in the secondary prevention of CHD events or in the angiographic progression of coronary atherosclerosis. In secondary analysis of the GISSI-Prevenzione trial, the authors did find a significant 20% reduction in all cardiovascular deaths (RR 0.80, 95% CI 0.65-0.99) and a 35% reduction in sudden cardiac deaths (RR 0.65, 95% CI 0.48-0.89). The ability to apply these results to a female population, however, is limited because of the low proportion of women (15% in CHAOS, 19% in GISSI, 25% in HPS) in the majority of these trials.

Similarly, the data for the role of vitamin E supplements in the primary prevention of CHD in women has also not been born out in randomized placebo-controlled studies. The HOPE and HOPE-TOO trials evaluated the role of 400 IU of Vitamin E from natural sources in the prevention of myocardial infarction (MI), stroke and death from cardiovascular causes over 4.5 years and 7 years of follow-up, respectively, in 2,545 women and 6,996 men who were at high risk for cardiovascular disease. These studies found no benefit of Vitamin E on the reduction of cardiovascular events (RR 1.05, 95% CI 0.95-1.16, $p = 0.33$). In subgroup analysis there was no difference in primary outcome when evaluating only the female subjects [45, 46]. Likewise, the Primary Prevention Project, a randomized controlled study of 4,495 high risk patients (2583 women) comparing placebo to 300 mg of synthetic Vitamin E supplementation on the rate of cardiovascular death, non-fatal MI and nonfatal stroke over a mean of 3.6 years of follow-up also found no benefit to Vitamin E supplementation (RR 1.07, 95% CI 0.74 – 1.56). This study, however, did not include a subgroup analysis based on gender [47].

The Women's Health Study evaluated the role of high dose vitamin E (600 IU every other day) in the primary prevention of CVD and cancer in 39,876 low risk women over ten years of follow-up. The authors found a non-significant 7% reduction in major cardiovascular events (non-fatal MI, non-fatal stroke, cardiovascular death) at the end of the trial (RR 0.93, 95% CI 0.82-1.05, $p = 0.26$). Although vitamin E had no effect on total MI or stroke, they did find a significant 24% reduction in cardiovascular death in the vitamin E group (RR 0.76, 95% CI 0.59-0.98), which was largely attributable to fewer sudden deaths in the vitamin E group. They also found a significant reduction in major cardiovascular events in the subgroup of women aged 65 years or older (RR 0.74, 95% CI 0.59-0.93, $p=0.009$) [48], suggesting a possible role in the primary prevention of CHD events in this elderly subset of women.

While the data regarding the use of antioxidant vitamins, specifically vitamin E, in the primary and secondary prevention of CHD have been contradictory; the bulk of the data does not support the use of vitamin E in the prevention of CHD in women. Randomized controlled trials have failed to show a significant benefit of any single vitamin supplement or combination of supplements in either the primary or secondary prevention of CHD death or non-fatal MI. In fact, several meta-analyses of the role of antioxidant vitamins in the prevention of CHD have failed to show a consistent benefit of antioxidant vitamins [38, 49] and at this point in time they should not be recommended for the primary or secondary prevention of CHD in women.

Is There a Role for Folic Acid or Vitamin B6 in the Prevention of CHD in Women?

Plasma homocysteine has been shown to be a strong, independent predictor of cardiovascular disease in both men and women. From country to country, there is a variation in homocysteine levels and with increasing levels of homocysteine there is a greater risk of cardiovascular mortality. The correlation between homocysteine and CVD mortality ($r = 0.71$) suggests that homocysteine may play an important role in determining CVD mortality between different populations [50]. Several plausible mechanisms by which homocysteine could increase risk of CHD (direct toxicity to endothelial cells, increased coagulation, decreased endothelial reactivity, and stimulation of smooth muscle cell proliferation [51]) have been previously elucidated.

Folate and vitamin B6 are important cofactors in the metabolism of homocysteine and changing the intake of folic acid and vitamin B6 can modify homocysteine levels. Accordingly, studies have shown that low dietary intake of vitamin B6 is also associated with increased risk of cardiovascular disease. Based on these observations, some investigators have hypothesized that lowering levels of homocysteine via folate and vitamin B6 supplementation would translate into a reduction in cardiovascular events. Support for this hypothesis in women was initially offered from observations from the Nurse's Health Study [51]. The authors found that the multivariate relative risk of CHD in the highest quintile of folate consumption (≥545 μg folate) was 0.69 (95% CI 0.55-0.87). The authors reported an 11% relative risk reduction of CHD events for each 200 μg increase in folate intake. Similar to folate intake, there was a 33% multivariate relative risk reduction in the women with the highest intake of vitamin B6 (median intake 4.6 mg) (RR 0.67, 95% CI 0.53-0.85) and a relative risk of 0.83 for each 2 mg increase in vitamin B6 consumption (95% CI 0.74-0.94). Because of the high correlation between folate and vitamin B6 intake (Spearman $r = 0.77$), the ability to assess the independent effects of the individual vitamins was limited.

The concern that the observed relation of homocysteine and vitamin B6/folate to CHD risk may actually represent unrecognized confounders rather than a true causal relationship has led to the development of randomized clinical trials. Therefore, in order to better understand the role of folate and vitamin B6 in the secondary prevention of cardiovascular disease, the NORVIT investigators [52]. randomized 3,749 patients (26% women) who had had an MI within the past 7 days, into four groups; folate (0.8 mg/day) plus vitamin B6 (40 mg/day), folate, vitamin B6, or placebo. These subjects were followed for an average of 3.5 years and were monitored for nonfatal and fatal MI and stroke. The investigators found that although the folate groups lowered plasma homocysteine levels by 28% (no significant change in homocysteine levels in the vitamin B6 group), there was no difference in the combined primary endpoint (folate RR 1.1, 95% CI 0.9-1.3, p = 0.3; vitamin B6 RR 1.1, 95% CI 1.0-1.3, p = 0.09). The authors found a trend towards increased risk in primary endpoint (MI and stroke) when folate and vitamin B6 were given in combination (RR 1.2, 95% CI 1.0-1.4, p = 0.03). The preliminary results from this study do not support a role for folate or vitamin B6 in the secondary prevention of CHD and suggest that these interventions may in fact be harmful. The role of these vitamins in the primary prevention of CHD, however, is still a question. Until a randomized, clinical trial addresses this issue, the routine use of these supplements in primary prevention of CHD in women is not recommended.

Is There a Role for Fish Oil (Omega-3 Fatty Acid) Supplementation in the Prevention of CHD in Women?

The observation that populations with a high intake of fish have a lower rate of cardiovascular disease initially led to the hypothesis that fish consumption may have a protective effect for atherosclerosis. Some of the proposed biological mechanisms that would explain this observation are: reducing susceptibility of the heart to ventricular arrhythmias, antithrombogenic properties of fish oil, lowering triglyceride levels, retardation of atherosclerotic plaque growth via reduced adhesion molecule expression, reducing platelet derived growth factor, acting as an anti-inflammatory mediator, and promoting nitric-oxide induced endothelial relaxation [53]. Several epidemiological prospective studies in men have lent support to this hypothesis. In the 30-year follow-up of the Chicago Western Electric Study, men who consumed 35 g or more of fish daily compared to those who ate none had a significant reduction in CHD death (RR 0.62) [53]. Similar risk reductions were also observed in women in the Nurse's Health Study cohort [54]. Using multivariate analysis the authors found that the risk of major CHD events in the women who consumed fish ≥5 times per week compared to the women who never ate fish was 0.69 (95% CI 0.52-0.93). They even found a 21% risk reduction in the women who only ate fish 1-3 times per month compared to those who ate fish < 1 time per month (RR 0.79, 95% CI 0.64-0.97). In addition, a similar reduction in CHD events was seen in the women who were in the highest quintile of omega-3 fatty acid supplement intake (0.24% of energy) compared to the lowest quintile (0.03% of energy), with a multivariate relative risk of 0.69 (95% CI 0.57-0.84). Although this epidemiologic data is compelling, to date there are no randomized controlled clinical trials to support the role of fish or fish oil in the primary prevention of CHD events in women. Currently the JELIS investigators [55] are following 10,796 postmenopausal women and 4,204 men who were free of CHD, in a trial of eicosapentaenoic acid (EPA), a component of fish oil, in addition to treatment with a statin in hyperlipidemic patients for 5 years. The primary end-points in this trial are major coronary events (sudden cardiac death, fatal and nonfatal MI, unstable angina, and coronary revascularization). The initial results of this trial, which were presented at the American Heart Association scientific session in 2005, revealed a 19% risk reduction in major cardiovascular events (RR 0.81, 95% CI 0.69-0.95) in the group treated with EPA plus statin therapy compared to statin therapy alone, and a 24% risk reduction in unstable angina (RR 0.76, 95% CI 0.62- 0.95).

In contrast to the dirth of data from randomized controlled trials on the role of fish oil in the primary prevention of CHD, there have been several observational trials as well as randomized controlled clinical trials showing a benefit of fish oil on the secondary prevention of CHD events. An observational trial of atherosclerosis progression in postmenopausal women revealed that the consumption of ≥ 2 servings of fish per week compared with < 2 servings per week was associated with significantly smaller increases in the percentage of stenosis (4.54 ± 1.37% versus – 0.06 ± 1.59%, $p < 0.05$) in diabetic women and fewer new stenoses (21% versus 34%, p = 0.02) [56]. Randomized clinical control trials have also supported the role of fish oil in the secondary prevention of CHD events. The first such trial, the DART trial [57] was published in 1989 and evaluated the role n-3 polyunsaturated fatty acids (PUFA) on the recurrence rate of CHD events over a 2 year period in men with a recent MI. This study found a 29% reduction in total mortality and in CHD deaths in the group who increased their dietary intake of n-3 PUFA to 0.5-1 g/day. The GISSI-Prevenzione trial [42] evaluated the role of n-3 PUFA and vitamin E in the secondary prevention of CHD events in 11,324 men and women (about 15% women). The authors found a 15% relative risk reduction in the rate of death, non-fatal MI and non-fatal stroke over 3.5 years of follow-up in the n-3 PUFA supplement group (RR 0.85, 95% CI 0.74-0.98). In secondary analysis the reduction in fatal events was almost entirely accounted for by a reduction in cardiovascular deaths (30% reduction in cardiovascular deaths, 95% CI 0.56-0.87). The low number of female subjects participating in these trials limits the applicability of the results to women.

Although the data is limited in women at this time, it is reasonable to recommend the use of n-3 omega fatty acids for the secondary prevention of CHD events in women who have recently had an MI. The recent results from the JELIS study also supports the recommendation of adding fish oil to the treatment of hyperlipidemics in the primary prevention of CHD events.

Aspirin Use in Women

The Debate over Aspirin in the Primary Prevention of CHD in Women

The role of aspirin in the secondary prevention of cardiovascular events is well established in both men and women. The role of aspirin in the primary prevention of cardiovascular disease in women, on the other hand, is not as clear. The Physician's Health Study, which was the first trial to uncover a significant 44% reduction in first myocardial infarction with aspirin use only included men in its subject population. Subsequent trials, however, have included women as well as men in their study population. The Hypertension Optimal Treatment Study (HOT) [58] evaluated the effect of blood pressure control and 75 mg of aspirin on the rate of major cardiovascular events (namely CV death, MI, stroke) in 9,907 men and 8,883 women over 3.8 years of follow-up. The authors found a significant 42% reduction in first MI in men (RR 0.58, 95% CI 0.41-0.81), which was similar to the results from the Physician's Health Study. However, there was only a non-significant 19% reduction in first MI in women (RR 0.81, 95% CI 0.49-1.31). In addition, there was a significant increase in non-fatal major bleeding in women randomized to aspirin therapy (2.7/1000 patient-years versus 1.3/1000 patient-years, p = 0.006). The Primary Prevention Project [47] evaluated the effect of 100 mg of aspirin on subsequent major cardiovascular events (cardiovascular death, non-fatal MI and non-fatal stroke) over 3.6 years of follow-up in 4,495 subjects (57% women) who had at least one cardiovascular risk factor. This study found a non-significant 29% reduction in combined endpoint (RR 0.71, 95% CI 0.48-1.04) and a significant reduction in cardiovascular death (RR 0.56, 95% CI 0.31-0.99). There was not a significant difference, however, in the rate of myocardial infarction (RR 0.69, 95% CI 0.38-1.23). The authors report that the direction and the size of the effects of aspirin on all of the predefined endpoints were similar in men and women when evaluated separately. This data, however, was not presented in the paper. The data from these two trials present a less than convincing argument for the use of aspirin in the primary prevention of MI in women.

The Women's Health Study [59] sought to finally answer this question. This study enrolled 39,876 women who were free of cardiovascular disease and had low risk cardiovascular profiles. The subjects were randomized to low dose aspirin (100 mg every other day) or to placebo and were followed for 10 years for a first cardiovascular event (non-fatal MI, non-fatal stroke or death from cardiovascular cause). The investigators found a non-significant 9% risk reduction in major cardiovascular events (RR 0.91, 95% CI 0.80-1.03), with no significant effect on fatal or non-fatal MI (RR 1.02, 95% CI 0.84-1.25). The authors did find, however, a significantly higher rate of bleeding complications in the aspirin group as compared to placebo (bleeding requiring transfusion RR 1.40, 95% CI 1.07-1.83, p 0.02). When evaluating the subgroup of women over the age of 65, however, they did find a significant reduction in major cardiovascular events (RR 0.74, 95% CI 0.59-0.92) and in MI (RR 0.66, 95% CI 0.44-0.97).

Based on these data there does not appear to a clear role for aspirin in the primary prevention of cardiovascular disease in women in the low-risk female population. There may be a benefit in the elderly female population. However, given the risk of bleeding complications, this needs to be further evaluated with a large-scale trial dedicated to answering this question.

Cholesterol and Inflammatory Biomarkers of CHD in Women

The Optimal Lipid Levels in Women for the Prevention of CHD

The role of LDL cholesterol in the development of atherosclerosis has been well established. However, the best lipid parameter for predicting CHD events in women continues to be an issue of some debate. In a nested case-control study from the Nurse's Health Study cohort [60], Shai et al preformed a multivariate assessment of the role of each lipid parameter in predicting future CHD events (non-fatal MI and fatal CHD) over 8 years of follow-up. In women without prior history of CHD, they found that an LDL cholesterol level of 132 mg/dL conferred a relative risk of future CHD events of 1.9 (95% CI 1.1-3.5) with 1 standard deviation (SD = 36 mg/dL) increase in LDL conferring a 40% increase in CHD risk (RR 1.4, 95% CI 1.1-1.7). LDL levels, however, did not completely predict CHD risk in women. In fact, one standard deviation (17 mg/dL) increase in HDL conferred a relative risk of CHD events of 0.5 (95% CI 0.4-0.7). Using the lipid index of total cholesterol/HDL-c provided an even better assessment of future CHD risk with one standard deviation corresponding to a relative risk of 1.8 (95% CI 1.5-2.1). When adding all of the lipid parameters to a step-wise model of CHD prediction (after accounting for age and smoking status), HDL-c was the primary contributor to the prediction model raising the ROC from 0.69 to 0.70, with LDL raising the ROC further to 0.72, suggesting that measurements of both LDL and HDL are essential in the prediction of CHD events. A similar contribution to the prediction model was seen when the ratio of total cholesterol/HDL was added (ROC increased to 0.72). This ratio reflects the proportion of atherogenic to antiatherogenic lipid fractions and appears to be a powerful tool for predicting CHD in postmenopausal women.

From this data it follows that lowering LDL cholesterol and raising HDL cholesterol should play a role in CHD prevention in women. Accordingly, the data from secondary prevention trials of statin therapy has shown reduced risks of CHD events in women placed on statin therapy. In subgroup analysis of the 4S trial [61], 827 postmenopausal women with known CHD and moderate hypercholesterolemia were randomized to either 20 mg of simvastatin or placebo and were followed over a mean of 5.4 years. They were monitored for all-cause mortality, CHD mortality, major coronary events (CHD death and non-fatal MI) and other acute atherosclerotic events. After 6 weeks of treatment the investigators found a mean 28% reduction in total cholesterol, 40% reduction in LDL cholesterol and 8% increase in HDL. They reported significant reductions in major coronary events (RR 0.66, 95% CI 0.48-0.91, p = 0.12), nonfatal MI (RR 0.64, 95% CI 0.47-0.98, p = 0.011), and revascularizations (RR 0.51, 95% CI 0.30-0.86, p = 0.012). These risk reductions were similar to those seen in the male population from the study. Because of the small number of events in women they did not find a significant decrease in overall or CHD mortality. A similar reduction in risk in CHD death and nonfatal MI was shown in the female subjects from the CARE trial [62]. This trial randomized 576 postmenopausal women (out of a total of 4,159 subjects) with a history of recent MI and an average cholesterol level (total cholesterol of < 240 mg/dL and LDL level between 115 to 174 mg/dL) to 40 mg of pravastatin or placebo. The subjects were followed for 5 years and were monitored for cardiac events. Similar to the 4S trial, the women treated with pravastatin had an average 20% reduction in total cholesterol level, a 28% reduction in LDL cholesterol and a 4% increase in HDL cholesterol levels. Women in the study experienced an overall risk reduction in combined coronary events of 46% (RR 0.54, 95% CI 0.48 – 0.78, p = 0.001) compared to a 20% reduction in events in men. In secondary analyses there were also significant reductions in nonfatal MI (RR 0.49, 95% CI 0.26 0.92, p = 0.028), and in revascularization rates (RR 0.47, 95% CI 0.30 – 0.74, p = 0.001) in the pravachol treatment group. The PROVE-IT –TIMI 22 trial [63], which included 22% women as subjects, has shown a significant reduction in recurrent CHD events in patients with a recent myocardial infarction who were treated with statins and achieved a mean LDL level of less than 70 mg/dL (2.7 vs. 4.0 events per 100 person years, p = 0.008). Based on observational and clinical trial data, the goal LDL in women with a history of CHD or diabetes should be ≤ 70 mg/dL.

Are There Other Markers of Inflammation that Are Predictive of CHD Events in Women?

In addition to LDL and HDL cholesterol, recent data has shown that various markers of inflammation are potent predictors of CHD events in women as well. Women in general have higher CRP levels compared to men [64] and black women have significantly higher CRP levels than white, Hispanic or Asian women [65]. These higher CRp levels may provide insight into the pathogenesis of angina in women with nonobstructive coronary disease and further aid in assessing CHD risk in women. Using the Nurse's Health Study cohort as a patient population, Ridker et al performed a nested-case control study to evaluate the role of inflammatory markers in the prediction of cardiovascular events (defined as death from CHD, nonfatal MI or stroke, or need for coronary revascularization) over 3 years of follow-up [66]. Four markers of inflammation (hs-CRP, serum amyloid A, IL-6, and sICAM-1) were univariate predictors of cardiovascular risk. Of these 4 markers, hs-CRP was the strongest predictor of future CHD events (RR 4.4, 95% CI 2.2-8.9 of highest [8.5 mg/L] to lowest [0. 6 mg/L] quartile) and the only independent predictor in multivariate analysis (RR associated with an increase of one quartile 1.5, 95% CI 1.1-2.1). In addition, they found that hs-CRP, IL-6, and amyloid A improved the prediction of cardiovascular events over the use of lipids alone. In fact when the authors performed a subgroup analysis of women with LDL < 130 mg/dL they found that the adjusted relative risk of cardiovascular events increased about 39% with each increase in quartile for hs-CRP (95% CI 13% to 89%, p= 0.03). In a subsequent analysis of the entire Nurse's Health Study cohort (27,939 women), Ridker et al compared the prognostic value of LDL cholesterol compared to CRP in the prediction of cardiovascular events over 8 years of follow-up [67]. Although CRP and LDL were both strong, independent predictors of cardiovascular events, the highest quintile of CRP (> 4.19 mg/L; RR 2.3, 95% CI 1.6-3.4) was a stronger predictor of events than the highest quintile of LDL (>153.9 mg/dL; RR 1.5, 95% CI 1.1-2.0). LDL and CRP, however, were not well correlated suggesting that each measurement identified different high-risk groups. Screening for both markers provided better information than either measurement alone. Additionally they reported that 77% of first cardiovascular events occurred in women with an LDL less than 160 mg/dL and 46% occurred in women with LDL less than 130 mg/dL. The addition of CRP measurements would have helped to identify at risk women that were missed by the standards set by the National Cholesterol Education Program. A prospective, randomized control study of the use of rosuvastatin in the primary prevention of cardiovascular disease in patients with low LDL cholesterol levels (<130 mg/dL) and elevated CRP levels (≥ 2 mg/L) is currently underway in the JUPITER trial [68]. Results of this study should be known in the next several years and should help in setting guidelines for the optimal management of women with normal LDL cholesterol levels but elevated CRP levels.

Diagnosis and Prognosis

Exercise Treadmill Testing – The Basics

Women generally manifest CHD about 10 years later than men [2], present more commonly with atypical chest pain or dyspnea, and have a lower prevalence of luminal obstructive coronary disease by angiography. However, when women do present with obstructive coronary disease, they have higher morbidity and mortality rates compared to age-matched men. It is therefore imperative not only to find effective primary and secondary prevention measures in women, it is also important to appropriately identify and risk stratify women with CHD. Historically, the non-invasive diagnostic work-up in women has been underutilized secondary to a lack of physician confidence in the accuracy of the test results

[69]. While exercise stress testing is the most commonly used non-invasive diagnostic modality for detecting coronary artery disease in men, many studies have demonstrated a low sensitivity and specificity of exercise treadmill testing in women. In a meta-analysis of 19 studies of exercise stress tests in 3,721 women, the mean sensitivity was 61%, mean specificity 70%, positive likelihood ratio (LR) 2.25 and negative LR 0.55. This is compared to a mean sensitivity of 68% and specificity of 77% in a meta-analysis of exercise testing in 24,074 men [70]. In fact, women are 5 to 20 times more likely to have a false positive exercise ECG compared to men.

Why Is Exercise Treadmill Testing Less Accurate in Women?

Several mechanisms for the reduced specificity of exercise ECG testing in women have been proposed. These mechanisms include a lower achieved workload, the digoxin-like effect of estrogen, an inappropriate catecholamine response to exercise in women, a higher incidence of mitral valve prolapse, and different chest wall anatomy [68]. In addition, it is important to note that the standards for abnormal exercise ECG test were developed in a male population. In order to better elucidate the role of estrogen and progesterone on the sensitivity and specificity of the exercise ECG to detect CAD in postmenopausal women, Bokhari et al retrospectively examined the ability of exercise ECG to detect CAD in 140 postmenopausal women who were either on ERT, HRT or no hormone therapy. Myocardial perfusion imaging (MPI) was the gold standard for comparison. When comparing women on ERT to HRT to no hormone therapy, they found that there was no significant difference in sensitivity (56% vs. 57% vs. 54%). However, there was a significant decrease in specificity in women on ERT alone compared to women on no hormone therapy or on combined estrogen/progestin therapy (46% vs. 78% vs. 80%, respectively) [71]. These finding support the observation that estrogen leads to an unacceptably high rate of false positives, which is counterbalanced by the addition of progesterone.

Does Perfusion Imaging Improve Diagnostic Accuracy in Women?

As a result of the high false positive rate in exercise ECG testing in women, various imaging modalities have been evaluated in the diagnosis and risk stratification of CHD in women. Myocardial perfusion imaging has been shown to have a significantly higher sensitivity and specificity for detecting CAD in men. However the small size of the left ventricle in women and breast artifact have led to some doubt regarding its utility in women. In an effort to evaluate the utility of MPI in the diagnosis of CAD in women, Taillefer et al compared the diagnostic accuracy of Tl-201 and Tc-99m sestamibi SPECT imaging in detecting CAD in 85 women with suspected CAD who were already scheduled for coronary angiography [72]. This study revealed that the overall sensitivity for detection of CAD ($\geq$50% stenosis) was 75% for Tl-201 and 71.9% for Tc-99m sestamibi with a specificity of 61.9% vs. 85.7%, respectively ($p = 0.07$). For the detection of stenosis $\geq$70% the sensitivity was 84.3% vs. 80.4% and the specificities were 58.8% vs. 82.4%, for Tl-201 and Tc-99m respectively ($p = 0.01$). The use of gated SPECT Tc-99m imaging resulted further improvement in the specificity of the test for detecting both ≥50% and ≥70% stenoses as compared to Tl-201 (70.6% vs. 94.1% $p=0.002$ and 67.2% vs. 92.2% $p=0.004$, respectively).

The addition of myocardial perfusion imaging to treadmill testing provides for a significant improvement in both the sensitivity and specificity in the detection of CAD in women regardless of the imaging agent used. However, for the greatest specificity Tc-99m gated SPECT imaging appears to be the ideal imaging agent.

How Does Stress Echocardiography Compare with ETT?

Exercise echocardiography has also been shown to be an accurate modality to non-invasively diagnose CAD in men. There have, however, been conflicting reports regarding its utility in women, with specificities ranging from 46% to 93% [73]. In order to determine whether there is a cost efficient role for exercise echocardiography in the detection of CAD in women (defined as ≥50% occlusion of a major epicardial artery), Marwick et al evaluated 161 women referred for exercise echocardiography and coronary angiography for an evaluation of cardiac symptoms. This study found that the sensitivity of exercise echocardiography for detecting CAD was 80%, the specificity was 81%, the positive predictive value was 71% and the negative predictive value was 87%. Compared to the exercise ECG, stress echocardiography had significantly higher specificity (80% vs. 56% $p \leq 0.0004$), accuracy (81% vs. 64% $p < 0.005$), and positive predictive value (74% vs. 54%, $p < 0.05$) whereas the sensitivity (81% vs. 77%, $p = 0.5$) and the negative predictive value (86% vs. 78%, $p = 0.19$) were comparable [71]. The authors concluded that exercise echocardiography was a cost efficient initial first test for the detection of coronary artery disease, especially in women with an intermediate pre-test probability of CAD.

Based on these studies it is clear that exercise ECG is a less than ideal test for detecting CAD in women, with a very high false positive rate which leads in turn to many unnecessary invasive coronary angiograms. The addition of Tc-99m sestamibi or echocardiography to exercise ECG provides for an effective and cost efficient way to diagnose women with suspected CAD without a high rate of false positives.

Is There a Role for Electron Beam Tomography in the Detection of CAD in Women?

Although myocardial perfusion imaging and stress echocardiography greatly increased the specificity of stress testing over exercise ECG, the sensitivity did not substantially improve. Electron beam tomography (EBT) has been offered as a possible non-invasive modality that would improve the sensitivity of detection of CAD in women. Budoff et al established the sensitivity, specificity and predictive value of EBT in 387 symptomatic women and 733 symptomatic men, using coronary angiography as the gold standard (significant CAD defined as a stenosis > 50%) [74]. Using a coronary calcium score cut-off of zero, the authors found that the sensitivity of EBT in detecting significant CAD in both men and women was 96%. The specificity, however, was significantly higher in women (57%

vs. 41%, $p < 0.001$). By using a receiver operator curve (ROC) the authors found that using a calcium score cutoff of 34 yielded the optimal sensitivity (81%) and specificity (81%).

Although EBT using a calcium score cutoff of 34 does offer a modest advantage in sensitivity over myocardial perfusion imaging, the specificity is still less than that seen in Tc-99m gated SPECT imaging or stress echocardiography. A combination of EBT and stress imaging may offer the best combination of sensitivity and specificity for non-invasively detecting CAD in women. See table 4 for a summary of these non-invasive diagnostic modalities.

Table 4. Stress Testing and Cardiac Imaging in Women

Test	Sensitivity	Specificity
ETT	61%	70%
Tl-201 MPI	75%	61.9%
Tc-99m MPI	71.9%	85.7%
Gated-Tc-99m MPI	n/a	94.1%
Exercise echo	80%	81%
EBT (cutoff 34)	81%	81%

What Is the Prognostic Utility of Stress Testing in Women?

Both myocardial perfusion imaging as well as stress echocardiography have been evaluated for their roles in risk stratification of women with suspected CAD. Hachamovitch et al explored the gender related differences in the prognostic value of exercise dual isotope stress testing in identifying men and women at risk for cardiac death or nonfatal myocardial infarction [75]. The authors retrospectively studied 2,742 men and 1,394 women for a mean 20 ± 5 months for the above endpoints. The women included in this study were significantly older, had more atypical symptoms and had more cardiac risk factors compared to the men who more frequently had a history of prior myocardial infarction and more frequently presented without symptoms. The overall event rates were similar between the men and the women (3.5% vs. 3.2% p = NS). The authors found that the event rate in both men and women increased as a function of the perfusion scan abnormality. Women with a definitely abnormal scan, however, had a greater than twofold higher event rate compared to men with a similar scan result (13.9% vs. 6.6% $p = 0.001$). Accordingly, the perfusion scan result was better able to risk stratify women than men. The odds ratio for an event with an abnormal versus a normal scan in women was 22.8, as compared to the odds ratio of 4.4 for men ($p < 0.0001$). This effectiveness was independent of patient characteristics and ECG test results. The nuclear scan information added 17% and 37% additional prognostic information in men and women, respectively.

In order to address the question of whether pharmacologic perfusion imaging adds incremental prognostic value over clinical predictors, Berman et al retrospectively examined the rate of cardiac death over a follow-up of 27 ± 8.8 months in 2,656 women and 2,677 men who had undergone adenosine dual isotope MPI [76]. Cardiac death occurred in 4.4% of women and 6.1% of men over the follow-up time period. Similar to the results in exercise MPI, the annual rate of cardiac death rose as a function of worsening sum stress score. With a normal scan the annual mortality rate was 0.6% and 0.9% for men and women respectively, while a severely abnormal scan conferred an annual cardiac mortality rate of 5.5% in men and 7.0% in women ($p < 0.001$). As in exercise myocardial perfusion imaging, the scan data added incremental prognostic value to the clinical predictors of cardiac death.

Exercise and dobutamine stress echocardiography have also been proven beneficial in risk stratifying both men and women. In a study of 3,322 men and 2,476 women who were prospectively followed for 3.2 years, exercise induced wall motion abnormality on exercise echocardiogram was independently associated with increased risk of cardiac events (defined as nonfatal myocardial infarction and cardiac death) with a relative risk in women 1.49 (95% CI 1.14-1.94, p 0.003) and a relative risk in men 1.53 (95% CI 1.32-1.77, $p = 0.0001$) [77]. These results were confirmed in a long-term prospective study in 4,234 women and 6,898 men. In both exercising patients and patients who underwent dobutamine stress echocardiography, extent of ischemia was an independent predictor of time to cardiac death, with a relative risk of 1.45 (95% CI 1.20-1.74, $p < 0.0001$) in exercising patients and a relative risk of 1.27 per vascular territory in patients undergoing dobutamine stress (95% CI 1.07-1.52, $p = 0.007$).

Based on these studies both exercise and pharmacologic myocardial perfusion imaging and stress echocardiography are valuable tools in women for risk stratification. The choice of imaging modality will need to be based on each individual woman's risk factors and body habitus.

Conclusion

Cardiovascular disease in women is a health problem of epidemic proportions throughout the world. The battle to properly diagnose, treat and prevent CVD in women is just beginning. While the majority of the data we have to guide our diagnostic and treatment decisions are based on trials done primarily in men, there is an emerging database that specifically addresses these important issues in women. In fact, a recent series of articles published in the Journal of American College of Cardiology have focused on the gender differences in the presentation, diagnosis and pathophysiology of CHD [78, 79]. Based on the data available to date several primary and secondary prevention strategies should be implemented in women. Women should be counseled about the importance of diet and exercise in the prevention of CHD. They should be encouraged to maintain a BMI less than 23, a waist to hip ratio of less than 0.72 and a waist circumference of less than 71 cm. In order to achieve these beneficial physical dimensions, women should be encouraged to eat a diet high in cereal fiber, foods with a low glycemic index and high in polyunsaturated fat. The consumption of trans-fatty acids and saturated fats should be avoided. Women of all sizes should be encouraged to walk briskly 3 hours per week or exercise vigorously for 1.5 hours per week. LDL cholesterol and HDL cholesterol, in addition to the index of total cholesterol/HDL and CRP levels should be used to guide statin therapy to optimize primary and secondary risk reduction of CHD in women. Currently, there is no role for postmenopausal hormone replacement, antioxidant vitamins or folate/Vitamin B6 therapy in either the primary or secondary prevention of CHD in women. In addition, aspirin should not be recommended for the primary prevention in low risk women but can be supported in diabetics, high-risk patients or in elderly women. There appears to be a role for fish oil supplementation in both the primary and secondary prevention of CHD in women. As ongoing and future trials in women are completed, novel approaches tailored towards eradicating the epidemic of CHD in women appears likely.

REFERENCES

[1] A Race Against Time: The Challenge of Cardiovascular Disease in Developing *Economies*. Available at: http://www.earthinstitute.columbia.edu /news/2004/images/raceagainsttime_FINAL_410404.pdf. Accessed January 15, 2006.

[2] Heart Disease and Stroke Statistics – 2005 Update. American Heart Association.

[3] Mosca L, Mochari H, Christian A et al. National Study of Women's Awareness, Preventive Action, and Barriers to Cardiovascular Health. *Circulation*. 2006; 113: 525-534.

[4] Rich-Edwards JW, Manson JE, Hennekens CH, and Buring JE. The Primary Prevention of Coronary Heart Disease in Women. *N. Eng. J. Med.* 1995; 332(26): 1758-1766.

[5] Marrugat J, Sala J, Masia R et al. Mortality Differences Between Men and Women Following First Myocardial Infarction. *JAMA*. 1998;280(16):1405-9.

[6] Daly C, Clemens F, Lopez-Sendon JL et al. Gender Differences in the Management and Clinical Outcome of Stable Angina. *Circulation*. 2006; 113: 490-498.

[7] Mendelsohn ME and Karas RH. The Protective Effects of Estrogen on the Cardiovascular System. *N Eng J Med.* 1999; 340 (23): 1801-11.

[8] The Postmenopausal Estrogen/Progesterone Interventions (PEPI) Trial: the Writing Group for the PEPI trial. Effects of Estrogen or Estrogen/Progestin regimens on heart disease risk factors in postmenopausal women. *JAMA*. 1995; 273: 199-208.

[9] Mosca L, Collin P, Herrington DM et al. Hormone Replacement Therapy and Cardiovascular Disease. A Statement for Healthcare Professionals From the American Heart Association. *Circulation*. 2001; 104: 499-503.

[10] Cushman M, Legault C, Barrett-Connor E et al. Effect of Postmenopausal Hormones on Inflammation-Sensitive Proteins. The PEPI Study. *Circulation*. 1999; 100: 717-722.

[11] Ridker PM, Hennekens CH, Rifai N, Buring JE, and Manson JE. Hormone Replacement Therapy and Increased Plasma Concentration of C-Reactive Protein. *Circulation*. 1999; 100: 713-716.

[12] Low AK, Russell LD, Holman HE et al. Hormone Replacement Therapy and Coronary Heart Disease in Women: A review of the evidence. *Am J Med Sci*. 2002; 324 (4): 180-4.

[13] Hulley S, Grady D, Bush T et al. Randomized Trial of Estrogen Plus Progestin for Secondary Prevention of Coronary Heart Disease in Postmenopausal Women. *JAMA*. 1998; 280: 605-613.

[14] Grady D, Herrington D, Bittner V et al for the HERS Research Group. Cardiovascular Disease Outcomes During 6.8 Years of Hormone Therapy. Heart and Estrogen/Progestin Replacement Study Follow-Up (HERS II). *JAMA*. 2002; 288(1): 49-57.

[15] The ESPRIT Team. Oestrogen therapy for prevention of reinfarction in postmenopausal women: a randomized placebo controlled trial. *Lancet*. 2002; 360: 2001-8.

[16] Clarke SC, Kelleher J, Lloyd-Jones H, Slack M, Schofield PM. A study of hormone replacement therapy in postmenopausal women with ischaemic heart disease: the Papworth HRT Atherosclerosis Study. *BJOG*. 2002; 109: 1056-62.

[17] Manson JE, Hsia J, Johnson KC et al for the Women's Health Initiative Investigators. Estrogen plus Progestin and the Risk of Coronary Heart Disease. *N Eng J Med*. 2003; 349: 523-34.

[18] Writing Group for the Women's Health Initiative Investigators. Risks and Benefits of Estrogen Plus Progestin in Healthy Postmenopausal Women. *JAMA*. 2002; 288(3): 321-333.

[19] The Women's Health Initiative Steering Committee. Effects of Conjugated Equine Estrogen in Postmenopausal Women with Hysterectomy. *JAMA*. 2004; 291(14): 1701-1712.

[20] Miller VM, Clarkson TB, Harman M et al. Women, hormones, and clinical trials: a beginning, not an end. *J. Appl. Physiol.* 2005; 99: 381-383.

[21] Harman SM, Brinton A, Cedars M et al. KEEPS: The Kronos Early Estrogen Prevention Study. *Climacteric*. 2005; 8: 3-12.

[22] Pradhan AD, Skerrett PJ, and Manson JE. Obesity, diabetes, and coronary risk in women. *J Cardiovasc Risk*. 2002; 9: 323-330.

[23] Willett WC, Manson JE, Stampfer MJ et al. Weight, Weight Change, and Coronary Heart Disease in Women: Risk Within the 'Normal' Weight Range. *JAMA*. 1995; 273(6): 461-465.

[24] Li TY, Manson JE, Willett WC et al. Obesity as Compared with Physical Activity in Predicting Risk of Coronary Heart Disease in Women. *Circulation*. 2006; 113: 499-506.

[25] Rexrode KM, Carey VJ, Hennekens CH et al. Abdominal Adiposity and Coronary Heart Disease in Women. *JAMA*. 1998; 280: 1843-1848.

[26] Kip KE, Marroquin OC, Kelley DE et al. Clinical Importance of Obesity versus the Metabolic Syndrome in Cardiovascular Risk in Women. A report from the Women's Ischemia Syndrome Evaluation (WISE) Study. *Circulation*. 2004; 109:706-713.

[27] Hu FB, Stampfer MJ, Manson JE et al. Dietary Fat Intake and the Risk of Coronary Heart Disease in Women. *N. Eng. J. Med.* 1997; 337: 1491-1499.

[28] Liu S, Willett WC, Stampfer MJ et al. A prospective study of dietary glycemic load, carbohydrate intake and risk of coronary heart disease in US women. *Am J. Clin. Nutr.* 2000; 71: 1455-1461.

[29] Joshipura KJ, Hu FB, Manson JE et al. The Effect of Fruit and Vegetable Intake on Risk for Coronary Heart Disease. *Ann. Intern. Med.* 2001; 134:1106-1114.

[30] Wolk A, Manson JE, Stampfer MJ et al. Long-term Intake of Dietary Fiber and Decreased Risk of Coronary Heart Disease among Women. *JAMA*. 1999; 281(21): 1998-2004.

[31] Fung TT, Willett WC, Stampfer MJ, Manson JE, Hu FB. Dietary Patterns and the Risk of Coronary Heart Disease in Women. *Arch. Intern. Med.* 2001;161: 1857-1862.

[32] Howard BV, Van Horn L, Hsia J et al. Low-Fat Dietary Pattern and Risk of Cardiovascular Disease. The Women's Health Initiative Randomized Controlled Dietary Modification Trial. *JAMA*. 2006; 295: 655-666.

[33] De Lorgeril M, Salen P, Martin JL et al. Mediterranean Diet, Traditional Risk Factors, and the Rate of Cardiovascular Complications after Myocardial Infarction. *Circulation.* 1999; 99: 779-785.

[34] Manson JE, Hu FB, Rich-Edwards JW et al. A Prospective Study of Walking as Compared with Vigorous Exercise in the Prevention of Coronary Heart Disease in Women. *N. Eng. J. Med.* 1999; 341:650-658.

[35] Hu FB, Stampfer MJ, Solomon C et al. Physical Activity and Risk for Cardiovascular Events in Diabetic Women. *Ann. Intern. Med.* 2001; 134: 96-105.

[36] Manson JE, Greenland P, LaCroix AZ et al. Walking Compared with Vigorous Exercise for the Prevention of Cardiovascular Events in Women. *N. Eng. J. Med.* 2002; 347: 716-725.

[37] Stampfer MJ, Hu FB, Manson JE, Rimm EB, Willett WC. Primary Prevention of Coronary Heart Diase in Women through Diet and Lifestyle. *N. Eng. J. Med.* 2000; 343: 16-22.

[38] Morris CD, Carson S. Routine Vitamin Supplementation to Prevent Cardiovascular Disease: A Summary of the Evidence for the U.S. Preventive Services Task Force. *Ann. Intern. Med.* 2003; 139: 56-70.

[39] Stampfer MJ, Hennekens CH, Manson JE et al. Vitamin E Consumption and the Risk of Coronary Disease in Women. *N. Eng. J. Med.* 1993; 328: 1444-1449.

[40] Kushi LH, Folsom AR, Prineas RJ et al. Dietary Antioxidant Vitamins and Death from Coronary Heart Disease in Postmenopausal Women. *N. Eng. J. Med.* 1996; 334: 1156-1162.

[41] Stephens NG, Schofield PM, Cheeseman K, Mitchinson MJ, Brown, MJ. Randomised controlled trial of vitamin E in patients with coronary disease: Cambridge Heart Antioxidant Study (CHAOS). *Lancet.* 1996; 347: 781-786.

[42] GISSI-Prevenzione Investigators. Dietary supplementation with n-3 polyunsaturated fatty acids and vitamin E after myocardial infarction: results of the GISSI-Prevenzione trial. *Lancet.* 1999; 354: 447-455.

[43] Heart Protection Study Collaborative Group. MRC/BHF Heart Protection Study of antioxidant vitamin supplementation in 20,536 high-risk individuals: a randomized placebo-controlled trial. *Lancet.* 2002; 360: 23-33.

[44] Waters DD, Alderman EL, Hsia J et al. Effects of Hormone Replacement Therapy and Antioxidant Vitamin Supplements on Coronary Atherosclerosis in Postemenopausal Women. A randomized controlled trial. *JAMA.* 2002; 288: 2432-2440.

[45] The Heart Outcomes Prevention Evaluation Study Investigators. Vitamin E Supplementation and Cardiovascular Events in High Risk Patients. *N. Eng. J. Med.* 2000; 342:154-60.

[46] The HOPE and HOPE-TOO Trial Investigators. Effects of Long-term Vitamin E Supplementation on Cardiovascular Events and Cancer. *JAMA.* 2005; 293:1338-1347.

[47] Collaborative Group of the Primary Prevention Project. Low-dose aspirin and vitamin E in people at cardiovascular risk: a randomized trial in general practice. *Lancet.* 2001; 357:89-95.

[48] Lee IM, Cook NR, Gaziano JM et al. Vitamin E in the Primary Prevention of Cardiovascular Disease and Cancer. The Women's Health Study: A Randomized Controlled Trial. *JAMA.* 2005; 294: 56-65.

[49] Eidelman RS, Hollar D, Hebert PR, Lamas GA, Hennekens CH. Randomized Trials of Vitamin E in the Treatment and Prevention of Cardiovascular Disease. *Arch. Intern. Med.* 2004; 164: 1552-1556.

[50] Alfthan G, Aro A, Gey KF. Plasma homocysteine and cardiovascular disease mortality. *Lancet.* 1997; 349: 397.

[51] Rimm EB, Willett WC, Hu FB et al. Folate and Vitamin B6 from Diet and Supplements in Relation to Risk of Coronary Heart Disease among Women. *JAMA.* 1998; 279: 359-364.

[52] NORVIT study group. Randomised trial of homocysteine-lowering with B vitamins for secondary prevention of cardiovascular disease after acute myocardial infarction. The Norwegian Vitamin Study (NORVIT). European Society of Cardiology Meeting. 2005.

[53] Kris-Etherton PM, Harris WS, Appel LJ. Fish Consumption, Fish Oil, Omega-3Fatty Acids and Cardiovascular Disease. *Circulation.* 2002; 106: 2747-2757.

[54] Hu FB, Bronner L, Willett WC et al. Fish and Omega-3 Fatty Acid Intake and Risk of Coronary Heart Disease in Women. *JAMA.* 2002; 287: 1815-1821.

[55] Yokoyama M, Origasa H. Effects of eicosapentaenoic acid on cardiovascular events in Japanese patients with hypercholesterolemia: rationale, design, and baseline characteristics of the Japan EPA Lipid Intervention Study (JELIS). *Am. Heart J.* 2003; 146: 613-620.

[56] Erkkila AT, Lichtenstein AH, Mozaffarian D, Herrington DM. Fish intake is associated with a reduced progression of coronary artery atherosclerosis in postmenopausal women with coronary artery disease. *Am. J. Clin. Nutr.* 2004; 80: 626-632.

[57] Schmidt EB, Arnesen H, Christensen JH et al. Marine n-3 polyunsaturated fatty acids and coronary heart disease. Part II: clinical trials and recommendations. *Thrombosis Research.* 2005; 115: 257-262.

[58] Kjeldsen SE, Kolloch RE, Leonetti G et al. Influence of gender and age on preventing cardiovascular disease by antihypertensive treatment and acetylsalicylic acid. The HOT study. *J. of Hypertension.* 2000; 18: 629-642.

[59] Ridker PM, Cook NR, Lee IM et al. A Randomized Trial of Low-Dose Aspirin in the Primary Prevention of Cardiovascular Disease in Women. *N. Eng. J. Med.* 2005; 352: 1293-1304.

[60] Shai I, Rimm EB, Hankinson SE et al. Multivariate Assessment of Lipid Parameters as Predictors of Coronary Heart Disease among Postmenopausal Women: Potential Implications for Clinical Guidelines. *Circulation.* 2004; 110: 2824-2830.

[61] Miettinen TA, Pyorala K, Olsson AG et al. Cholesterol Lowering Therapy in Women and Elderly Patients with Myocardial Infarction or Angina Pectoris. *Circulation.* 1997; 96: 4211-4218.

[62] Lewis SJ, Sacks FM, Mitchell JS et al. Effect of Pravastatin on Cardiovascular Evetns in Women After Myocardial Infarction: The Cholesterol and Recurrent Events (CARE) Trial. *J. Am. Coll. Cardiol.* 1998; 32: 140-146.

[63] Ridker PM, Cannon CP, Morrow D et al. C-Reactive Protein Levels and Outcomes after Statin Therapy. *N. Eng. J. Med.* 2005; 352: 20-28.

[64] Wong ND, Pio J, Valencia R, Thakal G. Distribution of C-reactive protein and its relation to risk factors and coronary heart diease risk estimation in the National Health and Nutrition Survey (NHANES) III. *Prev. Cardiol.* 2001; 4: 109-114.

[65] Albert MA, Glynn RJ, Buring J, Ridker PM. C-reactive protein levels among women of carious ethnic groups living in the United States (from the Women's Health Study). *Am. J. Cardiol.* 2004; 93: 1238-1242.

[66] Ridker PM, Hennekens CH, Buring JE, Rifal N. C-Reactive Protein and Other Markers of Inflammation in the Prediction of Cardiovascular Disease in Women. *N. Eng. J. Med.* 2000; 342:836-843.

[67] Ridker PM, Rifal N, Rose L, Buring JE, Cook NR. Comparison of C-Reactive Protein and Low-Density Lipoprotein Cholesterol Levels in the Prediction of First Cardiovascular Events. *N. Eng. J. Med.* 2002; 347:1557-1565.

[68] Ridker PM on behalf of the JUPITER study group. Rosuvastatin in the Primary Prevention of Cardiovascular Disease among Patients with Low Levels of Low-Density Lipoprotein Cholesterol and Elevated High-Sensitivity C-Reactive Protein: Rationale and Design of the JUPITER trial. *Circulation.* 2003; 108: 2292-2297.

[69] Bigi R, Cortigiani L. Stress testing in women: sexual discrimination or equal opportunity? *European Heart Journal.* 2005; 26:423-425.

[70] Kwok Y, Kim C, Grady D, Segal M, Redberg R. Meta-Analysis of Exercise Testing to Detect Coronary Artery Disease in Women. *Am. J. Cardiol.* 1999;83: 660-666.

[71] Bokhari S, Bergmann SR. The Effect of Estrogen Compared to Estrogen Plus Progesterone on the Exercise Electrocardiogram. *J. Am. Coll. Cardiol.*. 2002; 40: 1092-1096.

[72] Taillefer R, DePuey G, Udelson JE et al. Comparative Diagnostic Accuracy of Tl-201 and Tc-99m Sestamibi SPECT Imaging (perfusion and ECG-Gated SPECT) in Detecting Coronary Artery Disease in Women. *J. Am. Coll. Cardiol.* 1997; 29:69-77.

[73] Marwick TH, Anderson T, Williams MJ et al. Exercise Echocardiography Is an Accurate and Cost-Efficient Technique for the Detection of Coronary Artery Disease in Women. *J. Am. Coll. Cardiol.* 1995; 26: 335-341.

[74] Budoff MJ, Shokooh S, Shavelle RM, Kim T, French WJ. Electron beam tomography and angiography: sec differences. *Am. Heart J.* 2002; 143: 877-882.

[75] Hachamovitch R, Berman DS, Kiat H et al. Effective Risk Stratification Using Exercise Myocardial Perfusion SPECT in Women: Gender-Related Differences in Prognostic Nuclear Testing. *J. Am. Coll Cardiol.* 1996; 28:34-44.

[76] Berman DS, Kang X, Hayes SW et al. Adenosine Myocardial Perfusion Single-Photon Emission Computed Tomography in Women Compared with Men. Impact of Diabetes Mellitus on Incremental Prognostic Value and Effect on Patient Management. *J. Am. Coll. Cardiol.* 2003: 41: 1125-1133.

[77] Arruda-Olsen AM, Juracan EM, Mahoney DW et al. Prognostic Value of Exercise Echocardiography in 5,798 Patients: Is there a gender difference? *J. Am. Coll. Cardiol.* 2002; 39:625-631.

[78] Shaw LJ, Merz NB, Pepine CJ et al. Insights from the NHLBI-Sponsored Women's Ischemia Syndrome Evaluation (WISE) Study. Part I: Gender Differences in Traditional and Novel Risk Factors, Symptom Evaluation, and Gender-Optimized Diagnostic Strategies. *J. Am. Coll. Cardiol.* 2006; 47: 4S-20S.

[79] Merz NB, Shaw LJ, Reis SE et al. Insights from the NHLBI-Sponsored Women's Ischemia Syndrome Evaluation (WISE) Study. Part II: Gender Differences in Presentation, Diagnosis, and Outcome with regard to Gender-Based Pathophysiology of

Atherosclerosis and Macrovascular and Microvascular Coronary Disease. *J. Am. Coll. Cardiol.* 2006; 47: 21S-29S.

In: World Heart Research Yearbook. Volume 1
Editors: Franz Halberg and R. B. Singh
ISBN: 978-1-60741-881-8

Magnetic Resonance Imaging Methods in Cardiovascular Imaging: Experimental and Clinical Applications with Limitations

Rakesh Sharma*
Division of Cardiology, Department of Medicine, Columbia University, New York, NY, US

Introduction

Nuclear magnetic resonance (NMR) has emerged a powerful tool after its discovery by Felix Bloch and Edward Purcell [1]. Later NMR relaxation constants of tissues with possibility of NMR back-projection–reconstruction images and magnetic field inhomogeneity encoded locations of water and oil in small test tubes changed the scenario of magnetic resonance methods in disease detection [2, 3]. Based on the fact that specific radiowave excitations within magnetic field can induce different frequencies to generate spatial images by Fourier transformation became reality as present magnetic resonance imaging (MRI) [4]. Soon after, MRI of whole body was developed [5] with possibility of high speed echo-planar imaging (EPI) technique [6]. In recent years, cardiovascular imaging got momentum by experiments utilizing both multinuclear NMR spectroscopy and MR imaging to speculate myocardial metabolism and dynamic changes in the heart [7-8]. Other clinical application of cardiovascular MR (CMR) imaging to predict the myocardial viability and recovery encouraged the assessment of the myocardium [9]. Present time, efforts are continuing for faster acquisition, breadth-hold, 3D navigation, minimization of motion artifacts, real-time imaging and their robust automated 4D segmentation and registration analysis of whole cardiac cycle [10]. This present paper highlights the present state-of-the-art of cardiovascular MR (CMR) imaging methods and applications with their limitations.

CMR Spectroscopy and Imaging Techniques

Several approaches of radiofrequency pulse sequences and magnetic field gradients show the generation of cardiovascular MRI images and flow measurement (see Table 1). Current

* Address correspondence to: Rakesh Sharma, Department of Chemical and Biomedical Engineering, FAMU-FSU College of Engineering, A 160, 2525 Pottsdamer Street, Florida State University, Tallahassee, Florida 32310 Email: rs2010@columbia.edu.

trend is toward faster imaging sequences and the reduction of motion artifacts. However, routine clinical use of these sequences on the major clinical imagers is still in infancy and needs the development of user-friendly robust analysis software.

CARDIAC MRI LOCALIZATION TECHNIQUES

The clinical application of CMR requires the 3D localization of the observed MRI signals from *in situ* myocardium without contamination of surrounding pleural tissues. Initially the CMR was limited to myocardium metabolism and energy metabolites by P-31 MR spectroscopy. With advancements in 3D and 4D localization methods, localized cardiac MR imaging and spectroscopy could be possible by H-1, P-31, C-13 and Na-23 nuclei [10, 11, 12]. These localization techniques use the imaging gradients to define an excitation volume of interest (VOI) in single volume, and then gradients are turned off during the subsequent acquisition in multiple volumes (see Table 2).

Single-volume techniques generate image as cylinder of excitation using the lateral planes of a surface coil. In the perpendicular direction to the plane of the surface coil, applied spatial localization acquires CMR signal at different distances from the surface coil. Therefore, the diameter of the surface coil provides in-plane localization parallel to the surface coil to generate multiple volume sites. These multi-volume techniques are the most widely used clinical methods within the cardiovascular tissue by the use of several gradients.

Table 1. Comparison of common clinical imaging sequences

MR Imaging pulse sequence	Contrast information	Limitations
Spin echo sequence for dark blood images		
Excitation 90û and refocusing 180û pulse synchronized with cardiac cycle	Ventricles appear darker 180û pulse refocuses susceptibility artifacts	One echo generated per pulse Slow, long scan time
Gradient-recalled echo (GRE) sequence for bright blood images		
Gradients refocus dephasing spins Low flip angle, short TR	Blood pool high signal as "bright blood" Faster imaging speed	Increased T2* sensitivity Susceptibility effects persist
Fast Spin Echo (FSE) for fast imaging		
Single radiofrequency excitation followed by 180û pulse train for multiple echoes; T1 recovers many times before next 90û pulse	High signal noise ratio (SNR) Bulk inhomogeneities refocused Fast image acquisition	Rf power disposition
Multi-shot Echo-planar imaging (MEPI) and EPI images		
Rapid gradient switching after one 90û excitation pulse	Very fast with temporal resolution Fast image generation by >2 excitations	Sensitive to motion, flow & magnetic field inhomogeneity
Steady-State Free Precession (SSFP) images		
Gradient waveform applied in each TR for coherent steady-state magnetization	T2* and T1 weighted contrast, cine MRI Insensitive to breath motion and speed Fast, high contrast of blood & endocardium	Sensitive to motion and flow
3D Navigation and VENC real-time images		
Spiral acquisition of k-space during one TR	Velocity and real-time flow measurement	Sensitive to motion & MRI gradients
Sensitivity and velocity encoded (SENSE) cine MRI images		
Sensitivity coding with velocity encoded	Faster flow quantitation	Sensitive to flow & motion

Table 2. Single-volume and multivolume cardiac spectroscopic imaging localization techniques

Spectroscopic imaging localization	Advantages	Disadvantages	Ref.
Single-volume localization:			
Point-resolved spectroscopy(PRESS)			[11]
Spectra acquired from one voxel	High SNR for uncoupled metabolites with long T2	Long acquisition time	
Stimulated echo acquisition mode (STEAM)			[12]
Faster acquisition of high SNR by short TR Stimulated echoes used	High SNR of ^{13}C coupled spins	No quantitation	
Depth–resolved surface coil spectroscopy(DRESS)			[13]
Acquired Spectra from contiguous slices parallel to surface coil	Cardiac metabolism	Magnetic field sensitive	
Image-selected in vivo spectroscopy(ISIS)			[14]
Single sensitive volume selected by 3 orthogonal inversion pulses anywhere within coil	Multiple volumes query Sequential volume	No localized info Motion sensitive	
Multivolume localization:			
1D, 2D or 3D Chemical shift imaging (CSI) Muti-slices, volumes in one VOI or many VOI are used	Choice of slices/VOI	Sensitive to shim	[15]
Spatial localization with optimal point-spread function(SLOOP)			[16]
Spatial response function defined VOI determines the point-spread function to weigh MR spectral contribution; Combined with chemical shift imaging	Good for irregular VOI Accurate quantitation	*a priori* metabolite peaks Outer volume bleeding	
4D Segmentation and Registration			[17]
Non-rigid registration performs to deform elastically a cardiac atlas	End-diastolic time frame constructed		

Chemical Shift Imaging

Pulsed phase-encoding gradients control the localization of the signals using Fourier transform MRI method for chemical shift imaging (CSI). The grid was placed across the heart to reconstruct the metabolite chemical shift image of the beating heart by stimulated echo acquisition mode (STEAM) method [12]. Depth-resolved surface-coil improved the voxel size selection suitable for left ventricle [13]. Another approach of Image-selected in vivo spectroscopy (ISIS) uses the shape of the VOI (as cube with steep edges) representing the sensitive volume in CSI by the spatial response function (SRF). The SRF represents the contribution of amplitude and phase of each point existing in space. The shape of the SRF looks as sinc function in raw ISIS images [14]. So, CSI displays high sensitivity of different metabolites in different VOI locations [15]. However, several factors such as drifted non-static magnetic field can cause artifacts in measurements on CSI images and localization of region of interest (ROI) [16]. The CSI spectral maps mostly suffer from outer volume contamination outside the region of interest, motion artifacts, poor magnetic field sensitivity and linear combination of chemical shift signals at different time points throughout the image acquisition. Recently, advanced software techniques such as patient positioning protocols, high SNR sensitive coil design, and quicker parameter optimization has improved the spectral peak resolution and metabolite spatial resolution within reasonable acquisition time.

EXPERIMENTAL CARDIAC MRI IMAGING APPLICATIONS

Experimental MRI studies focused on isolated rat heart using patch and clamp method to achieve metabolic screening and contractile functions of beating heart [18, 19]. Main focus of isolated heart MRI was establishing relationship of MRI visible metabolites or their NMR peaks with cardiac and myocardial time-series events. P-31 MR spectroscopy and C-13 MR spectroscopy have attracted attention in this direction due to their capability of speculating PCr, ATP, pH distribution in tissue and source of ATP i.e. components of Tricarboxylic acid cycle [19].

At author's lab, new approach of rat heart sodium Na-23 MRI was developed focusing on evaluation of cardiac ischemia based on intracellular sodium MRI signals by modified spin echo pulse sequences [20]. The optimized inversion time, blood concentration of injected Gd-DTPA and shift contrast agents further enhanced the capability of isolating intracellular sodium distribution as shown in Figure 1. Other approach of enhanced intracellular sodium Na-23 heart images used Dysprosium (Dys) delayed enhancement using triple filtered quantum sequences at low level of myocardial intensity in areas of infarction or scar irreversible damage [21, 22] (Figure 1).

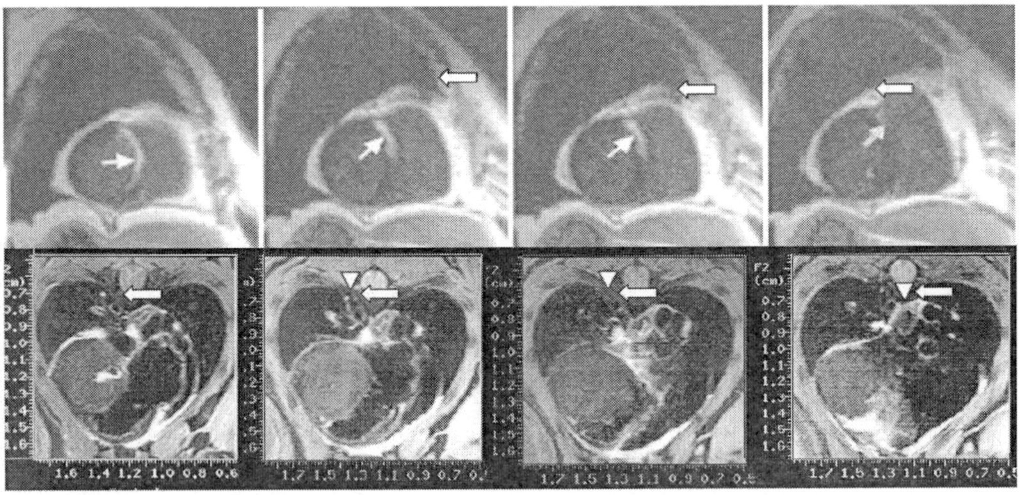

Figure 1. Delayed contrast short-axis views of the heart 30 minutes after contrast injection. The inversion time was optimized TI = 25 ms to null the normal myocardium and the area of infarction showing as a bright region. The arrows indicate the regions of contrast enhancement in sagittal view (top row) and transaxial view (bottom row).

Recent studies have significantly improved the novelty of isolated heart MRI time series monitoring approach to assess the myocardial viability and its functional recovery [23]. High magnetic field MRI may further enhance potentials of the time series metabolic imaging and spectroscopy of vulnerable regions such as left ventricles and walls to determine biochemical cause of myocardial viability [24].

Recently, cine-fluoroscopy using high-speed real-time imaging MR methods demonstrated the catheter tracking and placing in position to perform catheter-guided cine-angiography at high resolution, with the potential to characterize 3D imaging of swine heart [25]. Due to their invasive nature, still catheter methods remain less popular.

CLINICAL CARDIAC MRI IMAGING APPLICATIONS

Routine clinical use currently awaits the full implementation of fast and motion-insensitive imaging techniques. Angiography, myocardial contrast enhancement and flow imaging techniques mainly serve the purpose of myocardial viability and contractile function evaluation to some extent.

Magnetic Resonance Angiography

Distal radiofrequency (RF) emission visualized the cardiovasculature by using MRA signal of flowing blood spin labeling to determine vascular blood velocity [26]. Presently, several approaches using paramagnetic contrast agents, rapid and high-resolution imaging are in practice of cardiovasculature imaging without catheter-based angiography [27].

Myocardial-Viability Assessment: Delayed Contrast Enhancement

Myocardial viability evaluation depends upon the measurement and identification of subendocardial inferior wall thickness and apex in hibernating myocardium in order to assess the revascularization benefits on left ventricular function. Non-viable myocardial tissues in infarcted or scarred myocardium with ischemia retain the administered Gadolinium-diethylene-amine penta-acetate (Gd-DTPA) and generate delayed contrast enhanced images using an inversion-recovery pulse sequence [28]. Still paucity of information on optimal dose of Gd-DTPA, inversion time and signal optimization for accurate assessment of the nonviable or scar tissue warrants further investigation before this technique may become a routine clinical tool.

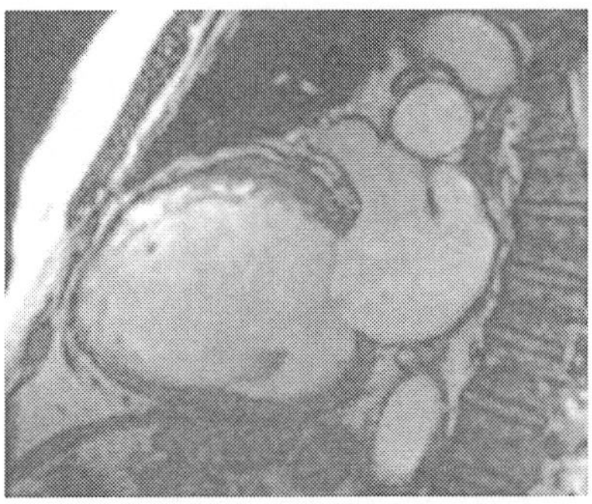

Figure 2. Anatomical detail of the heart using single radiofrequency excitation followed by 180° pulse train for multiple echoes to achieve high signal noise ratio (SNR) by fast spin echo at 1.5 T MRI.

Myocardial Contractile Function

MRI methods may assess regional and global contractile functions. MRI images offer dimensional accuracy, high resolution, and 3D signal properties to evaluate the contractile ventricular function on right or left at regional and global levels (see Figure 2). Other potentials of MRI methods are assessment of ejection fraction for left ventricular systolic function to evaluate cardiac end-systolic and end-diastolic volumes. The ejection fraction measured ventricular volumes in noninvasive, reproducible manner and the calculated cardiac output and stroke volume [29].

Radiofrequency Tagging and Phase Tracking Contrast

Radiofrequency pulses acquire the 'radiofrequency tag line' in 3D planes appearing as orthogonal view through the imaged tissue where the net magnetization differs due to underlying tissue motion. Various tagging schemes have been proposed such as stacks of parallel lines, grids and radial stripes as a function of time [30-32]. These radiofrequency tags can compute the local Lagrangian strain tensor (description of motion around a given point in the tissue) as it traverses through time and space. The strain tensors determined the extent of myocardial tissue contraction as determination of myocardial viability [33].

Myocardial strain monitoring of myocardial deformation has attracted the value of phase information by Lagrangian strain tensor measurements of relative myocardial tissue velocity of the myocardial tissue on a pixel-by-pixel basis [34]. The local gradient of the velocity field at a specific spatial location computes the Eulerian strain rate tensor. In a phase-contrast image, the changes in phases of the net magnetization inside each pixel correlate to the velocities of the underlying tissue in the parallel direction to the applied magnetic field gradient with reference to the original phase of image. Each pixel represents its motion measurement to reconstruct 3D motion map [35]. Displacement encoding with stimulated echoes (DENSE) was reported to generate black-blood high-resolution myocardial-displacement mapping [36]. Velocity encoding by gradient moments was reported to reduce the motion-related artifacts in size and number [37].

Cine MRI Technique

Cine MRI acquires images of one location at multiple time points throughout the cardiac cycle as repeated movie loop, gated with ECG, R-R intervals to generate one image per cardiac phase. Cine MRI complements with MRA by providing hemodynamic and functional data of vascular lesions. Cine gradient echo pulse sequences combine the aspects of 2D TOF MRA and Cine MRI to distinguish bright laminar blood flow from dark turbulent flow in heart valve dysfunctions and flow quantitation by velocity-encoding (VENC). However, border pixels of vessel peripheries always cause artifacts due to their skewed phase offsets. Recently, cine MRI technique was used to evaluate coronary artery stents with MR using both navigator echo and cine gradient echo sequences. These techniques visualized the stents on left anterior descending coronary artery as signal void with GE, and all but one with NE [38].

Image-Guided Catheter Placement

New developments are in progress using high-speed real-time imaging MR methods to track and place the catheter in position to perform catheter-guided cine-angiography at high resolution, with the potential to characterize 3D plaque imaging [39]. Due to their invasive nature, still catheter methods remain less popular.

Coronary MR Angiography

Coronary MR angiography of the moving heart for the imaging of the coronary arteries is still in development phase (Figure 3). Present time, main emphasis is focused on the development of higher-speed standard or spiral techniques for imaging of bypass graft patency and congenitally anomalous coronary arteries [40].

Our recent study (please see in this issue) demonstrated that the left main, the left anterior descending, and the right coronary arteries were well visualized on multicontrast MRI images [41]. The circumflex coronary artery was adequately visualized but less frequently. The technique has potential to enhance resolution of secondary branches and stenotic portions of the coronary arteries. The CMRA seems to be a safe and promising technique for non-invasive evaluation of coronary stents.

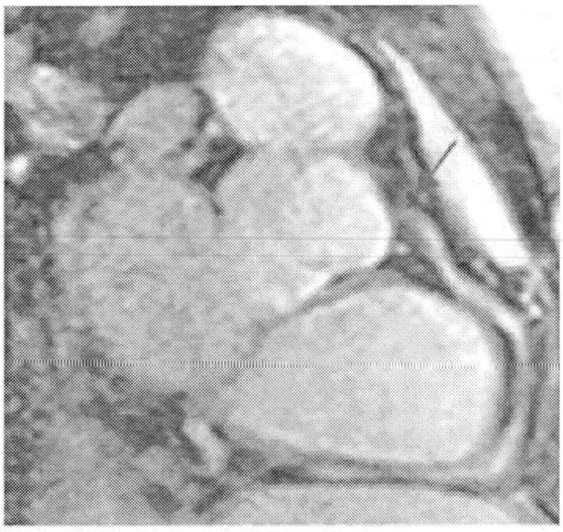

Figure 3. Gradients refocus dephasing spins at low flip angle, short TR show blood pool with high signal "bright blood" and increased T2* sensitivity was achieved by gradient-recalled echo (GRE) sequence for MRI of the right main coronary artery as shown by arrow.

Plaque Imaging and Characterization

MRI can visualize the carotid and coronary arteries in cross section for the plaque and wall morphology and its characterization. Recently author determined the constituents of the plaque in the larger carotid and coronary vessels using both co-registered MRI and histology images. Calcium was not visible (creating a region without signal), lipids and fibrosis had differences in relaxation properties [42, 43]. Plaque composition and % stenosis by MRI evaluated the plaque stability and vulnerability to predict future occlusive events [42, 43]. Routine clinically relevant coronary arterial plaque imaging still needs substantial MRI magnet technical development and robust image processing software development.

QUANTIZATION AND CHARACTERIZATION OF PLAQUE

Extent of stenosis and thrombus size measurement of coronary artery both have recently attracted the attention to evaluate vulnerability and instability of plaques. To some extent, plaque quantitation has given hope to evaluate the cardiovascular risk in advance based on MRI and histology correlation [43]. 3D plaque volume measurement still remains a unsolved problem and poses threat of wrong evaluation using irregular shaped plaque voluming robust techniques available in present time [44]. Clinical application of plaque quantitation remains far from reality and may take long time to implement as routine clinical modality.

Myocardial-Perfusion Imaging

Paramagnetic (e.g., gadolinium) or superparamagnetic (e.g., Fe^{2+}) MRI contrast agents can visualize their perfusion track through the myocardium after intravenous injection at rest and with a vasodilator (e.g., adenosine). Myocardial-perfusion MRI imaging generates higher spatial resolution free from attenuation loss [45]. However, it suffers from the motion artifacts within the interventricular septum between two ventricles [46].

Time Series MRI as ^{31}Phosphorus Stress Test

^{31}P MR chemical shift peaks represent the high-energy phosphates i.e. ATP, phosphocreatine (PCr), and inorganic phosphates. PCr decreases in myocardial ischemia. ATP is more stable during ischemic insults. So, PCr/ATP ratio measurement can track the ischemic insults clinically at 1.5 tesla imagers using 3D CSI and ISIS with low resolution. Recently, high field trio- (i.e., 3 tesla) whole-body system measured the intracellular low pH based on inorganic phosphates (Pi) in myocardial insult due to acidic environment detectable by the "chemical shift" of the Pi spectral peak after handgrip exercise in patients with ischemia consequent to disease of the left anterior descending coronary artery [47]. However, the application of this method remains limited for the anterior wall of the left ventricle in left anterior descending coronary artery disease. The future of ^{31}P-NMR spectroscopy depends on high field clinical scanners, coil developments, and pulse sequences that can generate a uniform excitation volume to examine the entire left ventricle in one session.

Sodium-23 MRI of Myocardial Sarcolemmal Integrity

Sodium-23 is NMR-sensitive. It can detect the sodium accumulation in myocardium territories having inadequate cell membrane function. For sodium-23 MRI imaging, paramagnetic dysprosium shift reagents readily differentiate the intra- and extracellular sodium populations. The author reported intracellular sodium imaging without shift agents as safer for 4.23 T clinical applications with possibility of the development of sodium imaging an ideal clinical tool using optimized inversion recovery pulse sequence set-up [48].

Single-, double-, triple- and quadruple quantum filtering pulse sequence techniques can distinguish intra- from extracellular sodium [49]. These methods resolve the resonances on the basis of ion motion and restriction experienced in the intracellular environment [50-53]. The author reported optimized inversion recovery pulse sequence set-up required their way into routine clinical practice without the toxicity of the currently available shift reagents [54].

Myocardial Intracellular Lipid Content

Myocardial ischemic insult accumulates myocardial amphiphilic lipids as a result of metabolic shift from aerobic lipids (fatty acids) to anaerobic lipids (glycolysis). Such myocardial lipids were visualized by H-1 MRI spectroscopic imaging to examine their effects on myocardial function and conduction at different locations in the interventricular septum after a myocardial ischemic insult [55]. The method suffers from adjacent adipose tissue that surrounds the myocardium. Higher-resolution MRI imaging may detect the lipids in nonseptal myocardium after ischemic insult.

Imaging Applications in Future

Diffusion Weighted Myocardial Imaging

Diffusion weighted myocardial imaging overcomes the motion artifacts. However, the resolution remained poor due to diffusion of water in the myocardium follows the muscle fibers [56]. The orientation of the fibers can be visualized though the use of diffusion tensor MR imaging (DTMRI). Cardiac motion further plagues the multiexponential diffusion behavior characteristics of the intracellular environment vs. extracellular environment of myocardial edema associated with the loss of ionic homeostasis [57]. Still problem persists due to larger cardiac motion than the MRI pulse sequence sensitive diffusion distances in diffusion tensor imaging (7-9 micrometers) to evaluate the myocardial structure and viability of heart [58]. The future depends on development of time-series gating and robust automated registration methods.

Nanoparticle Targeted Contrast Agents

Very tiny lipid spheres (100–200 nm size) with a fluorochemical core is made of two main components. The first component has a target antibody fragment, and a small receptor peptide molecule to direct delivery of the particle [59, 60]. The second component has a contrast agent in high local concentration. Such targeted molecules detect the delivery and monitoring of site-specific therapeutic agents [61, 62]. Labeling of either stem cells or macrophages with superparamagnetic iron oxide (SPIO) particles is under investigation at using cardiomyocyte cells at author's lab. However, reduced image intensity in the presence of SPIO labeled cells can limit their clinical applicability.

Cardiac ^{17}Oxygen MRI imaging

^{19}F MR chemical shift peak represents the oxygenated blood substitute and determines the percent oxygenation in heart. The perfluorochemical composition and percent oxygen both within the core of the targeted nanoparticle contrast-agents may determine the regional oxygen content using targeting of cell-specific markers [63].

Other MRI visible paramagnetic $^{17}O_2$ shows the possibility of the mitochondrial electron transport evaluation. It is based on the fact that oxygen is reduced to water ($H_2{}^{17}O$) by mitochondrial electron transport to generate ATP, while the protons bonded to the ^{17}O result in broadening of the spectral peaks.

However, the signal-to-noise ratio suffers from poor sensitivity. The amount of spectral peak broadening is directly proportional to the amount of reduced oxygen that serves as an independent measure of oxygen consumption and resultant ATP production in the heart [64-65].

MRI Susceptibility Imaging

The ferrous iron in hemoglobin is diamagnetic in oxygenated hemoglobin but it becomes paramagnetic in deoxygenated hemoglobin. Blood oxygen level–dependent (BOLD) imaging uses the same principles to determine the regional oxygen consumption by measuring the tissue perfusion and the quantitation of the deoxyhemoglobin content [66].

Molecular and Metabolic Imaging Applications

Localized Carbon-13 MR Spectroscopy

The ^{13}C MR spectroscopy is very less sensitive but provides some insight of the glycolysis and the tricarboxylic acid (TCA) cycle inside the myocardium. At the present time, low sensitivity of ^{13}C NMR spectroscopy limits it to only laboratory investigations [67]. Development of high field clinical MRI systems with the use of novel pulse sequences may improve the MRI sensitivity for detection of ^{13}C-enhanced compounds. Other options of cross-polarization ^{1}H[^{13}C]-NMR spectroscopy, heteronuclear multiple-quantum coherence (HMQC) spectroscopy, and heteronuclear chemical shift correlation (HETCOR) strategies may improve the SNR and sensitivity of the ^{13}C nucleus detection based on the transfer of magnetization from the carbon to the proton.

Table 3. Recently reported cardiac magnetic resonance imaging techniques under development

Cardiac MRI and MR spectroscopy [reference]	Potential of the technique	Limitation of technique
Olhafen M et al. 2006 [72]	Assessing arterial blood flow and	Real-time zonal phase contrast
Travin MI et al. 2005 [73)	area	Metabolites and LV
Francone M et al. 2005	Assessment of myocardial viability	dysfunction
[74]	Real-time cine MRI of septal motion	Ventricle filling artifacts
Cuocolo A et al. 2005 [75]	Myocardial perfusion techniques	Quantitation poor
Ichikawa Y, et al. 2005	Wall thickness by delayed Gd MRI	In chronic stage, unpredictable
[76]	Myocardial viability assessment	Irreversible or reversible
Bogaert J et al. 2005 [77]	Real time cardiac physio-monitoring	damage
Stainsby JA et al. 2005	Multicentric MRI approach of LVF	Limited scan localization
[78]	Newer displacement encoded MRI	Limited systolic LVF
Hoffmann R et al. 2005	Manganese enhanced contrast	assessment
[79]	Manganese enhanced contrast	Possibility of 3D motion
Gilson WD et al. 2005 [80]	Coronary blood flow measurement	encoding
Hu TC et al. 2004 [81]	Myocardial viability in LV	Simultaneous assessment of
Wendland MF et al. 2004	dysfunction	LV, infarction size and
[82]	Biplane area-length measured for	viability
Sakuma et al. 2004 [83]	atrial volumes by TrueFISP	Dynamic imaging of heart
Thomas B et al. 2004 [84]	Myocardial heterogeneity of end-	Motion artifacts
Sievers B et al. 2004 [85]	systole & end-diastole by Cine MRI	Gadolinium contrast based-
Sievers B et al. 2004 [86]	LV ejection fraction measurement	assessment of sinus rhythm
Swingen C et al. 2004 [87]	3D VENC MRI for mitral valve flow	Limited evaluation,
	Rapid pulse wave velocity measured	Automated but biased method
Lalande A. et al. 2004 [88]	Delayed contrast at optimized TI	Limited accuracy and
Westenberg JJ et al.2004	Free breath radial cardiac	reproducibility
[89]	acquisitions	Multisite flow displacement
Shao X et al. 2004 [90]	Computational cardiac anatomy	Limited value in infarct
Gupta A et al. 2004 [91]	Automated rectilinear cine MRI	imaging
Mc Leish et al. 2004 [92]	No artifact generating echoes	Unpredictable
Beg MF et al. 2004 [93]	3D motion and phase contrast MRI	Limited to morphology
Crowe ME et al. 2004 [94]	New active appearance motion model	Unreliable self gating
Epstein FH et al. 2004 [95]	Automated SENSE cine MRI	Possibility of 3D motion
Kvitting JP et al. 2004 [96]	Adenosine stress MR perfusion MRI	encoding
Vander Geest et al.2004	Automated 3D isotropic MRI	Limited 3D motion assessment
[97]	Pacemaker compatible MRI trial	Time series of LV boundaries
Kostler H et al. 2004 [98]	Gd enhanced R1 cardiac mapping	Cardiac cine imaging
Paetsch I et al. 2004 [99]	Gd enhanced cardiac tissue kinetics	Unpredictable
Sorensen TS et al. 2004	Fibrin labeled MRI of thrombi	Operator independent
[100]	Contrast-enhanced MRI review	Pacemaker safety unreliable
Martin ET et al. 2004 [101]		Unreliable
Kiss P. et al. 2006 [102]		Ischemia-perfusion evaluation
Suranyi P et al. 2007 [103]		Myocardial tissue perfusion
Spuentrup E et al. 2007		Cardio-pulmonary embolism
[104] Saraste et al. 2008		Myocardial viability
[105]		

Cardiac TCA Cycle Kinetics

Due to low NMR sensitivity of ^{13}C nuclei, the possible detection of TCA metabolites is limited to the concentration of 100 μM or greater while the concentrations of the intermediates in the TCA cycle are too low in myocardium. However, in myocardium, the intracellular glutamate is present in concentrations of 1.5 to 4 mM and α-ketoglutarate is in rapid exchange with the intracellular glutamate pool [68]. Recently, ^{13}C MR spectroscopy estimated of TCA cycle turnover from the incorporation of ^{13}C from energy substrates (such as glucose, or free fatty acids) into the glutamate pool. The TCA cycle supports the primary means for energy-metabolism. So, the incorporation rates of ^{13}C from energy substrates into glutamate served as an indirect estimate of oxygen consumption more sensitive than ^{31}P spectroscopy for the detection of myocardial ischemia in animal models [69].

LIMITATIONS AND FUTURE OF CARDIAC MR

Enhancement of high SNR ratio achieved at higher magnetic fields may remain attractive to increase both imaging speed and spatial resolution. In recent years, imaging atherosclerotic plaque, characterization of coronary artery walls, cardiac morphology, myocardial perfusion, myocardial function, metabolic ischemia, and rapid heart viability evaluation still remain as main focus of future cardiovascular MRI as cost effective means to detect and therapeutic monitoring of ischemic heart disease (see Table 3). Perfusion and myocardial viability at high spatial resolution may improve further the cardiac imaging with possibility of MR spectroscopy. Current trend is towards automated techniques, myocardium metabolic and molecular imaging using MRI in the assessment of new therapeutics and their mechanisms of action [70-100]. Fast imaging speed MRI successfully reduced the motion and flow artifacts in real-time acquisition and display. 3D navigation and imaging of wall-motion abnormalities have been recent focus to achieve high SNR in a single breath-hold. High SNR and higher spin-lattice relaxation constants (T1) of cardiac wall simplified the regional wall motion analysis appearing as persistent RF tag-lines throughout the cardiac cycle. High magnetic field rapid MR imaging methods have improved cardiac tissue MRI signal intensity measurement with higher temporal resolution at higher dynamic range in the myocardial delayed non invasive contrast enhancement [49, 70]. In spite of these technique advancements cardiac imaging has limitations. Still, no promising approach exists to measure myocardial tissue perfusion without exogenous contrast agent or spin labeling, use of catheter interventional methods etc.

Cardiac Spectroscopic Imaging

Cardiac high resolution ^{31}P-MR spectroscopic imaging has improved the intracellular imaging capability for pH imaging using Pi /PCr as indicator of myocardial ischemia. High field MRI magnets may improve the weaker ^{13}C MR signal of ^{13}C nuclei strongly coupled by cross-polarization transfer and minimize the time of NMR signal transfer to adjacent protons lesser than imaging over volume of interest. Partial volume averaging and larger volume of interest (VOI) selection limit the accuracy of larger spectroscopic selection and localization methods such as ISIS and depth-resolved surface coil spectroscopy (DRESS) techniques. Turning off gradients during data acquisition remains current practice to reduce partial volume averaging and contamination of adjacent tissues around heart i.e. liver, ventricular blood pool and skeletal muscle. Spectroscopic imaging combined with echo-planar imaging may improve scanning speed [71]. Real-time arterial blood flow by sensitivity encoding and area assessment by zonal phase contrast is other emerging approach [72].

CONCLUSION

MRI has improved the present understanding of cardiovascular structural and functional information at molecular, cellular level and whole heart. There has been tremendous advancement in recent years in the cardiovascular application of MRI as functional and molecular imaging tool in present time. In future, new techniques may improve cardiovascular 3D information as powerful tool in cardiovascular therapy and management.

REFERENCES

[1] Bloch, F. Nuclear induction. *Physical Review (Physics).* 1946; 70:460-473 and Purcell, E., Torrey, H., and Pound, R. Resonance adsorption by nuclear magnetic moments in a solid. *Physical Review (Physics).* 1946; 69:37-38.

[2] Damadian, R.V. Tumor detection by nuclear magnetic resonance. *Science.* 1971; 171:1151-1153.

[3] Lauterbur, P. Image formation by induced local interactions: examples employing nuclear magnetic resonance. *Nature.* 1973; 242:190-191.

[4] Kumar, A., Welti, D., and Ernst, R.R. NMR Fourier zeugmatography. *J. Magn. Reson.* 1975; 18:69-83.

[5] Damadian, R., Goldsmith, M., and Minkoff, L. NMR in cancer. XVI. FONAR image of the live human body. *Physiol. Chem. Phys.* 1977; 9:97-100.

[6] Mansfield, P. 1977. Multi-planar image formation using NMR spin echoes. *J. Phys.* 1977; 10:L55-L58.

[7] Jacobus, W.E., Taylor, G.J.T., Hollis, D.P., and Nunnally, R.L. Phosphorus nuclear magnetic resonance of perfused working rat hearts. *Nature.* 1977; 265:756-758.

[8] Garlick, P.B., Radda, G.K., and Seeley, P.J. Phosphorus NMR studies on perfused heart. *Biochem. Biophys. Res. Commun.* 1977; 74:1256-1262.

[9] Goldman, M.R., Pohost, G.M., Ingwall, J.S., and Fossel, E.T. Nuclear magnetic resonance imaging: potential cardiac applications. *Am. J. Cardiol.* 1980; 46:1278-1283.

[10] Lorenzo-Valdes M., Sanchez-Ortiz G.I., Mohiaddin R., Rueckert D. Atlas-based segmentation of 4D cardiac MR sequences using non-rigid registration. *Med Image Anal.* 2004;8(3):255-65.

[11] Neubauer S. Cardiac magnetic resonance spectroscopy: potential clinical applications. *Herz.* 2000; 25(4):452-60.

[12] Weiss, R.G. ^{13}C-NMR for the study of intermediary metabolism. *MAGMA*. 1998; 6:132.

[13] Okada M, Mitsunami K, Inubushi T, Kinoshita M.1998. Influence of aging or left ventricular hypertrophy on the human heart: contents of phosphorus metabolites measured by ^{31}P MRS. *Magn Reson Med*. 1998; 39(5):772-82.

[14] Ljungberg M, Starck G, Vikhoff-Baaz B, Alpsten M, Ekholm S, Forssell-Aronsson E. The magnitude of signal errors introduced by ISIS in quantitative ^{31}P MRS. *MAGMA*. 2002; 14(1):30-8.

[15] Neubauer, S., Horn, M., Hahn, D., and Kochsiek, K. Clinical cardiac magnetic resonance spectroscopy: present state and future directions. *Mol. Cell. Biochem.* 1998; 184:439-443.

[16] Beer M, Seyfarth T, Sandstede J, Landschutz W, Lipke C, Kostler H, von Kienlin M, Harre K, Hahn D, Neubauer S. Absolute concentrations of high-energy phosphate metabolites in normal, hypertrophied, and failing human myocardium measured noninvasively with (31)P-SLOOP magnetic resonance spectroscopy. *J. Am. Coll. Cardiol.* 2002;40(7):1267-74.

[17] Sharma R.,Sharma A. Advances in magnetic Resonance Angiography Chapter 3, pp 114-187 in: *Handbook of Biomedical Image Analysis Volume 1: Segmentation Models Part A Series*: International Topics in Biomedical Engineering, Suri, Jasjit S.; Wilson, David; Laximinarayan, Swamy (Eds.) 2005, XVIII, 630 p. ISBN: 0-306-48550-8.

[18] von Kienlin, M. et al.2001. Advances in human cardiac 31P-MR spectroscopy: SLOOP and clinical applications. *J. Magn. Reson. Imaging.* 2001; 13:521-527.

[19] Schmidt, O. et al. Artifacts in CSI-measurements caused by the drift of the static magnetic field. *MAGMA.* 2000; 10:167-170.

[20] Dizon J, Burkhoff D, Tauskela J, Whang J, Cannon P, Katz J Metabolic inhibition in the perfused rat heart: evidence for glycolytic requirement for normal sodium homeostasis.AJP *Am. J. Physiol.* 1998;274(4 Pt 2):H1082-9.

[21] Navon G, Werrman JG, Cohen S. Triple quantum filtered ^{23}Na NMR of intracellular sodium in workingt and ischemic isolated hearts:effect of specific inhibition of Na+/H+ exchange. *Mag. Reson. Med.* 1993; 1:362.

[22] Allis JL, Seymour AML, Radda GK. Absolute quantification of intracellular Na+ using triple quantum filtered sodium-23 NMR. *J. Mag. Reson.* 1991; 93: 71-76.

[23] Kim, R.J., Hillenbrand, H.B., and Judd, R.M. Evaluation of myocardial viability by MRI. *Herz.* 2000; 25:417-430.

[24] Forder JR, Povost GM. Cardiovascular nuclear magnetic resonance basic and clinical applications. *J Clin invest.* 2002; 111(11) 1630-39.

[25] Spuentrup, E. Ruebben A, Schaeffter T, Manning WJ, Gunther RW, Buecker A. Magnetic resonance: guided coronary artery stent placement in a swine model. *Circulation.* 2002; 105:874-879.

[26] Chapon C, Lemaire L, Franconi F, Marescaux L, Legras P, Denizot B, Le Jeune JJ. Assessment of myocardial viability in rats: Evaluation of a new method using superparamagnetic iron oxide nanoparticles and Gd-DOTA at high magnetic field. *Magn Reson Med.* 2004;52(4):932-6.

[27] Mahrholdt, H. Wagner A, Holly TA, Elliott MD, Bonow RO, Kim RJ, Judd RM. Reproducibility of chronic infarct size measurement by contrast-enhanced magnetic resonance imaging. *Circulation.* 2002; 106:2322-2327.

[28] Brucks S, Little WC, Chao T, Kitzman DW, Wesley-Farrington D, Gandhi S, Shihabi ZK. 2005 Contribution of left ventricular diastolic dysfunction to heart failure regardless of ejection fraction. *Am. J. Cardiol.* 2005; 95(5):603-6.

[29] Castillo E, Lima JA, Bluemke DA. Regional myocardial function: advances in MR imaging and analysis. *Radiographics.* 2003;23 Spec No:S127-40.

[30] Ryf, S., Spiegel, M.A., Gerber, M., and Boesiger, P. Myocardial tagging with 3D-CSPAMM. *J. Magn. Reson. Imaging.* 2002; 16:320-325.

[31] NessAiver M, Prince JL. Visualization of myocardial motion using MICSR trinary checkerboard display. *Inf. Process Med. Imaging.* 2003;18:573-85.

[32] Drangova, M., Zhu, Y., Bowman, B., and Pelc, N.J. In vitro verification of myocardial motion tracking from phase-contrast velocity data. *Magn. Reson. Imaging.* 1998; 16:863-870.

[33] Selskog P, Heiberg E, Ebbers T, Wigstrom L, Karlsson M. Kinematics of the heart: strain-rate imaging from time-resolved three-dimensional phase contrast MRI. *IEEE Trans Med Imaging.* 2002 Sep;21(9):1105-9.

[34] Wen, H. Mapping the velocity vector onto the spin vector: two-dimensional velocity-selective spin excitation for MR flow imaging. *Magn. Reson. Med.* 2001; 46:767-772.

[35] Aletras, A.H., Ding, S., Balaban, R.S., and Wen, H. DENSE: displacement encoding with stimulated echoes in cardiac functional MRI. *J. Magn. Reson.* 1999; 137:247-252.

[36] Watzinger N, Lund GK, Saeed M, Reddy GP, Araoz PA, Yang M, Schwartz AB, Bedigian M, Higgins CB. Myocardial blood flow in patients with dilated cardiomyopathy: Quantitative assessment with velocity-encoded cine magnetic resonance imaging of the coronary sinus. *J. Magn. Reson. Imaging.* 2005;21(4):347-53.

[37] Dora SK, Kumar VK, Bhat A, Tharakan JA. Venogram-guided extrathoracic subclavian vein puncture. *Indian Heart J.* 2003;55(6):637-40.

[38] Spuentrup E, Ruebben A, Mahnken A, Stuber M, Kolker C, Nguyen TH, Gunther RW, Buecker A. Artifact-free coronary magnetic resonance angiography and coronary vessel wall imaging in the presence of a new, metallic, coronary magnetic resonance imaging stent. *Circulation.* 2005;111(8):1019-26.

[39] Yang PC, Nguyen P, Shimakawa A, Brittain J, Pauly J, Nishimura D, Hu B, McConnell M. Spiral magnetic resonance coronary angiography-direct comparison of 1.5 Tesla vs. 3 Tesla. *J Cardiovasc Magn Reson.* 2004;6(4):877-84.

[40] Sharma R, Singh RB. MRI of coronary artery atherosclerosis in rabbits: Histopathology-MRI correlation and atheroma characterization. *Thromb. J.* 2004;2(1):5.

[41] Morrisett J, Vick W, Sharma R, Lawrie G, Reardon M, Ezell E, Schwartz J, Hunter G, Gorenstein D. Discrimination of components in atherosclerotic plaques from human carotid endarterectomy specimens by magnetic resonance imaging ex vivo. *Magn. Reson Imaging.* 2003;21(5):465-74.

[42] Sharma R. MRI in carotid artery atherosclerosis plaque characterization. *Magn. Reson. Med. Sci.* 2002; 1(4): 217-232.

[43] Schroeder S, Kuettner A, Leitritz M, Janzen J, Kopp AF, Herdeg C, Heuschmid M, Burgstahler C, Baumbach A, Wehrmann M, Claussen CD. Reliability of differentiating human coronary plaque morphology using contrast-enhanced multislice spiral computed tomography: a comparison with histology. *J. Comput. Assist. Tomogr.* 2004;28(4):449-54.

[44] Zenovich, A., Muehling, O.M., Panse, P.M., Jerosch-Herold, M., and Wilke, N. Magnetic resonance first-pass perfusion imaging: overview and perspectives. *Rays.* 2001;26:53-60.

[45] Doyle M, Fuisz A, Kortright E, Biederman RW, Walsh EG, Martin ET, Tauxe L, Rogers WJ, Merz CN, Pepine C, Sharaf B, Pohost GM. The impact of myocardial flow reserve on the detection of coronary artery disease by perfusion imaging methods: an NHLBI WISE study. *J. Cardiovasc. Magn. Reson.* 2003 Jul;5(3):475-85.

[46] Buchthal, SD, den Hollander JA, Merz CN, Rogers WJ, Pepine CJ, Reichek N, Sharaf BL, Reis S, Kelsey SF, Pohost GM. Abnormal myocardial phosphorus-31 nuclear magnetic resonance spectroscopy in women with chest pain but normal coronary angiograms. *N. Engl. J. Med.* 2000; 342:829-835.

[47] Sharma,R. Clinical brain imaging by Sodium MRI at 4.23 Tesla and Inversion Recovery pulse sequence: *Slovenia Medical Informatica.* 2003; 3(3): 112-123.

[48] Katz J, Cannon PJ. Use of sodium-23 for cardiac magnetic resonance imaging and spectroscopy. In: Cardiac Imaging: A Companion to Brauwald's Heart Disease, Marcus ML, Skorton DJ, Schelbert M, Wolf GL, Editors, Braunwald E, consulting editor. Saunders Company, Philadelphia, 1992;pp 828-840.

[49] Navon, G., Shinar, H., Eliav, U., and Seo, Y. Multiquantum filters and order in tissues. *NMR Biomed.* 2001; 14:112-132.

[50] Jerecic, R., Bock, M., Wacker, C., Bauer, W., and Schad, L.R. ^{23}Na-MRI of the human heart using a 3D radial projection technique. *Biomed. Tech. (Berl.)* 2002; 47(Suppl. 1):458-459.

[51] Sandstede JJ, Hillenbrand H, Beer M, Pabst T, Butter F, Machann W, Bauer W, Hahn D, Neubauer S. 2004 Time course of 23Na signal intensity after myocardial infarction in humans. *Magn. Reson. Med.* 2004;52(3):545-51

[52] Horn, M Weidensteiner C, Scheffer H, Meininger M, de Groot M, Remkes H, Dienesch C, Przyklenk K, von Kienlin M, Neubauer S. Detection of myocardial viability based on measurement of sodium content: a ^{23}Na-NMR study. *Magn. Reson. Med.* 2001; 45:756-764.

[53] Kim RJ. Judd RM, Chen EL, Fieno DS, Parrish TB, Lima JA. Relationship of elevated ^{23}Na magnetic resonance image intensity to infarct size after acute reperfused myocardial infarction. *Circulation.* 1999; 100:185-192.

[54] Reeves, R.C., Evanochko, W.T., Canby, R.C., McMillin, J.B., and Pohost, G.M. Demonstration of increased myocardial lipid with postischemic dysfunction ("myocardial stunning") by proton nuclear magnetic resonance spectroscopy. *J. Am. Coll. Cardiol.* 1989;13:739-744.

[55] Hsu, E.W., and Henriquez, C.S. 2001. Myocardial fiber orientation mapping using reduced encoding diffusion tensor imaging. *J. Cardiovasc. Magn. Reson.* 3:339-347.

[56] Dou, J., Reese, T.G., Tseng, W.Y., and Wedeen, V.J. 2002. Cardiac diffusion MRI without motion effects. *Magn. Reson. Med.* 48:105-114.

[57] Tseng, W.Y., Reese, T.G., Weisskoff, R.M., Brady, T.J., and Wedeen, V.J. 2000. Myocardial fiber shortening in humans: initial results of MR imaging. *Radiology.* 216:128-139.

[58] Flacke S, Fischer S, Scott M.J., Fuhrhop R.J., Allen J.S., McLean M., Winter P., Sicard G.A., Gaffney P.J., Wickline S.A., Lanza G.M. 2001. Novel MRI contrast agent for

molecular imaging of fibrin: implications for detecting vulnerable plaques. *Circulation.* 104:1280-1285.

[59] Lanza, G.M., Wickline S.A. 2001. Molecular imaging and targeted drug delivery with a novel, ligand-directed paramagnetic nanoparticle technology. *Acad. Radiol.* 9(Suppl. 2):S330-S331.

[60] Wickline, S.A., and Lanza, G.M. 2002. Molecular imaging, targeted therapeutics, and nanoscience. *J. Cell. Biochem. Suppl.* 39:90-97.

[61] Wickline, S.A., and Lanza, G.M. 2003. Nanotechnology for molecular imaging and targeted therapy. *Circulation.* 107:1092-1095.

[62] Zhu, X.H., Merkle, H., Kwag, J.H., Ugurbil, K., and Chen, W. 2001. 17O relaxation time and NMR sensitivity of cerebral water and their field dependence. *Magn. Reson. Med.* 45:543-549.

[63] Zhu, X.H. et al.2002. Development of (17)O NMR approach for fast imaging of cerebral metabolic rate of oxygen in rat brain at high field. *Proc. Natl. Acad. Sci. USA.* 99:13194-13199.

[64] Mateescu, G.D. 2003. Functional oxygen-17 magnetic resonance imaging and localized spectroscopy. *Adv. Exp. Med. Biol.* 510:213-218.

[65] Knuuti J, Sipola P. 2005 Is it time for cardiac innervation imaging? *Q J Nucl Med Mol Imaging*. 2005; 3.

[66] Ziegler A, Zaugg CE, Buser PT, Seelig J, Kunnecke B. Non-invasive measurements of myocardial carbon metabolism using in vivo ^{13}C NMR spectroscopy. *NMR Biomed.* 2002;15(3):222-34.

[67] Lloyd S, Brocks C, Chatham JC Differential modulation of glucose, lactate, and pyruvate oxidation by insulin and dichloroacetate in the rat heart. *Am J Physiol Heart Circ Physiol.* 2003;285(1):H163-72.

[68] Des Rosiers C, Lloyd S, Comte B, Chatham JC. A critical perspective of the use of (13)C-isotopomer analysis by GCMS and NMR as applied to cardiac metabolism. *Metab. Eng.* 2004;6(1):44-58.

[69] Barr RL, Lopaschuk GD Methodology for measuring in vitro/ex vivo cardiac energy metabolism. *J Pharmacol Toxicol Methods*. 2000;43(2):141-52.

[70] Elkington AG, Gatehouse PD, Prasad SK, Moon JC, Firmin DN, Pennell DJ. Combined long- and short-axis myocardial perfusion cardiovascular magnetic resonance. *J. Cardiovasc. Magn. Reson.* 2004;6(4):811-6.

[71] Klocke FJ. Cardiac magnetic resonance imaging: what can it add clinically in 2004? *Am. Heart Hosp J.* 2004;2(2):97-9.

[72] Oelhafen M, Schwitter J, Kozerke S, Luechinger R, Boesiger P. Assessing arterial blood flow and vessel area variations using real-time zonal phase-contrast MRI. *J. Magn. Reson. Imaging.* 2006 Mar;23(3):422-9.

[73] Travin MI, Bergmann SR. Assessment of myocardial viability. *Semin. Nucl. Med.* 2005;35(1):2-16.

[74] Francone M, Dymarkowski S, Kalantzi M, Bogaert J. Real-time cine MRI of ventricular septal motion: a novel approach to assess ventricular coupling. *J. Magn. Reson. Imaging*. 2005;21(3):305-9.

[75] Cuocolo A, Acampa W, Imbriaco M, De Luca N, Iovino GL, Salvatore M. The many ways to myocardial perfusion imaging. *Q. J. Nucl. Med. Mol. Imaging.* 2005;49(1):4-18.

[76] Ichikawa Y, Sakuma H, Suzawa N, Kitagawa K, Makino K, Hirano T, Takeda K. Late gadolinium-enhanced magnetic resonance imaging in acute and chronic myocardial infarction: improved prediction of regional myocardial contraction in the chronic state by measuring thickness of nonenhanced myocardium. *J. Am. Coll. Cardiol.* 2005;45(6):901-9.

[77] Bogaert J, Dymarkowski S. Delayed contrast-enhanced MRI: use in myocardial viability assessment and other cardiac pathology. *Eur. Radiol.* 2005;15 Suppl 2:B52-8.

[78] Stainsby JA, Sussman MS, Flexman ML, Wright GA. Real-time magnetic resonance with physiologic monitoring for improved scan localization. *Magn. Reson. Med.* 2005;53(4):954-959.

[79] Hoffmann R, von Bardeleben S, ten Cate F, Borges AC, Kasprzak J, Firschke C, Lafitte S, Al-Saadi N, Kuntz-Hehner S, Engelhardt M, Becher H, Vanoverschelde JL. Assessment of systolic left ventricular function: a multi-centre comparison of cineventriculography, cardiac magnetic resonance imaging, unenhanced and contrast-enhanced echocardiography. *Eur. Heart J.* 2005;26(6):607-16.

[80] Gilson WD, Yang Z, French BA, Epstein FH. Measurement of myocardial mechanics in mice before and after infarction using multislice displacement-encoded MRI with 3D motion encoding. *Am. J. Physiol Heart Circ. Physiol.* 2005;288(3):H1491-7.

[81] Hu TC, Bao W, Lenhard SC, Schaeffer TR, Yue TL, Willette RN, Jucker BM. Simultaneous assessment of left-ventricular infarction size, function and tissue viability in a murine model of myocardial infarction by cardiac manganese-enhanced magnetic resonance imaging (MEMRI). *NMR Biomed.* 2004;17(8):620-6.

[82] Wendland MF. Applications of manganese-enhanced magnetic resonance imaging (MEMRI) to imaging of the heart. *NMR Biomed.* 2004;17(8):581-94.

[83] Sakuma H, Higgins CB. Magnetic resonance measurement of coronary blood flow. *Acta Paediatr*. Suppl. 2004;93(446):80-5.

[84] Thomas B, Tavares NJ. A protocol to evaluate myocardial viability in ischemic left ventricular dysfunction using magnetic resonance imaging and a gadolinium-based contrast agent. *Rev. Port Cardiol.*2004;23(11):1421-7.

[85] Sievers B, Kirchberg S, Addo M, Bakan A, Brandts B, Trappe HJ. Assessment of left atrial volumes in sinus rhythm and atrial fibrillation using the biplane area-length method and cardiovascular magnetic resonance imaging with TrueFISP. *J. Cardiovasc. Magn. Reson.* 2004;6(4):855-63.

[86] Sievers B, Brandts B, Franken U, Trappe HJ. Single and biplane TrueFISP cardiovascular magnetic resonance for rapid evaluation of left ventricular volumes and ejection fraction. *J. Cardiovasc Magn Reson.* 2004;6(3):593-600.

[87] Swingen C, Wang X, Jerosch-Herold M. Evaluation of myocardial volume heterogeneity during end-diastole and end-systole using cine MRI. *J. Cardiovasc. Magn. Reson.* 2004;6(4):829-35.

[88] Lalande A, Salve N, Comte A, Jaulent MC, Legrand L, Walker PM, Cottin Y, Wolf JE, Brunotte F. Left ventricular ejection fraction calculation from automatically selected and processed diastolic and systolic frames in short-axis cine-MRI. *J. Cardiovasc. Magn. Reson.* 2004;6(4):817-27.

[89] Westenberg JJ, Danilouchkine MG, Doornbos J, Bax JJ, van der Geest RJ, Labadie G, Lamb HJ, Versteegh MI, de Roos A, Reiber JH. Accurate and reproducible mitral

valvular blood flow measurement with three-directional velocity-encoded magnetic resonance imaging. *J. Cardiovasc. Magn. Reson.* 2004;6(4):767-76.

[90] Shao X, Fei DY, Kraft KA. Rapid measurement of pulse wave velocity via multisite flow displacement. *Magn. Reson. Med.* 2004;52(6):1351-7.

[91] Gupta A, Lee VS, Chung YC, Babb JS, Simonetti OP. Myocardial infarction: optimization of inversion times at delayed contrast-enhanced MR imaging. *Radiology.* 2004; 233(3):921-6.

[92] McLeish K, Kozerke S, Crum WR, Hill DL. Free-breathing radial acquisitions of the heart. *Magn. Reson. Med.* 2004; 52(5):1127-35.

[93] Beg MF, Helm PA, McVeigh E, Miller MI, Winslow RL. Computational cardiac anatomy using MRI. *Magn. Reson. Med.* 2004; 52(5):1167-74.

[94] Crowe ME, Larson AC, Zhang Q, Carr J, White RD, Li D, Simonetti OP. Automated rectilinear self-gated cardiac cine imaging. *Magn. Reson. Med.* 2004; 52(4):782-8.

[95] Epstein FH, Gilson WD. Displacement-encoded cardiac MRI using cosine and sine modulation to eliminate (CANSEL) artifact-generating echoes. *Magn. Reson Med.* 2004; 52(4):774-81.

[96] Kvitting JP, Ebbers T, Engvall J, Sutherland GR, Wranne B, Wigstrom L. Three-directional myocardial motion assessed using 3D phase contrast MRI. *J. Cardiovasc Magn Reson.* 2004; 6(3):627-36.

[97] van der Geest RJ, Lelieveldt BP, Angelie E, Danilouchkine M, Swingen C, Sonka M, Reiber JH. Evaluation of a new method for automated detection of left ventricular boundaries in time series of magnetic resonance images using an Active Appearance Motion Model. *J. Cardiovasc. Magn. Reson.* 2004; 6(3):609-17.

[98] Kostler H, Beer M, Ritter C, Hahn D, Sandstede J. Auto-SENSE view-sharing cine cardiac imaging. *MAGMA.* 2004; 17(2):63-7.

[99] Paetsch I, Jahnke C, Wahl A, Gebker R, Neuss M, Fleck E, Nagel E. Comparison of dobutamine stress magnetic resonance, adenosine stress magnetic resonance, and adenosine stress magnetic resonance perfusion. *Circulation* 2004; 110(7):835-42.

[100] Sorensen TS, Korperich H, Greil GF, Eichhorn J, Barth P, Meyer H, Pedersen EM, Beerbaum P. Operator-independent isotropic three-dimensional magnetic resonance imaging for morphology in congenital heart disease: a validation study. *Circulation.* 2004; 110(2):163-9.

[101] Martin ET, Coman JA, Shellock FG, Pulling CC, Fair R, Jenkins K. Magnetic resonance imaging and cardiac pacemaker safety at 1.5-Tesla. *J. Am. Coll. Cardiol.* 2004; 43(7):1315-24.

[102] Kiss P, Suranyi P, Simor T, Saab-Ismail NH, Elgavish A, Hejjel L, Elgavish GA. In vivo R1-enhancement mapping of canine myocardium using ceMRI with Gd(ABE-DTTA) in an acute ischemia-reperfusion model. *J Magn Reson Imaging.* 2006; 24(3):571-9.

[103] Surányi P, Kiss P, Ruzsics B, Brott BC, Simor T, Elgavish A, Baker RA, Saab-Ismail NH, Elgavish GA. In vivo myocardial tissue kinetics of Gd(ABE-DTTA), a tissue-persistent contrast agent. *Magn Reson Med.* 2007;58(1):55-64.

[104] Spuentrup E, Katoh M, Buecker A, Fausten B, Wiethoff AJ, Wildberger JE, Haage P, Parsons EC Jr, Botnar RM, Graham PB, Vettelschoss M, Günther RW. Molecular MR imaging of human thrombi in a swine model of pulmonary embolism using a fibrin-specific contrast agent. *Invest Radiol.* 2007;42(8):586-95.

[105] Saraste A, Nekolla S, Schwaiger M. Contrast-enhanced magnetic resonance imaging in the assessment of myocardial infarction and viability. *J Nucl Cardiol.* 2008;15(1):105-17.

In: World Heart Research Yearbook. Volume 1
Editors: Franz Halberg and R. B. Singh

ISBN: 978-1-60741-881-8

PHYSICAL PARAMETERS ARE GOOD PREDICTORS OF CARDIORESPIRATORY FITNESS IN MALE COLLEGE STUDENTS OF INDIA

Amit Bandyopadhyay*
School of Health Sciences
University Sains Malaysia
Kelantan, Malaysia

ABSTRACT

The study assess to explore the relationship between cardiorespiratory fitness (expressed in terms of Physical Fitness Index or PFI) and physical parameters and also to establish suitable norms for predicting PFI from physical parameters in young sedentary Indians. 110 students between 20 to 24 years of age were randomly sampled from the Institute of Dental Sciences, Bareilly, India. They were subdivided into "study group" (N=70) and "control group" (N=40). PFI was determined by modified Harvard step test (HST). Significant correlation of PFI with body weight (r=0.59), body height (r=0.73) and body surface area or BSA (r=0.71) depicted the following prediction norms for PFI:

PFI=1.50xBody weight–21.96, (r = 0.59, P<0.001, SEE = 5.61)
PFI=1.30xBody height–151.57, (r = 0.73, P<0.001, SEE = 4.75)
PFI=82.24xBSA–70.16 (r = 0.71, P<0.001, SEE = 4.79)
PFI= 0.80x Body Height + 40.54x BSA –135.13 (R=0.72, R^2=0.52, P<0.001, SEE =4.52)

Among these norms, prediction of PFI from body height was considered as the most valid and reliable one because of the highest value of correlation coefficient between body height and PFI, as well as for the minimum standard error of estimate (4.75). The simple equation established from body height is therefore recommended as the most reliable and valid to predict PFI in the young sedentary Indian males; and multiple regression equation is also recommended for cross-checking the value.

Keywords: PFI, body weight, body height, body surface area

---

* Author for Correspondence: Dr. Amit Bandyopadhyay M.Sc., Ph.D., FICN , School of Health Sciences, University Sains Malaysia, 16150 Kubang Kerian, Kelantan, Malaysia. E-mail: bamit74@kb.usm.my, bamit74@india.com Phone: + 609 7663982; Fax : + 609 7647884.

Introduction

Physical fitness index or PFI is an accepted and widely used parameter for assessing an individual's cardiorespiratory fitness populations are available [1-5], but none of those literatures provides any comprehensive analysis on the relationship of PFI with different physical parameters (e.g., body weight, body height and BSA). Furthermore, attempt to establish prediction norms of PFI from physical parameters in Indian subjects are also unavailable.

Therefore, the purpose of the present investigation was to assess the relationship between PFI and physical parameters, and also to establish norms for prediction of PFI from physical parameters among sedentary young males of India.

Methods

Selection of Subjects

One hundred and ten (110) healthy young sedentary male students between 20 to 24 years of age from the middle-class socio-economic background were selected on the basis of simple random sampling from Institute of Dental Sciences at Bareilly, Uttar Pradesh, India. Out of the 110 subjects, 70 individuals were further randomly separated as 'Study Group' on which tests were carried out in order to examine the relationship between PFI and physical parameters and also to compute regression norms for PFI from physical parameters. Later on, the 40 remaining subjects, termed as 'Control Group', were tested to evaluate the validity of the norm obtained from the 'Study Group'.

Written consent was taken from the subjects and their age was calculated to the nearest year from the date of birth as obtained from the Institute's records. Body weight and body height were measured with the use of a standard calibrated scale with height attachment (Avery India Ltd., India). Body surface area (BSA) was calculated from the equation of DuBois and DuBois [6].

Preparation of Subjects [7]

The experiments were conducted in the morning, i.e., 2 to 3 hours after the breakfast of the volunteers who abstained from any strenuous activity during that period. The experimental procedure was explained to the subjects and they were asked to rest at least for half an hour.

Determination of Physical Fitness Index

Physical fitness index (PFI) was measured by HST [1-5, 8] which was performed on a stool of 18 inches height at the rate of 30 cycles per minute, which was set by a metronome. The maximum duration of the exercise was 5 minutes or up to exhaustion of the subject. After exhaustion or completion of the exercise, the subject was asked to rest on chair and three recovery heart rates were measured from carotid pulse during 1–1.5 min, 2–2.5 min and 3–3.5 min of the recovery period. The following equation was used to calculate the PFI score:

$$PFI = \frac{(\text{Duration of Exercise in Seconds x 100})}{\{2 \text{ x } (\text{Sum of the three recovery heart rates})\}}$$

The necessary permission was taken from the ethical committee and the study was performed at a room temperature varying from 27 to 29^{0}C and at a relative humidity ranging between 70 and 85 per cent.

Statistical Analysis

Student's t-test, Pearson's product moment correlation, Bland and Altman's analysis for limit of agreement [9] and simple and multiple regression analysis were used.

RESULTS

Physical parameters (viz., body weight, body height, BSA) and PFI of the study group and the confirmatory group are presented in table 1.

The PFI values obtained in both groups corroborated with the previous reports on young Indians [2, 3, 5]. Prediction equations of PFI from corresponding physical parameters were applied in the control group. Such predicted values of PFI showed insignificant variation from the directly measured value of PFI.

Table 1. Physical parameters and PFI of subjects

Parameters	Study Group (n = 70)	Confirmatory Group (n = 40)
Age (Years)	22.03 ±1.77	22.10 ±1.09
Body Weight (kg)	59.43 ±2.72	59.82 ±3.74
Body Height (cm)	168.27 ±3.90	169.04 ±2.94
BSA (m^2)	1.67 ±0.06	1.68 ±0.07
PFI	67.18 ±6.95	68.14 ±3.33

All values are expressed as Mean ± SD.

DISCUSSION

All the physical parameters exhibited significant ($P<0.001$) correlation with PFI indicating dependence of the latter on physical parameters. In the present study BSA exhibited higher value of correlation coefficient with PFI than body weight but the highest value of correlation coefficient was obtained between PFI and body height. Hence body height was considered as the most valuable predictor of PFI among all the physical parameters in the examined population. The prediction equations are as follows:

PFI = 1.50 x Body weight – 21.96
(r = 0.59, P < 0.001, SEE = 5.61)

PFI = 1.30 x Body height – 151.57
(r = 0.73, P < 0.001, SEE = 4.75)

PFI = 82.24 x BSA – 70.16
(r = 0.71, P < 0.001, SEE = 4.79)

BSA was computed from body weight and body height, therefore, application of BSA as an independent variable for prediction of PFI appeared a bit complicated than using body weight or height. The SEE of PFI while predicting from the currently established norms, were found to be substantially low (4.75 to 5.61) to consider all these parameters, viz., body height, body weight and BSA as good predictors of PFI in the currently examined population.

However, for having the maximum value of correlation coefficient (r=0.73) with PFI and lowest standard error of estimate (SEE = 4.75), body height was considered as the best predictor of PFI among all the physical parameters. In the confirmatory group, application of Bland and Altman's limit of agreement analysis depicted that the mean difference between directly measured PFI score (68.19 ± 3.38) and predicted value of PFI from body height (68.34 ± 3.27) was considerably low (0.05) (Figure 1).

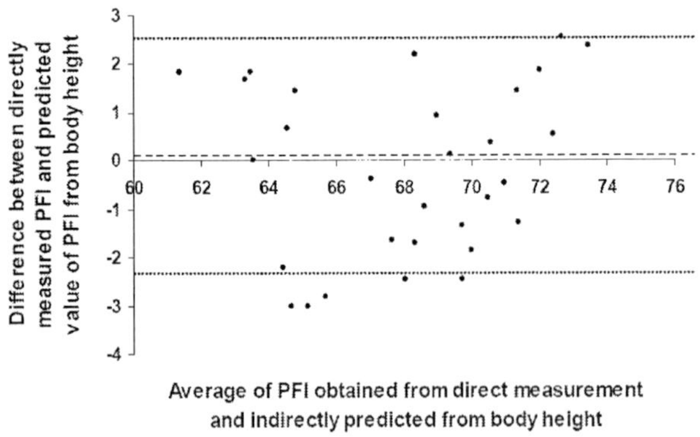

..........Mean. --------Mean ± 2 SD

Figure 1. Plotting of difference between directly measured PFI Value and predicted PFI value from body height.

As both body height and BSA were highly correlated with PFI, hence prediction of PFI from these two physical parameters were also attempted and revealed the following norm in the form of multiple regression equation:

PFI = 0.80 x Body Height + 40.54 x BSA – 135.13
($R = 0.72$, $R^2 = 0.52$, $P<0.001$, SEE =4.52)

This multiple regression equation is more complicated than the simple ones but depicted lower value of SEE than those of the simple regression equations. Therefore, beside the simple prediction equation for PFI from body height, the multiple regression equation with considerably lower value of SEE was also found reliable in this aspect.

From the present investigation it may be concluded that body weight, body height and BSA are good predictors of PFI in young sedentary subjects of India; but body height is the best among them. Therefore, the norm established from body height is recommended as the most reliable, valid and well applicable to predict PFI in the studied population. In addition, multiple regression equation is also recommended for the assessment of PFI or cross-checking the predicted value of PFI in young sedentary Indian males.

REFERENCES

[1] Banerjee PK, Chatterjee S. Harvard step test as a measure of physical fitness in adolescent boys. *Indian J. Med. Res.* 1983, 79: 413-417.

[2] Das SK, Ray A. Evaluation of physical fitness in boys. *Indian J. Physiol. and Allied Sci.* 1990, 42: 39-42.

[3] Chatterjee S, Bandyopadhyay A, Chatterjee P, Mukherjee PS. Short term training induced changes in recovery cardiac cost and physical fitness index of smoker and non-smoker university students. *Indian J. Physiol. and Allied Sci.* 2002, 56: 16 – 24.

[4] Bandyopadhyay B, Chattopadhyay H. Assessment of physical fitness of sedentary and physically active male college students by a modified Harvard step test. *Ergonomics* 1981, 24: 15-20.

[5] Mandal A, Thakur B. A comparative study of physical fitness of some hard working populations. *Indian J. Physiol. and Allied Sci.* 2004, 58 : 20-26.

[6] DuBois D, DuBois EF. Clinical Calorimetry: A formula to estimate approximate surface area if height and weight be known. *Arch. of Intern. Med.* 1916, 17 : 863-871.

[7] Chatterjee S, Chatterjee P, Mukherjee PS, Bandyopadhyay A. Validity of Queen's College step test for use with young Indian men. *Br. J. Sports Med.* 2002, 38: 289-291.

[8] Sloan AW. Physical fitness and body build of young men and women. *Ergonomics* 1969, 12 : 25– 35.

[9] Bland JM, Altman DG. Statistical method for assessing agreement between two methods of clinical measurements. *Lancet* 1986, 1: 307 – 310.

In: World Heart Research Yearbook. Volume 1
Editors: Franz Halberg and R. B. Singh
ISBN: 978-1-60741-881-8

Human Coronary Artery Lesions: Magnetic Resonance Imaging, NMR Spectroscopy, Histopathology and Oxidative Stress Markers

Rakesh Sharma*[*,1] and Ram B. Singh[2]

[1]Department of Medicine, Columbia University, New York, US

[2]Heart Research Medical Center, Moradabad, India

Abstract

Aim: Magnetic resonance imaging (MRI) techniques measured the dimensions of atheroma and stenosis in human coronary plaque disruption and lipid disorder due to oxidative stress. *Hypothesis:* Coronary atheroma is a lipid disorder and MRI visible. *Materials and Methods*: Contiguous cross-sectional T2-weighted fast spin echo MRI images were point-by-point compared with coronary histopathology for quantitation of coronary wall and plaque features. Coronary atheroma tissues were used for NMR spectroscopy and oxidative stress content analysis.

Results: MRI images showed distinct measurable wall thickness and vessel radii. The quantitative comparison of lumen areas and wall thickness in endarterectomy specimens using MRI images and histology images showed mean difference 5.0 % for lumen area and 4.5 % for wall thickness. MRI data correlated with the histopathology for aortic wall thickness (R^2=0.92, $P < 0.0001$), plaque size (R^2=0.99, $P < 0.0001$) and vessel radii (R^2=0.79, $P < 0.0001$). MRI images and histological sections showed intraluminal thrombus and plaque disruption. High-resolution NMR peaks suggested the lipid-rich nature of coronary plaque due to presence of triglycerides, phospholipids, sterols and fatty acids. Oxidative stress markers were higher in plaque bearing coronary artery homogenates than the normal coronary artery homogenates. Ex vivo, MRI reliably determined the presence, location, and size of the thrombus and % stenosis in coronary artery atherosclerosis and histopathology defined the plaque composition. *Conclusion*: The study demonstrates the utility of MRI for *in vivo* measurement of % stenosis and distinguishes different components of coronary thrombus *ex vivo* suggesting the coronary artery plaque as a result of lipid disorder and oxidative stress.

Keywords: Coronary artery disease; atherosclerosis; MRI; thrombosis; plaque; oxidative, stress

[*] Correspondence: Rakesh Sharma, Ph.D Department of medicine, Columbia University, New York, NY 10032; Email: rs2010@columbia.edu; icn@mickyonline.com

INTRODUCTION

Atherothrombosis is a systemic disease of the coronary vessel wall that causes coronary artery lesions appearing heterogeneous in morphology and chemical constitution. Disrupting or vulnerable plaques in the coronary arteries exhibit a thin fibrous cap (fibrous cap thickness 65 to 150 μm) with a large lipid core, as defined by American Heart Association AHA plaque type V-Va [1]. Acute coronary syndromes often result from disruption of a modestly stenotic vulnerable plaque. Coronary artery vulnerable plaques occasionally show high likelihood of thrombotic complications and rapid progression of lipid content and a thin fibrous cap [2]. Coronary arteries are thin but their measurements speculate important clinical correlates [3]. Quantitation of the high-risk plaque lipid components and degree of stenosis is state-of-art approach but difficult [4]. However, MRI measures lumen volume, wall thickness, thrombus size, total plaque volume and characterize the composition of the plaques. Noninvasive MRI is emerging tool for identification of flow-limiting coronary stenoses, calcified plaques, imaging of the atherothrombotic lesions, measurement of atherosclerotic burden, and *ex vivo* characterization of the coronary plaque components. This combined information for degree of stenosis and the plaque composition, may predict cardiovascular risk, atherothrombosis progression and its response to therapy for the assessment of subclinical disease [5]. The segmentation of coronary plaque MRI images serves to generate plaque feature maps as morphological correlates suggesting heterogeneous nature of coronary plaque [6]. Coregistration of MRI images with histopathology stereotactic match may provide validity of quantitation. Oxidative stress causes accumulation of oxidants viz. lipid peroxides and hydroperoxides during atherothrombosis due to lipid disorder [4, 6]. The present report focused on application of MRI in stenosis and plaque composition. We measured inner / outer wall perimeters and their radii, plaque features using MRI and histology coregistration to calculate wall thickness, thrombus area, lumen size and % stenosis in support of MRI and histological data as possible predictors of stress (higher % stenosis, elevated oxidative stress markers with NMR visible lipid peaks) in different branches due to coronary lipid disorder. We report new approaches of measurement of *in vivo* plaque burden at different branches; better stereotactic visualization of coronary lesion components.

MATERIALS AND METHODS

Ex Vivo MRI and High-Resolution NMR Spectroscopy of Coronary Plaque

10 male human (mean age 45 $\pm$ 4 years) with 30 % - 80 % lumen stenosis participated. 14 coronary artery endarterectomy samples were obtained within 4 hours of cardiac surgery. Severe atherosclerosis and cardiac death were exclusion criteria to select the endarterectomy specimens [3, 6]. The area of dissection was defined as a position including right coronary aorta, left anterior descending and circumflex coronary arteries about 10 mm away from the anterior descending artery. The specimens were placed in a device surrounded by phased array surface coil and fast spin echo (FSE) images were acquired at GE Horizon 1.5 T clinical MRI system physiological temperature 37 ^{0}C as described elsewhere [7]. All research protocols complied with human ethical committee of clinical research. Optimized scan

parameters were used to achieve T1, T2 and proton density images of contiguous slices as described elsewhere [8]. Segmentation using SNAKE algorithm was used to quantify wall thickness and coronary artery lumen areas [9]. Segmentation method used delineation and recognition of region and boundaries of vessels in a given scene [10]. To validate the surrogate of truth for comparison, coronary inner and outer wall perimeters were delineated. Adding up plaque or wall areas from 1 mm thick stacked slices provided quantification of plaque constituents [10]. % stenosis and thrombus size was measured as reported elsewhere [10].

High resolution 1-H NMR peaks were obtained in lipid extracts on a Varian VXR500 magnet housed at Albert Einstein College of Medicine, operating at frequency of 500 Hz (11.5 T) after water peak (4.6 ppm) suppression by selective Rf saturation; internal standard $CHCl_3$ (7.24 ppm); TR =10 sec; number of FID 64; Fourier Transformed using 16 K points; line broadening 1 Hz; acquisition delay 10 μsec. Peaks were identified on spectra of lipid extracts from coronary plaque tissue based on *a priori* knowledge of their chemical shifts (fatty acid ω-CH_3 at ca. 0.86 ppm; -$(CH_2)n$ 1.27 ppm; =CH-CH2- methylene at 2.0-2.2 ppm; =CH-CH_2-HC= methylene at 2.75 ppm; vinyl -CH=CH- protons at 5.3 ppm; choline head group -$N(CH_3)_3$ at 3.3 ppm of phospholipids; sterol methyl 18-CH_3- at 0.4 ppm as previously reported [10,11].

Coronary Wall and Plaque Measurements

Using in vivo MRI images, outer and inner vessel radii measure wall thickness and atheroma size as following and described elsewhere [7]. Wall thickness T can be measured as difference of radii (outer R and inner r) as following equation 1:

$$T = R - r \tag{1}$$

where atheroma size may be calculated based on atheroma length L, atheroma rich area B, and vessel radii as following equation 2.

$$V_{(atheroma)} = L(2R+r).B/6 \tag{2}$$

Histology of Plaque

Endarterectomy tissue blocks were fixed by immersion in 10 % neutral formalin. Four-micrometer sections comprising all layers of the ventricular wall were stained with Hematoxylin and Eosin with pentachrome [11]. Of the multiple sections of each endarterectomy, one section was randomly analyzed for further morphometric measurements. Optimas 6.5 Image analysis software digitized all arterial segments.

The inner perimeter was defined as the difference of borderlines between lumen and outer vessel wall. Further dividing it by 2π, yielded the inner vessel radius. The outer perimeter was defined by the borderline between tunica media and adventitia. The outer vessel radius was obtained by dividing outer perimeter with 2π. Wall thickness was computed as the difference between outer vessel radii and inner vessel radii.

Oxidative Stress Markers

Angiotensin, insulin, beta-carotene, TBARS, malonaldehyde (MDA), vitamin E and C, diene conjugates measured oxidative stress in tissue homogenates of coronary artery segments and control coronary artery segments without plaques as described elsewhere [12].

Results

Ex Vivo MRI of Coronary Artery Endarterectomy Specimens

The endarterectomy specimens placed in the close proximity of maximum influence of phased array surface coil magnetic field generated high signal-to-noise (SNR) ratio. The wall and plaque constituents were distinct on serial MRI images as shown in Figure 1.

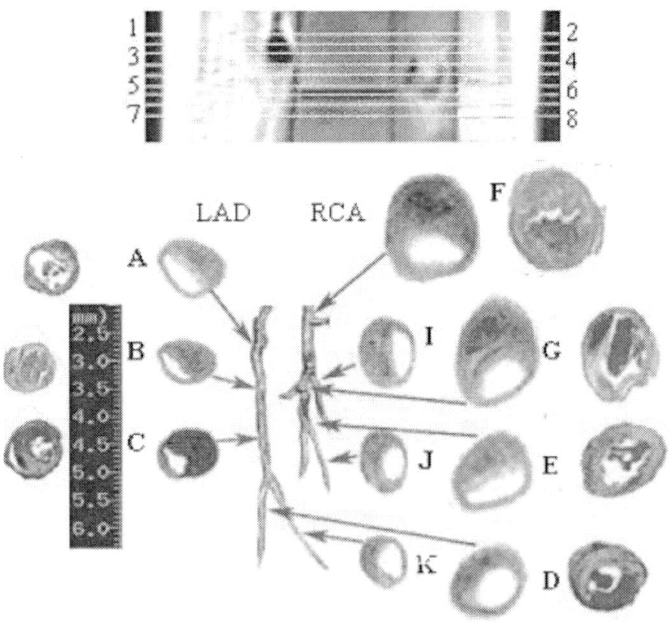

Figure 1. A representative *ex vivo* MRI axial view is shown at different levels (1-8) for coronary endarterectomy coronary artery specimens (panel on top) placed in the close proximity of maximum magnetic field influence of phased array surface coil on its both sides to generate high signal to noise ratio. Notice the different branches of RCA, LAD and LCx coronary arteries showed distinct wall thickening and MRI visible plaque constituents on serial sagittal images in two columns at bottom. RCA branch (D-K) show maximum thickening (right panels at bottom) while LCx and LAD branches (A-C) show lesser thickening (left 3 specimens on left column). For comparison, each coronary image is matched with corresponding histology section shown by side. Notice the histology processing reduces the measurement due to coronary tissue shrinkage.

Table 1. Comparison of histomorphometric measurements and ex vivo MRI visible coronary artery thrombus features of coronary artery serial segments. % aorta wall thickness (mm), atheroma size (mm²) and total plaque volume (mm³) were measured by superimposed delineation of area on both histology and MRI images in Figure 1

Patient slice[a] Patient segment[b] % difference	Coronary artery perimeter			Wall thickness (mm)	Wall radius (mm)	% stenosis	Thrombus area (mm^2)
	Outer (mm^2)	Lumen (mm^2)	Lumen Area (mm^2)				
A_1	17.40	16.33	42.47	0.12	2.78	30.47	12.94
A_seg0.5	17.34	16.02	40.85	0.11	2.76	31.6	12.91
% difference	0.35	1.9	3.8	8.3	0.72	3.5	0.23
B_4	18.10	16.65	44.12	0.23	2.88	29.63	13.10
B_seg1.5	17.84	15.96	40.53	0.30	2.84	32.44	13.15
% difference	1.44	4.14	8.14	23.3	1.39	8.66	0.4
C_3	19.80	17.09	46.31	0.44	3.15	31.3	14.50
C_seg1.5	17.60	15.20	36.80	0.38	2.80	37.5	13.80
% difference	11.1	11.05	20.53	13.6	11.1	16.0	4.82
D_6	20.60	15.08	36.19	0.88	3.28	42.14	15.25
D_seg1.0	20.35	13.82	30.41	1.04	3.24	49.49	15.05
% difference	1.21	8.35	15.9	15.4	1.22	14.9	1.31
E_2	20.73	15.70	39.27	0.80	3.30	46.34	18.20
E_seg2.0	20.10	15.08	36.19	0.80	3.20	50.15	18.15
% difference	3.04	3.95	7.84	0.0	3.0	7.58	0.28
F_4	22.11	16.02	40.85	0.97	3.52	53.36	21.80
F_seg2.5	21.67	15.70	39.27	0.95	3.45	55.13	21.65
% difference	1.99	1.99	3.86	2.06	1.98	3.21	0.69
G_6	16.96	11.62	21.50	0.45	2.70	42.79	9.20
G_seg2	16.02	11.31	20.35	0.75	2.55	41.27	8.40
% difference	5.54	2.66	5.34	40.0	5.55	3.55	8.69
H_8	16.65	9.11	13.21	1.20	2.65	72.67	9.60
H_seg4	15.70	8.80	12.31	1.10	2.50	71.08	8.75
% difference	6.30	3.40	6.81	8.33	1.87	2.18	8.85
I_4	13.19	6.79	7.33	1.02	2.10	62.07	4.55
I_seg2.5	12.88	6.28	6.28	1.05	2.05	70.06	4.40
% difference	2.35	7.51	14.32	2.85	2.38	11.4	1.10
J_10	14.45	10.05	16.08	0.70	2.30	41.98	6.75
J_seg3.0	14.13	10.18	16.49	0.63	2.25	39.72	6.55
% difference	2.22	1.28	2.48	10.0	2.17	5.38	2.96
K_12	15.70	8.73	12.14	1.11	2.50	82.37	10.00
K_seg3.5	15.39	8.86	12.49	1.04	2.45	78.94	9.86
% difference	1.97	1.49	2.80	6.30	2.0	4.16	1.40
L_14	16.65	9.39	15.09	1.10	2.65	51.68	7.80
L_seg4.0	16.40	9.36	13.95	1.12	1.49	46.95	6.55
% difference	1.50	0.30	7.55	1.78	43.8	9.15	16.0
M_3	12.25	9.74	15.09	0.40	1.95	34.46	5.20
M_seg1.5	12.06	9.43	14.13	0.42	1.50	36.09	5.10
% difference	1.55	3.18	6.36	4.76	23.0	4.51	1.92
N_5	11.62	10.05	16.08	0.25	1.85	19.90	3.20
N_seg2.0	11.24	9.67	15.48	0.25	1.54	20.35	3.15
% difference	3.27	3.78	3.73	0.0	15.6	2.21	1.56

[a] Coronary specimen number and magnetic resonance microimage slice number(1 mm thick).
[b] Speciman number and coronary tissue segment containing corresponding MRM slice(5 mm thick).

Wall thickness and wall radii were calculated by measuring outer wall and lumen perimeters as presented in the Table 1. Lumen area and thrombus area were delineated and % lumen stenosis was calculated as [area of thrombus / (area of lumen) x 100%]. Outer vessel radius ranged from 1.0-3.5 mm and wall thickness from 0.1-1.0 mm. Wall thickness, % stenosis and vessel radius comparison is shown in Table 1 and Figure 5 as regression plots indicating linear relationship. The standard error was 6 % above or below the fitted curve. This relationship was more valid in the large vessels. However, some variation of measurements was also due to anatomical variability of coronary arteries. Coronary artery MRI image mainly defined three morphometric features i.e. lumen area, wall area and plaque area. However, several plaque features viz. lipid core, thrombus, atheroma, calcification, were distinct but not definitive as shown in Figure 2. Using SNAKE algorithm, wall thickness was measured as shown in Figure 3.

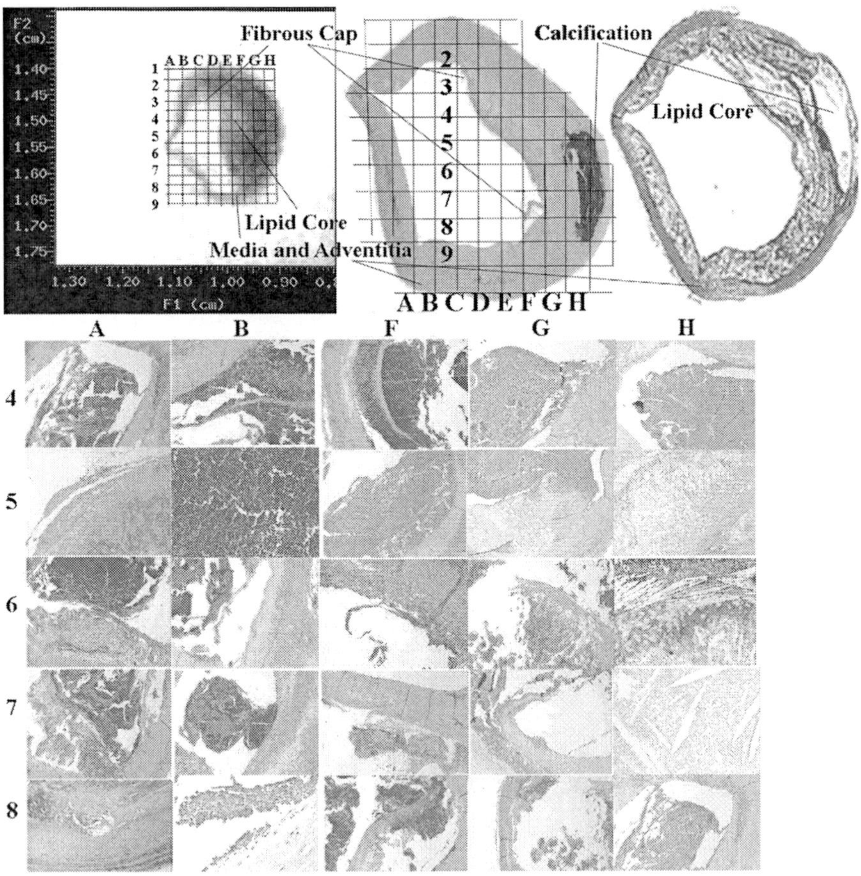

Figure 2. A representative coronary artery T2 weighted MRI image is shown with distinct darker calcification, isotense lipid core and media-adventitia layers seen on MRI image(left panel on top row) for comparison with corresponding histology sections stained with H and E(middle panel on top row) and pentachrome(right panel on top row). A method of point-by point match in different high power fields (hpf) numbered as A-H horizontally and 1-9 vertically on histology sections is shown to establish MRI visible coronary artery wall features. Notice distinct fibrous cap rupture(F-6,G-6), calcification (H-6,H-7), lipid deposits(F-5,G-5), cholesterol accumulation (F-4, G-4), media damage (A-8), extracellular matrix (B-6, A-7), necrosis (A-5, A-6), atheroma formation (B-5), collagen (F-7,F-8) on different panels at bottom.

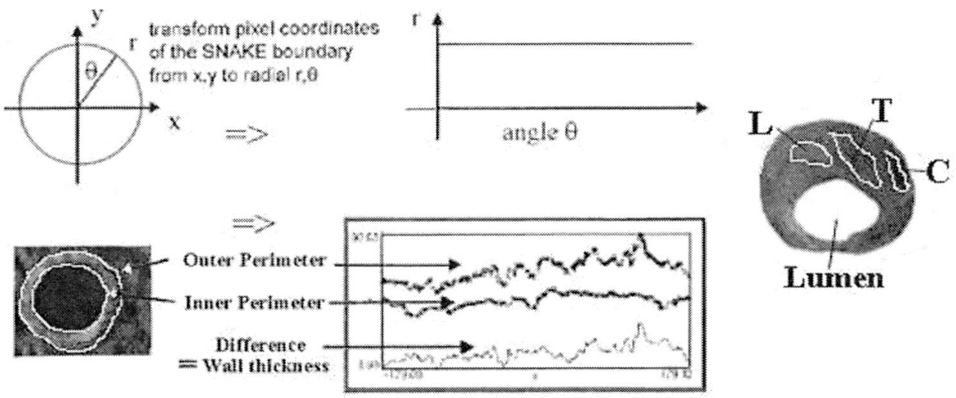

Figure 3. The delineation of outer and inner perimeters is shown to measure wall thickness at different points in a coronary artery ex vivo MRI image using SNAKE algorithm (left panel). The delineation of plaque features isointense atheroma (T), darker calcification (C), gray lipid core (L) is shown in a *ex vivo* MRI image is shown (right panel).

Different levels of MRI image slices showed the *in vivo* measurements of right coronary aorta (RCA), left anterior descending (LAD) and circumflex (LC_x) coronary arteries as shown in Figure 4 and Table 2 indicating RCA at higher risk. Plaque features viz. necrotic core, lipid core, atheroma and wider wall thickness were distinct on MRI images and represented high percent stenosis as shown in Figure 4. Different wall perimeters, lumen area, wall thickness and thrombus size measurements and their correlation with plaque stability are shown in Figure 5.

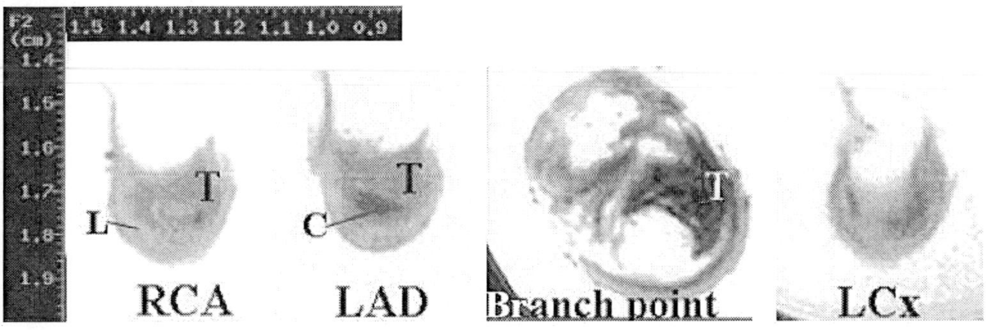

Figure 4. *Ex vivo* MRI transverse images of right coronary artery (RCA), left anterior descending (LAD), left circumflex artery (LCx) and branch point of coronary arteries show wall thickness (cm) , media narrowing and distinct plaque features. Lumen area, wall thickness and plaque area were compared (see Table 2). Note the thick wall, atheroma (T) and lipid (L) and calcification (C) damage and deposits show up as distinct features.

Histopathology

The endarterectomy coronary artery tissues were white with smooth surface. However, permanent fixation in formalin reduced its size due to shrinkage. The histology sections stained with trichrome-Mason showed microscopic distinct features. The coregistration method using 'edge detection' for lumen size, wall thickness, wall radii, and plaque constituents showed % differences by using MRI and histology methods as shown in Table 1 and Figure 6. Histopathology characterized the coronary plaque tissue point-by-point stereotactic match with their MRI signal intensities. On histology sections, lipids, calcification, atheroma, elastin, collagen were main plaque features with fibrous cap, inner wall disruption as shown in different high power fields in Figure 2.

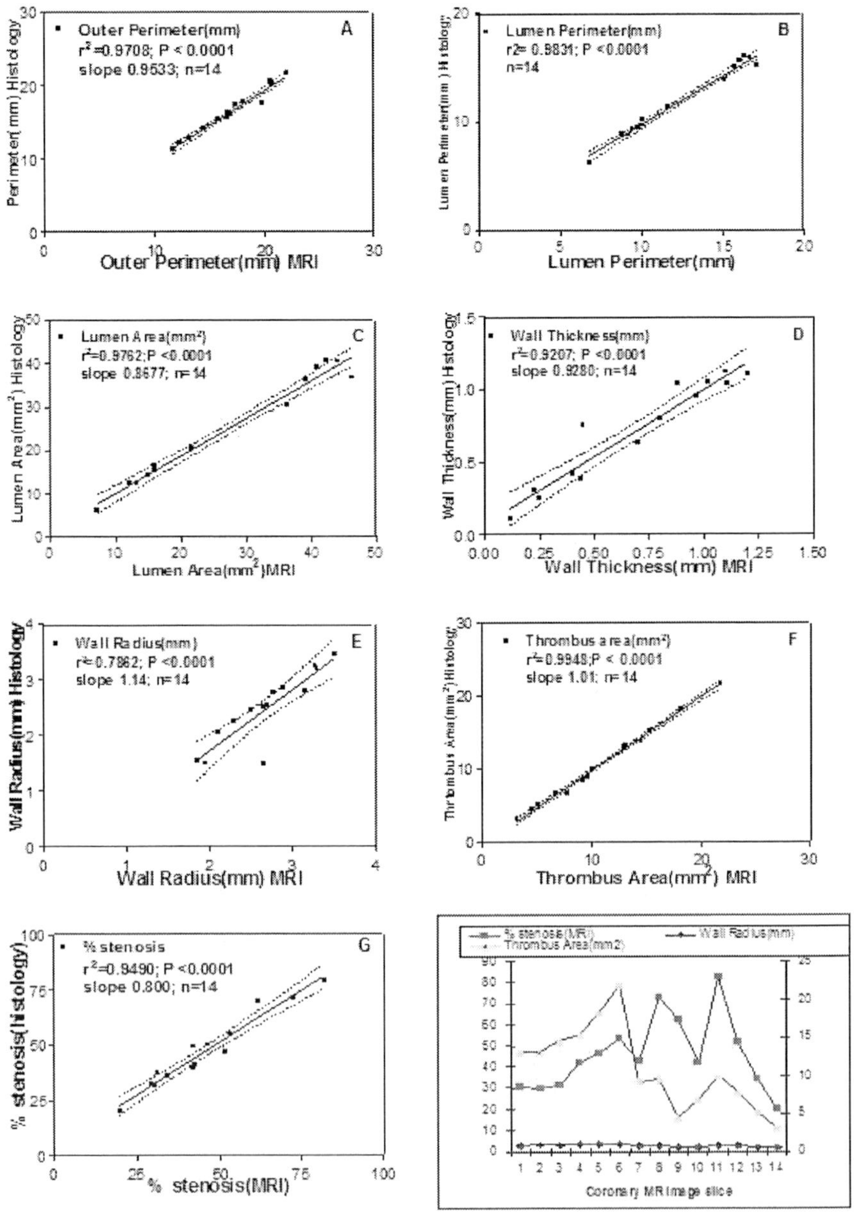

Figure 5. Regression plots are shown for outer and inner perimeters, lumen area, wall thickness, vessel radius, % stenosis and thrombus size to show linear correlation between *ex vivo* MRI and histology data (panels A-G). Note the better correlation of thrombus area and % stenosis than wall radius (right panel at bottom).

Table 2. Lateral difference in RCA, LCx and LAD coronary artery area measurements of a representative endarterectomy specimen # C (see Figure 4) for lumen, wall and plaque are shown

Plaque feature	RCA	LC_x	LAD
Lumen area (mm^2)	40.85	16.08	15.09
Wall area (mm^2)	36.95	5.32	8.77
Plaque area(mm^2)	21.80	3.2	5.2
Lipid core area(mm^2)	6.5	--	2.1
Atheroma area(mm^2)	12.8	1.2	2.3
Calcification area(mm^2)	4.5	--	--
Fibrous tissue area(mm^2)	5.5	0.75	0.3

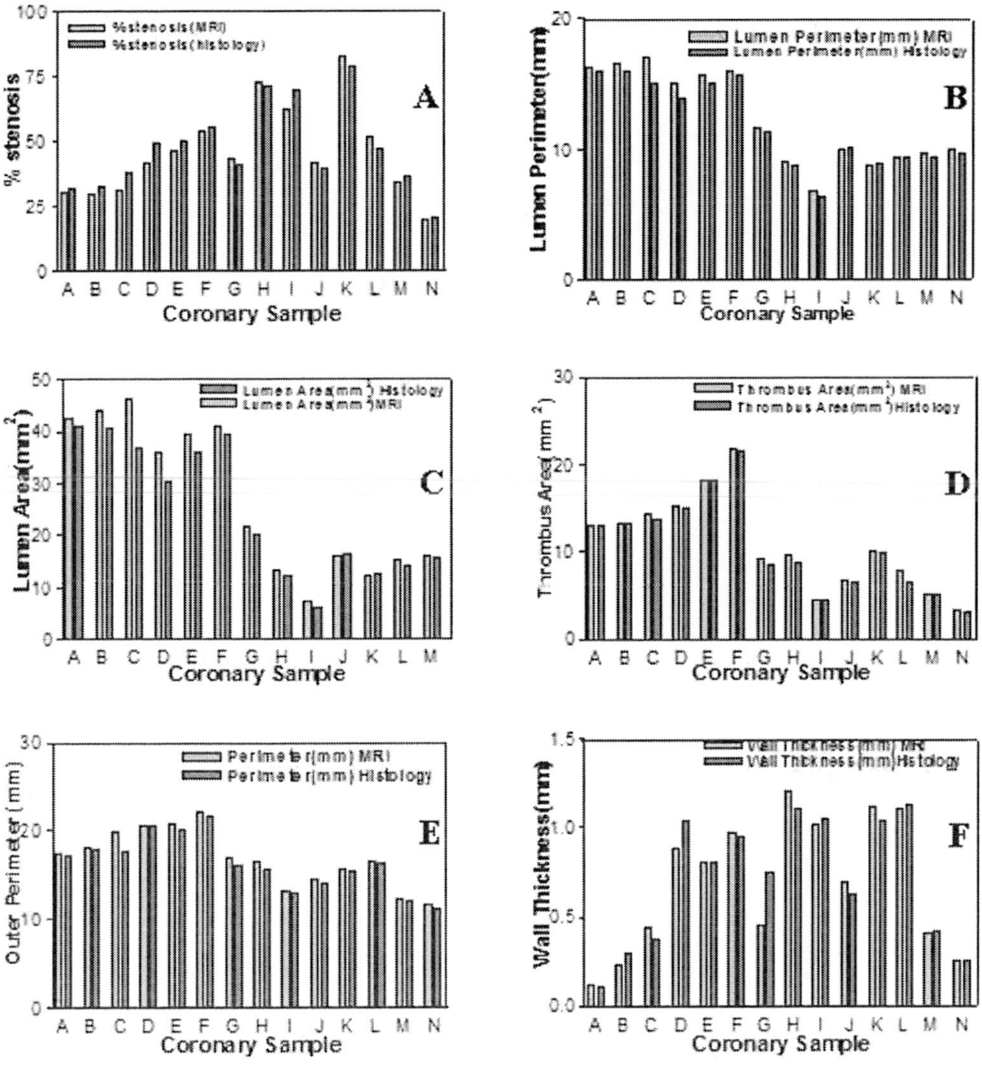

Figure 6. Different histogram bars (1-6) represent ex vivo MRI data and histology data (A-L) of different coronary artery tissues as shown in Table 1. Comparison is shown in % difference for different measurements.

Table 3. High-resolution NMR spectroscopy peak assignments are shown in chloroform extracts of coronary plaque tissues 1-4 (#C,#D,#I and #L). Distinct peak heights at different chemical shift positions suggest protons of specific chemical groups in the lipid-rich plaque constituents as finger prints

Lipid NMR peaks	Plaque 1 (% stenosis >60%)	Plaque 2 (% stenosis<50%)	Plaque 3 (% stenosis >70%))	Plaque 4 (% stenosis >50%)
ω $-CH_3$	12.3	8.2	12.7	10.0
-(CH2)n	>15	14	>15	15
$=CH-CH_2-$	4.1	1.3	2.9	2.0
$=CH-CH_2-HC=$	3.5	-	-	0.7
$=CH-CH_2-HC=$	2.5	1.5	3.0	1.8
$-N(CH_3)_3$	1.1	0.5	10.0	-
$18-CH_3-$	7.2	4.5	6.4	5.8

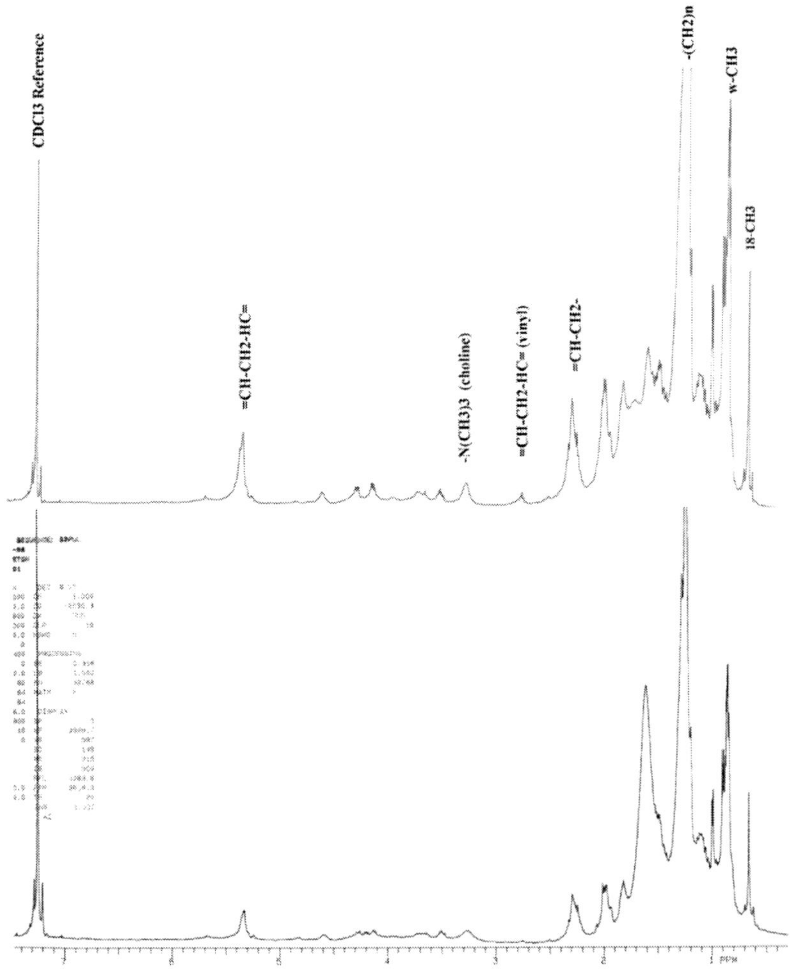

Figure 7. High-resolution NMR spectroscopy peak assignments are shown in chloroform extracts of coronary plaque tissues (#G and #L). Distinct peak heights at different chemical shift positions suggest the lipid-rich plaque constituents as finger prints. However, some NMR peaks remained unidentified.

High-Resolution NMR Spectroscopy of Coronary Plaques

Fatty acid moieties of triglycerides, phospholipids, and cholesterol esters were prominent contributors to the observed proton resonances peaks identified on spectra of lipid extracts from coronary plaque tissue.

The peaks showed chemical shifts (fatty acid ω-CH_3 at 0.86 ppm; -$(CH_2)_n$ 1.27 ppm; =CH-CH_2- methylene at 2.0-2.2 ppm; =CH-CH_2-HC= methylene at 2.75 ppm; vinyl =CH-CH_2-HC=protons at 5.3 ppm; choline head group -$N(CH_3)_3$ at 3.3 ppm of phospholipids; sterol methyl 18-CH_3- at 0.65 ppm based on *a priori* knowledge of these peak positions as shown in Figure 7. However, other unidentified peaks at 0.95, 1.5, 2.0, 4.1 and 4.2 were also accountable as shown in Figure 7.

Oxidative Stress Markers

Coronary artery normal tissues and atheroma bearing tissue homogenates showed distinct and comparable high values of angiotensin, insulin, beta-carotene, vitamins C and E, TBARS, MDA, diene conjugates contents as shown in Table 4.

Table 4. Oxidative stress marker atheroma constituents are shown in normal and atheroma in coronary tissues. These constituents are represented in international units for comparison

Oxidative stress constituent	% difference from Normal Coronary aorta	Coronary atheroma
Angiotensin	+ 25.5	45.8 ± 13.7
Beta-carotene	- 38.5	0.6 ± 0.09
TBARS	+ 55	1.58 ± 0.30
Cholesterol	+ 35	4.2 ± 0.39
Triglycerides	+ 42	2.84 ± 0.33
MDA	+ 39	2.45 ± 0.55
Diene conjugates	+ 58	30.8 ± 2.97
Insulin	+ 13.8	0.18 ± 0.11
Vitamin C	- 14	1.05 ± 0.14
Vitamin E	- 25.5	2.15 ± 0.44

However, cholesterol and triglycerides were similar in both homogenates as shown in Figure 8. Very often, high % stenosis > 60 % and bigger atheroma size were associated with -$(CH_2)_n$, 18-CH_3- sterol peak, choline head group -$N(CH_3)_3$ NMR peaks and higher oxidative stress markers viz. TBARS, MDA, diene conjugates in cholesterol rich plaques common in RCA tissues. Less vulnerable plaques however showed =CH-CH_2- methylene, =CH-CH_2-HC= NMR peaks with comparable oxidative markers common in LAD and LC_x tissues. However, it did not rule out the possibility of other plaque lipids.

Discussion

Coronary atheroma is the consequence of lipid disorder and continuous oxidative stress that leads to plaque disruption. We believe that the size of atheroma and % stenosis serve as morphometric indices measured as wall thickness and lumen area. Further, plaque features such as disruption, fibrous cap, calcium and lipid deposits earlier highlighted the physiochemical processes in coronary wall [1-4, 14, 15]. In same direction, the present study demonstrated the enhanced power of MRI as tool of MRI-visible coronary vessel morphomteric measurements and plaque constituents to evaluate degree of stenosis and thrombosis. It highlighted the use of phased array coil to get combined T1 weighted, T2 weighting and proton-density weighted images in wall visualization and validated the multicontrast MRI signal intensities of different coronary plaque components at various locations.

Multicontrast MR Plaque Imaging

MR microimaging is emerging as the potential noninvasive *ex vivo* MR imaging modality. MR techniques differentiate plaque components on the basis of biophysical and biochemical coronary tissue properties such as chemical composition, chemical concentration, water content, physical state, molecular motion, or diffusion. In present study, *ex vivo* MR coronary artery imaging utilized a multi-contrast approach with high-resolution black blood spin echo- and fast spin echo (FSE)-based MR sequences [13]. The signal from the blood flow is rendered black through preparatory pulses (e.g. radiofrequency spatial saturation or inversion recovery pulses) to improve the image of the adjacent vessel wall. However, bright blood imaging by 3D Fast time-of-flight pulse sequence was also employed in assessing fibrous cap thickness and morphological integrity of the coronary artery. This sequence enhanced the signal from flowing blood and a mixture of T2* and proton density contrast weighting highlighting the fibrous cap. Atherosclerotic plaque composition by MRI is generally based on the signal intensities and morphological appearance of the plaque on T1 weighted, proton density-weighted, and T2-weighted images as previously validated [14, 15]. Optimized scan parameters and combined weighting generate good contrast for coronary artery features. However, this weighting scheme for imaging may suffer from plaque semi liquid phase and its fatty esters in cholesterol-rich moiety whose saturated/unsaturated lipid ratio determines the severity of disease and plaque stability [12, 18]. Therefore, delineation and feature visual identification of coronary vessel constituents may serve the purpose to some extent.

Ex Vivo MR Imaging of Human Coronary Arteries and Aorta Histopathology Correlation

Adventitia and thin layer of innermost media were poorly visible in coronary specimens. These observations corroborate with earlier report on thin fibrous cap, respiratory motion, and poor lipid rich moiety as factors for T2-weighted MRI visibility or Contrast Noise Ratio

(CNR) of lumen narrowing [14, 15]. In present study, short T2 plaque components were MR visible such as calcification and thrombus. These components were quantified *in vivo* before surgery procedure and correlated with coronary artery lesion size obtained *ex vivo* after surgery. The quantification of lesion size, detection of media thickness and fibrous cap 'integrity' evaluations were main focus. In present study, the images were acquired with a resolution of 0.25 x 0.25 x 2.0 to 0.4 x 0.4 x 3.0 mm^3 by use of a coronary phased-array coil to improve signal-to-noise ratio and image resolution. A recent report reviewed the data on coronary aorta composition and atheroma size with the use of T1-weighted, T2-weighted, and proton density-weighted images at a resolution of 0.8 x 0.8 x 5.0 mm^3 using a phased array coil-high-resolution imaging or contrast-enhanced MRA by gadolinium-based contrast agents for plaque neovascularization, necrotic core and fibrous tissue [15].

In present study, SNAKE contour algorithm demarcated the distinct lumen and artery wall boundaries in less time to measure all of the coronary artery size. Coronary artery wall thickness and areas in CAD were greater than normal coronary artery. Different branches of coronary artery showed similar relationship. The correlation of coronary artery wall and plaque measurements by MRI and histology methods offered comparison as % difference < 6 % and demonstrated the thrombus area as better plaque stability indicator over wall thickness. It supported other previous report [13].

The plaques features such as lipids, calcification, atheroma, elastin and collagen were main plaque features. Fibrous cap, inner wall disruption were quite distinct on histology sections but on MRI images only different signal intensities suggested presence of different components due to limited MRI resolution. So, we suggest combined information on wall morphology and plaque features offer better sensitivity and specificity with possibility of cardiovascular risk.

Sensitivity and Specificity of Coronary MRI (Stenoses: > 50%)

The present study suggested the % stenosis based on our new technique [7] to measure wall radii and lumen size as possible cardiovascular risk marker (no risk with 30-39 % stenosis; prone to risk with 40-50 % stenosis; mild risk with 50-69 % stenosis; unstable or vulnerable plaque with 70-79 % stenosis; high risk with 80 % stenosis or above). However, wall thickness also appeared as better risk correlate. Our results support the previous investigations predicting >50 % stenosis as considerable risk [13, 19]. The current state-of-art using several modified MR pulse sequences suggested further improvement in specificity and sensitivity of techniques used.

Coronary Plaque Lipids with High Resolution NMR Spectroscopy

Saturated and mono- or polyunsaturated (ω-3 or ω-6 esters) of fatty acid rich phospholipids and triglycerides as major coronary lipids have been reported by high resolution NMR as fingerprints [17, 18] and partial lack of lipid molecule mobility was attributed for their accumulation around coronary wall. It is a disadvantage in clinical time-dependent assessment of lipids during plaque progression. Presence of high-saturated lipids and free cholesterol contents reduce the plaque stability or cause adverse consequence [5, 18].

Coronary Oxidative Stress Markers

Triglycerides, cholesterol, insulin and angiotensin converting Enzyme in the atheroma are believed as indicators of plaque severity and extent of atherosclerosis. Malonaldehyde, TBARS, and diene conjugates serve as indicators of free radical damage in artery. Beta-carotene, vitamin E and C decrease with increased free radical damage and plaque severity indicates coronary artery at high risk of atheroma.

The increased atheroma biochemical precursors and NMR lipid peaks in artery homogenates indicated the coronary artery disease as consequence of lipid accumulation in walls or plaques within arteries. Both NMR and oxidative stress data suggested atherosclerosis as a lipid disorder [16,17,18]. Moreover, it gave a window to understand further the possible role of oxidative stress in atheroma formation. In control coronary tissue homogenates, indirect measures of oxidatively damaged lipids indicated the lesser free radical stress or no stress [5].

Higher concentrations of TBARS indicating high oxidative activity have been observed in coronary artery disease [6]. Higher triglyceride concentrations compared to cholesterol in CAD tissue homogenates may be due to less hydrolysis of triglycerides into fatty acids.

Limitation of This Study

Limitation of this study was that *ex vivo* investigations of endarterectomy coronary artery material changed the morphometric data during fixation and tissue processing such as shrinkage artifacts during dehydration. Other factors were limited lipid discrimination on MRI images due to vessel small size, hypercontracture of vessels and wall tension considerations while evaluating plaque vulnerability.

Some notable improved blood suppression methods are reported for accurate coronary plaque imaging by dual-inversion 3D FSE imaging sequence with real-time navigator technology for high-resolution, free- breathing black-blood CMRA [20], delineation of coronary artery by echoplanar imaging [21],MRA and TrueFISP imaging [22,23].

CONCLUSION

Multicontrast MR imaging may measure dimension of coronary stenoses in different branches. MRI may visualize the coronary plaque disruption and atherosclerotic lesion components, measuring atherosclerotic burden comparable with histological features. Relationship of outer vessel radius and wall thickness, plaque atheroma size and % stenosis might serve as clinical correlates of cardiovascular risk, its response to therapy and assessment of subclinical disease.

These results indicate possibility of coronary stenosis and thrombsis due to oxidative stress and lipid disorder.

ACKNOWLEDGMENTS

First author acknowledges the atherosclerosis training and methods adopted for MRI images in Figures 1, 3, and 4 as pilot experiments with Atherosclerosis Division, Baylor College of Medicine, Houston. Authors acknowledge the help of Dr. Niaz MA for the oxidative stress analysis and histology experiments at Heart Research Laboratory, Moradabad, India and Dr. Raj K. Gupta for NMR experiments at Albert Einstein College of Medicine, Bronx, New York.

REFERENCES

[1] Naghavi M, Libby P, Falk E, et al. From vulnerable plaque to vulnerable patient: a call for new definitions and risk assessment strategies: Parts I and II. *Circulation.* 2003;108(15):1764-78.

[2] Erbel R, Ge J, Gorge G, Baumgart D, Haude M, Jeremias A, von Birgelen C, Jollet N, Schwedtmann J. Intravascular ultrasound classification of atherosclerotic lesions according to American Heart Association recommendation. *Coron Artery Dis.* 1999;10(7):489-99.

[3] Podesser BK, Neumann F, Neumann M, Schreiner W, Wollenek G, Mallinger R. Outer radius-wall thickness ratio, a postmortem quantitative histology in human coronary arteries. *Acta Anat* (Basel). 1998;163(2):63-8.

[4] Witztum, J.L. The oxidative hypothesis of atherosclerosis. *Lancet* 1994; 344:793-796.

[5] Singh RB, Dubnov G, Niaz MA, Ghosh S, Singh R, Rastogi SS, Manor O, Pella D, Berry EM. Effect of an Indo-Mediterranean diet on progression of coronary artery disease in high risk patients(Indo-Mediterranean Diet Heart Study): a randomised single-blind trial. *Lancet.* 2002; Nov 9;360(9344):1455-61.

[6] Niato C., Kawamura, M., Yamamoto, Y. Lipid peroxides as the initiating factor of atherosclerosis. *Annual NY Medical Science* 1993; 676: 27-45.

[7] Sharma, R. A device for MR imaging of atherosclerosis plaque in carotid endarterectomy specimens ex vivo. *Journal of Magnetic Resonance in Medical Science 2002.*1(1),116-124.

[8] Morrisett, J., Vick, W., Sharma, R., Lawrie,G,, Reardon, M., Ezell, E., Schwartz,J., Hunter,G., Gorenstein D. Discrimination of components in atherosclerotic plaques from human carotid endarterectomy specimens by MRI in vivo. *Magn Reson Imaging* 2003; 21(5): 468-474.

[9] Sharma R, Singh R.B. and Gupta R.K. A Segmentation method for Carotid Artery Atherosclerosis Plaque for MRI contrast and Oxidative Stress markers in plaque. *Proceedings 16th IEEE Symposium on Computer-Based Medical Systems* June 26 - 27, 2003 Mt Sinai Hospital, New York, New York Ed. Krol M. 2003: 16: 323-328.

[10] Cline HE, Thedens DR, Irarrazaval P, Meyer CH, Hu BS, Nishimura DG, Ludke S. 3D MR coronary artery segmentation. *Magn. Reson. Med.* 1998;40(5):697-702.

[11] Pearlman JD, Zajicek J, Merickel MB, Carman CS, Ayers CR, Brookeman JR, Brown MF. High-resolution 1H NMR spectral signature from human atheroma. *Magn. Reson. Med.* 1988;7(3):262-79.

[12] Singh RB, Shinde SN, Chopra RK, Niaz MA, Thakur AS, Onouchi Z. Effect of coenzyme Q10 on experimental atherosclerosis and chemical composition and quality of atheroma in rabbits. *Atherosclerosis.* 2000;148(2):275-82.

[13] Worthley SG, Helft G, Fayad ZA, Fuster V, Rodriguez OJ, Zaman AG, Badimon JJ. Cardiac gated breath-hold black blood MRI of the coronary artery wall: an in vivo and ex vivo comparison. *Int. J. Cardiovasc. Imaging.* 2001;17(3):195-201.

[14] Yuan C, Hatsukami TS, Obrien KD. High-Resolution magnetic resonance imaging of normal and atherosclerotic human coronary arteries ex vivo: discrimination of plaque tissue components. *J. Investig. Med.* 2001;49(6):491-9.

[15] Fayad ZA, Choudhury RP, Fuster V. Magnetic resonance imaging of coronary atherosclerosis-Review. *Current Atheroscler. Report* 2003;5(5):411-7.

[16] Duerinckx AJ. Imaging of coronary artery disease-Review. MR. *J. Thorac. Imaging.* 2001;16(1):25-34.

[17] Zajicek J, Pearlman JD, Merickel MB, Ayers CR, Brookeman JR, Brown MF. High-resolution proton NMR spectra of human arterial plaque. *Biochem. Biophys. Res. Commun.* 1987;149(2):437-42.

[18] Pella D, Dubnov G, Singh RB, Sharma R, Berry EM, Manor O. Effects of an Indo-Mediterranean diet on the omega-6/omega-3 ratio in patients at high risk of coronary artery disease: the Indian paradox. *World Rev. Nutr. Diet.* 2003;92:74-80.

[19] Fayad ZA, Fuster V, Nikolaou K, Becker C. Computed tomography and magnetic resonance imaging for noninvasive coronary angiography and plaque imaging: current and potential future concepts. *Circulation.* 2002;106(15):2026-34.

[20] Botnar RM, Stuber M, Kissinger KV, Kim WY, Spuentrup E, Manning WJ. Noninvasive coronary vessel wall and plaque imaging with magnetic resonance imaging. *Circulation.* 2000;102(21):2582-7.

[21] Deshpande VS, Li D. Contrast-enhanced coronary artery imaging using 3D trueFISP. *Magn. Reson. Med.* 2003;50(3):570-7.

[22] Stehning C, Boernert P, Nehrke K. Advances in coronary MRA from vessel wall to whole heart imaging. *Magn Reson Med Sci.* 2007;6(3):157-70.

[23] McCarthy RM, Deshpande VS, Beohar N, Meyers SN, Shea SM, Green JD, Liu X, Bi X, Pereles FS, Finn JP, Davidson CJ, Carr JC, Li D. Three-dimensional breathhold magnetization-prepared TrueFISP: a pilot study for magnetic resonance imaging of the coronary artery disease. *Invest Radiol.* 2007;42(10):665-70.

In: World Heart Research Yearbook. Volume 1
Editors: Franz Halberg and R. B. Singh
ISBN: 978-1-60741-881-8

HUMAN CAROTID ARTERY: SEGMENTATION METHODS IN ATHEROSCLEROSIS IMAGING

***Rakesh Sharma**[*1], **Bharati D. Shrinivas**[2] and **Avdhesh Sharma**[3]*

[1] Department of Medicine, Baylor College of Medicine, Houston, TX, US
[2] Department of Zoology, RTM Nagpur University, Nagpur, India
[3] Department of Electrical Engineering, Maharana Pratap A&T University, Udaipur, Rajasthan, India

ABSTRACT

Objective: Carotid artery stenosis measurement evaluates the cardiovascular risk and vascular disease.

Hypothesis: Automated robust 3D segmentation offers display of vascular morphology as well as measurement of carotid plaque constituents.

Results: 3D segmentation methods of carotid artery in vivo MRI images were used in vascular feature characterization by: 1. parametric deformable models, 2. feature contour map and contrast enhancement methods. Segmentation was done by object delineation and recognition using surrogate vascular marker. T1 weighted and T2-weighted segmentation methods used parametric color-coded feature maps and 3D reconstruction rendered images to display different plaque and vascular wall features. Segmented carotid wall thickness, lumen area and carotid plaque constituents appeared as significant cardiovascular risk indicators.

Conclusion: Carotid artery segmentation and contrast enhancement distinguished carotid plaque features by spatial transformation and image 3D reconstruction.

Keywords: 3D segmentation, atherosclerosis, carotid artery imaging, magnetic resonance, carotid plaque

INTRODUCTION

Atheromatous plaques develop in the walls of large and medium carotid arteries. Carotid artery displays 80% risk of Atherosclerosis in the US population especially on high risk of stenosis. Common carotid artery bifurcates into two internal and external branches.

[*] Corresponding Address: Rakesh Sharma, Ph.D. 200 Wadsworth Avenue #2, New York, NY 10033. Email: rs2010@columbia.edu.

Progressive enlargement of carotid plaques narrows the arterial lumen, causing vascular stenosis and occlusion. Atherosclerosis may remain acute and asymptomatic when an unstable atheromatous plaque ruptures. The contents of ruptured plaque are highly thrombogenic, causing arterial occlusion 'emboli' and lead to the development of aneurysm. These cause tears longitudinally in the arterial wall. Later, these tears in carotid artery wall allow blood to escape from their vessel lumen. Vascular magnetic resonance imaging (MRI) imaging helps to define the nature and extent of vascular disease and statin therapy monitoring for progression or reoccurrence after therapy. Automated image processing is used to extract information from carotid artery vascular imaging. Carotid artery segmentation differentiates the wall features and locates the incidence of atheroma formation near to bifurcation region. The main reason of atheroma formation and plaque development at the point of bifurcation is blood flow across bifurcation either as pulsatile, laminar or vertex flow. The defective blood flow initiates the slow deposited blood lipid components mainly saturated fats through diet and lipid rich plaques can be classified according to AHA classification of plaque MRI features and scored criteria of atherosclerosis disease burden [1]. In this direction, Glagov et al. [2] classified and defined morphological segments of common carotid (CC1 CC2), bifurcation (B), external and internal branches (E1,2 and I1,2) as shown in Figure 1. Atherosclerosis in vivo evaluation mainly depends on accurate carotid segmentation for vessel wall, plaque chemical composition and lumen measurement. However, many controversial questions in vascular imaging are important such as: isolated plaque or multiple lesions, % occlusion or narrowing of lumen in vascular segment, site of occlusion either distal or proximal to the lesion, presence of collateral vessels to provide blood flow around lesion, abnormal blood flow patterns.

In present paper, 3D segmentation method is demonstrated based on algorithms of object delineation and object recognition of atherosclerosis vascular wall and plaque features. Our focus was to perform segmentation of carotid artery *in vivo* MRI and *ex vivo* MRI images of endarterectomy specimen to visualize carotid artery MRI features and plaque constituents as possible cardiovascular risk predictors such as % stenosis.

THEORY

Vascular Image Segmentation

Classifiers and segmentation algorithms extract out features and characteristics of image primitives or a priori information. This a priori information is boundary-based and region-based edge-detection approximate gray-level values of carotid vessel wall tissue, spatial location of bifurcation to initialize a threshold-based or spatial transformation or boundary detection and interpretation of wall layers. Segmentation depends on thresholding that suffers from noise and sampling artifacts. Deformable models minimize these problems in segmentation. Deformable models are 'curves' or 'surfaces' defined within image domain that can move under the influence of internal forces within the curve or surface itself and external forces that are computed from the image data.

Deformable Models as SNAKES or Active Contours

Parametric deformable models use 'snakes' and 'curves'. Snakes show direct interaction with the model and lead to fast-real time implementation. These 'snakes' are also known with other names such as balloons, surfaces etc. Deformable models may be geometric models. Parametric deformable models may be two types: 'energy minimizing formulation' and a 'dynamic force formulation'. Energy minimization Formulation: It finds a parameterized curve with minimum internal energy (tension or the smoothness of contour) and potential energy (local minima at the image intensity edges occurring at object boundaries). Curve may be defined as X(s) = (X(s), Y(s)), s E[0,1] which moves through the spatial domain of an vascular image to minimize the following energy functional component:

$$E(X)=S(X)+P(X) \quad (1)$$

Dynamic Force Formulation

The force formulation represents the external force as dynamic formulation as represented by dynamics of a contour $X_{(s,t)}$ as following:

$$\mu d^2X/dt^2=F_{damp}(X)+F_{in}(X)+F_{ext}(X), \quad (2)$$

where μ=0 (in segmentation) is coefficient that has mass unit and F_{damp} is the damping (or viscous) force defined as –y*dX/dt with y being the damping coefficient. Several external forces are now applicable to deformable contours and surfaces such as multiscale Gaussian potential force, pressure force, distance potential force, Gradient vector flow, dynamic distance force, interactive force. Deformable models generate 'contours' by finite difference method, dynamic programming, greedy algorithm, marching algorithm [3].

Interpretation of Features from Segmentation

Color-coded feature classification aims to the specific identification of plaque components. Descriptions of regions may be either "Contour-based" or "Region-based (in terms of effective diameter, circularity and projection) [4].

Classification vs. Representation

Color-coded feature based classification of plaque tissue represents the compositional and dimensional properties of atherosclerosis lesions. However, question of diffuse or semi-solid, fibous, collagenous or elastic, still remains a problem into one of a finite number of mutually exclusive classes. A 'classifier' needs to designate and separate points representing distinct 'classes' with assumption that matching points tend to be closer with each other away from other points. The subset of features yielding minimum P(e) represents best set and parametric classifier (Bayes method) uses probability structure data class-by-class to generate 'feature set' or class decision for a given sample. If data is insufficient, non-parametric classifier methods (ANN, KNN) are used [5].

Quantitative Analysis of Segmented Images and Algorithms

The typical segmentation goals are identification of accurate vessel morphology, topology (angles and curvatures), correct plaque labeling and voluming. It is accomplished by measurement of wall thickness, lumen and plaque size. Automatic segmentation requires robust and quick methods to perform accurate separation and identification of vascular structure with minimal amount of user interaction. This allows the selective visualization (region of interest display), and quantitation of vascular function. *a priori* knowledge based image segmentation depends on *a priori* knowledge. It may involve knowledge of approximate gray-level value of a tissue class to initialize a threshold based method, spatial location of tissue or organs for automated selection of training points for a classifier, or shape of object. Training points design the spatial transformations and constraints for the boundary detection algorithms [6].

This information can be used to improve the specificity and sensitivity of the low-level segmentation algorithms.

Vasculature Assessment (Object Extraction) Algorithm

Extraction of bifurcation segment starts from operator-choice of seed point. The segment is 3D portion of vasculature. Using seed point, image intensity ridges are extracted out approximately same vessel dimensions utilizing *a priori* information supplied. The vessel dimensions can be measured proportional to the scale as following [6].

1. Geometry-based semi-automatic segmenta- tion of MRA volume to extract bifurcation segment in the region of interest;
2. Comparison of extracted vessel segments with maximum intensity projection of MRI data in the region of interest. If bifurcation segment is missing, repeat step 1;
3. Iterative construction of carotid artery bifurcation segment;
4. 3D visualization and interactive editing of resulting bifurcation artery segment.

Artery Visualization and Suppression of Overlapping Veins

Algorithm: Vessel segmentation uses automated process after operator selects two points (start and end points) of vessel. At the start point location, a search for the vessel borders is performed by dynamic programming in a plane perpendicular to the vessel segment (two interactively marked points). Dynamic programming identifies approximately elliptic border of artery cross-section and a centroid of vessel region is calculated as new centerline point. It is mapped to the next plane of vessel segment in the direction of segment end [7].

1. Maximum intensity projection of bifurcation region of interest in 3D
2. Interactive identification of start and end points of adjacent veins, and their removal;
3. Interactive generation of targeted MIP image
4. Bifurcation segment labeling
5. Repetition of steps 2, 3, 4 until resulted bifurcation MIP image.

SNAKES Algorithm

Snakes are deformable active contour models attracted to image features such as edge, lines, contours etc. Snake is a energy-minimizing spline guided by internal constraint forces and influenced by external forces that pull it towards image features. These snakes pass by edges. It behaves as balloon and skips high intensity points and passes over edges that are weaker intensity points. The starting point for SNAKES algorithm is manually chosen as a single seed point at common carotid artery (centroid). Further, application of 3 x 3 Sobel edge detector mask to carotid MRA images enhances the speed of snake energy minimization. At optimized settings of edge force, expansion force and use of constants, several node points approximate a contour. The vertices of the obtained contours are placed in areas with significant values of the image gradients. The algorithm is the equation determining vertex movement. Equation (3) defines the new iterative process for finding the SNAKE location. A contour by a set of points v(s)=(x(s), y(s)) on an image parameterized with respect to the contour arc length s. The total energy of the active contour is the integration of local energies along its normalized contour, which is written as

$$E_{snake} = \int_0^1 E_{int} + E_{ext} ds \quad (3)$$

E_{int} represents the internal energy of the snake that measures the continuity and smoothness of the contour. The internal energy can be defined as $E_{int} = a(s)|v_s(s)|^2 + b(s)|v_{ss}(s)|^2$, where v_s and v_{ss} are the first and second derivative of v by the arc length s. E_{ext} are external forces, which can be lines, edges and terminations derived from the image.

$$E_{ext}(v) = -\int_{\Omega} g_0(|f_M * I| + D * I)\, ds = -\int_{\Omega} F(v)\, ds \quad (4)$$

where f_M represents the Macleod operator, I denotes the raw image, g_o is the gravity constant, A is a positive weighting factor, and represents the convolution operator. In addition, Ω defines a local area in which the gravity is assumed to be effective to current position v. Depending on positive or negative value of f_M the contour vertices move forward or backward along their normal vectors n. Function f in Equation (4) looks along the vector n for the maximum value of dot product between image gradient and vector n. The neighborhood of radius b (in one dimensional space) maxima point can be searched. The search step is set to a fractional part of a pixel. The gradient computed value gives an intensity difference on a similar distance. The image intensity is calculated by means of bilinear interpolation. If the maximum gradient is found on the outer side of the contour, function f obtains a positive value and the vertex moves towards till the maxima point inside is searched. At maxima point inside the contour, the vertex moves in the opposite direction. The SNAKES algorithm enables the user to change the radius b as one of the parameters' control the distance of the contour edge located in the expected location. In this algorithm, snake vertices oscillate near the sharpest edge based on the assumption that the initial contour for locating the intima always lies above the sub-intima region. So the iterative process must be stopped after a certain number of iterations (usually ten iterations). If the function f_M is set to zero in Equation (4) the algorithm can be used for contour smoothing by using the sequence of ten iterations of the full snake algorithm, five iterations of smoothing and again five iterations of the snake algorithm. The smoothing phase avoids spurious edge for the smooth curved object shape.

Tracking the Carotid Aorta

This method produces surface as a set of voxels with user supervision during the segmentation process and sometimes parameter correction [9]. The algorithm is completed in the procedure for aorta tracking based on connectivity as following:

1. Initialization in one of the slices (just under the aortic arch) and automatically finding starting point and performs segmentation for other slices;
2. Find the descending aorta in all slices under the initial one. three additional features in comparison to the method used for a single slice;
3. The initial point in the next slice is determined as an average position of all snake points in the previous slice;
4. The parameter associated with pixel intensity is corrected for each slice, so that the product p and av is constant, where p is the balloon parameter, av is an average pixel value computed for certain neighborhood of the initial point; and
5. Segmentation must be repeated only for the skipped slices. A maximum number of iterations is done that is acceptable for a contour approximation. If the contour exceeds this number, its average position is not used as an initial point for the next slice. In that case the last regular snake is used to compute the initial point. This feature is used to track the aorta, in cases when a single image can destroy an entire set by moving the initial point completely out of the desired area of the aorta.

Dynamic Programming Algorithm

It computes optimal paths in a graph for searching boundaries in one direction based on the principle that "an optimal policy has the property that whatever the initial state and initial decision are, the remaining must constitute an optimal policy with regards to the state resulting from the first decision"[10]. So, the choice of a transition from n_j to n_{j+1} can be based on only the cost of optimal path to n_j and the local cost associated with a move from n_j to n_{j+1}. The strategy is following:

1. Positioning of the region of interest according to the location of an image marker that was inserted during image acquisition.
2. Separation of near and far borders, detection of an appropriate vessel centerline in a low resolution image.
3. Dynamic programming based determina-tion of approximate near and far wall borders.
4. Dynamic programming based determina-tion of final positions of near wall media-adventitia NWMA border (trailing edges) and far wall media-adventitia FWMA border (leading edges) in full resolution.
5. Dynamic programming based determina-tion of final positions of the near wall-lumen-intima NWLI border (leading edges). Far wall lumen-intima FWLI border is determined (leading edges).

Both border detection searches are performed in small bands along the approximate border positions in full resolution data.

Contrast Enhancement Methods

In vivo MRI imaging evaluation of 1-mm thick carotid artery image slice with plane resolution of 0.1 mm visualizes atheroma tissue components appearing as dark, brighter and gray areas. Carotid artery wall mainly consists outer layer intima, outlined by epithelium collagen embedding media which is the seat of connective tissue components like elastin, collagen, fibrous muscles, blood capillaries and deposits including thrombus, plaque etc.

Two important plaque components are atheromatous core and fibrous cap generate contrast by selecting different TE and TR values [11]. Apparently the major presence of water hydrogen atoms in the core in comparison with lipids allows better NMR signal by frequency selective methods. T2 weighted sequences using broad range of TE and TR provide good contrast between plaque components with lesser effect of noise, motion artifacts, acquisition time demand and longer TE.

The contrast enhancement is accomplished by segmentation and image processing. The raw images may be processed by automatic or manual delineation of boundaries, edges, contours. Further, image processing may be used to train data set and color-coded feature maps of each carotid artery and wall structure. T1 and T2 parametric segmentation methods display a unique opportunity of distinguishing carotid artery wall and plaque components at all different angles throughout 360° by automated tracking of outer boundaries of artery.

Using segmentation of in vivo MRI images of carotid artery has recently replaced the ambiguity of pre-surgical clinical judgement of the disease based on enhanced contrast on carotid wall and plaque evaluation. A non-invasive, *in vivo* imaging method to identify, quantify, and characterize carotid plaques enables monitoring plaque changes over time and assessment of how these changes relate to clinical events. MRI serves inherently powerful imaging technology, capable of displaying different soft tissues with high contrast. Recently MRI techniques have been used either alone or together with molecular imaging techniques to demonstrate the presence of different components in atherosclerotic lesions. Since the MR image intensity of a tissue is determined by its relaxation times, T1, T2, and its proton density

(PD), unique combinations of these parameters may uniquely characterize a particular tissue component. A good account of recent clinical trials such as NASCET and ESCET clinical studies have demonstrated the need to measure the degree of carotid stenosis in order to determine the clinical usefulness of carotid endarterectomy in symptomatic patients (11). Measurements of stenosis on projectional MR angiograms further have been used to correlate well with conventional angiographic techniques. However, standard projectional MRA studies tend to overestimate the degree of lumen stenosis for lesions that exceed 70% diameter because of signal loss due to a complex flow pattern. More recent efforts of several groups have been directed toward identifying MRA methods that are insensitive to signal loss from complex flow (11). More importantly, the cross-sectional information regarding vessel lumen diameter available from MRA source images is likely to measure the actual luminal area than do the conventional projection techniques. Evaluating the clinical impact of area measurements of these MRA images on patient outcome may be difficult since NASCET data were all based upon projectional angiograms (11). However, MR studies of arterial specimens ex vivo over several years demonstrated various aspects of atherosclerotic plaque structure by segmentation such as feature extraction, morphometry, shape, texture and chemical constitution of plaque and carotid artery wall. In vivo MR imaging of the carotid arterial wall and atherosclerotic plaque can be quite challenging due to i) the artery's small size, ii) its pulsatile motion, and iii) blood flowing in its lumen. Accordingly, an effective in vivo MRI methodology must provide high resolution, small field-of-view (FOV) images, and suppression of artifacts caused by vessel wall motion and blood flow. For imaging the plaque itself, recent results using chemical shift imaging and lipid suppression techniques have provided valuable information about plaque morphology. In contrast to ultrasonography, MRI images of plaques are not limited by calcium deposits.

In recent past, custom made phased-array surface coils have enhanced the capability of in vivo MRI to study the carotid arteries of a patient with significant stenosis one day before endarterectomy, and the plaque constitutional analysis that was resected at surgery. The strategy of contrast determination depends on combination of different MRI weighting. The *in vivo* study may reveal a plaque at the carotid artery bifurcation, and a distinct region of low signal within the plaque, most likely corresponds to calcification while the plaque microstructure can be examined histologically. Differentiation of the plaque from the rest of the vessel wall may appear clear on the PD weighted images. Based on this preliminary assumption, The present study was designed for optimal imaging protocol to visualize and quantifying carotid plaques in vivo using T1-weighted, T2-weighted, and spin echo (SE)-weighted imaging sequences.

Object Delineation

Five possible choices of the vascular surrogate of truth for delineation are outlined below.

Manual Delineation

It is easier but it is not exact. Suppose, corresponding to a given set T of scenes for the application domain <X, Y, Z>, manual delineation in either of these forms produces a set T_{td}

of scenes representing the fuzzy objects defined by the same object represented in the scenes in T. Manual 'delineation' produces a hard set 0 for each scene C Є T, which is later converted to a fuzzy object. There are several ways of averaging the results to get binary scenes, T_{td}. The binary objects (0) segmented in each scene C Є T in multiple trials may be averaged first and then the fuzzy object may be computed using Adobe Photoshop or MedEX®.

Automated Delineation

Automated delineation of vessel boundaries and edge identification assesses carotid artery stenosis. An example of automated contour delineation of vascular boundaries and measurement of wall thickness by using SNAKE algorithm is demonstrated in present report (see Figure 12). In this approach, transform pixel coordinates of SNAKE boundary from x, y to radial r, θ are used to delineate the outer and inner boundaries of the vessel to measure wall thickness.

Simulated Scenes

3D Deformations: 3D deformations generate simulated scenes to capture variations for segmentation. The same method was applied for manual segmentation. The complete set of scenes (original $\pm$ deformed) in this case constitutes T, and the complete set of segmentations represents T_{td}.

Simulated Scenes

Cutoff Regions: Another method to simulate vascular scenes first creates an ensemble of "cut-outs" of object regions from actual acquired scenes. In second step, these "cut-outs" of object regions get buried realistically in different scenes. Each cut-out may be segmented by appropriate segmentation method viz. validated, seed growth, supervised etc. The cut-out regions contain the object region with a background tissue region only without any other confounding tissue regions the resulting scenes and the segmentations constitute T and T_{td}, respectively.

Contour Delineation

A semi-automatic contour delineation technique by Ladak et al. [8] was based upon the discrete dynamic contour (DDC). A DDC is a poly-line, a sequence of points connected by straight-line segments that deforms to fit features in an image. DDC drives outwards through a balance of image-derived forces (which define the edges of the vessel), internal forces (which keep the DDC smooth in the presence of noise), and damping forces (which keep the

DDC stable during deformation). The image-derived forces are based on edges. So, it is necessary to initialize the DDC by drawing an approximate outline of the object.

In this approach, an operator first identifies and then crops out the vessel of interest in the given image. The operator then draws an approximate outline of the inner arterial wall in the form of a polygon with four to six vertices. The DDC is then deformed towards the inner (lumen/wall) boundary, with additional points automatically introduced to maintain a fixed spacing (patching) between points. In case of unsuccessful segmentation (e.g., if part of the contour undershoots an edge due to overdamping), individual points on the DDC can be manipulated, and the DDC is deformed again. Once the algorithm successfully finds the inner boundary of the arterial wall, this inner contour is saved and then inflated by approximately 626 m (i.e., two pixels at the standard 16-cm FOV, and roughly equal to the wall thickness of a normal carotid) to create a 'second contour' as the initial approximation for the outer arterial wall boundary. This second contour is then automatically deformed and saved to fit the outer arterial wall boundary in the same manner as described for the inner contour.

Object Recognition

In evaluation approaches, the overall vascular volume delineated by segmentation may not match with segmentation truth i.e. some areas of a vessel may be missed regions in delineation. If it is a crucial landmark area, such as a location of lesions, vascularization then missing or overestimating could affect important clinical-decision making for the location of vital regions such as vulnerable plaque fibrous cap. It highlights the algorithm's recognition performance. Prerequisites of object recognition: Plaque as true surrogate needs reliable information for assessing accuracy of segmentation. It needs a priori information related to the object (recognition) based on the following strategy.

1) Compile a list of features/landmarks that are vital for <X, Y, Z> through help from a set of experts (radiologists, surgeons, cardiovascular-anatomists).
2) Each expert assigns a score to each feature to indicate its level of importance in <X, Y, Z>.
3) Compute an average of the scores. Normalize these to the range [0, 1]. It generates a feature vector F whose components have values in [0, 1].
4) Experts locate and delineate the critical plaque area of these features in scenes in T repeatedly.
5) Use the mean location and spread information and the mean vector F to generate a scene Ctr, (for each scene C Є T) which is a composite of the Gaussian weighted scores for all features in the set. In this composite scene C_{tr} = (C, f_{tr},), a high value $f_{tr}(c)$ for a voxel c Є C indicates that c is both close to the mean location for a particular feature.

It generates a scene e_{tr} for each feature i in F or make C_{tr}, a vectorial scene. Alternatively, these individual scenes e_{tr} may be combined into a composite scene C_{tr}, as indicated above by taking an average or a fuzzy union. In any case, let S_{tr}, denote the set of resulting scenes containing information about truth in object recognition. Object recognition measurements may be done by segmented contours. Other approach may be using the inner and outer contours (C_{in} and C_{out}), to compute six measures: 1) arterial wall area (A_w); 2) average radius of C_{in} (R_{in}); 3) average radius of C_{out} (R_{out}); 4) signal difference to noise ratio (SDNR) at the inner wall-blood interface ($SDNR_{in}$); 5) SDNR at the tissue-outer wall interface ($SDNR_{out}$); and 6) SNR within the wall.

Using this approach, wall area was calculated by subtracting the area enclosed by C_{in} from the area enclosed by C_{out}. Since the computed wall areas are dependent on both C_{in} and C_{out}, R_{in} and R_{out} were calculated to characterize the effects of resolution and noise on these contours individually [12]. R_{in} was calculated by finding the average distance between C_{in} and its centroid. R_{out} was calculated similarly from C_{out}.

For 'edge detection' algorithm, a particularly convenient and appropriate measure is the SDNR difference at the inner wall-blood interface ($SDNR_{in}$) and the tissue-outer wall interface ($SDNR_{out}$) to detect the edge between the regions. SDNR serve as objective measure of quality for interfaces. It is calculated by taking the ratio of the signal difference at the interface of interest and the standard deviation (SD) of pixel values with in an area of no signal. Each inner-outer wall boundary contour pair (C_{in} and C_{out}) from a given image generates two additional contours automatically: a deflated inner boundary contour (C_{def}) was created by moving the nodes of the inner boundary contour 626 μm inward in a direction normal to C_{in} while an inflated outer contour (C_{inf}) was created by moving the nodes of C_{out} 626 μm outward in a direction normal to C_{out}. It calculates $SDNR_{in}$ by subtracting the mean pixel value of the wall region (bounded by C_{in} and C_{out}) from the mean pixel value of the blood boundary region (bounded by C_{def} and C_{in}) and dividing by the SD of pixel values in the blood-core region (enclosed by C_{def}). In same way, $SDNR_{out}$ is subtraction of the mean pixel value of the tissue-boundary region (bounded by C_{in} and C_{out}) from the mean pixel value in the wall region (bounded by C_{inf} and C_{out}) and dividing by the SD of pixel values in the blood-core region. Mean pixel value of the wall region (bounded by C_{in} and C_{out}) divided by the SD of pixel values in the blood-core region gives SNR. So, both $SDNR_{in}$ and $SDNR_{out}$ are measures of "interface quality" associated with the C_{in} and C_{out} contours.

3D Reconstruction and 3D Rendering Analysis

Three-dimensional analysis of stacked gray scale images or of stacked binary image is performed on computer as geometrical transformations (rotation, translation and zooming) by use of the "reslicing" and "projective imaging" tools of the NIH-Image 1.63 software [12]. Volumetric analysis can be done after 3-D reconstruction in rotating frame using Vision 2.5 software as described with example in the following results. 3D reconstruction is done by use of contour image series of the specimen surfaces and of the internal structures display. Marching cube algorithms generate three-dimensional models based on feature vectors and cluster partitioning for geometrical transformation, projection, hidden-part removal and shading. These models can be viewed from all angles and can be animated for enhanced 3D effect using the "Vascular Display" module of the image Vision 2.5 software. Commonly available methods of rendering are z-buffer technique, ray-casting, 'surface approximation' and 'voxel projection' in vascular 3D rendering based on distinct blocks of different translucencies (opacity) of each binary scene (vascular regions at plaque interface) at various angles. In other words, different density of each voxel shows distinct opacity and color.

Table 1. Table represents scan imaging parameters of the different pulse sequences for image acquisition with different T1/T2/proton density weighting for carotid artery bifurcation

Plane(weight)	Slices	Pulse sequence	PSD	Flip Angle	TR /TE	Gated	BW	Thick/Sp	FOV	Matrix	NEX
Sagittal(PDW)	11	FSE, ETL=12	-	90	2000/26		64	4/4	24x24	512x512	1
2D TOF	50	GRE, ETL=12	2D TOF	60	24/5		64	1.5/0	16x12	256x232	1
Axial(PDW)	6	FSE, ETL=8	-	90	2200/32	2RR	64	3/0	13x13	512x384	2
Axial(T1W)	5	FSE, ETL=3	-	90	550/16		32	3/0	13x13	512x384	2
Axial(T2W)	6	FSE, ETL=18	FSE-XL90	90	2500/108	3RR	62	3/0	13x13	512x256	3

MATERIALS AND METHODS

Image Acquisition for Carotid Artery Bifurcation

The patients (n=24) presenting for bilateral endarterectomy (AHA class III plaques) underwent MRI before and after each procedure (4 scans each over 18 weeks). Patients were receiving following statin dose at the time of unilateral endarterectomy.

Low dose group 0.2 mg; n=30 (5 scans each over 18 months).

High dose group 0.8 mg; n=30 (5 scans each over 18 months).

All study data was immediately stored in PACS system. As soon as possible image data was DICOM transferred over existing network to lab server. The *in vivo* MRI images (n=24) of carotid artery were used for segmentation and registration. These MRI images of patients with atherosclerosis were earlier acquired as pilot study using 1.5 T GE Signa Lx Horizon® attached Cardiac Imaging system at Methodist Hospital, Houston, TX with ECG gating and following MRI scan parameters (see Table 1) to get images with it or nearly same phase of cardiac cycle as part of a pilot study [11].

Multicontrast Protocol

With a multicontrast protocol using T1-, proton density-, and T2 weighted images generated distinct area of carotid artery with different tissue features due to their different Larmor frequencies of plaque constituents resulting with specific T1 and T2 values and signal intensities [12, 13].

T1 Parametric Contrast Method

Two 3D image analysis algorithms, one a nearest-neighbor (ANN) tissue segmentation algorithm, the other a 'surface modeling' algorithm, were applied to serial MR images. The algorithms operate on different principles to determine tissue volume: the nearest-neighbor approach used manually identified 'tag' points to assist in classifying tissue types while 'boundary' and 'volumes' are calculated automatically. The surface-modeling algorithm relied on manual segmentation while volume determination was automated. Volumes of contrast enhancement and rates of volumetric change were determined by both algorithms. The tissue segmentation algorithm was used to create 3D maps [14].

T2 Parametric Imaging for Segmentation and Quantification of Plaque Components

T2 parametric segmentation was based on their TE and TR values as earlier described elsewhere [15]. It separated out different tissue classes of plaque components using 'tag' points on nearest-neighbor approach.

Supervised Semi-automated Parametric Color coded Segmentation Method

Color-coding segmentation by using k-nearest neighbor algorithm (k-NN) was utilized to create a stack of color-coded segmented image slices. It discards seed points. Connectivity algorithm classifies the color coded features. The method was based on color-coded pixel intensity probability distribution [16]. Similarly, voxel-coding probability provides a voxel-by-voxel parametric for automated structure parameterization. A supervised classifier was used to derive binary map. In each 2D slice a fast algorithm propagates a distance field from image exterior to interior. Local maxima distances are identified. The second shortest voxel paths to exterior were also identified. A third distance field is traversed to establish object connectivity between slices, and resulting voxel set was uniformly re-parameterized and triangulated as described in detail elsewhere [17].

3D Reconstruction Display

Volume rendering was done by using Volume J a java image processing program for DICOM multi-slice stacked images. For surface rendering, VISION 5.4 and VTK software generated 3D graphic view of vascular frame [18]. Plaque volume may be calculated from the outer wall radius (R) and inner wall radius (r) and length of plaque rich segment as:

$$V_{(maximum)} - V_{(minimum)} = L(2R+r).B/6 \tag{5}$$

where B is small plaque-rich region on MR image of the plaque. The difference in outer and inner wall volumes comes out as plaque volume as validated elsewhere [19] and shown in Figure 10.

RESULTS

The patients showed in vivo wall thickness as shown in Figure 1. Data (digital format) showed following max, min, and mean carotid wall thickness; max, min, and mean lumen area; max, min, and mean plaque area for left and right sides as shown in Table 2.

3D TOF FSE images showed distinct quantifiable wall boundaries, however, different flow rates appeared visibly to artifact these image signal intensities (see Figure 1). Wall thickness and atheroma size were main distinct features to assess plaque stenosis and vulnerability (see Table 2).

Multislice comparison showed good agreement between segmentation truth and post-segmented delineated wall measurements of inner and outer wall perimeters, lumen size and plaque curves at the bifurcation landmark on in vivo MRI images (see Figures 2-4). Interestingly, at different levels of carotid vessel after supervised multiparametric color-coded feature maps of the lumen size and wall thickness gave an estimate of extent for % stenosis and plaque tissue proton density with distinct color (see Figures 5). For true estimate of dimensions, intact plaque and its histology section with plaque features are shown (see Figure 6).

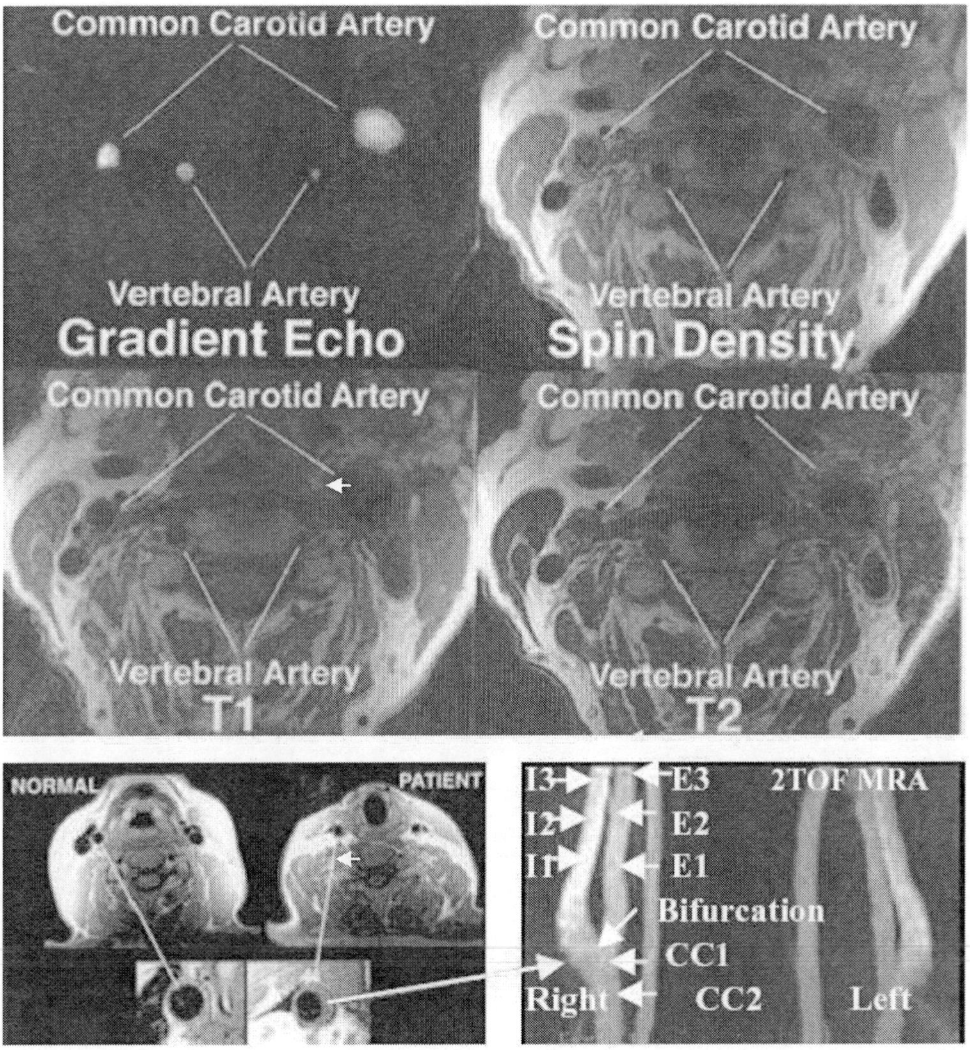

Figure 1. 3D TOF and FSE images of carotid artery at the level of bifurcation show distinct plaque sites (see arrow).

T1 Parametric Contrast

T1 values of images provided less information than T2 values or proton density images. Due to dependence of T1 and T2 relaxation times upon magnetic field, it might not allow same MRI criteria. It needed appropriate TE and TR choice for in vivo microimaging application using 1.5 T MRI clinical imager. However, wall measurement in post-segmented carotid arteries was better due to sharp edges (see Figure 7) while plaque features were poorly measurable.

T2 Parametric Contrast

Specifically, spin-spin relaxation time T2 of image micro-dissected necrotic core at different sets of TE settings, overcome the problem of observed darker T2 images than actual low signal of plaque components e.g. fibrocellular and thrombus contents. On other hand, the wall measurement was not as good as measured by T1 parametric segmentation (see Figure 8).

Table 2. The manual measurement is shown for right carotid artery external, internal and common (RCCA, RCEA, RCIA) and left carotid artery external, internal and common (LCCA, LCEA, LCIA) branches for lumen area (mm^2)* and wall thickness (mm)$^\#$ shown in Figure 1

	Observations (n)	Lumen Area*	Wall Thickness#		Observations (n)	Lumen Area*	Wall Thickness#
LCCA	28	30.34	1.02	RCCA	27	34.29	1.13
LCCA	21	26.23	1.07	RCCA	20	32.20	1.02
LCCA	24	35.69	0.95	RCCA	32	33.52	0.99
Average		30.75	1.01	Average		33.34	1.05
SD		4.75	0.06	SD		1.06	0.07
LECA	12	36.26	0.96	RECA	9	38.28	1.01
LECA	12	33.42	0.84	RECA	9	42.87	0.98
LECA	12	33.75	0.87	RECA	9	41.63	0.91
Average		34.14	0.89	Average		40.93	0.97
SD		0.98	0.06	SD		2.37	0.05
LICA	11	21.26	1.04	RICA	10	19.00	1.12
LICA	11	22.65	0.86	RICA	10	16.67	0.93
LICA	11	19.84	0.96	RICA	10	18.70	0.94
Average		21.25	0.95	Average		18.12	1.00
SD		1.41	0.09	SD		1.27	0.11

Multiparametric Contrast

Combined T1/T2/proton density multipara-metric approach allowed interactive segmentation by color cluster statistics (as 3D histograms) and tracking stereo display of different tissue constituents (see Figure 9) [15].

3D Reconstruction

3D reconstruction of staked DICOM images showed as contiguous display. The plaque *in situ* 3D features were distinct and plaque volume measurement was based on using curvature and outer and inner radii (see Figure 10).

Volume Rendering and 3D Display

NIH Image J interfaced with Volume J was used for 3D graphic display and staked cross-sectional 3D display was obtained by VTK software. The minimum intensity projection (MIP) stacked slices demonstrated the calcification on transverse sites while 3D surface rendering demonstrated features in longitudinal sites along the wall (see Figure 11).

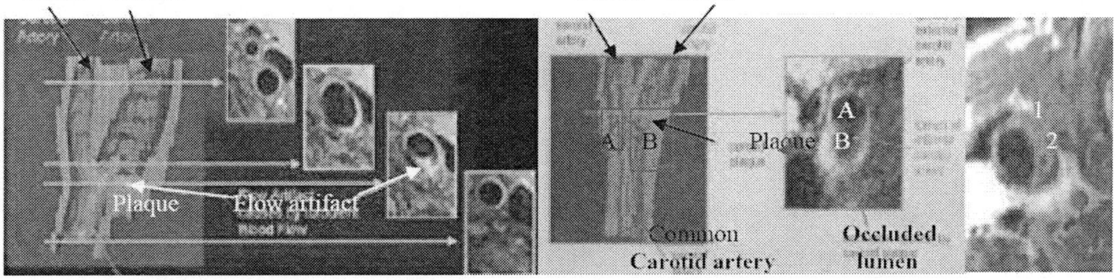

Figure 2. An *in vivo* post-segmented carotid artery plaque at the bifurcation shows the distinct wall thickness at different levels in different slices (see arrows in left panel) and delineated wall boundaries (middle panel) representing different wall thickness in one slice (right panel).

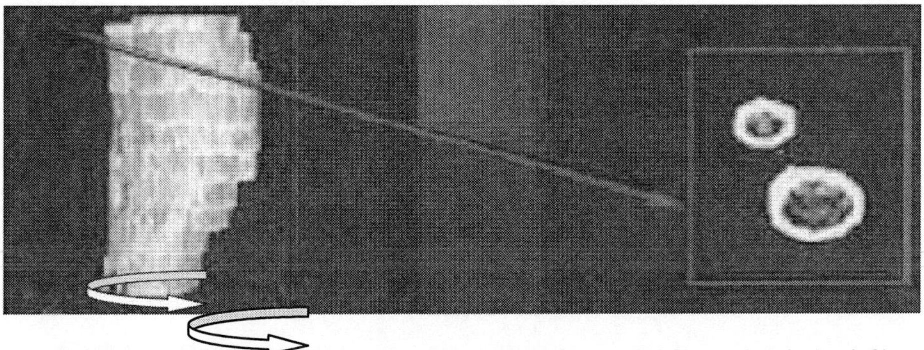

Figure 3. The method of 3D multislice in vivo stereographic display at different levels (on left) and wall delineation by SNAKES algorithm demonstrates the measurement of outer and inner wall radii (right panel).

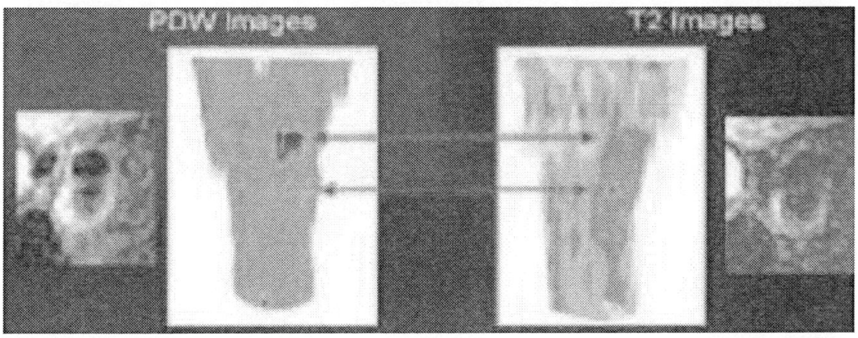

Figure 4. Supervised multiparametric color-coded feature maps show lumen size and wall thickness. Contours are shown with different signal intensities of different plaque consituents (on right panel). Notice the distinct plaque visibility and contrast on *in vivo* PDW and T2 weighted images. PDW and T2 weighted images provide different contrast for plaque components.

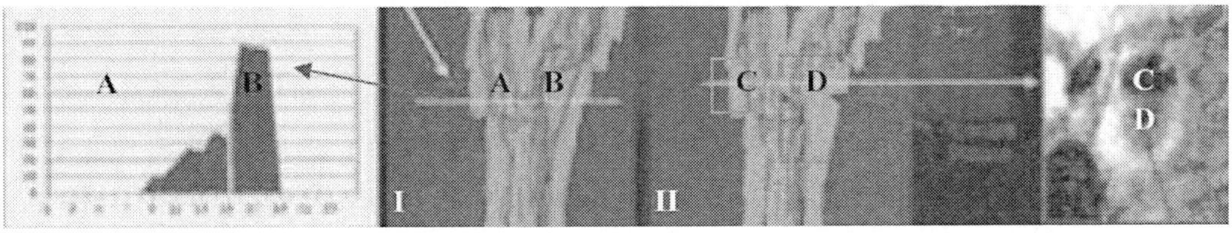

Figure 5. A sagittal semiautomated thresholding method of delineation is shown on PDW (on left I panel) and T2 weighted (on right II panel) to extract out plaque region. Using plaque size as index, at different distances graph (x axis) demonstrates the measurement of % stenosis (>70 on B) (on leftmost panel). The T2 weighted image better contrast of the external (C) and internal (D) lumen size on in vivo image (on rightmost panel).

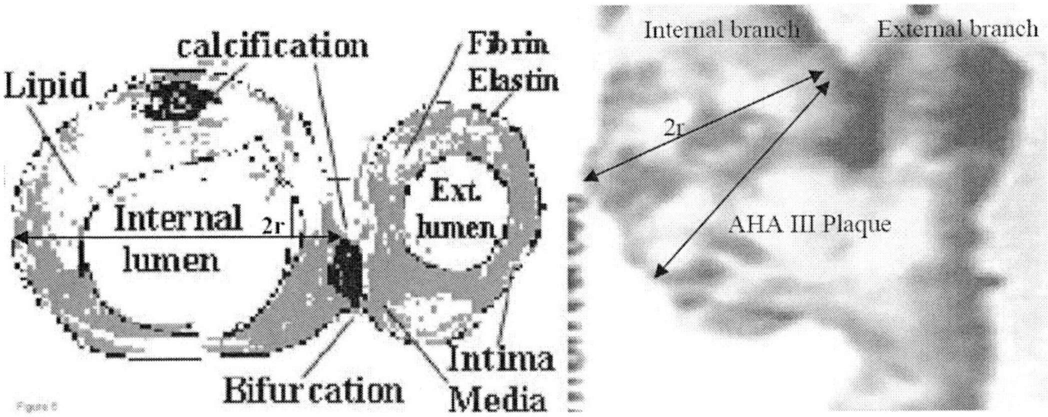

Figure 6. A comparison of excised plaque histology digital image mask (AHA type III on left) and endarterectomy specimen (on right) shows true wall thickness and plaque features as surrogate markers for MRI segmentation.

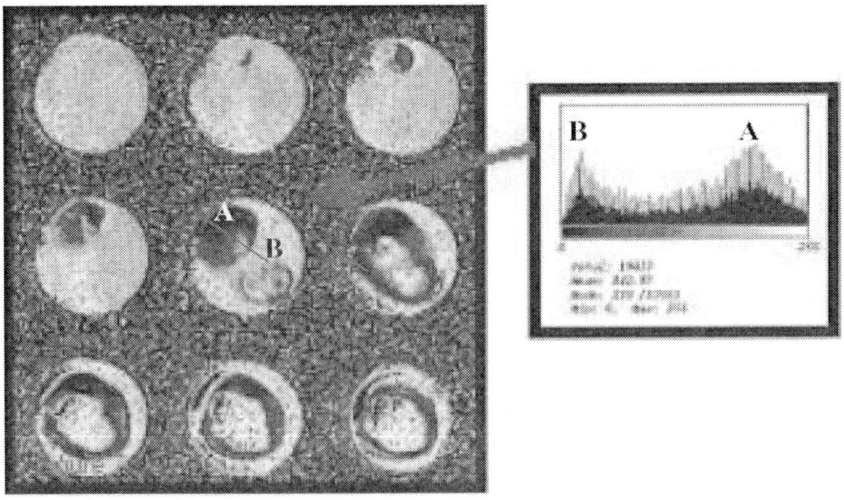

Figure 7. The *ex vivo* T1 parametric segmentation is shown to highlight wall thickness at various segments as contiguous post-segmented images of carotid endarterectomy sample. The post-segmented color-coded LUT histogram graphic presentation shows distinct signal intensities of plaque region A, thin wall region B and lumen.

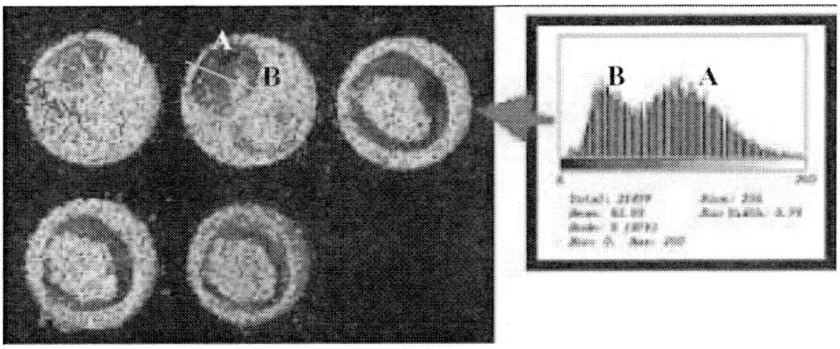

Figure 8. The *ex vivo* T2 parametric segmentation method is shown at same T1 parametric level to highlight wall thickness at various plaque segments in contiguous post segmented wall images of carotid endarterectomy sample. Notice the histogram LUT graphs show better contrast of wall on T2 and distinct measurable wall, lumen and plaque regions (see the different heights in graph).

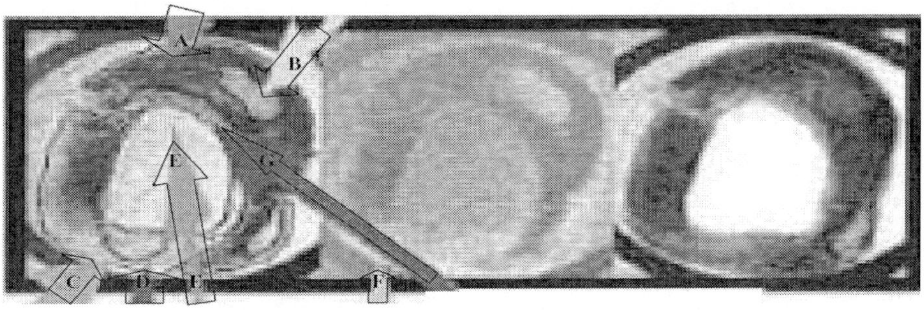

Figure 9. Multicontrast *ex vivo* MR images of a carotid endarterectomy sample shows distinct features of plaque on T1-weighted (left); proton density-weighted (in center); and T2-weighted (right) images. Plaque delineated features are shown with arrows. Different calcified intima/media(A), necrotic core(B), media(C) lipid core(D), luman(E), thick intima/media(F), and fibrous cap(G) constituents of plaque are shown by matching with their T1 and T2 relaxation constants.

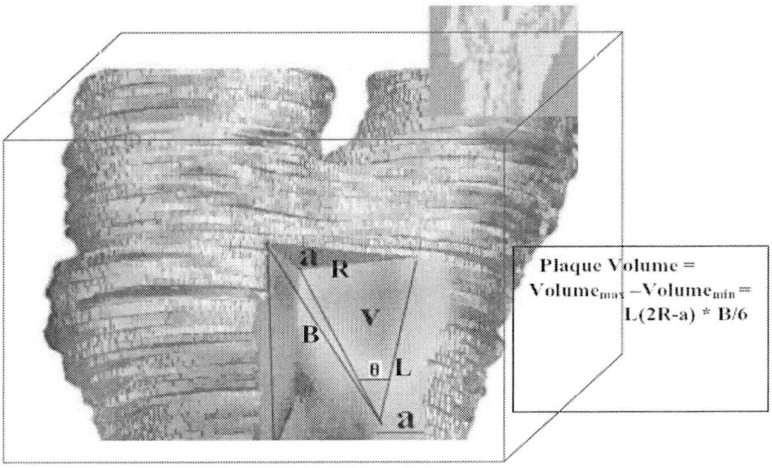

Figure 10. A 3D rendered conconstruct set was generated out of post-segmented stacked carotid endarerectomy in vivo MRI images shows reconstructed 3D display. The display demonstrated the plaque size V and wall area 'a' features at various angles θ. The insert on top, shows the plaque dimension in one vertical cross-section. The plaque volume may be calculated using equation. (see reference 19).

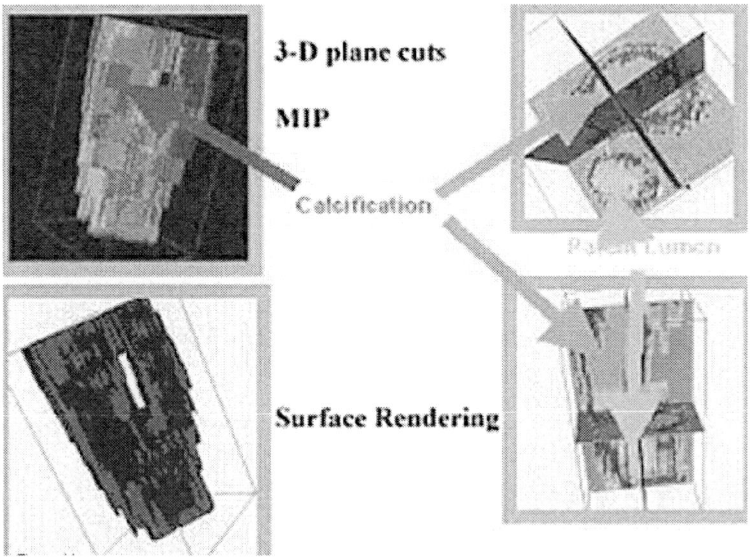

Figure 11. Continuous 3D display of in vivo carotid artery endarterectomy sample shows the 3D reconstructed MIP images (left on top); 3D plane cut to show calcification in transverse plane (right on top); surface rendering in 3D box (left at bottom); and 3D plane cut to show calcification in longitudinal plane (right on bottom). The 3D display enhances the possibility of shape analysis.

Deformable Models and SNAKES for Wall Thickness Segmentation

Deformable parametric models of contours of outer and inner walls generated automated wall thickness curves at different levels of carotid artery (see Figure 12). The SNAKES as contours were pixel transformations at different angle. The semi-automated method of delineation in contiguous image slices may be summed up to measure total plaque burden (see Figure 13). The measurement accuracy of outer and inner wall is demonstrated in in vivo MRI image (see Figure 14).

Evaluation of Segmentation

Deformable models extracted out the carotid plaque boundaries from MRI images and generated parametric curve and parametric surface by object delineation (plaque and lumen size) and bifurcation landmark as surrogate marker. Object recognition was accomplished by distinct T1, T2 and proton density signal intensities of plaque features and clear edges of carotid vessel wall.

Color-coded Feature Maps

Non-parametric trained data sets of feature maps showed the measurable lumen size and wall thickness at various transverse image sections. These could be used as indicators of tissue composition (see Figure 14).

Plaque Voluming

Outer and inner radii and size of plaque rich segment, volume of plaque from *in vivo* MR images was measured. However, other method of plaque volumetry used by summing up of all plaques areas in every contiguous image slice (see Figure 10).

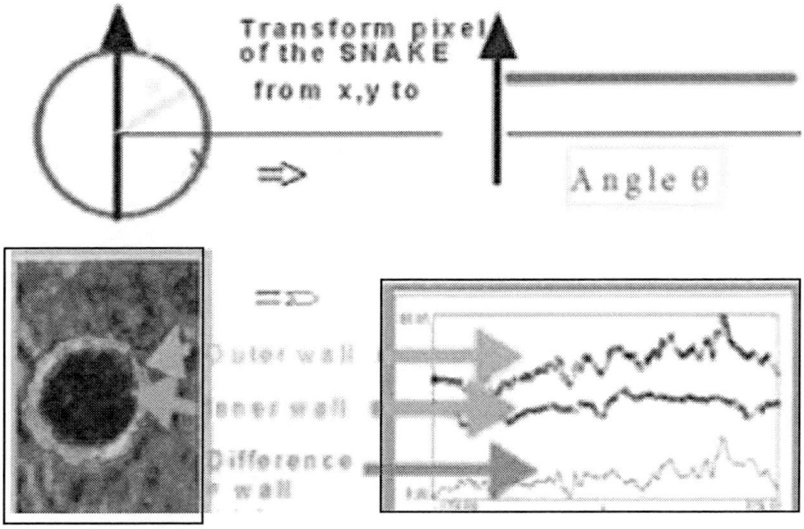

Figure 12. Deformable model and SNAKES parametric method shows the contours on outer and inner walls to measure wall thickness (right panel at bottom). Notice the continuous tracking of outer and inner walls to measure the total wall area in all directions using transformation of pixels in x, y directions.

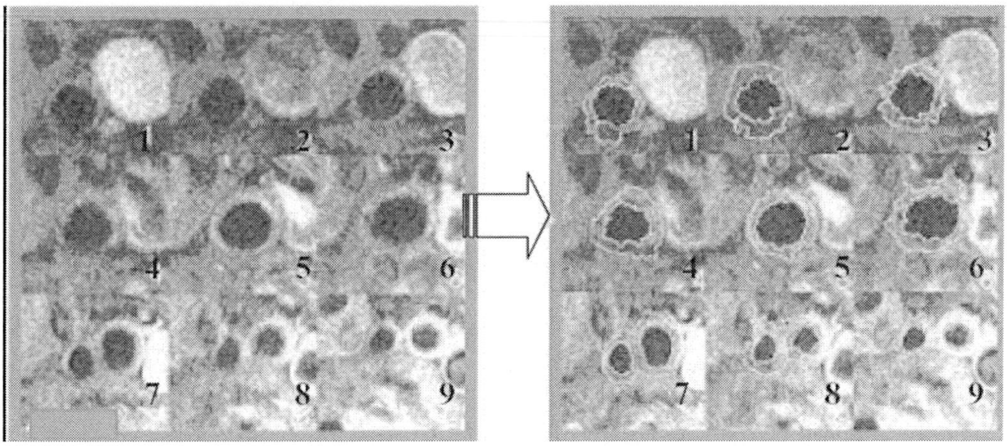

Figure 13. A set of contiguous serial image slices is shown before delineation (left panels). For comparison, a semi-automated delineation segmentation method shows the outer and inner boundaries of carotid walls on *in vivo* contiguous MRI slices of a patient (right panels).

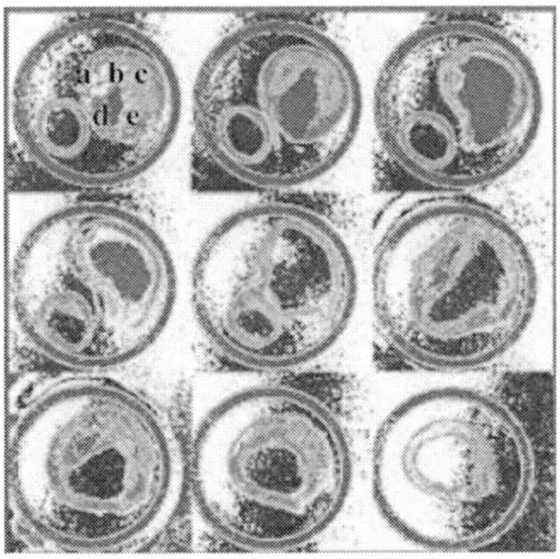

Figure 14. A set of carotid artery endarterectomy specimen in tube is shown as *ex vivo* MRI transverse color-coded post-segmented feature map of an atherosclerosis plaque AHA type III at different levels. Notice that each image set represents distinct plaque constituent with distinct color with wall size and lumen size at each level of increasing 1 mm height of artery. Combining distinct areas (a,b,c,d,e) at different heights may calculate the vascular wall composition as shown distinct colors of different plaque features.

DISCUSSION

Carotid artery atherosclerosis imaging is investigated as important clinical-decision making modality for plaque vulnerability. 3D segmentation techniques are in developing stage but very promising in tissue classification using in vivo MRI methods. 2D/3D time-of-flight FSE or GRE methods are now available for fast vascular imaging. So, segmentation plays crucial role and as challenge due to its several trade-offs. Main emphasis was focused in recent years on dimensionality and quantification of carotid artery morphology features. However, success was limited but encouraging for parametric and non-parametric segmentation on one hand while 3D voluming and surface or volume rendering showed window for time-dependent dynamic angiography applications. Present time interest in plaque constituents and feature analysis at different levels of carotid bifurcation image slices was reported as good indicator of plaque instability and vulnerability [20]. Of specific mention, these images of carotid artery on multicontrast (using T1, T2 and proton density) protocol visualize better segmentation and contrast information on these three image sets. In our previous report, T1/T2/proton density multiparametric approach allowed interactive segmentation by color cluster statistics (as 3D histograms) and tracking stereo display of different tissue constituents [21]. Carotid artery bifurcation is used as a landmark for overall vessel segmentation process. 3D skeleton build-up is important approach as guide map for segmentation. From quantification point of view, center of vessel and *a priori* knowledge of carotid artery is important for segmentation tasks such as artery-vein separation, object extraction. Most of times, image acquisition suffers from partial volume effects, intensity non-uniformities. From quantitative point of view, several following segmentation methods overcome these non-uniformities. Of special mention are following methods: 1.thresholding (shape-based histogram techniques, optimal thresholding either by non-parametric optimal or parametric optimal, Maximum Likelihood methods); Edge-based, border tracing, graph searching, dynamic programming, advanced border detection, Hough transforms, are used. Other methods are: region-based segmentation (region growing, region splitting and merging, connected component labeling) and classification (clustering algorithm-parallelepiped, minimum distance, K-means ISODATA, Fuzzy C-means, Bayes classifiers, Perzan window (by k-NN, Adaptive fuzzy c-means with INU estimation, decision trees, ANN-Feed forward ANN, Kohonen ANN), Contextual classifiers [22]. In this study, the display of three-dimensional angiograms used *a priori* knowledge of quantitative shape features such as tangent and curvature of the centerline of vessels. These could be obtained in previous reports from a curve-like skeleton representation [23]. If connectivity and topology were preserved, and if geometrical constraints such as smoothness and centeredness were satisfied, it was possible to estimate length, orientation, curvature, and torsion (see Figure 2).

An efficient robust method for the identification of such shape components was developed. First, a suitable representation was obtained using a voxel-coding approach to yield connected and labeled unit-thick paths. The desired features were estimated from a smoothed version of the skeleton produced by a moving average filter [24]. Previously, most investigators reported standard fast spin-echo sequences for atherosclerotic plaque distinct MRI signals appearing as darker lipid rich core and lighter fibro-cellular tissue by T2-weighted sequences [9-10]. These factors were highlighted in this study showing further the need of T1-weighting using frequency selective sequences with very short TE for achieving good contrast between atheroma and fibrous tissue. In recent studies, monitoring of progression or regression of atherosclerotic lesions of carotid aorta and lumen stenosis or wall thickening in serial images and use of 2-D/3-D fast spin-echo proton density weighted images improved the contrast–to-noise ratio and discriminated lumen, peri-adventitial fat and plaque. Common carotid intima-media thickness and atherosclerotic lipid-rich plaque characterization at carotid bifurcation served as unique indicators of generalized atherosclerosis. Other approach of enhancing in-plane resolution was based upon using short TE, T2 weighting MR imaging to define better plaque region by Morrisett et al. [11]. In that study, intravascular T2-weighted imaging generated better MR contrast resolution. It served well by placing phased array coils closer to carotid artery wall using short TE for 'high spatial resolution' weighted images. The present report supports previous multicontrast approach of selection (T1/ T2 and proton density weighted MRM) to acquire maximum signal-to-noise ratio (SNR) for better segmentation of plaque components in 1 mm thick MRM slice. Differentiation of plaque components by T2 contrast resolution at 9.4 T generates discriminated plaque structural components after segmentation to distinguish calcification, fibrous, collagen, elastin, hemorrhage, crystalline cholesterol, other lipids based upon different MR signal intensities due to their MR visible distinct proton species. Atheroma and fibrous cap in plaque images are generally considered to represent plaque instability and generate optimized contrast by selecting TE and TR values [11]. Parametric imaging of segmentation and quantification of plaque components based on their TE and TR values could be accomplished with high degree of sensitivity and specificity on T1 parametric and T2 parametric segmentation. T1 parametric segmentation was better for vessel geometry and T2 parametric segmentation was better for classification. These values appear to provide information of noninvasive in vivo application of MRI criteria. Specifically, T2 values micro dissected necrotic core at different sets of TE values, overcome the problem of observed darker T2 images than actual low signal of plaque thrombus and fibrous components. T1 weighted images provide less information than T2 weighted images or proton density weighted images. So, it needs appropriate TE and

TR choice for in vivo microimaging application. In supervised semiautomatic parametric segmentation generated color-coded feature maps for each plaque features that measures the composition of plaque. Interestingly, stacked image slices and the inclusion of T1 based images, as a third input, produced significant improvement in the delineation and curvatures of carotid vessel wall and it supports earlier reports [25, 26]. Volumetric segmentation techniques visualize 3D to 2D projections such as object-based approach to reconstruct the artery but less known and future hope [27-33]. However, these help to calculate the plaque size quantification directly from MRI image by iterative dilatation approach by starting distal artery end traveling in proximal direction along the center of vessels, determining the lumen boundaries [18]. 3D reconstruction and surface and volume rendering techniques promise for cross-sectional multislice axial, coronal and sagittal comparisons and a future hope of 3D registration of multi-session studies for drug or therapy monitoring [12, 20, 21, 27, 28-33]. The present study has limitations due to its preliminary evidence to demonstrate the possibilities of less known robust segmentation power of different algorithms to be applied in clinical studies. Segmented images, however, evaluated the wall thickness, lumen size, plaque volumes, diagnosis, location of pathology, vascular anatomical structure, treatment planning, partial volume correction of vascular dynamic imaging data, and computer integrated endarterectomy surgical procedure.

Conclusion

Segmentation algorithms may be applied to in vivo MRI images of carotid artery vessels to estimate carotid artery atherosclerosis plaque burden and its feature identification. Segmented images can be used in femoral and other major vessels to evaluate the risk of atherosclerosis.

References

[1] Naghavi M, Libby P, Falk E, et al. From vulnerable plaque to vulnerable patient: a call for new definations and risk assessment strategies: *Part I. Circulation.* 2003; 108(14): 1764-72.

[2] Glagov S., Bassiouny HS, Masawa N. Sakaguchi, Giddens DP, Zarins CK. *Cerebrovascular Disease*: A Pathologist's View. In Syndromes of Athero-sclerosis: Correlation of Clinical Imaging and Pathology, Ed. Fuster V., Futura Publishing Company Inc. Armonk, NY. 1996, pp 161-180.

[3] Liang Q, Wendelhag I, Wikstrand J, Gustavsson T (2000) A mutiscale dynamic programming procedure for boundary detection in ultrasound carotid artery images *IEEE Trans Med Imaging* 2000: 19(2):127-42.

[4] Chao H, Kerwin WS, Hatsukami TS, Hwang JN, Yuan C. Dynamic contours: Detecting objects in image sequences using rule based control in an active contour model. *IEEE Trans Biomed. Eng*. 2003; 50(6):705-10.

[5] Makowski P, Sorensen TS, Therkildsen SV, Materka A, Stodkilde Jorgensen H, Pedersen EM. Twophase active contour method for semiautomatic segmentation of the

heart and blood vessels from MRI images for 3D visualization. *Comput Med Imaging Graph.* 2002;26(1):917.

[6] Pizer SM, Eberly DH, Morse BS, Fritsch DS, Zoom invariant vision of figural shape: The mathematics of cores, "Computer Vision and Image Understanding, 1998; 69: 55-71.

[7] Wink O, Niessen W, Viergever M. Fast quantification of abdominal aortic aneurysms from cta volumes, "in *Medical Image conference and Computer Assisted Interventions*(MICCAI'98), Berlin, pp 138-145, Springer Verlag, 1998.

[8] Ladak HM, Milner JS, Steinman DA. Rapid threedimensional segmentation of the carotid bifurcation from serial MR images. *J. Biomech. Eng.* 2000; 122(1):969.

[9] Troussaint JF, LaMuraglia GM, Southern JF, Fuster V, Kantor HL. Magnetic Resonance Images: lipid, fibrous, calcified, hemorrhagic, and thrombotic components of human atherosclerosis in vivo. *Circulation* 1996; 94(5):932-938.

[10] Shinner M, Fallon JT, Wehrli S. The diagnostic accuracy of ex vivo MRI for human atherosclerotic plaque characterization. *Arteriovascular. Thromb. Vasc. Biol.* 1999; 19: 27562761.

[11] Morrisett J, Vick W,Sharma R, Lawrie G, Readon M, Ezell E, Schwartz J, Hunter G, Gorenstein D. Discrimination of components in atherosclerotic plaques from human carotid endarterectomy specimens by magnetic resonance imaging ex vivo. *Magn. Reson. Imaging* 2003; 21:465-474.

[12] Vinitski S. Gonzalez CF, Knobler R, Andrews D, Iwanaga T, Curtis M. Fast tissue segmentation based on a 4D feature map in characterization of intracranial lesions. *J. magn Reson Imaging*. 1999; 9(6): 768-76.

[13] Beltrame F, Fato M, Raposio E, Sobel I Recent results in color compositing of three parameter magnetic resonance scans as a preoperative aid to the management of upper limb sarcomas. *MAGMA.*1997; 5(4):289-298.

[14] Ishimori Y, Kimura H, Uematsu H, Matsuda T, Itoh H. Dynamic T1 estimation of brain tumors using double echo dynamic MR imaging. *J. Magn. Reson Imaging* 2003; 18(1) 113-120.

[15] Helms G. T2 based segmentation of periventricular paragraph sign volumes of quantification of proton magnetic paragraph sign resonance spectra of multiple sclerosis lesions. *MAGMA* 2003; 16(1): 1016.

[16] Yi D, Hayward V. Skeletonization of volumetric angiograms for display. *Comput Methods Biomech. Biomed. Engineering*. 2002; 5(5):329-41.

[17] Woods RP, Grafton ST, Watson JD, Sicotte NL, Mazziotta JC. "Automated Image Registration": Intersubject validation of linear and nonlinear models, *J. Computer Assisted Tomography*, 1998; 22(1):153-165.

[18] Ashburner J, Friston KJ "Nonlinear spatial normalization basis functions," *Human Brain Mapping*. 1999; 7(4):254-66.

[19] Sharma R. A device for MR imaging of atherosclerosis plaque in carotid endarterectomy specimens ex vivo. *Mag. Res. Med. Sci.* 2002; 1(2):129-136.

[20] Zhang S, Cai J, Luo Y, Han C, Polissar NL, Hatsukami TS, Yuan C. Measurement of carotid wall volume and maximum area with contrastenhanced 3D MR imaging: initial observations. *Radiology*. 2003 Jul;228(1):2005.

[21] Long Q, Ariff B, Zhao SZ, Thom SA, Hughes AD, Xu XY.Reproducibility study of 3D geometrical reconstruction of the human carotid bifurcation from magnetic resonance images. *Magn. Reson. Med.* 2003 Apr;49(4):665-74.

[22] Dawant BM, Zijdenbos AP. Image Segmentation, Chapter 2 in: Hand Book of Medical Imaging Volume 2. *Medical image processing and analysis,* Editors: Sonka M, Fitzpatrick JM 2000, SPIE Press Wash. USA pp 711-28.

[23] Yuan C, Lin E, Millard J, Hwang JN.Closed contour edge detection of blood vessel lumen and outer wall boundaries in black blood MR images. *Magn. Reson. Imaging.* 1999;17(2):257-66.

[24] Goubergrits L, Affeld K, Fernandez-Britto J, Falcon L.Geometry of the human common carotid artery. A vessel cast study of 86 specimens. *Pathol. Res. Pract.* 2002; 198(8):543-51.

[25] Clarke SE, Hammond RR, Mitchell JR, Rutt BK.Quantitative assessment of carotid plaque composition using multicontrast MRI and registered histology. *Magn. Reson. Med.* 2003 Dec;50(6):1199208.

[26] Cai JM, Hatsukami TS, Ferguson MS, Small R, Polissar NL, Yuan C.Classification of human carotid atherosclerotic lesions with in vivo multicontrast magnetic resonance imaging. *Circulation.* 2002; 106(11):1368-73.

[27] Merickel MB, Carman CS, Brookeman JR, Mugler JP 3rd, Brown MF, Ayers CR. Identification and 3D quantification of atherosclerosis using magnetic resonance imaging. *Comput. Biol. Med.* 1988; 18(2):89-102.

[28] Hänni M, Lekka-Banos I, Nilsson S, Häggroth L, Smedby O. Quantitation of atherosclerosis by magnetic resonance imaging and 3-D morphology operators. *Magn Reson Imaging* . 1999;17(4):585-91.

[29] Clarke SE, Hammond RR, Mitchell JR, Rutt BK.Quantitative assessment of carotid plaque composition using multicontrast MRI and registered histology. *Magn Reson Med* . 2003;50(6):1199-208.

[30] Adame IM, van der Geest RJ, Wasserman BA, Mohamed MA, Reiber JH, Lelieveldt BP.Automatic segmentation and plaque characterization in atherosclerotic carotid artery MR images. *MAGMA* . 2004;16(5):227-34.

[31] Yang F, Holzapfel G, Schulze-Bauer C, Stollberger R, Thedens D, Bolinger L, Stolpen A, Sonka M. Segmentation of wall and plaque in in vitro vascular MR images. *Int J Cardiovasc Imaging*. 2003;19(5):419-28.

[32] Auer M, Stollberger R, Regitnig P, Ebner F, Holzapfel GA.3-D reconstruction of tissue components for atherosclerotic human arteries using ex vivo high-resolution MRI. *IEEE Trans Med Imaging* . 2006; 25(3):345-57.

[33] Anderson RW, Stomberg C, Hahm CW, Mani V, Samber DD, Itskovich VV, Valera-Guallar L, Fallon JT, Nedanov PB, Huizenga J, Fayad ZA. Automated classification of atherosclerotic plaque from magnetic resonance images using predictive models. *Biosystems.* 2007;90(2):456-66.

* Author was post doc scientist working with Professor Joel Morrisett for the presented human carotid data in this paper during the year 1999-2000.

In: World Heart Research Yearbook. Volume 1
Editors: Franz Halberg and R. B. Singh
ISBN: 978-1-60741-881-8

LARGER CIRCADIAN AMPLITUDE OF HEART RATE ASSOCIATED WITH ACTIVE PRAYER IN HINDU INDIANS IN ASIA

***Ram B. Singh*[1], *Germaine Cornélissen*[2], *Adarsh Kumar*[3], *Srilakshmi Bathina*[2] *and Franz Halberg*[2*]**

[1]Halberg Hospital and Research Institute, Moradabad, India
[2]Halberg Chronobiology Center, University of Minnesota, Minneapolis, MN, US
[3]Government Medical College (G.M.D. Hospital), Amritsar, India

ABSTRACT

To determine whether praying had any influence on blood pressure (BP) and/or heart rate (HR) variability, these variables were measured around-the-clock for up to 7 days and interpreted in the light of a detailed questionnaire about lifestyle, nutrition and other habits. The circadian amplitude of HR was found to be larger among Hindus who prayed as compared to Hindus who did not pray ($P<0.05$). Longitudinal studies are needed to determine whether active prayer may offer cardiovascular protection, as a decreased HRV has been associated with an elevated risk of coronary artery disease.

INTRODUCTION

An elevated heart rate (HR) has been related to a higher cardiovascular disease risk, notably in men, and to high arterial rigidity in both normotensives and hypertensives [1, 2]. A deficient HR variability (HRV) has also been associated with an increase in the risk of cardiac arrhythmias, unstable angina, myocardial infarction, progression of heart failure and atherosclerosis. Meditation, relaxation techniques, and prayer have all been associated with beneficial effects in terms of cardiovascular health [3]. Few studies, however, relied on automatic around-the-clock measurements of blood pressure (BP) and HR interpreted chronobiologically (time-structurally) [4, 5].

* Address correspondence to: Franz Halberg, MD, Halberg Chronobiology Center, University of Minnesota, MMC 8609. 420 Delaware St. SE, Minneapolis, MN 55455, USA, Tel 612.624.6976 Fax 612.624.9989. E-mail halbe001@umn.edu.

Subjects and Methods

The study involved 209 subjects (142 men and 67 women) 42.4 ± 18.0 years of age living in Moradabad, India. Their BP and HR were measured using the ambulatory monitor TM-2421 from AandD (Tokyo, Japan). Data were collected at 30-minute intervals (with interruptions) for up to 7 days. Information was also recorded for each subject regarding religion (Hindu or Muslim) and praying habits, among other items including food consumption. Each BP and HR data series was analyzed by cosinor [6-8], yielding estimates of the MESOR (M, midline estimating statistic of rhythm, a rhythm-adjusted mean), double circadian amplitude (2A, a measure of the extent of predictable change within a day), and acrophase (ϕ, a measure of the timing of high values recurring each day). Associations between circadian characteristics of BP and HR and praying were sought, using correlation and linear regression analyses.

Results

HRV, gauged by HR-2A, was higher among Hindus who prayed (11.8 beats/min, N=53) as compared to Hindus who did not pray (8.1 beats/min, N=33) (Student t=2.186, P=0.032). A similar difference is observed among Muslims but there were only few Muslims who did not pray in this study. When results are pooled between the two religions, the difference in HR-2A is statistically significantly larger among prayers (11.7 ± 0.7 beats/min, N=113) than among non-prayers (8.5 ± 0.9 beats/min, N=40) (t=2.411, P=0.017), Figure 1. A similar result applies to the standard deviation (SD) of HR (14.7 ± 0.4 vs. 13.8 ± 0.7 beats/min), but statistical significance is not reached in this case (P=0.230).

Discussion and Conclusion

Unexpectedly, important negative results were reported in a study of the effects of intercessory (passive) prayer in behalf of cardiac bypass patients [9]. Patients from 6 US hospitals were randomly assigned to one of three groups; patients in two groups were or were not prayed for after being informed that they might or might not be prayed for, whereas patients in the third group were certain that they would be prayed for. While no difference in complications within 30 days of the surgery was observed between the first two groups, among patients who were prayed for, there were 7% more complications in patients certain to receive intercessory prayer [9]. The present study focused, however, on active rather than passive prayer.

Other studies have reported an increase in HRV associated with meditation. In particular, one study concluded that endeavors such as yoga mantras that involve breathing at six breaths per minute induce favorable psychological and possibly physiological effects, associated notably with an increase in baroreflex sensitivity [10]. Work at the Institute of HeartMath in Boulder Creek, California, determined that the rhythmic pattern of heart activity is associated with the subjective activation of distinct emotional states [11]. More specifically, HRV is viewed as a measure of neurocardiac function that reflects heart-brain interactions and the autonomic nervous system dynamics. Patterns associated with similar amounts of HRV can differ depending on emotions, being erratic in the presence of negative emotions such as anger or frustration, or "coherent" (in the sense of being synchronized at a frequency of about one cycle in 10 s) in the presence of positive emotions such as appreciation [11].

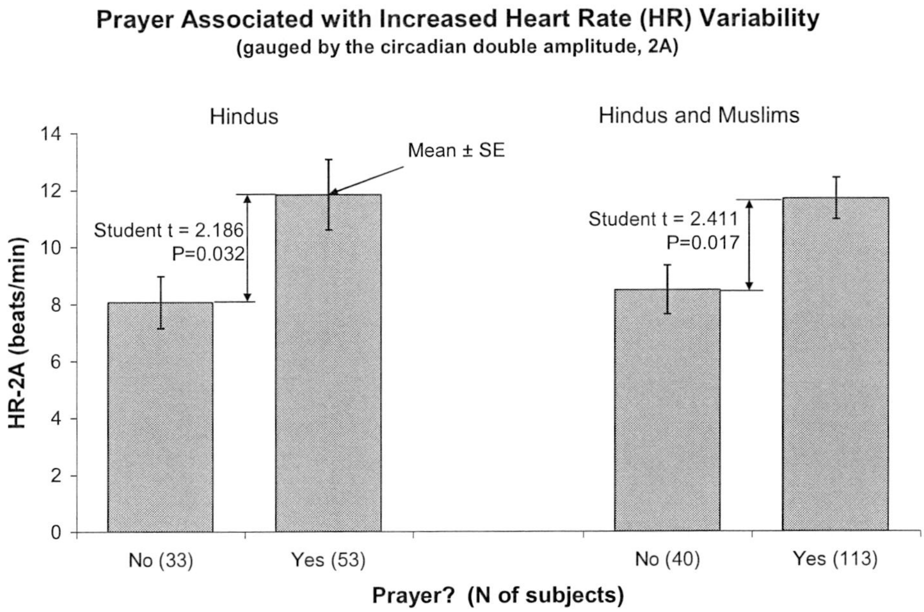

Figure 1. The circadian HR-2A in up to 7-day-long records is a measure of HR variability over a span longer than usual. In this study, it detects an effect based on a sinusoidal waveform in noisy data. (The overall variation is usually estimated by the SD, which in the case of HR was found to be a more sensitive gauge of cardiovascular disease risk than HR-2A. Statistical significance, however, was not reached for HR-SD [P=0.230], even if, like HR-2A, it was larger among prayers than among non-prayers.) Methodologically noteworthy is the need to distinguish HR-2A from HR-SD in assessing HR variability. © Halberg.

The results herein are based on a transverse rather than longitudinal design, the effect of prayer being assessed on a population basis rather than separately for each subject before, during and after praying. The variance used for testing is thereby inflated, notably since the study included patients with heart disease and clinically healthy subjects. The fact that a difference in circadian HR-2A is detected nonetheless suggests that the effect of prayer is rather strong.

REFERENCES

[1] Gupta M, Singh N, Verma S. South Asians and cardiovascular risk: what clinicians should know. *Circulation* 2006; 113: e924-e929.

[2] Dyer AR, Persky V, Stamler J. Oglesby P, Shekelle RB, Berkson DM, Lepper M, Schoenberger JA, Lindberg HA. Heart rate as a prognostic factor for coronary heart disease and mortality: findings in three Chicago epidemiologic studies. *Am. J. Epidemiol.* 1980; 112: 736-749.

[3] Paul-Labrador M, Polk D, Dwyer JH, Velasquez I, Nidich S, Rainforth M, Schneider R, Bairey Merz N. Effects of a randomized controlled trial of transcendental meditation on components of the metabolic syndrome in subjects with coronary heart disease. *Arch. Intern. Med.* 2006; 166: 1218-1224.

[4] Cornélissen G, Halberg F, Otsuka K, Singh RB, Chen CH. Chronobiology predicts actual and proxy outcomes when dipping fails. *Hypertension* 2007; 49: 237-239.

[5] Halberg F, Cornélissen G, Halberg J, Schwartzkopff O. Pre-hypertensive and other variabilities also await treatment. *Am. J. Medicine* 2007; 120: e19-e20.

[6] Halberg F. Chronobiology: methodological problems. *Acta. Med. Rom.* 1980; 18: 399-440.

[7] Cornélissen G, Halberg F. Chronomedicine. In: Armitage P, Colton T (eds). *Encyclopedia of Biostatistics,* 2nd ed. Chichester, UK: John Wiley and Sons Ltd; 2005. p. 796-812.

[8] Refinetti R, Cornélissen G, Halberg F. Procedures for numerical analysis of circadian rhythms. *Biological Rhythm Research* 2007; 38: 275-325.

[9] Benson H, Dusek JA, Sherwood JB, Lam P, Bethea CF, Carpenter W, Levitsky S, Hill PC, Clem DW, Jain MK, Drumel D, Kopecky SL, Mueller PS, Marek D, Rollins S, Hibberd PL. Study of the Therapeutic Effects of Intercessory Prayer (STEP) in cardiac bypass patients: A multicenter randomized trial of uncertainty and certainty of receiving intercessory prayer. *Am. Heart J.* 2006; 151: 934-942.

[10] Bernardi L, Sleight P, Bandinelli G, Cencetti S, Fattorini L, Wdowczyc-Szulc J, Lagi A. Effect of rosary prayer and yoga mantras on autonomic cardiovascular rhythms: comparative study. BMJ 2001; 323: 1446-1449.

[11] McCraty R, Atkinson M, Tomasino D, Bradley RT. The coherent heart. *Heart-brain interactions, psychophysiological coherence, and the emergence of system-wide order.* Institute of HeartMath, California, 2006.

Support: US Public Health Service (GM-13981; FH), University of Minnesota Supercomputing Institute (GC, FH)

In: World Heart Research Yearbook. Volume 1
Editors: Franz Halberg and R. B. Singh
ISBN: 978-1-60741-881-8

SEPARATE CARDIOVASCULAR DISEASE RISKS: CIRCADIAN HYPER-AMPLITUDE-TENSION (CHAT) AND AN ELEVATED PULSE PRESSURE

***Germaine Cornélissen*[*,1], *Franz Halberg*[1], *Kuniaki Otsuka*[2] *and Ram B. Singh*[3]**
[1] University of Minnesota, Minneapolis, MN, US
[2] Tokyo Women's Medical University, Tokyo, Japan
[3] Halberg Hospital and Research Institute, Moradabad, India

ABSTRACT

Prospective data from 297 patients, interpreted in the context of outcomes on >2,750 patients providing >140,000 measurements, assess relative risks (RR) of elevated pulse pressure (EPP), diastolic CHAT, and decreased heart rate variability (DHRV), singly or combined. Cardiovascular morbidity assessed every 6 months for 6 years is increased in association with each risk factor. Risk is higher when EPP and D-CHAT coexist or when all three conditions are present than when D-CHAT, EPP, or DHRV is present singly. That EPP, D-CHAT and DHRV are to some degree additive deserves further scrutiny on larger samples.

INTRODUCTION

In a 6-year prospective study of 297 patients [1-5], the three highest risk factors among all tested were a pulse pressure (PP) above 60 mmHg, a circadian amplitude (A) of diastolic blood pressure (BP) above the upper 95% prediction limit for clinically healthy subjects matched by gender and age (CHAT), and a decreased heart rate variability (DHRV), gauged by the 48-hour standard deviation (SD) of heart rate (HR) in the lowest 7th percentile. CHAT and DHRV were found to constitute separate and additive risks [6]. CHAT was found to be associated with a statistically significant increase in risk, notably of cerebral ischemic events and nephropathy, even in the absence of an elevated blood pressure MESOR (*midline estimate statistic of rhythm,* a rhythm-adjusted mean value, or rather a mean value adjusted for a broad time structure or chronome) [4].

* Address for correspondence: Germaine Cornélissen, Halberg Chronobiology Center, University of Minnesota, MMC 8609. 420 Delaware Street SE. Minneapolis, MN 55455, USA. Tel: 612-624-9989. Fax: 612-624-9989. E-mail: corne001@umn.edu.

By contrast to the linear relation existing between cardiovascular disease risk and the 48-hour mean value of BP, risk relates nonlinearly to the circadian BP-A or to the circadian HR-SD, Figure 1 [7]. The nonlinear relation between risk and indices of variability in BP and HR is found not only in this 6-year prospective study of 297 patients, but also in another independent study of over 1,000 patients also contributing an estimate of left ventricular mass index, used as surrogate outcome measure, Figure 2 [7]. Risk increases only when the circadian BP-A exceeds the upper 95% prediction limit for this parameter, which is derived from data on clinically healthy subjects matched by gender and age, or when the HR-SD drops below a critical level, also determined from archives obtained in clinical health.

In order to diagnose the presence of CHAT, around the clock monitoring of BP is needed, preferably for a week or longer when abnormality is found, to accommodate large day-to-day changes in circadian rhythm characteristics seen in some people. By comparison, a reliable assessment of an elevated PP may perhaps be achieved with less extensive monitoring since its circadian variation is less prominent [8]. An estimate of HRV could also be obtained without the need for an arm cuff, which many subjects find uncomfortable and/or embarrassing. If the cardiovascular disease risk associated with CHAT would overlap that associated with an elevated PP or a decreased HRV, it might be possible to dispense with or reduce the required duration of the monitoring. In order to address this question, the data from the 6-year prospective study on 297 patients are re-analyzed, focusing on the relative risk of the three risk factors present alone or in combination.

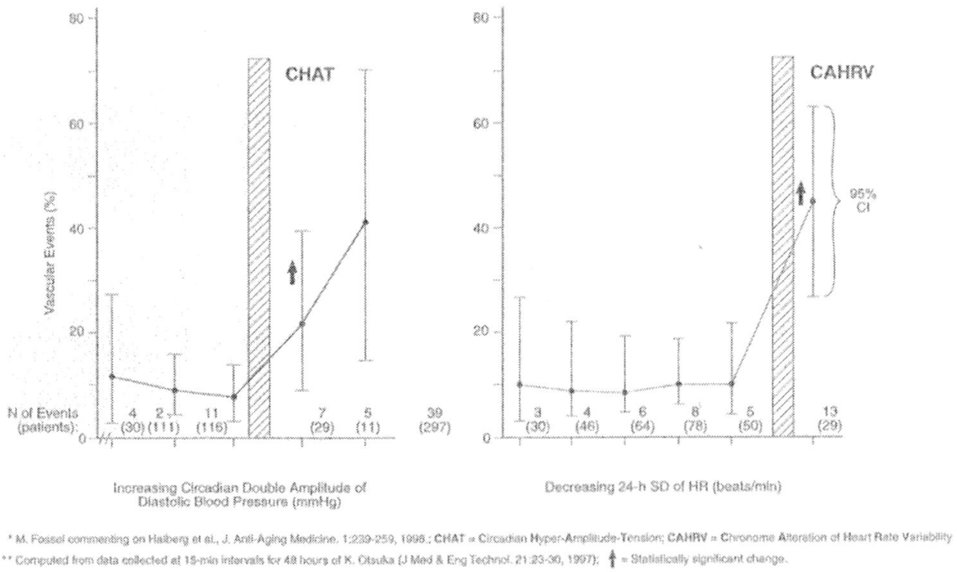

Figure 1. Risk of morbid event as a function of increasing circadian DBP-A (left) and decreasing (HR-SD) based on 48-hour profile (right). Data are provided by 297 patients in a 6-year prospective study in Tokyo, Japan. The relationship is nonlinear in each case. For a wide range of DBP-A or HR-SD values there is no change in morbidity incidence. Risk increases sharply, however, when the DBP-A increases above a threshold or when the HR-SD decreases below a critical value, as ascertained by chi-square test (shown by arrow when difference in percent morbidity is statistically significantly elevated). Thresholds can be determined from archives of BP and HR profiles from clinically healthy subjects classified by gender and age. © Halberg.

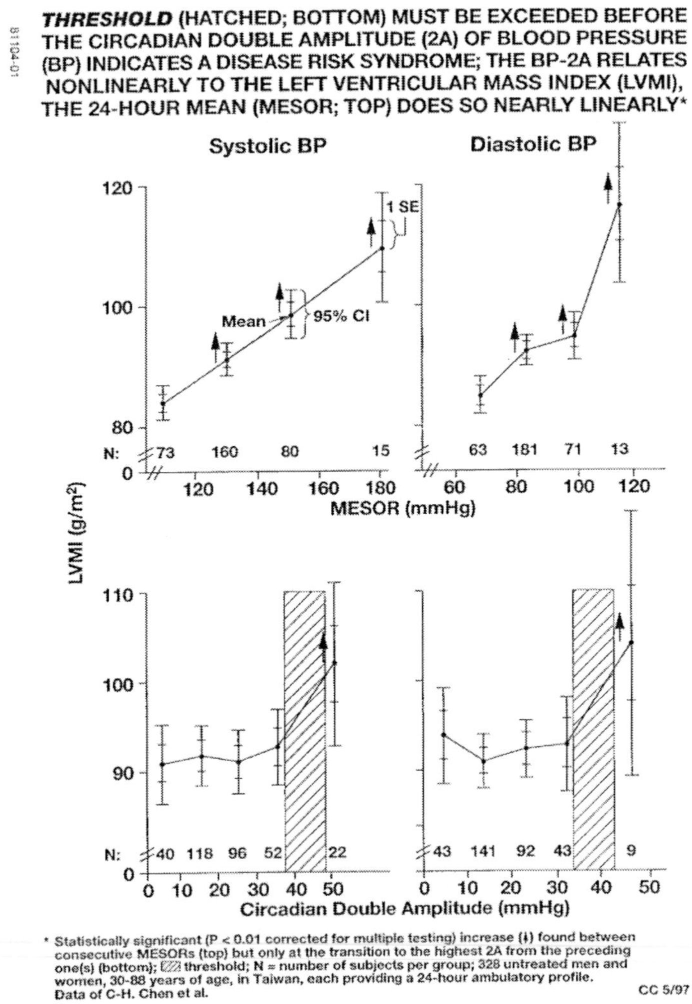

Figure 2. Confirmation of the nonlinear relation of cardiovascular disease risk as a function of the circadian SBP-2A (bottom left) and DBP-2A (bottom right). Risk is gauged by the left ventricular mass index (LVMI), used as a surrogate outcome measure, available for each of the 328 untreated men and women in this study in Taiwan. For comparison, risk (LVMI) steadily increases as a function of the 24-hour average BP-MESOR (top). © Halberg.

SUBJECTS AND METHODS

From October 1987 to September 1988, 145 women and 152 men 30-72 years of age entered the study, which took place in Tokyo, Japan. There were 121 MESOR-normotensive subjects and 176 treated MESOR-hypertensive patients. None of the volunteers had complications such as diabetes mellitus. At the start of study, BP and HR were automatically measured around the clock at 15-min intervals for 48 hours with an ambulatory monitor from Colin Medical Instrument (Komaki, Japan). The incidence of coronary artery disease, cerebral ischemic events, nephropathy, and retinopathy was assessed in 6-monthly follow-ups over 6 years, from October 1987 to September 1993.

Each data series was analyzed by single cosinor, which consists of fitting by least squares a 24-hour cosine curve to the data [9, 10]. Estimates were thus obtained for the MESOR (M), the double amplitude (2A), a measure of the extent of predictable change within a day, and the acrophase (ϕ), a measure of the timing of overall high values recurring each day. The 48-hour SD of HR was also computed. The PP was calculated as the difference between the MESORs of systolic (S) and diastolic (D) BP.

Patients with a circadian DBP-A above the previously established upper 95% prediction limit of gender- and age-matched healthy peers were diagnosed as having diastolic CHAT (D-CHAT). A PP above 60 mmHg was defined as being excessive (EPP). A 48-hour HR-SD below the lowest 7th percentile characterized a decreased HR variability (DHRV). After 6 years of follow-up, the incidences of angina pectoris (with coronary artery disease), ischemic stroke (including transient ischemic attack), nephropathy (with proteinuria and an increase in serum creatinine above 1.0 mg/dL) and retinopathy (with retinal bleeding) were assessed. All events were cumulated to distinguish between patients presenting without or with such morbid events after 6 years. The relative risk (and 95% confidence interval, CI) of subjects with D-CHAT, EPP, or DHRV singly or in combination was computed by comparison with subjects not presenting with any of the three risk factors under investigation herein [11]. Linear regression analyses were also applied to examine whether there was any association among the circadian parameters (DBP-A, PP, and HR-SD).

RESULTS

Risk is invariably increased in association with each risk factor, Table 1.

Risk is further increased when EPP and D-CHAT coexist, by comparison to D-CHAT or EPP alone. The presence of all three risk factors also raises the relative risk by comparison to each risk factor present alone, Table 1. The results are presented in Figure 3.

In the reference population of 214 patients presenting none of the three risk factors, morbidity was found in 8 cases (3.7%) (Figure 3, top left). The presence of DRHV or EPP alone raises the incidence of morbidity to 30.8% (Figure 3, top middle). When these two risks are both present, morbidity is doubled (66.7%) (Figure 3, top right). The presence of CHAT (Figure 3, bottom) invariably increases the incidence of morbidity, from 3.7% to 23.5% in the absence of the other two risk factors (Figure 3, bottom left), from 30.8% to 50% or 100% when either DHRV or EPP is also present (Figure 3, bottom middle), or from 66.7% to 100% when all three risk factors are present (Figure 3, bottom right).

No correlation is found between PP and DBP-A ($r = 0.08$; $P = 0.18$) or between HR-SD and DBP-A ($r = 0.06$; $P = 0.29$). A weak linear relation is found, however, between PP and HR-SD ($r = -0.27$; $P < 0.001$).

Further tests by analysis of variance of patients subdivided by two of the three risk factors indicate that PP is elevated among patients with both D-CHAT and DHRV ($F=2.91$; $P=0.035$) and that HR-SD is decreased among patients with EPP ($F=7.11$; $P<0.001$). No difference in BP-A is found, however, among patients classified by PP and HR-SD ($F=0.64$; $P=0.59$).

Table 1. Relative Risk (RR) and 95% Confidence Interval (CI) of Diastolic Circadian Hyper-Amplitude-Tension (D-CHAT), Decreased Heart Rate Variability (DHRV), and Excessive Pulse Pressure (EPP), Alone or in Combination*

Group 1: Reference (N_1)	Group 2: Test (N_2)	RR	[95%	CI]
Risk?	Risk?			
None (214)	D-CHAT (17)	6.294	[2.108;	18.794]
None (214)	DHRV (13)	8.231	[2.847;	23.797]
None (214)	EPP (39)	8.231	[3.600;	18.819]
None (214)	D-CHAT & DHRV (2)	13.375	[2.857;	62.621]
None (214)	D-CHAT & EPP (3)	26.750	[13.554;	52.795]
None (214)	DHRV & EPP (6)	17.833	[7.364;	43.189]
None (214)	D-CHAT & DHRV & EPP (3)	26.750	[13.554;	52.795]
D-CHAT (17)	D-CHAT & DHRV (2)	*2.125*	*[0.417;*	*10.840]*
D-CHAT (17)	D-CHAT & EPP (3)	4.250	[1.804;	10.013]
D-CHAT (17)	D-CHAT & DHRV & EPP (3)	4.250	[1.804;	10.013]
DHRV (13)	DHRV & D-CHAT (2)	*1.625*	*[0.325;*	*8.113]*
DHRV (13)	DHRV & EPP (6)	*2.167*	*[0.803;*	*5.846]*
DHRV (13)	D-CHAT & DHRV & EPP (3)	3.250	[1.438;	7.345]
EPP (39)	EPP & D-CHAT (3)	3.250	[2.030;	5.204]
EPP (39)	EPP & DHRV (6)	2.167	[1.038;	4.523]
EPP (39)	D-CHAT & DHRV & EPP (3)	3.250	[2.030;	5.204]

*Assessed in population of 297 patients, among whom 39 had a morbid event during the following 6 years. RR is computed as ratio of incidence of morbid event in Group 2 versus that of Group 1. A 95% CI not overlapping 1 indicates statistically significant increase in risk in Group 2 versus Group 1. D-CHAT is defined as circadian DBP-A above the upper 95% prediction limit of clinically healthy peers matched by gender and age; DHRV is defined as 48-hour HR-SD in the lowest 7th percentile of distribution; EPP is defined as a pulse pressure (SBP-M – DBP-M) above 60 mm Hg, where M (MESOR) is a chronome-adjusted mean value.

DISCUSSION

The question is often raised whether too small a circadian BP-A may also constitute a risk factor. 'Non-dipping' has been defined as a day-night ratio less than 10% [12]. This condition has been associated with an increase in cardiovascular disease risk in some patient populations [12]. As shown in Figure 4, 'non-dipping' only increases the risk of women and not that of men in the present study. Even in women, the risk associated with 'non-dipping' is much less than that of CHAT.

Moreover, it should be noted that diabetes mellitus was an exclusion factor in the present study. Some patients with non-insulin-dependent diabetes mellitus (NIDDM) develop circadian 'ecphasia', that is their circadian BP-ϕ occurs by night instead of in the afternoon, whereas their circadian HR- ϕ is unaltered [13]. There is evidence suggesting that ecphasia is found among NIDDM patients with an impaired autonomic nervous system, who also have a decreased HRV [14]. The day-night ratio of such patients would be less than 10% in view of the ecphasia rather than due to reduced circadian amplitude.

When patients in an independent study are classified by their day-night ratio in three rather than two classes, further distinguishing between a day-night ratio that is small but positive (between 0 and 10%) and one that is negative, the risk elevation is seen only for the latter group [15], Table 2. This result suggests that the risk associated with 'non-dipping' may relate in part to ecphasia rather than a reduced circadian variation. Reliance on the relatively simple computation of a circadian amplitude and acrophase may thus be preferred to the use of the day-night ratio. The latter is often not adjusted to the subject's own rest-activity schedule, and also ignores any phase shift in the usual circadian BP pattern as well as changes in the circadian BP waveform as a function of age.

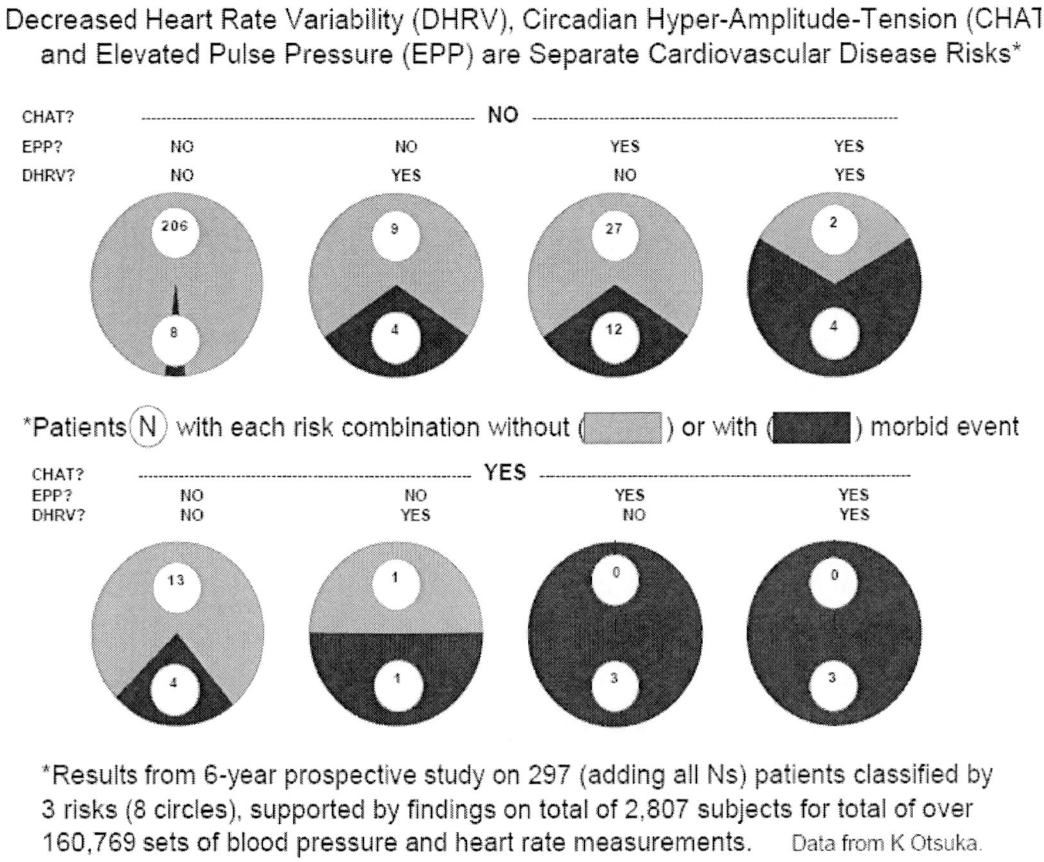

Figure 3. Incidence of morbid events in population of 297 patients followed-up prospectively for 6 years is assessed in relation to risk factors involving the variability in BP and HR. The three conditions considered are diastolic CHAT (circadian DBP-A above the upper 95% prediction limit for clinically healthy subjects), decreased HR variability (48-hour HR-SD in the lowest 7th percentile), and an elevated PP (difference in SBP-M and DBP-M above 60 mmHg). As compared to the reference population (patients with none of the three conditions), each risk factor is associated with a statistically significant increase in risk (incidence of morbidity within 6 years of monitoring). Moreover, risk is further statistically significantly increased when two or all three conditions are present concomitantly (see Table 1 for relative risks and the corresponding 95% confidence intervals, indicating statistical significance when the latter do not overlap one, representing equal risk). © Halberg.

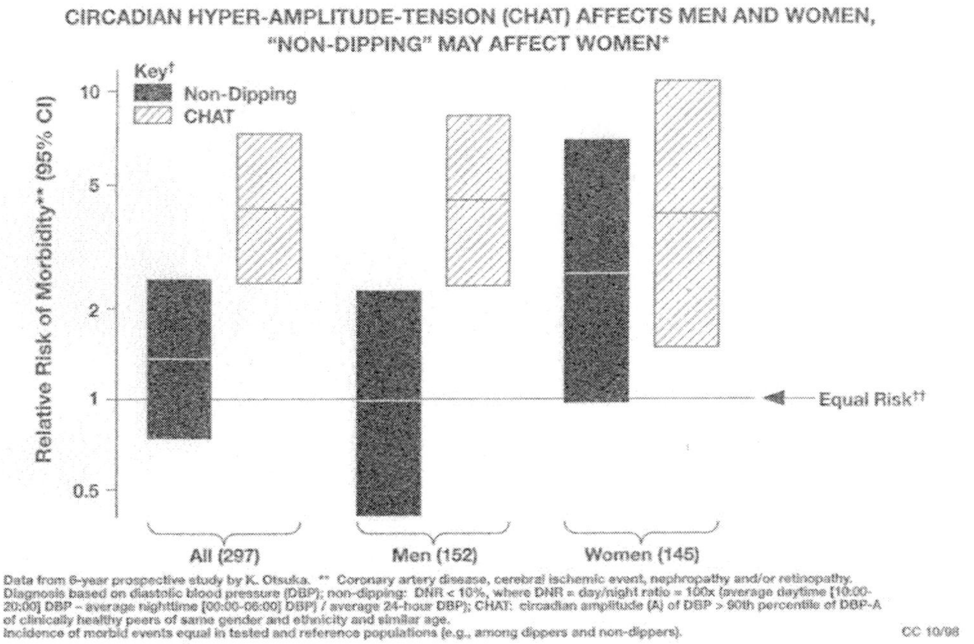

Figure 4. The relative risk (RR) of morbidity occurring within 6 years of monitoring of 297 patients in Tokyo, Japan, associated with diastolic CHAT is statistically significant for men and women, as well as overall, as evidenced by the 95% confidence intervals of RR values not overlapping one (equal risk). By contrast, the relative risk associated with 'non-dipping' (day-night ratio less than 10%) is only marginally elevated, and only so for women and not for men. © Halberg.

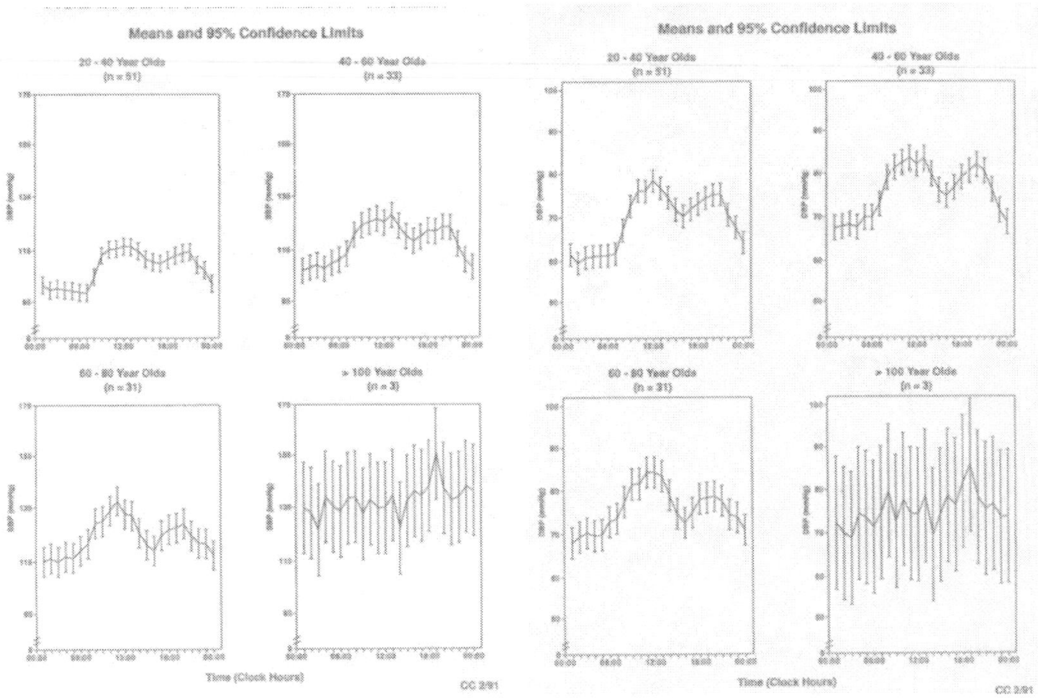

Figure 5. (Continued).

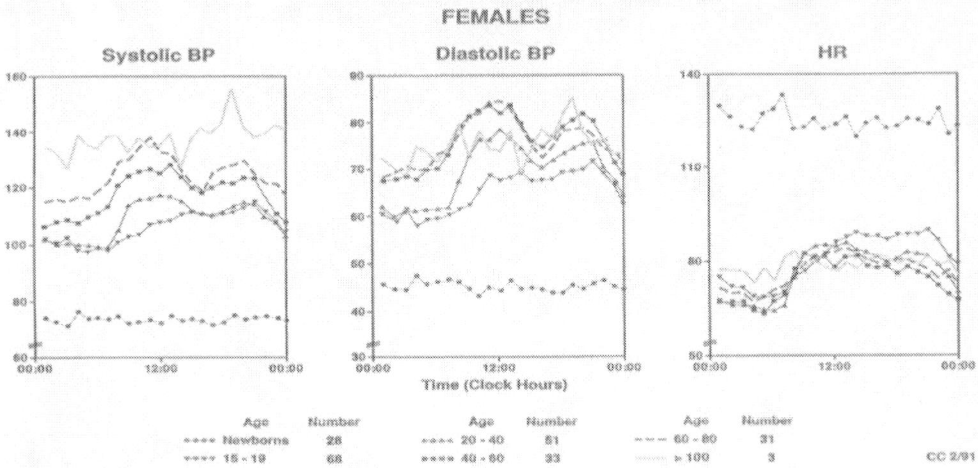

Figure 5. Changes as a function of age in the circadian waveform of SBP (top left) and DBP (top right) of Caucasian women classified in four age groups. Changes in the circadian waveform from womb to tomb shown for SBP, DBP, and HR (bottom). © Halberg.

This includes a more pronounced post-prandial dip resulting in a reduced day-night ratio in older individuals, Figure 5.

The results presented herein strongly suggest the desirability to routinely assess BP variability in addition to HR variability. Indeed, except for a weak relation between PP and the HR-SD, the three risk factors considered herein are mostly separate and additive. The diagnosis of CHAT is also important for MESOR-normotensive subjects, who also are at an increased cardiovascular disease risk [1-5]. Once diagnosed, CHAT can be successfully treated [16-18]. Whereas the number of morbid events and the number of patients in this study are small, the results are supported by several other prospective and retrospective chronobiological investigations by us (Table 3) as well as others [19].

Table 2. CHAT (circadian hyper-amplitude-tension) rather than 'non-dipping' is associated with an increase in left ventricular mass index (LVMI) An elevated LVMI is observed only in subjects showing a reversal of their circadian blood pressure variation (DNR<0), and is statistically significant only for women*

LVMI (g/m2): Mean ± SE

Variable	Gender		CHAT			DNR	(%)	
		No	Yes	P	>10	0-10	<0	P
SBP	Men	89.0±0.8	99.4±4.2	0.016	88.4±1.1	89.4±1.2	93.7±3.3	0.140
DBP	Men	89.1±0.8	94.1±3.8	0.189	89.0±1.0	90.0±1.5	89.5±3.1	0.883
SBP	Women	87.2±0.9	100.0±3.2	<0.001	88.5±1.3	85.2±1.2	94.6±2.5	0.001
DBP	Women	87.0±0.9	100.8±3.3	<0.001	87.7±1.1	86.0±1.4	94.0±2.6	0.018

Results from Student t-test (CHAT) or one-way analysis of variance (DNR) comparing all three groups: the LVMI of women with a (SBP or DBP) DNR < 0 is larger than that of women with a DNR > 10% or a positive DNR < 10% (P<0.05), whereas no difference is seen between positive DNR values less than or greater than 10% (P>0.05). By contrast, the LVMI of men with a negative DNR of SBP is only slightly larger than that of dippers (P=0.057). DNR: Day-night ratio ('non-dipping' is defined as DNR < 10%). SBP: Systolic Blood Pressure; DBP: Diastolic Blood Pressure.

Table 3. Outcomes of chronobiological screens of blood pressure and heart rate*

N of patients (ref)	N at follow-up	Sampling	N measurements: Total (outcomes)	Finding
10 (1)	10 (up to 5 years)	5/day daily	Up to 9,125 (only partially analyzed)	Among P. Scarpelli's patients, the 4 who died with malignant hypertension had a larger circadian BP amplitude than the 6 who were still alive (SBP: t=1.84; P=0.103; DBP: t=2.99; P=0.017)
63 (2, 3)	21 after 28 years	~q4h for 2 days	756 (252)	9 of 10 subjects without CHAT are alive while 7 of 11 subjects with CHAT are dead 28 years later (chi-square=6.390; P<0.01)
56 (4)	56: Concomitant LVMI	q15 min for 24 h	5,376 (5,376)	Classification by Y. Kumagai of patients by LVMI (<100; 100-130; >130 g/m^2) reveals elevation of circadian amplitude at LVMI in 100-130 range whereas MESOR elevation occurs only at LVMI >130.
221 (5, 6)	221 (time of delivery)	q1 h/48 h in each trimester of pregnancy (336 profiles)	16,128 (16,128)	In addition to an 8 mm Hg difference in mean value between women who will or will not develop complications (gestational hypertension, preeclampsia) already observed during the first trimester of pregnancy, the occurrence of complications is also associated with BP profiles characterized by an elevated circadian BP amplitude. In particular, one case (JK) of CHAT where warning was not heeded, was followed 8 weeks later by severe pre-eclampsia, premature delivery and 26 months of hospitalization of offspring at a cost of about $1 million
297 (7-12)	297 after 6 years	q15 min for 48 h	57,024 (57,024)	CHAT or a reduced circadian standard deviation of heart rate, or an excessive pulse pressure (>60 mm Hg) are large risk factors (larger than hypertension) for cerebral ischemic events, nephropathy and coronary artery disease, even when the blood pressure is within acceptable limits.
2039 (13-15)	2039 Concomitant LVMI	Hourly averages for 24 h	48,936 (48,936)	LVMI is increased in patients with CHAT, a reduced circadian standard deviation of heart rate, or an elevated pulse pressure. The relation between LVMI and the circadian endpoints is nonlinear.

Table 3. (Continued)

N of patients (ref)	N at follow-up	Sampling	N measurements: Total (outcomes)	Finding
23 (16)	12 after 7 years	q15 min for 9 days	19,872 (10,368)	10 of 20 patients with no consistent BP abnormality are alive and well; 2 of 3 patients with consistent BP abnormality reported an adverse vascular event (P=0.015 by Fisher's Exact Test).
80 (17, 18)	80 Response to treatment administered 2 h before daily BP peak vs. control group treated 3 times a day	q4 h for 24 h before and on treatment	960 (960)	With smaller doses of medications, BP was lowered by R. Zaslavskaya to a larger extent and treatment was accompanied by fewer complications. Treatment: propranolol, clonidine, or alpha-methyldopa ($P<0.05$ for each effect)
18 (19)	18 (12 weeks)	q30 min (≥24h) on 3 regimens	≥2592 (≥2592)	Treating CHAT may prevent adverse vascular events: As compared to placebo, nifedipine (1 mg b.i.d. at 08 & 20) increases and benidipine (4 mg/day at 08) decreases the circadian amplitude of blood pressure. The resulting increase vs. decrease in the incidence of CHAT on nifedipine vs. benidipine may account for the corresponding difference between the number of stroke events of 7.6 vs. 3.5 and the total number of cardiovascular events of 20.4 vs. 8.8 per 1,000 person-years.
Totals:				
2,807	2,754		160,769 (>141,636)	

*SBP and DBP: Systolic and Diastolic blood pressure; HR: heart rate; CHAT: Circadian Hyper-Amplitude-Tension, a condition defined by a circadian amplitude exceeding the upper 95% prediction limit of acceptability (in healthy peers matched by gender and age); LVMI: left ventricular mass index. By comparison with several classical studies, the number of measurements in chronobiological work completed thus far is likely to be larger, and confounding by inter-subject variability smaller (20).

CHAT, as a vascular variability disorder (VVD), can coexist with other VVDs to form a vascular variability syndrome (VVS) that can detect not only pre-hypertension [15] but also pre-diabetes [14, 20].

MESOR-hypertension also constitutes a VVD that is best diagnosed on the basis of 24-hour, or preferably 7-day or longer-span ABPM. It should be realized that treatment of MESOR-hypertension can on occasion result in iatrogenic CHAT, thus putting the patient at a risk higher than MESOR-hypertension itself [1-2, 4-5]. Such a situation can also often be readily remedied by adjusting the timing of treatment administration [16, 17].

REFERENCES

[1] Otsuka K, Cornélissen G, Halberg F. Predictive value of blood pressure dipping and swinging with regard to vascular disease risk. *Clin. Drug Invest.* 1996; 11: 20-31.

[2] Otsuka K, Cornélissen G, Halberg F, Oehlert G. Excessive circadian amplitude of blood pressure increases risk of ischemic stroke and nephropathy. *J. Medical Engineering and Technology* 1997; 21: 23- 30.

[3] Otsuka K, Cornélissen G, Halberg F. Circadian rhythmic fractal scaling of heart rate variability in health and coronary artery disease. *Clinical Cardiology* 1997; 20: 631-638.

[4] Halberg F, Cornélissen G, Halberg J, Fink H Chen C-H., Otsuka K, Watanabe Y, Kumagai Y, Syutkina EV, Kawasaki T, Uezono K, Zhao ZY, Schwartzkopff O. Circadian Hyper-Amplitude-Tension, CHAT: a disease risk syndrome of anti-aging medicine. *J. Anti-Aging Med.* 1998; 1: 239-259.

[5] Cornélissen G, Schwartzkopff O, Halberg F, Otsuka K, Watanabe Y. 7-day ambulatory monitoring for adults with hypertension and diabetes. *Am. J. Kidney Diseases* 2001; 37: 878.

[6] Cornélissen G, Otsuka K, Bakken EE, Halberg F, Siegelova J, Fiser B. CHAT (circadian hyper-amplitude-tension) and CSDD-HR (circadian standard deviation deficit of heart rate): separate, synergistic vascular disease risks? *Scripta medica* 2002; 75: 87-94.

[7] Cornélissen G, Otsuka K, Chen C-H, Kumagai Y, Watanabe Y, Halberg F, Siegelova J, Dusek J. Nonlinear relation of the circadian blood pressure amplitude to cardiovascular disease risk. *Scripta medica* 2000; 73: 85-94.

[8] Halberg F, Drayer JIM, Cornélissen G, Weber MA. Cardiovascular reference data base for recognizing circadian MESOR- and amplitude-hypertension in apparently healthy men. *Chronobiologia* 1984; 11: 275-298.

[9] Halberg F. Chronobiology. *Ann. Rev. Physiol.* 31: 675-725, 1969.

[10] Cornélissen G, Halberg F. Chronomedicine. In: Armitage P, Colton T (eds). Encyclopedia of Biostatistics, 2nd ed. Chichester, UK: John Wiley and Sons Ltd, 2005. p. 796-812.

[11] Agresti A. *Categorical Data Analysis*. John Wiley and Sons, New York, 1990.

[12] Verdecchia P, Schillaci G, Guerrieri M, Gatteschi C, Benemio G, Boldrini F, Porcellati C. Circadian blood pressure changes and left ventricular hypertrophy in essential hypertension. *Circulation* 1990; 81: 528-536.

[13] Nakano S, Ishii T, Kitazawa M, Kigoshi T, Uchida K, Morimoto S. Altered circadian blood pressure rhythm and progression of diabetic nephropathy in non-insulin dependent diabetes mellitus subjects: an average three year follow-up study. *J. Invest Med.* 1996; 44: 247-253.

[14] Sanchez de la Peña S, Gonzalez C, Cornélissen G, Halberg F. Chronomics: time structure (chronome) of blood pressure and heart arte in health and diabetes. Abstract 27, 2nd International Symposium: Workshop on Chronoastrobiology and Chronotherapy, Tokyo Kasei University, Tokyo, Japan, November 17, 2001.

[15] Chen C-H, Cornélissen G, Siegelova J, Halberg F. Does overswinging provide an early warning of cardiovascular disease risk when non-dipping may fail? A meta-analysis of 2039 cases. *Scripta medica* 2001; 74: 75-80.

[16] Halberg F, Cornélissen G, International Womb-to-Tomb Chronome Initiative Group: Resolution from a meeting of the International Society for Research on Civilization Diseases and the Environment (New SIRMCE Confederation), Brussels, Belgium, March 17-18, 1995: Fairy tale or reality? April 1995, 12 pp. text, 18 figures. http://www.msi.umn.edu/~halberg/

[17] Shinagawa M, Kubo Y, Otsuka K, Ohkawa S, Cornélissen G, Halberg F. Impact of circadian amplitude and chronotherapy: relevance to prevention and treatment of stroke. *Biomedicine and Pharmacotherapy* 2001; 55: 125-132.

[18] Watanabe Y, Cornélissen G, Watanabe M, Watanabe F, Otsuka K, Ohkawa S, Kikuchi T, Halberg F. Effects of autogenic training and antihypertensive agents on circadian and circaseptan variation of blood pressure. *Clin. and Exper. Hypertension* 2003; 25: 405-412.

[19] Scarpelli PT, Gallo M, Chiari G. Chronobiology of blood pressure. J of Nephrology 2000; 13: 197-204.

[20] Gupta AK, Greenway FL, Cornélissen G, Pan W, Halberg F. Prediabetes is associated with abnormal circadian blood pressure variability. *J. Human Hypertension 2008* (advance online publication; doi:10.1038/jhh.2008.32).

Support: US Public Health Service (GM-13981; FH), University of Minnesota Supercomputing Institute (GC, FH).

In: World Heart Research Yearbook. Volume 1
Editors: Franz Halberg and R. B. Singh
ISBN: 978-1-60741-881-8

HOME C-ABPM FOR PREVENTIVE AND CURATIVE HEALTH CARE AND TRANSDISCIPLINARY SCIENCE

Franz Halberg*[1], Germaine Cornélissen[1], Kuniaki Otsuka[2], Yoshihiko Watanabe[2], Ram B. Singh[3], Miguel Revilla[4], Salvador Sanchez de la Peña[5], Clicerio Gonzalez[6], Jarmila Siegelova[7], Pavel Homolka[7], Jiri Dusek[7], Michal Zeman[8], R. K. Singh[9], Dana Johnson[1] and Bohumil Fiser[7]

[1] University of Minnesota, Minneapolis, Minnesota, US
[2] Tokyo Women's Medical University, Daini Hospital, Tokyo, Japan
[3] Halberg Hospital and Research Institute, Moradabad, India
[4] University of Valladolid, Valladolid, Spain
[5] Escuela Nacional de Medicina y Homeopatía, IPN Mexico City, Mexico
[6] Centre de Diabetes A.C., Mexico City, Mexico
[7] Masaryk University, Brno, Czech Republic
[8] Comenius University, Bratislava, Slovakia
[9] Chhatrapati Shahuji Maharaj Medical University, Lucknow, India

ABSTRACT

The clinical everyday management of blood pressure (BP) and heart rate (HR) can be greatly improved by the mapping of time structures in home ambulatory BP and HR assessment. Thereby, we change focus from the BP and the HR to the dynamics of these variables. This change is achieved by computer-implemented chronomics, the mapping of chronomes, consisting of cyclicities (our concern herein) along with chaos and trends, in the service of cardiologists, general health care providers, the educated public, and transdisciplinary science. We here further illustrate the yield of chronomics in research on long BP and HR series covering years, some several decades long, and on archives of human sudden cardiac death revealing magnetoperiodisms, e.g., "years" longer than a calendar year, i.e., transyears. In this case of cardiac arrest, what we do not see, the 16- to 20-month transyear is prominent, in the absence of any signature of the calendar year, and so can be a cis-half-year of about 5 months.

* Correpondence: Franz Halberg, Chronobiology Center, University of Minnesota MMC 8609. 420 Delaware Street SE, Minneapolis, Minnesota 55455, USA. Tel. 612-624-6976, Fax. 612-624-9989, Email. halbe001@umn.edu.

BACKGROUND

The resolution of chronomes, Figure 1, and of their inferential statistical endpoints of variability, lifts a curtain of ignorance drawn over the physiological range by concepts such as a "true BP" (Figure 2 left). Chronomics reveal time structures, far beyond the photoperiodisms of the biological day and year (Figure 2 middle).

Magnetoperiodisms around us and their genetically preserved signatures in us abound (Figure 2 right, Figure 3, cf. Figure 1 for the broader picture that emerges with chaos in dense time series – not shown). These provide quantitative new endpoints derived, among others, from a spectrum of rhythms, already much broader than that in Figure 3.

Endpoints of each spectral component, Figures 4a and 4b, serve not only for medical research but can be placed immediately at the service of cardiologists, general health care providers and the educated public.

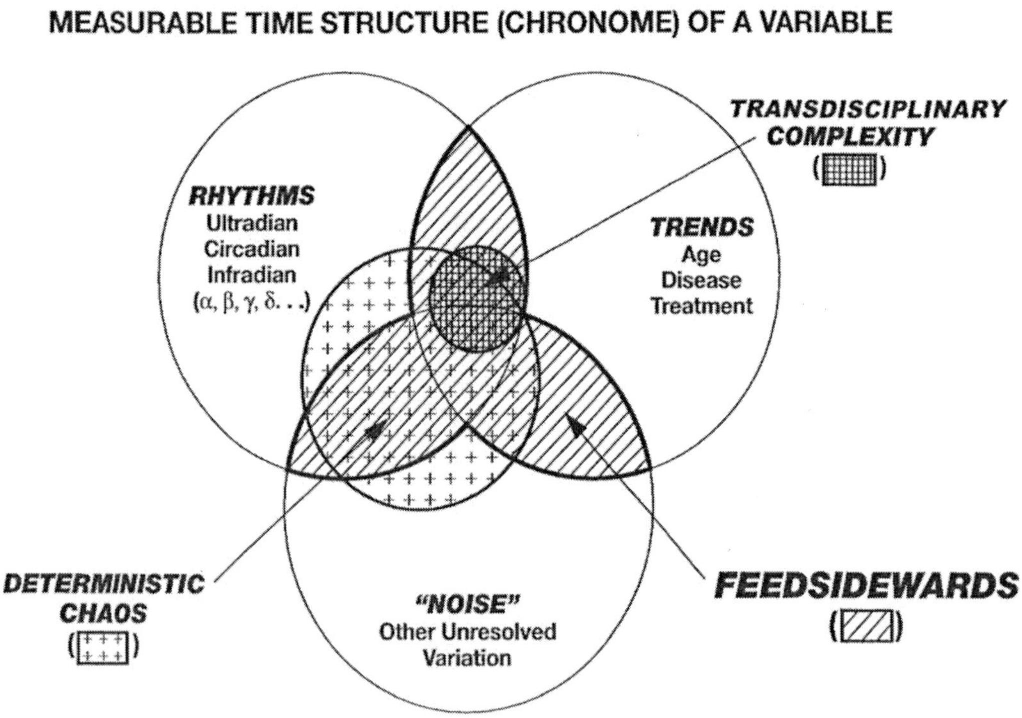

Figure 1. Chronomes consist of multifrequency rhythms and deterministic (or other) chaos, as well as trends in rhythmic and chaotic endpoints. © Halberg.

This is within the scope of chronobiology, the study of mechanisms underlying biological diversity in time, derived from genetics, concerned with diversity in space [1].

Genetics eventually required genomics, the mapping of genomes, while chronobiology led to chronomics [2], the mapping of time structures in us and in our environment, Scheme 1, with focus herein on the chronomics of BP and HR assessment.

Health care based on large randomized clinical trials Variabilities, a formidable foe and confounder when ignored [1], can be computer-resolved into chronomes -- clinically informative time structures [2, 3]. As yet, any ruleful variability is currently largely ignored in countries with resources. There, research on high BP is largely dominated by the pharmaceutical industry and the National Institutes of Health, providing funds for clinical trials and guidelines derived from these trials are used for the public at large (4). At entry into a trial, the BP of very many adults is usually measured without any recording of timing, without any specific consideration of age group or ethnicity, and often ignoring gender even at the most renowned clinics [4]. Measurements may be made only on a few occasions, if not only once.

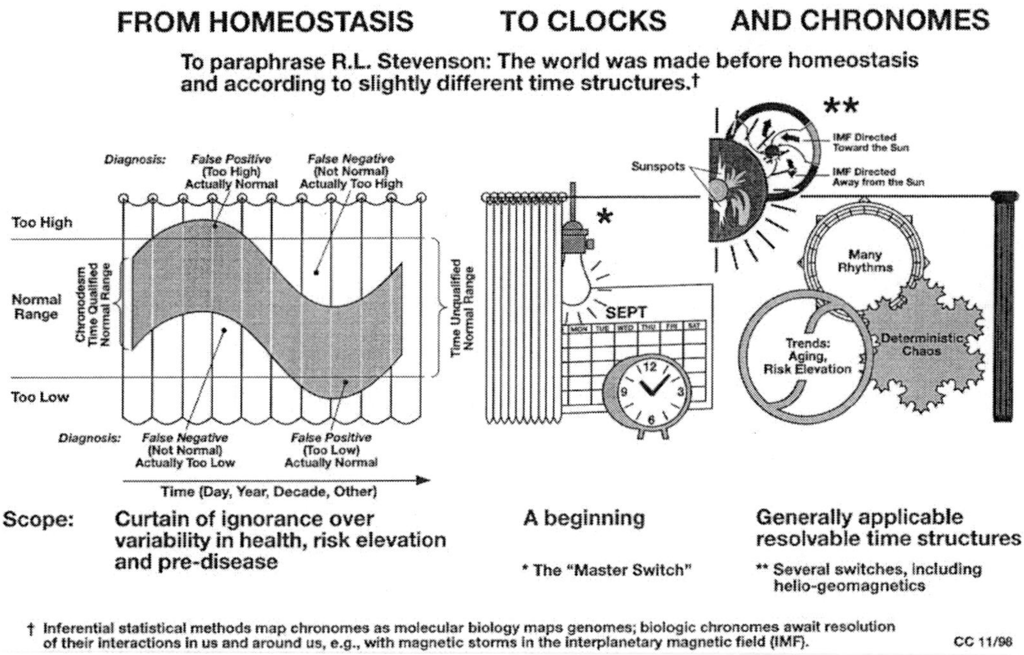

Figure 2. Variation within the physiological range can be resolved into meaningful information, including rhythms with frequencies covering 10 orders of magnitude, far beyond the circadian system and seasonal changes. Non-photic as well as photic influences of the sun have been genetically preserved in a set of photo- and magneto-periodicities from which much can be learned. © Halberg.

Unfortunately too often, this method of procedure and the resulting evidence are the guideline for clinical practice, notwithstanding the fact that it is spotcheck-evidence-based medicine. The procedure of spotchecks is carried over into practice, with the saying that "what is good enough for government-directed trials is good enough for my clinical practice".

Along this line of thinking, one forgets that in the trials, one or a few measurements are contributed by very many, usually thousands of people before conclusions (that may not be generally pertinent) are drawn. As an analogy only, accordingly for any one person one would actually need thousands of measurements to match the procedure of these trials.

To account for periodic variations, indeed one needs time series in practice, before one examines a patient, as recognized a century ago [5].

Another important point to consider is that chronomic time series-based N-of-5 [6], or preferably N-of-6, and in any event relatively small studies (7; cf. 8) also have their reason for implementation; they are cost-effective.

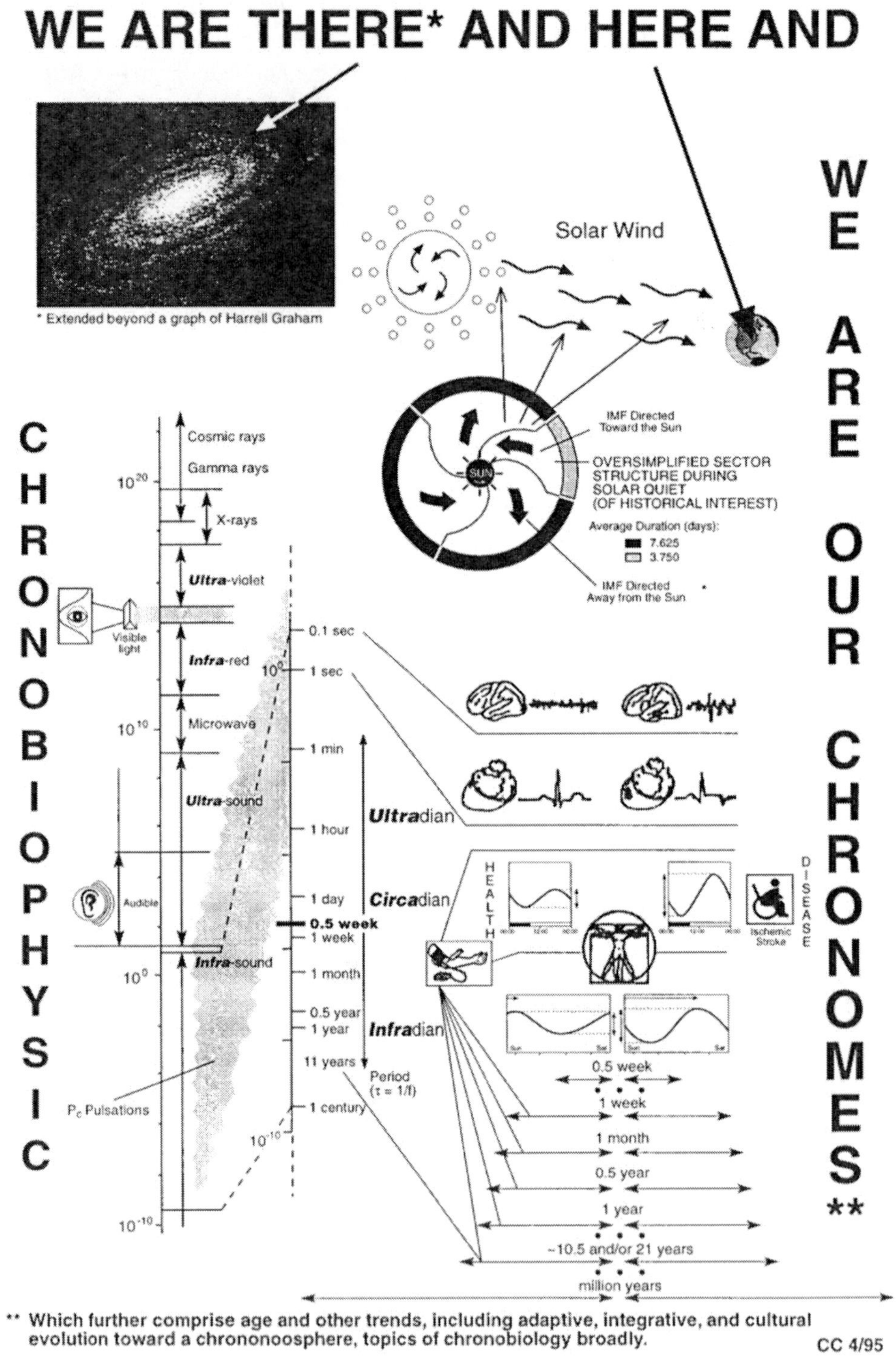

Figure 3. Frequency ranges of cycles in us and around us. © Halberg.

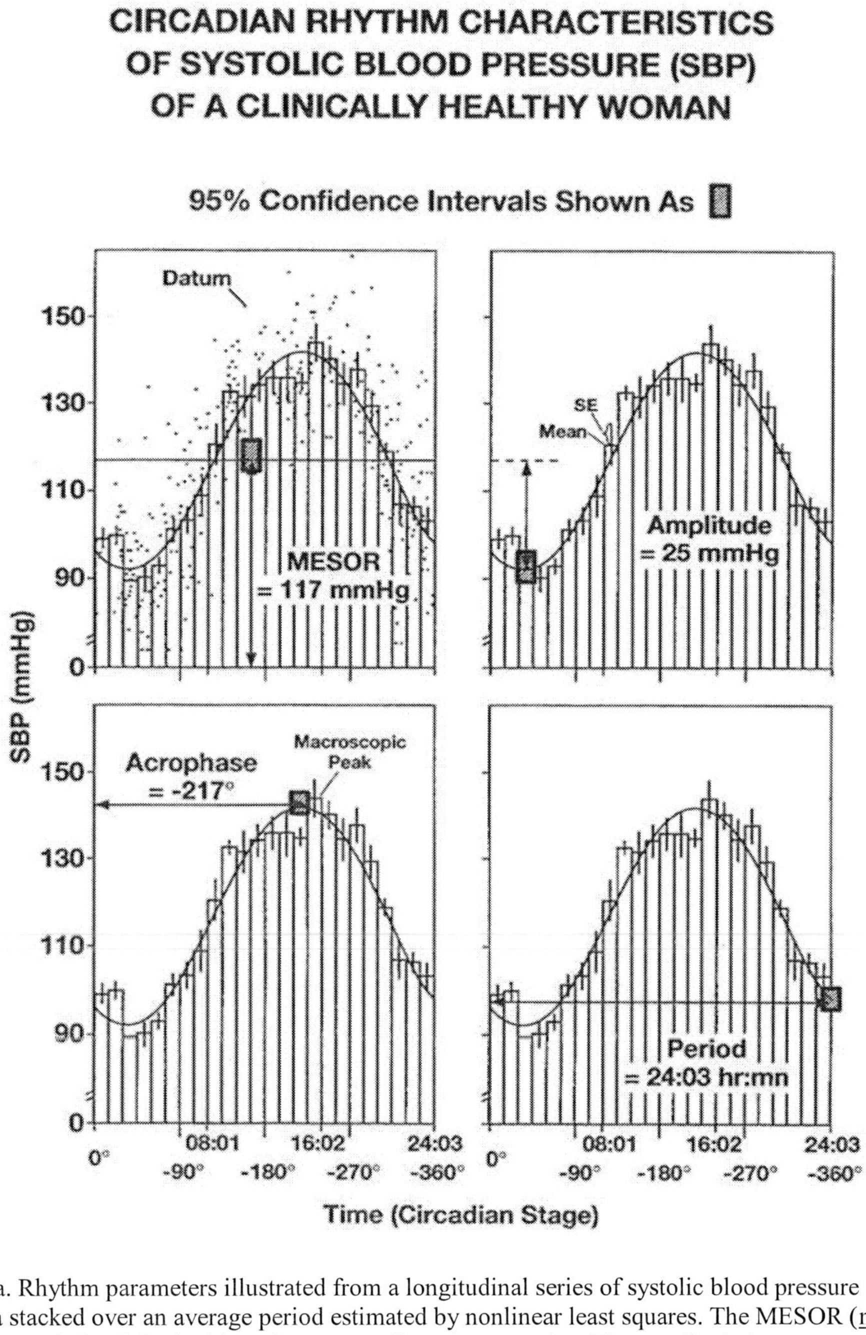

Figure 4a. Rhythm parameters illustrated from a longitudinal series of systolic blood pressure values, with data stacked over an average period estimated by nonlinear least squares. The MESOR (midline estimating statistic of rhythm) is a chronome-adjusted mean value. The amplitude is a measure of half the extent of change within a cycle, predictable by the fitted model consisting in this case of a 24:03-hour cosine curve (while it can be a magnitude when the extent of predictable change within a cycle is derived from a multiple component model). The acrophase is a measure of the timing of overall high values recurring in each cycle (determined in relation to a given reference time). The period is the duration of one cycle. Each parameter is estimated with a measure of uncertainty, the 95% confidence interval, shown as a shaded quadrangle. © Halberg.

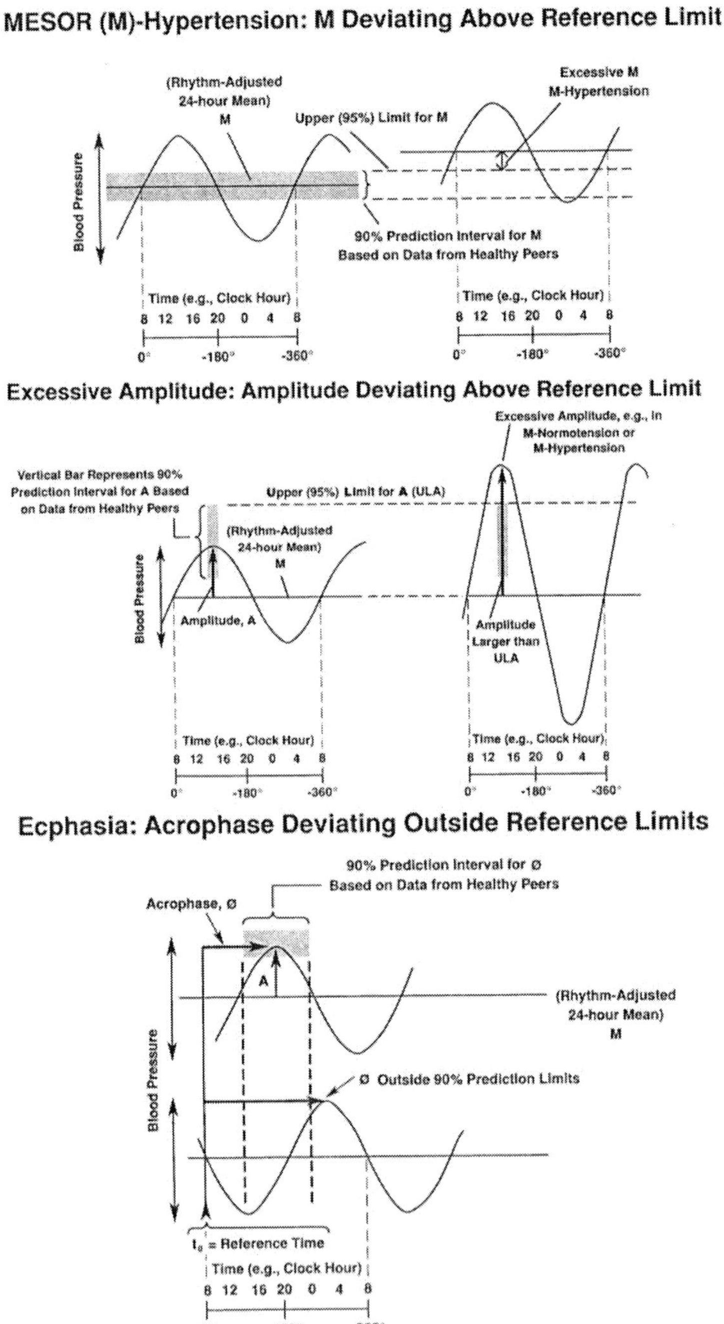

Figure 4b. Deviation from norms for each parameter provides diagnostic information applicable to blood pressure. When the patient's MESOR is above the upper 95% prediction limit for the BP MESOR of clinically healthy subjects of the same gender as the tested patient and a similar age, MESOR-hypertension is diagnosed. When the circadian amplitude exceeds the upper 95% prediction limit derived from data on clinically healthy peers matched by gender and age, circadian hyper-amplitude-tension (CHAT) is diagnosed. When BP peaks at an odd time, that is when the circadian acrophase occurs outside the 95% prediction interval in gender- and age-matched clinically healthy peers, ecphasia is diagnosed. Like MESOR-hypertension, CHAT and ecphasia are associated with an elevated cardiovascular disease risk. © Halberg.

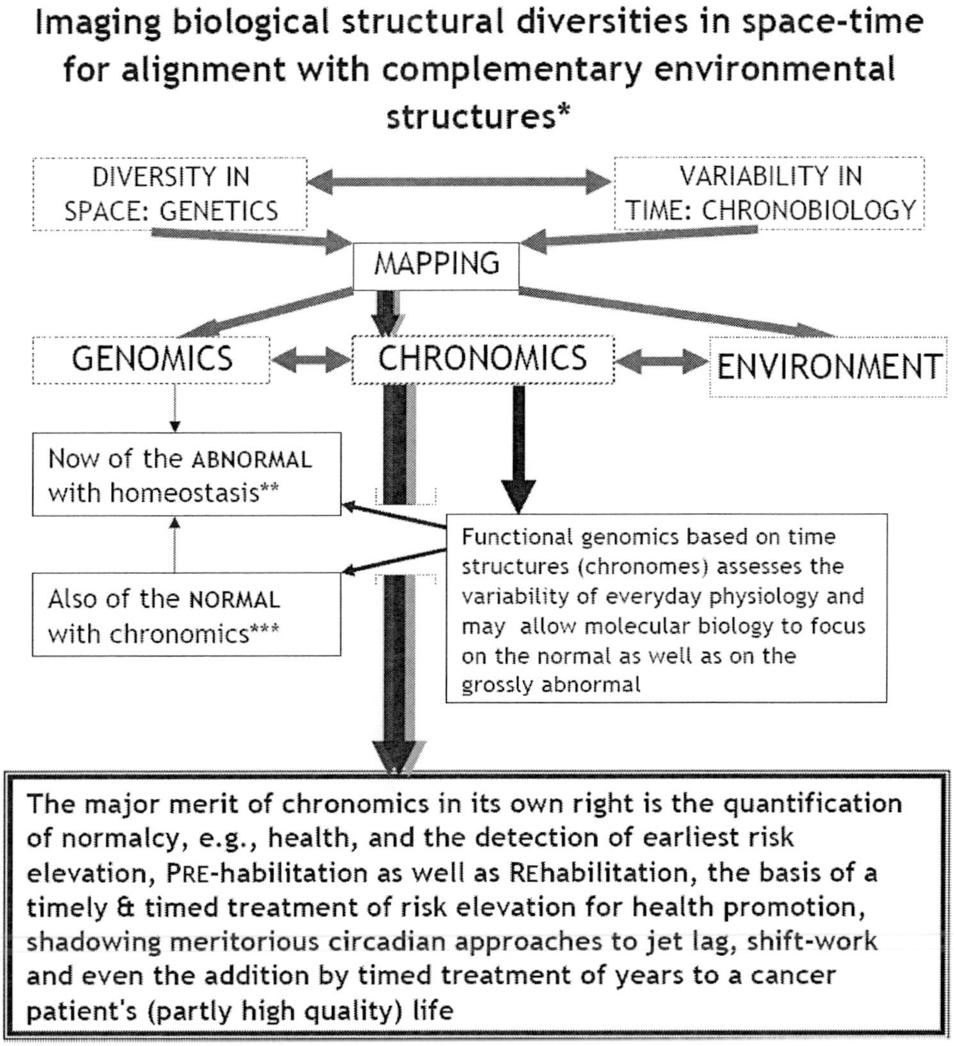

*An outcome of puzzles encountered in the 1950s (Halberg F, Visscher MB. Proc Soc exp Biol [N.Y.] 1950; 75: 846-847).

**Time- and otherwise-unspecified normal ranges close a curtain of ignorance over everyday physiology by homeostatic imaginary "baselines".

***Imaging time structures of rhythms, i.a., with frequencies covering over 10 orders of magnitude in and around us, opens the curtain of ignorance drawn over everyday physiology by time- and otherwise-unspecified normal ranges.

Scheme 1.

INTER- AND INTRA-INDIVIDUAL VARIABILITY

Whenever large inter-individual differences are demonstrated, the trials' results need not agree with those concerning the given individual, for instance, in the response to sodium [9, 10; cf. 11]. The N-of-1 study then becomes indispensable. An average population response to sodium will ignore that some individuals do show an increase in BP with an increase in sodium intake, while others do not show this response in the doses tested, and a third, admittedly very small group will show a decrease in BP with an increase in sodium intake in a highly controlled study on a metabolic ward at NIH (Figure 5).

Apart from such drastic inter-individual variability, the current large trials have a major shortcoming, notably in dealing with BP; they ignore intra-individual variability, which can involve, in beat-to-beat BP, recording a change of more than 30 mmHg during several seconds in a person at rest. Larger changes recur daily and smaller changes recur weekly, yearly and at other intervals, Figure 6a-f.

Consequences of Spotchecks

When the ruling-out of "hypertension"[1] is based on a single time-unqualified screening, cyclic and other variations in BP are ignored and false negative spotcheck-based diagnoses ensue. Hence, those who could greatly benefit from medication, may be left untreated until they suffer a stroke or other morbid event. These are patients with false negative diagnoses (of normotension) and with only chronomically detectable disorders, separate from or coexisting with MESOR-hypertension. When the ruling-in of "hypertension" is based on measurements at one or two more visits to a care provider's office, false positive diagnoses abound, notably when the person is seen in the afternoon, Figure 7a. By the same token, a white-coat hypertension in the morning may be a white-coat hypotension in the afternoon, Figure 7b. As a consequence of this clock-hour confounded diagnostic spotcheck approach, many millions of people in the developed world may be falsely labeled as "hypertensive" and treated, perhaps for a lifetime, without needing their stigma, the cost and possible side effects.

Sphygmochrons

An immediate alternative in everyday practice is obtained by a time-structural (chronomic) imaging of variability with computer analyses of systematically obtained BP and HR data, e.g., in a sphygmochron, Figures 8a-c. This comparison of a given series with reference values from clinically healthy peers, matched by age group, gender and, when possible, ethnicity, consists of a parametric and a non-parametric part. Automatic ambulatory BP and HR monitoring is an easy and useful approach, if and only if the data are also time-structurally (chronomically) computer-analyzed. In some cases chronomics are applicable to systematic self-measurements, even if in other cases these yield inconsistent results [12]. Certainly, one measurement is better than none. Equally, a systematic manually self-measured series is better than a spotcheck, if it is chronomically analyzed, but it is best replaced by such analysis on ambulatorily collected series, as soon as technology permits.

---

[1] The spotcheck-based diagnosis of high blood pressure is placed in quotes and is best replaced by a chronomic diagnosis, such as MESOR-hypertension, an elevation of the chronome-adjusted average, i.e., the MESOR, short for midline-estimating statistic of rhythm.

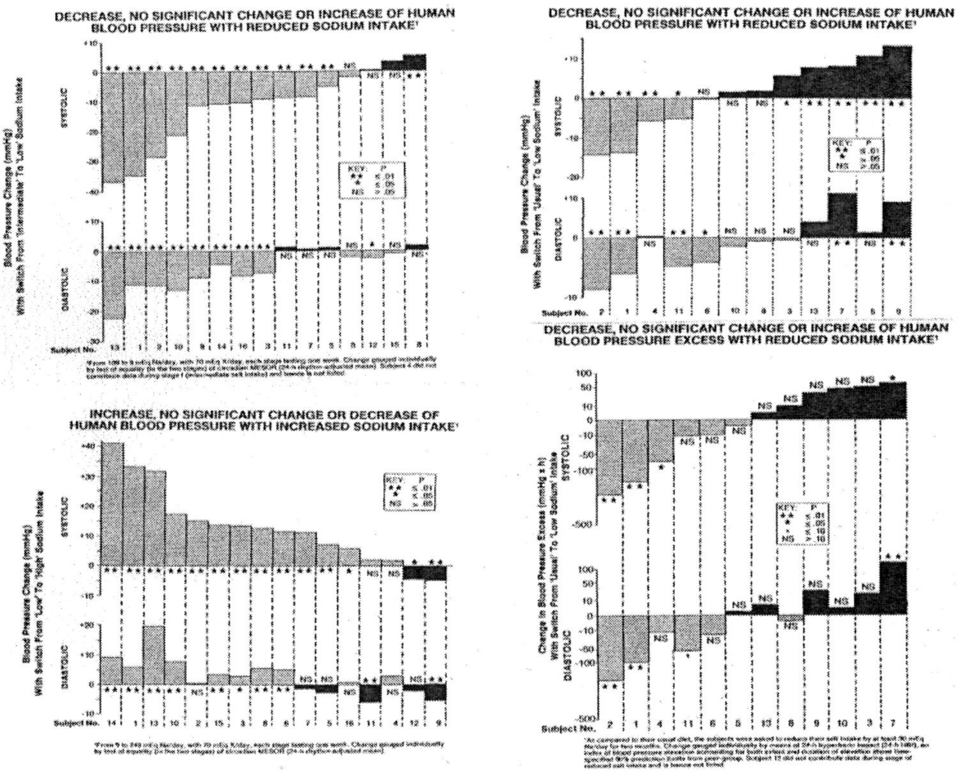

Figure 5. Increase in sodium intake in some cases can be associated with a decrease in blood pressure, whereas in other cases it is associated with an increase in blood pressure or with no statistically significant change in blood pressure. © Halberg.

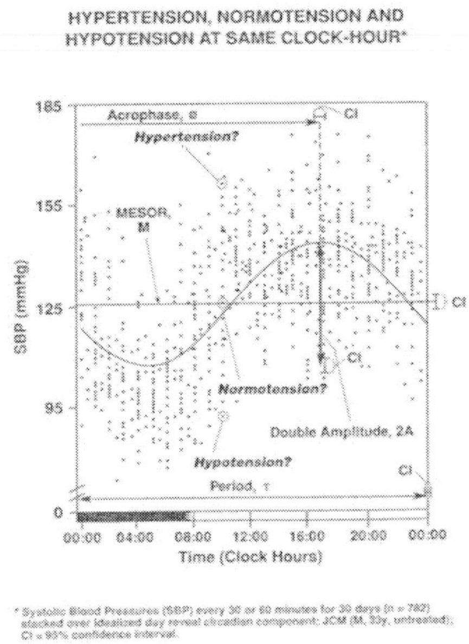

Figure 6a. Large intra-individual variation in blood pressure, seen in a 30-day record, with data stacked over an idealized 24-hour day. Some single measurements would qualify for contradictory diagnoses, from hypertension to normotension and even hypotension. © Halberg.

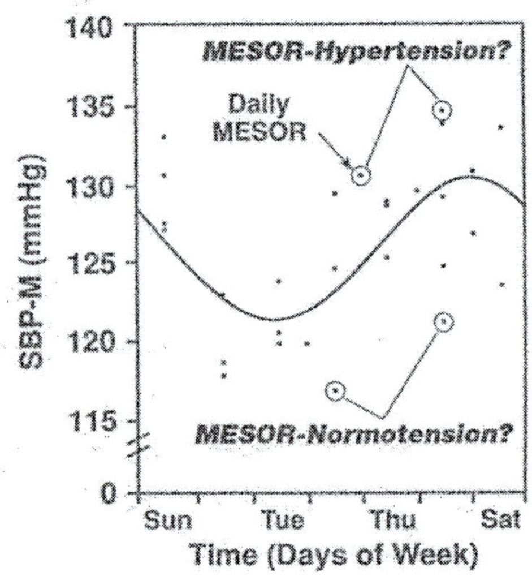

Figure 6b. Large intra-individual variation in blood pressure, seen in a 30-day record, shown as daily MESORs stacked over idealized 7-day week. Part of the variability in blood pressure can be accounted for by the prominent circadian variation ,as shown in Figure 6a, and, to a lesser extent by the about-weekly (circaseptan) variation. The fact that some daily averages correspond to the diagnosis of MESOR-hypertension, whereas others correspond to the diagnosis of MESOR-normotension, strongly support the desirability to monitor blood pressure around the clock for longer than a single 24-hour span, preferably for 7 days at the outset or longer as needed. © Halberg.

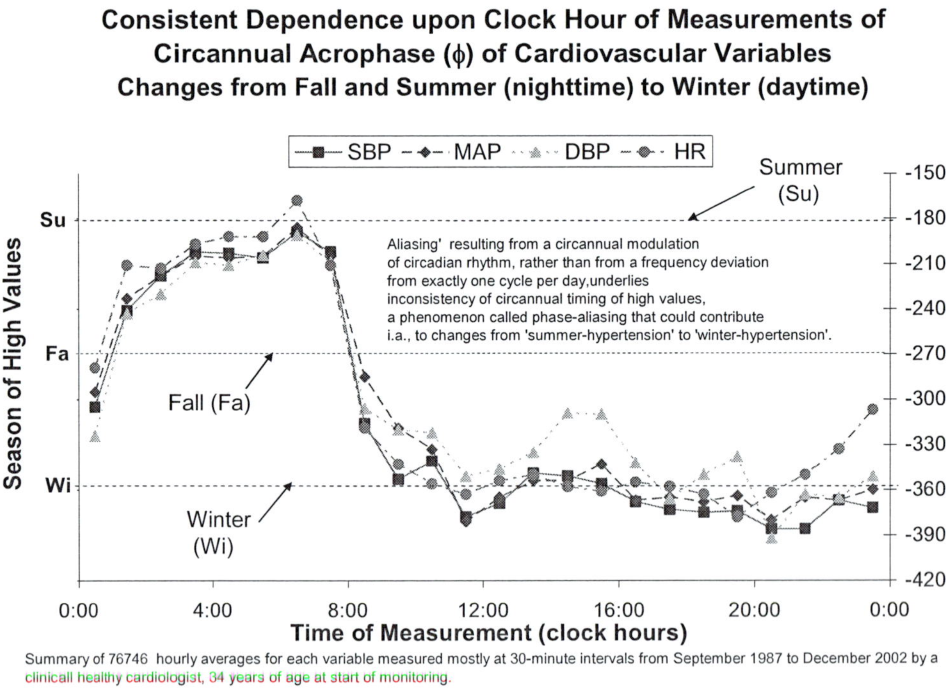

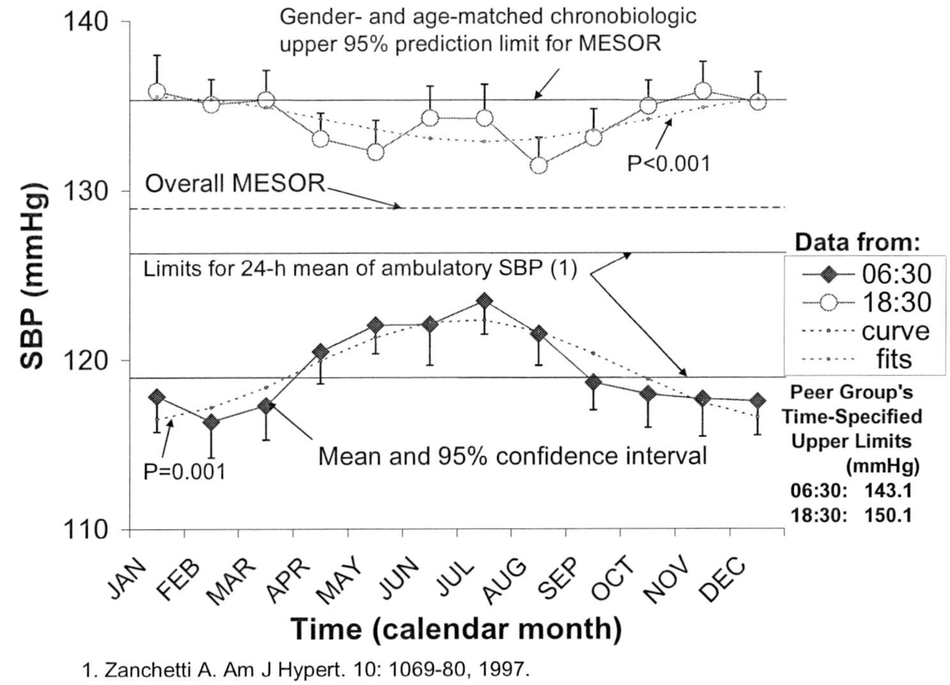

Figure 6c. Fallacy of "controlling" any effects of rhythms by fixing the time of day of measurements. Opposite conclusions concerning hypertension will be drawn from long-term consistent spotchecks at a fixed clock hour, even when the time series covers 15 years of daily values. © Halberg.

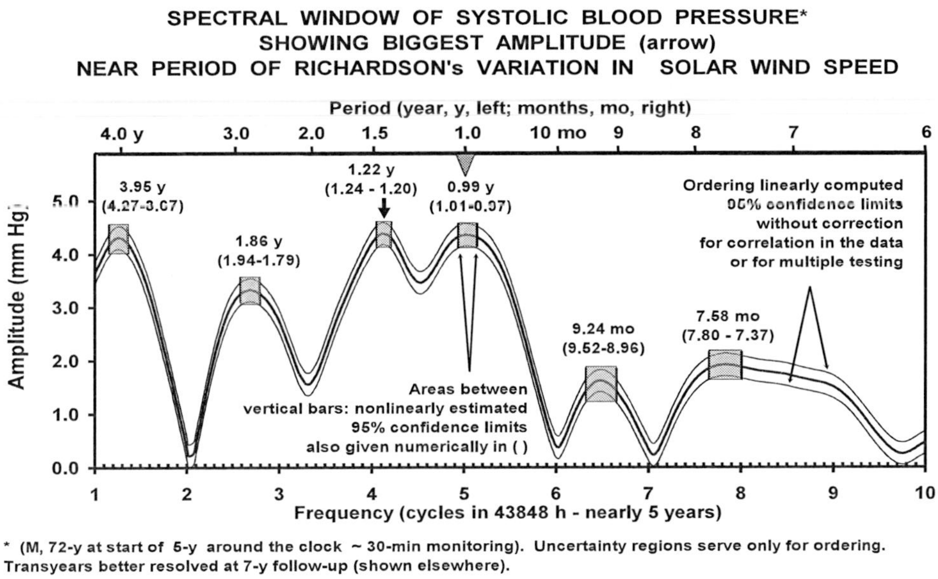

Figure 6d. Least squares spectrum of systolic blood pressure values taken around the clock at 30-min intervals over 5 years reveals the presence of an about 1.22-year component in addition to the about-yearly cycle related to the seasons. Both components have about the same prominence. Sampling over a short span shorter than 5 years may yield controversial results regarding the presence of any circannual variation, which is likely detected when the 1.22-year and the 1.0-year cycles are in phase, but not when they are out of phase and cancel each other out. © Halberg.

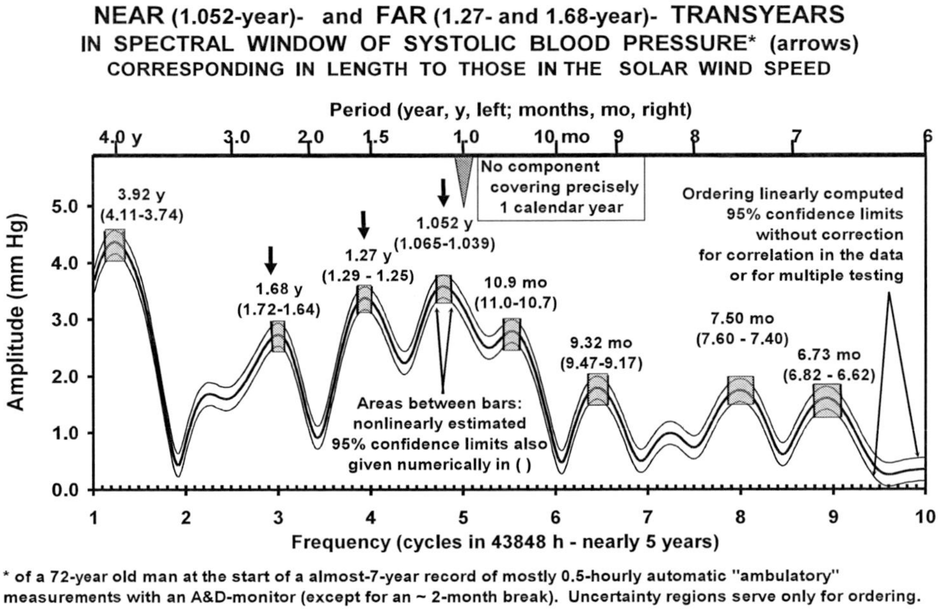

Figure 6e. At the 7-year follow-up, confirmation of the transyear with a period previously of about 1.22 years shown in Figure 6d, now of 1.27 years, a far-transyear. Note that the about-yearly component in Figure 6d is now resolved as a near transyear with a period of about 1.05 years. A second far-transyear of about 1.68 years is also resolved in the 7-year record. It is emphasized that the longer the record, the better is the resolution of its chronome. For any given person, the longest record analyzed by a gliding spectral window can reveal changes in time structure not readily seen in an average or global spectrum. © Halberg.

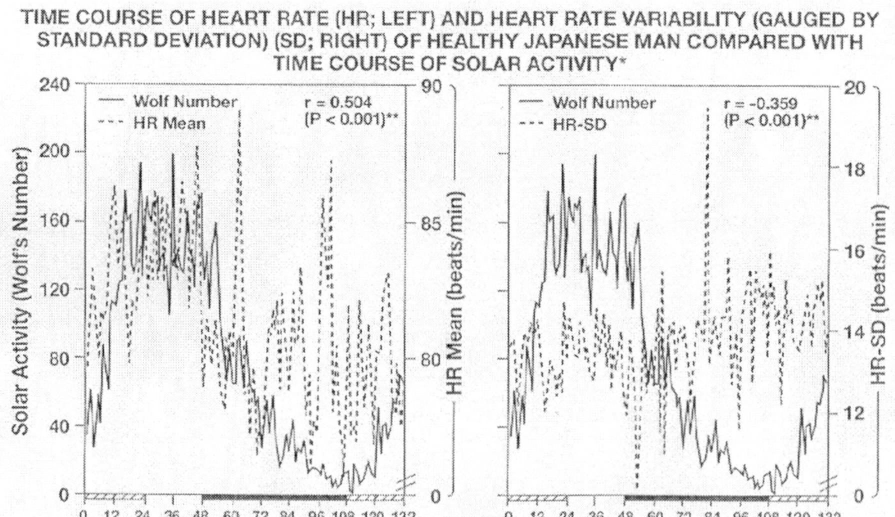

Figure 6f. Large intra-individual variation in heart rate variability on the scale of years. Heart rate variability was gauged by the monthly standard deviation of around the clock data at about 30-min intervals collected over 11 years. An about 10.5-year cycle is detected with statistical significance and resembles the solar activity cycle, albeit no conclusions (on hints) can be drawn from the similarity of time structures. © Halberg.

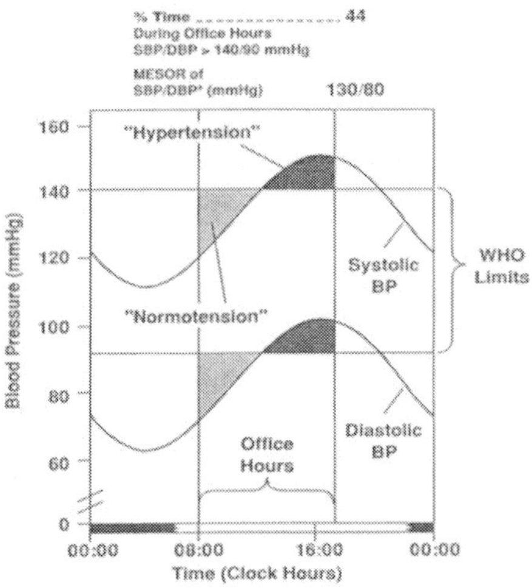

Figure 7a. Abstract demonstration that due to the usually large circadian variation in blood pressure, subjects with a wide range of average blood pressure values are likely to be diagnosed as normotensive in the morning and as hypertensive in the afternoon when blood pressure measurements are interpreted in the light of fixed thresholds, as is current ("spotcheck evidence"-based) practice. © Halberg.

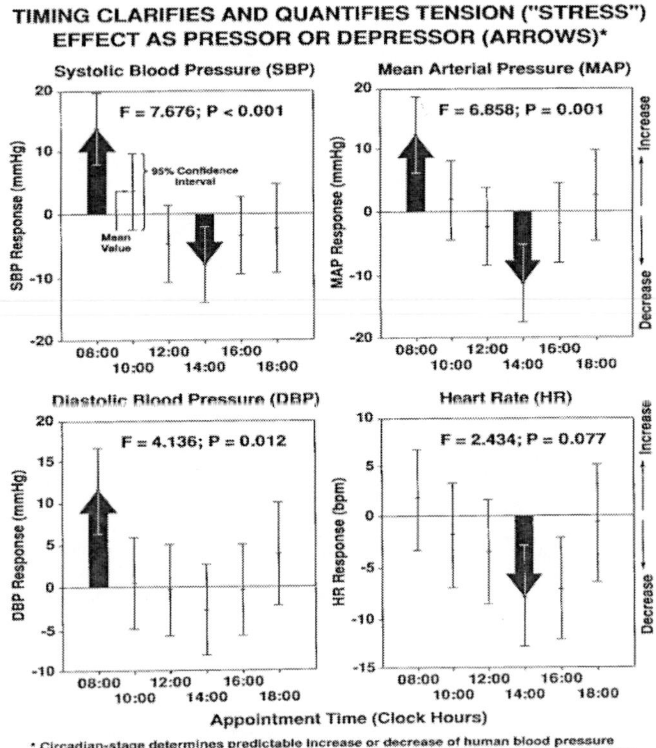

Figure 7b. In relation to periodontal surgery, the blood pressure and heart rate of patients treated in the morning tended to increase with statistical significance but tended to decrease with statistical significance for patients seen in the afternoon. The "white-coat hypertension" of the morning patients becomes a "white-coat hypotension for the afternoon patients. © Halberg.

Monitoring Profile Over Time;
Computer Comparison
with Peer Group Limits

SPHYGMOCHRON™-S (short form)

Blood Pressure (BP) and Related Cardiovascular Summary
(Circadian Sphygmochron; from sphygmo-, of or relating to the circulation, notably blood pressure, as well as pulse and chronos, time)

Name ______ Patient # ______ No. of Profiles: ______

Age ______ Sex [M] [F] Monitoring From ______ To ______, 19 ______

Time of Awakening (A) ______ (______) Falling Asleep (S) ______ (______)
Day of Profile (Habitually) Day of Profile (Habitually)

R_x: ______ Comments[1,2] ______

Chronobiologic Characteristics

	Systolic BP (mmHg)		Diastolic BP (mmHg)		Heart Rate (bpm)	
	Patient Value	Peer Group Reference Limits	Patient Value	Peer Group Reference Limits	Patient Value	Peer Group Reference Limits
Adjusted 24-h Mean (MESOR)		Range		Range		Range
Predictable Change (Double Amplitude)		Range		Range		Range
Timing of Overall High Values (Acrophase) (hr:min)		Range		Range		Range

Figure 8a. Sphygmochron (top part) summarizing the parametric results. © Halberg.

	STD (Min; Max)	STD (Min; Max)	STD (Min; Max)
Percent Time of Elevation			
Timing of Excess	(hr:min)	(hr:min)	(hr:min)
Extent of Excess During 24 Hours HBI	(mmHg x hour)	(mmHg x hour)	(mmHg x hour)
10-Year Cumulative Excess	(mmHg x hour) (in 1,000's units)	(mmHg x hour) (in 1,000's units)	(bpm x hour) (in 1,000's units)

Individualized bounded indices: (STD = Standard) (Min = Minimum) (Max = Maximum) (HBI = Hyperbaric Index)

Intervention Needed

☐ No
☐ Yes ☐ Drug ☐ Non-Drug

More Monitoring Needed

☐ Annually
☐ As soon as possible
☐ Other specify ______

Prepared By ______ Date ___ / ___ / ___

1) Unusually long standing or lying-down during waking; unusual activity, such as exercise, emotional loads, or schedule changes, e.g., shiftwork, etc.; 2) Salt, calories, kind and amount, other, etc.

© Chronobiology Laboratories, University of Minnesota, 5-187 Lyon Labs., 420 Washington Ave. S.E., Minneapolis, MN 55455
For questions, call F. Halberg or G. Cornélissen at 612-624-6976

Figure 8b. Sphygmochron (bottom part) summarizing the non-parametric results. © Halberg.

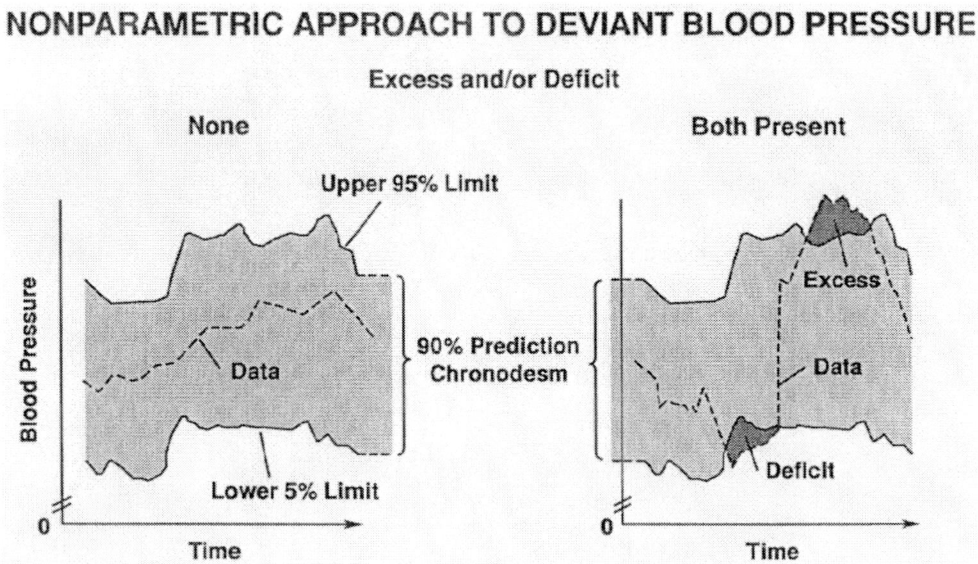

Figure 8c. Illustration of hyperbaric and hypobaric indices, the amounts of blood pressure excess and/or deficit approximated by the area of excess/deficit delineated by the individual's profile when it is deviant and the upper/lower 95% prediction limit itself. © Halberg.

Chronomics, the resolution of altered variability (Scheme 1), is important, first in its own right; it serves to detect novel conditions, i.e., a very high risk of stroke, myocardial infarction, kidney disease and blindness and of eclampsia during pregnancy, risks that for stroke are higher than that associated with hypertension, Figures 9a-c. Second, and important for very many people, as detailed under *Spotchecks* above, variability assessment by chronomics is critical to improve the diagnosis of a BP that on the average is too high or too low -- MESOR-hyper- or -hypotension -- but greatly variable, in order to guard against false diagnoses. Third, chronomics are important for transdisciplinary science [2, 13].

A chronobiologic approach to variability by sphygmochrons is already implemented in locations with limited resources, such as Armenia, China and India, with measurements beyond 24 hours, the target being 7-day records. By contrast, the (false) gold standard in countries with resources, namely a diagnosis based only on, say, half-hourly measurements during 24 hours and overall day- and nighttime means computed from such a profile can be misleading because of day-to-day BP variability in both the average and the dynamics, among others. A computation of ratios of mean values for the day and night is simple [14], can be useful for women [15], but incompletely approximates the dynamics confounding amplitude and phase. Indeed, everything should be rendered as simple as possible but not simpler [15-17].

As a start, one week of chronomically analyzed monitoring is preferable: half-weekly and one-weekly cycles provide additional diagnostic and prognostic information, and what is important, a 7-day record assesses the characteristics of day-night variation much more rigorously than a 24-hour snapshot. Assessing a daily cycle with a 24-hour profile is reminiscent of taking the pulse for one second, that is for only one cardiac cycle [18-20].

PRACTICABILITY

Automatic ambulatorily collectable oscillometric instrumentation is available to those 1. contributing to a chronomic data base 7-day series, properly specified by gender, age, ethnicity and health status (with names coded to guard privacy), and 2. benefiting from analyses based on the accumulating reference standards through the international imaging project on The BIosphere and the COsmos, briefly BIOCOS (corne001@umn.edu).

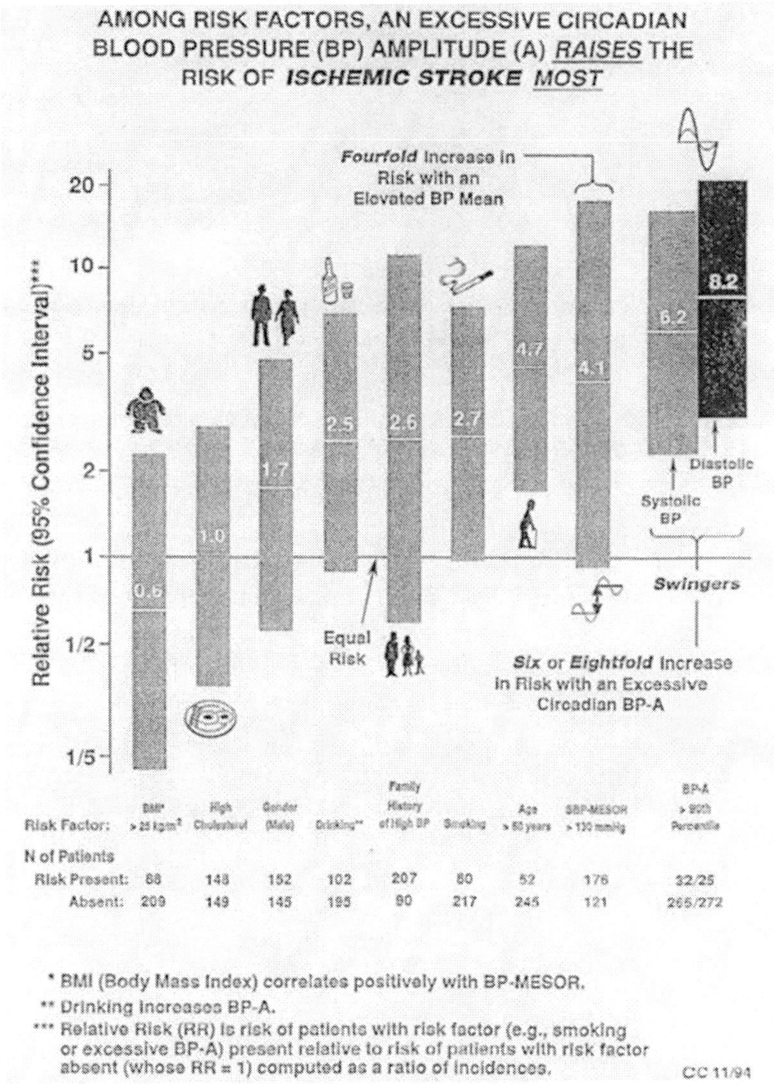

Figure 9a. Risk of cerebral ischemic event associated with different risk factors, assessed in a 6-year prospective study on 297 patients. Of all risk factors here considered, an excessive circadian amplitude of blood pressure (CHAT, short for circadian hyper-amplitude-tension) carries the highest risk, as shown by the relative risk much higher than unity and corresponding 95% confidence interval (vertical bar) non-overlapping equal risk (RR=1). © Halberg.

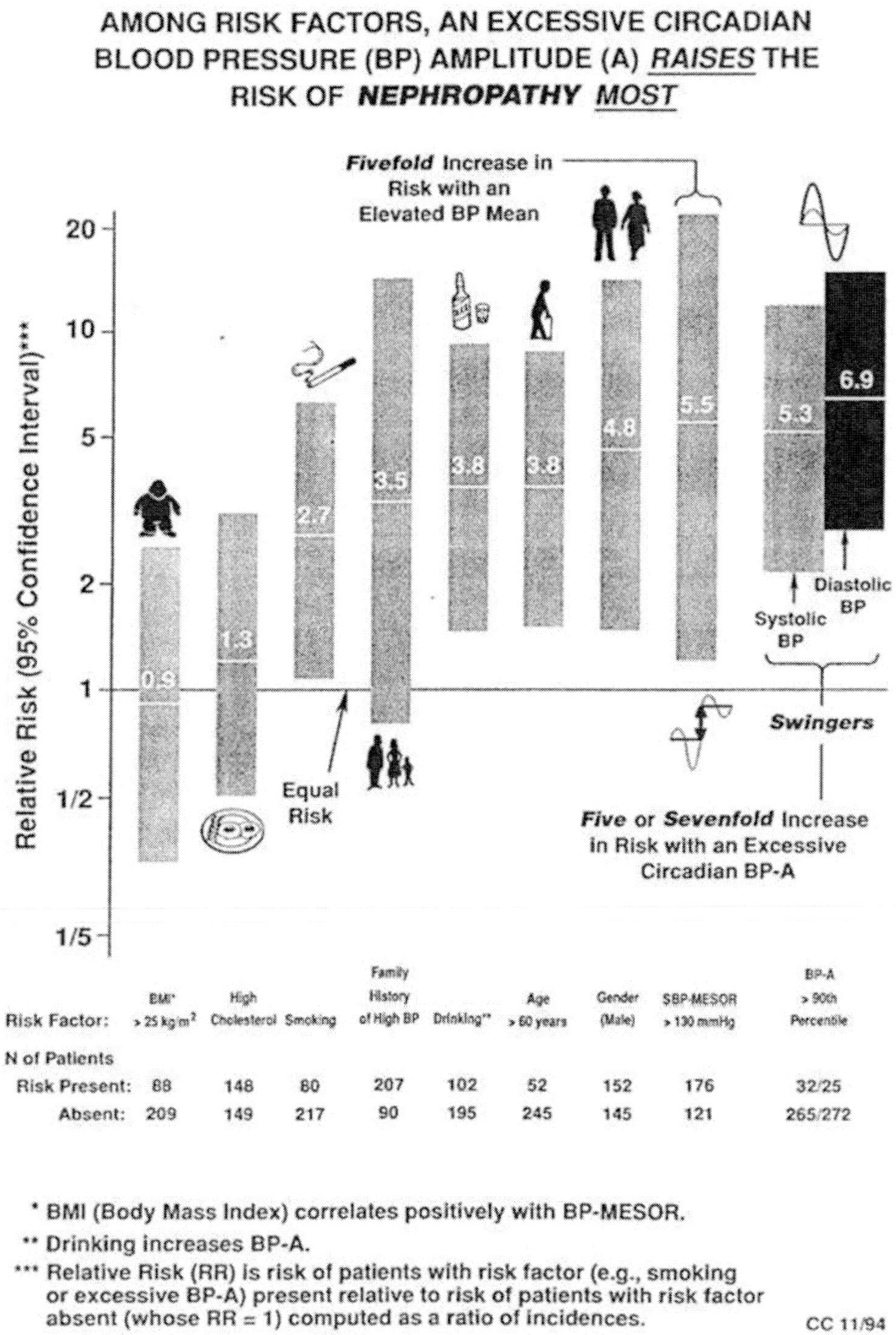

Figure 9b. Risk of nephropathy associated with different risk factors, assessed in a 6-year prospective study on 297 patients. Of all risk factors here considered, an excessive circadian amplitude of blood pressure (CHAT, short for circadian hyper-amplitude-tension) carries the highest risk, as shown by the relative risk much higher than unity and corresponding 95% confidence interval (vertical bar) non-overlapping equal risk (RR=1). © Halberg.

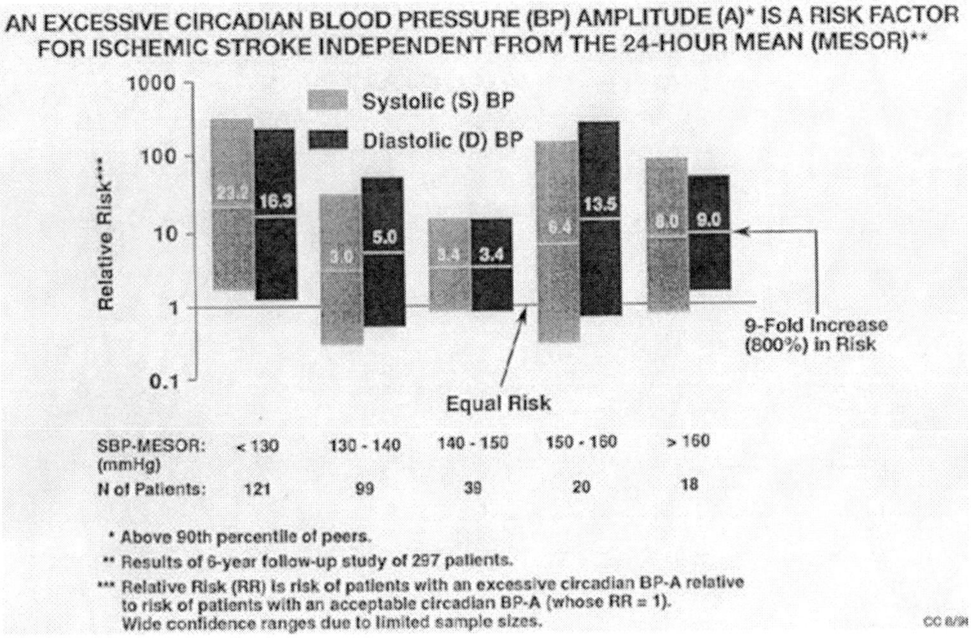

Figure 9c. Risk of cerebral ischemic event associated with CHAT (circadian hyper-amplitude-tension) is present irrespective of the presence or absence of MESOR-hypertension. © Halberg.

Via BIOCOS, a single monitor costs US $450 (rather than $2,250 on the open market), plus freight with an added $50 for editing and displaying software, paid only once, irrespective of the number of monitors purchased.

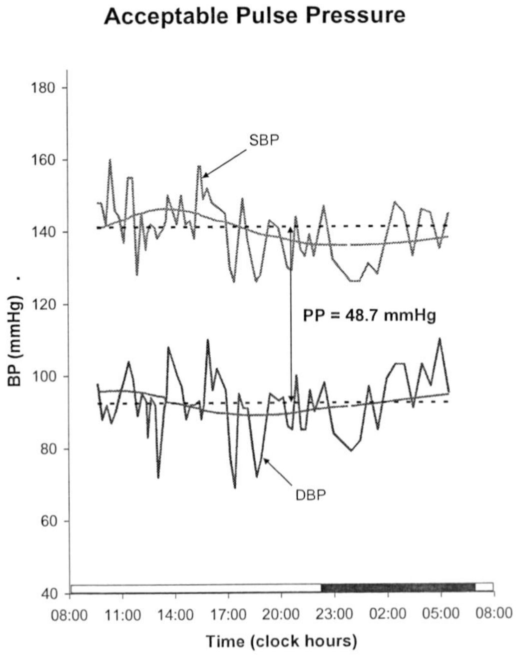

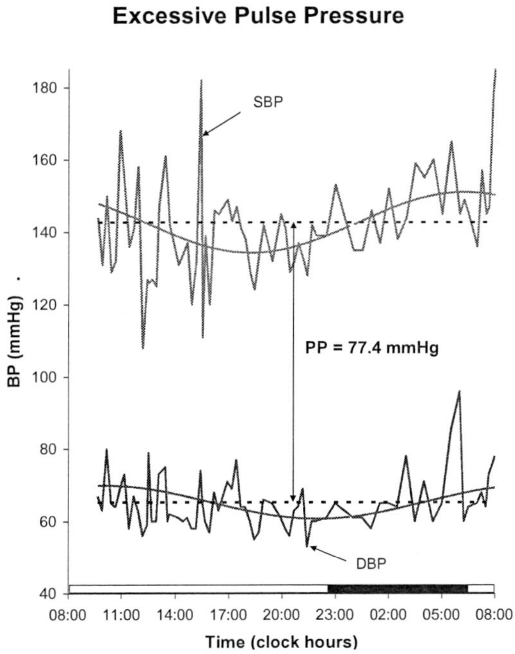

Figure 10. Circadian profiles of systolic and diastolic blood pressure from two patients with a similar MESOR of systolic blood pressure but different MESORs of diastolic blood pressure. Although the MESOR of diastolic blood pressure is lower for one patient (right) than for the other patient (left), the cardiovascular disease risk of the former patient may be higher than that of the latter in view of the excessive pulse pressure, seen in outcome studies to be associated with an elevated risk. © Halberg.

Chronomically analyzed week-long monitoring is cost-effective since, with a system of education and scheduling in self-help, it allows the collection of 1-week profiles for more than 50 people/year/instrument; if the instrument is used for 4 or 5 years, the cost/person/week is US $2.50 or $2.00, much cheaper than the $200/day charged in the U.S. for only 24-hour chronomically-*un*analyzed monitoring and certainly cheaper than coronary artery bypass graft surgery or care after a massive stroke, that the detection and treatment of high risks and certainly of the risk of a (less unreliably diagnosed) MESOR-hypertension will prevent.

BIOCOS currently provides cost-free chronomic computer analyses, indispensable for diagnosing certain vascular disease risks [2, 21, 22] such as a. an excessive within-day swing (CHAT, short for circadian hyper-amplitude-tension), Figures 9a-c; and/or b. excessive differences during 24 hours in BP when the heart contracts vs. when it dilates (a pulse pressure exceeding a circadian threshold), Figure 10; and/or c. an odd day/night timing (circadian ecphasia), Figure 11; and/or d. a reduced (under-circadian-threshold) HR variability, Figure 12. These separate conditions, notably if they coexist, indicate a great nonlinear risk (i.e., involving a threshold rather than a gradually increasing risk). Some of the conditions can be treated, Scheme 2 [21-24], sometimes only by changing the timing of medication, Figures 13a and 13b. As compared to an arithmetic mean, a more accurate or more precise estimate of the average BP, is also usually gained by a chronomic (time-structural) BP and HR imaging, Figure 14.

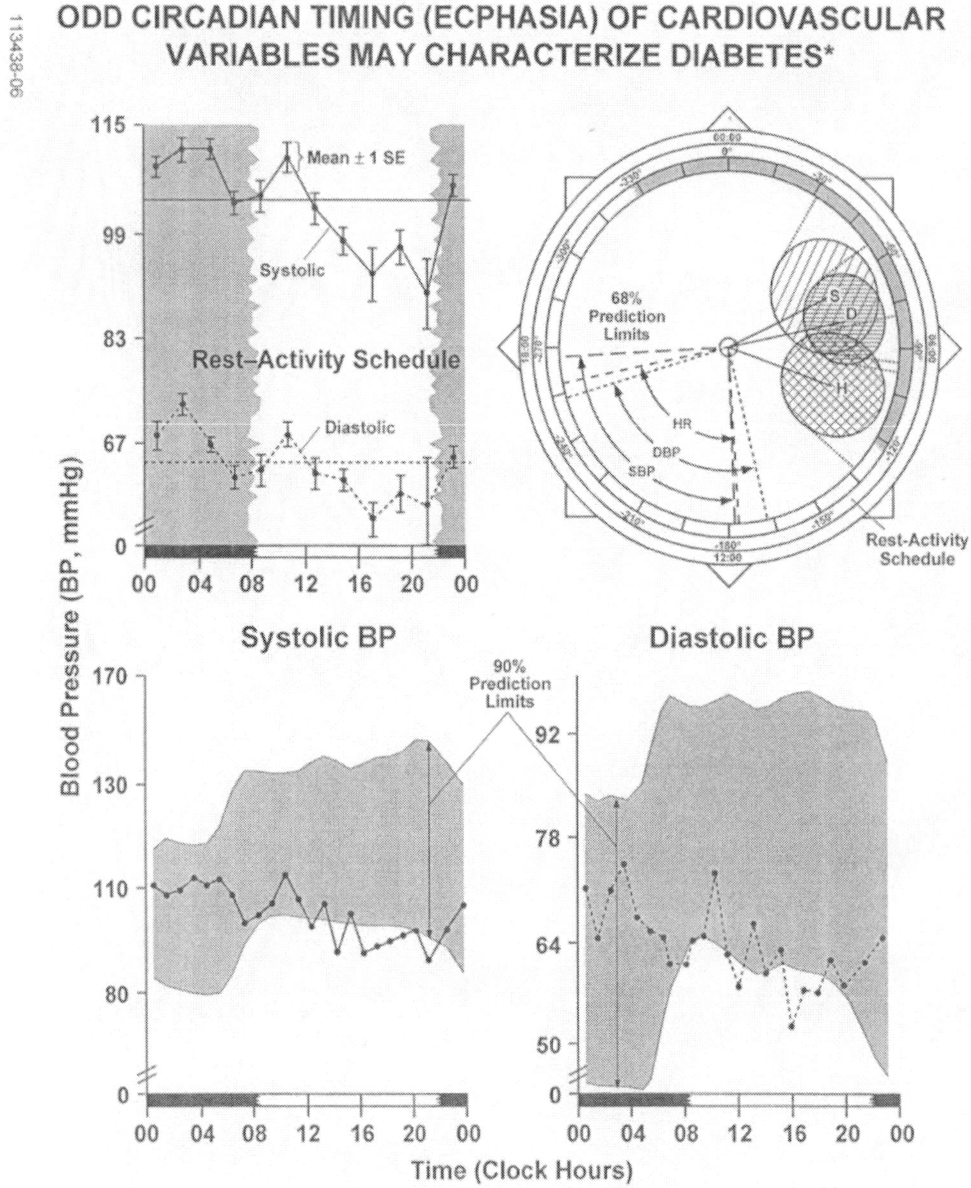

Patient's Characteristics

Variable	MESOR	Double Amplitude	Acrophase**	Reference Limits
SBP (mmHg)	104	14.8	-76°	-222° (-177; -265)
DBP (mmHg)	64	9.0	-63°	-206° (-167; -252)
HR (beats/min)	97	6.6	-108°	-209° (-176; -260)

* A case of diabetic pregnancy described in Chronobiologia 14: 201, 1987.
** 0° = local midnight; 360° = 24 hours (N = 131; P < 0.001 in each case).

CC 11/99

Figure 11. Ecphasia, that is an odd timing of the circadian variation in blood pressure, peaking during the night (rest span) instead of mid-afternoon, is observed in some patients with non-insulin-dependent diabetes mellitus who developed autonomic nervous dysfunction (not shown) or in pregnancies complicated by gestational diabetes (this figure). © Halberg.

It is necessary to educate the people on how to self-measure BP and HR by automatic monitoring rather than relying only on manual measurements that should be taken systematically several times a day, including one measurement in bed immediately after awakening and one in bed before retiring for sleep, along with at least 5 others, at intervals of 2 to 3 hours. The preferred self-use of automatic instruments, however, is easy to learn: one puts on a cuff and sets a switch just once, and measurements are taken automatically at preset intervals during waking and sleep, except for showering or exercising.

For these and certain other purposes, the switch is then reset and the cuff removed, and put on again upon completion of the task with the activation of the switch. In the very few cases where sleep is prevented by cuff inflation, the interval between consecutive measurements during the usual sleep span can be set to be longer than 30 minutes, and this simple maneuver usually enables falling sleep.

Reference standards adjusted for gender, age and certain ethnicities are used in BIOCOS for averages (MESORs), and for some dynamic characteristics, instead of values that are implied to apply to all people 18 years of age and older [4, 25]. Chronomic guidelines for care providers (or educated laypeople, for example teachers) are available [2, 21, 22, 26]. This time structure-imaging approach can be used for a timely diagnosis and, when needed, in combination with a timed treatment, preferably with continued surveillance by monitoring and e-mailed data assessment, by a BIOCOS center, until the desired effect is validated [21, 27, 28].

Centers now accumulating ethnicity-, age- and gender-specified reference data on mean BP, HR and their variability and in particular one summarizing these data from centers worldwide (corne001@umn.edu) while providing free analyses are functional in BIOCOS and, should be made WHO centers; they play an essential role in health promotion for prehabilitation. Thereby, the expenses for care after a massive stroke and of coronary artery bypass grafting and rehabilitation are reduced, a point critical for health care systems in all areas and in particular in those with limited resources, as stipulated by a consensus of many more than 10 international meetings [2, 29].

Chronomics for Medical and Other Science

The scope of chronomics is much broader than dealing with BP and HR in everyday health care for prevention, i.e., for prehabilitation to save the cost of rehabilitation [30]. In health research, a metabolic syndrome (MS) has been emphasized [31]. Figures 15a and 15b suggest the possibility of an early detection of a pre-metabolic syndrome (PMS), gauged by CHAT, as a more frequent condition, at the transition from MESOR-normotension to MESOR-hypertension [32]. CHAT is also found at the transition from normoglycemia to hyperglycemia, as in the case of glucose sensitivity [33, see also 34].

An as-yet basic recent finding by chronomics is a fartransyear, longer than a calendar year, namely a "year" of about 16 months (~1.3 calendar years) or an about 1.6-calendar-year, ~20-month "year" in BP. Figures 6d and 6e show spectral components corresponding in period length to changes described by physicists [35, 36] for the changes in speed of the solar wind measured by satellites.

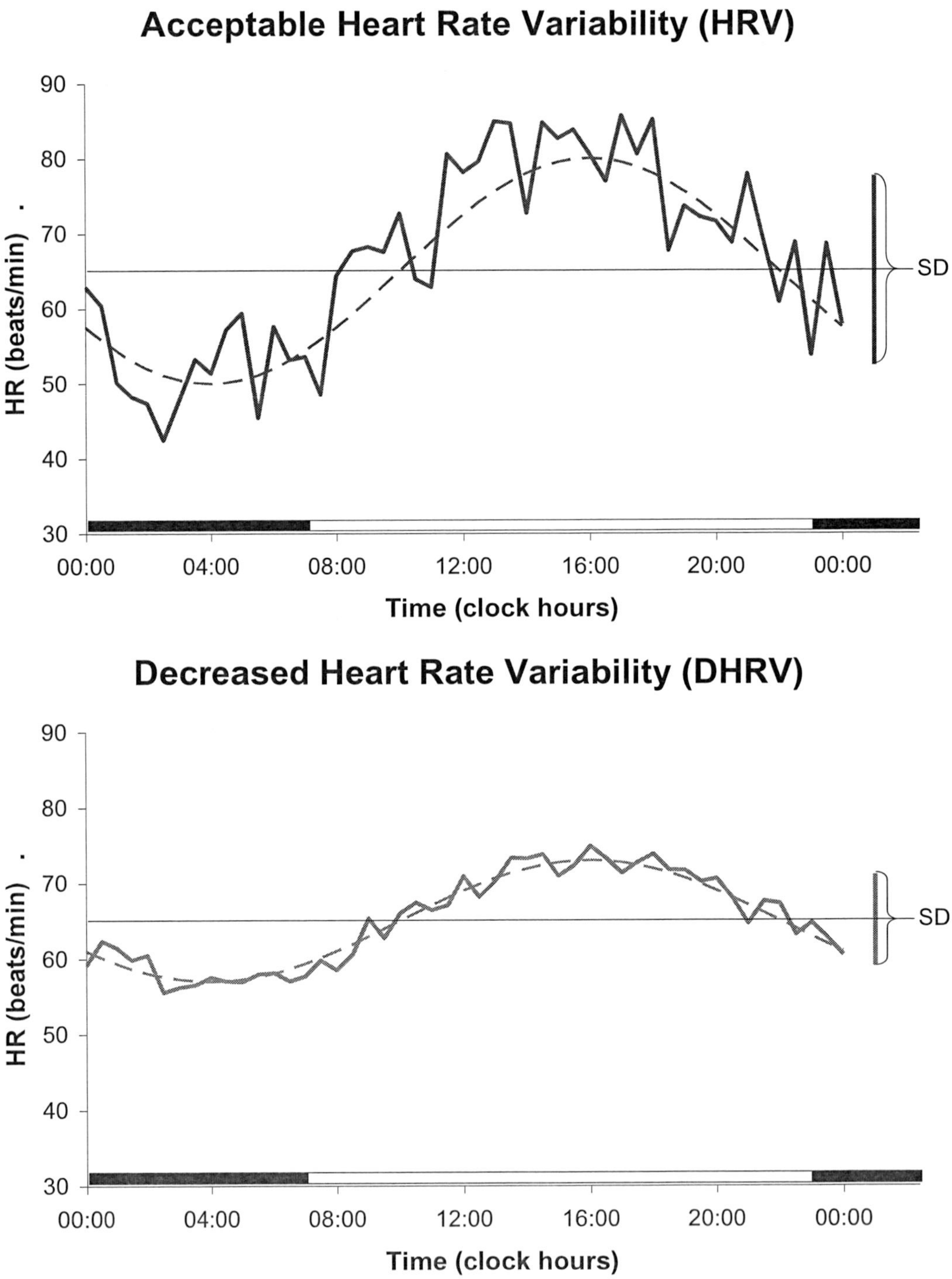

Figure 12. Abstract illustration of decreased heart rate variability, gauged by the circadian standard deviation of heart rate. © Halberg.

Toward multiply-individualized chronotherapy*
Different calcium channel blockers can have different effects on blood pressure (BP) and heart rate (HR) deviations associated with elevated vascular disease risk

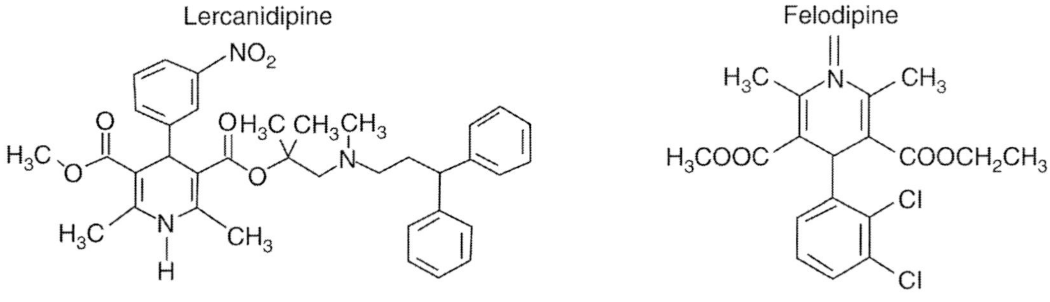

Lercanidipine	For a specific requirement, we ask of each drug:	Felodipine
NO	1. Does it reduce the circadian amplitude of BP ?	YES
YES	2. Does it increase the circadian HR variability (CHRV) ?	NO
YES	3. Does it reduce pulse pressure (PP) ?	YES
YES	4. Does it reduce the BP MESOR ?	YES

*Individualized by 1. kind of chronome alteration detected by a chronodiagnosis that recognizes risk elevation as well as disease (against a gender- and age-qualified standard), 2. kind of drug, i.a., with respect to the desired effect on variabilities of BP and/or HR, and 3. multiple considerations also of timing. For instance, decisions regarding drug choice can be based on a chronodiagnosis using felodipine in the presence of CHAT (circadian hyper-amplitude-tension) (1), with MESOR-hypertension (2) and/or an elevated PP, but not with a decreased CHRV; or using lercanidipine in the presence of a deficit in CHRV, with MESOR-hypertension and/or an elevated PP, but not with CHAT. In each case, individualization is further desirable in relation to the timing of any BP or HR alteration, including the timing of blood pressure excess (1, 2). Evidence thus far for the above drugs is available only in MESOR-hypertension. In MESOR-normotension, non-drug approaches are indicated first, and the action in MESOR-normotension remains to be explored.

1. Halberg F, Cornélissen G, Schack B. Self-experimentation on chronomes, time structures; chronomics for health surveillance and science: also transdisciplinary civic duty? Behavioral and Brain Sciences, http://www.bbsonline.org/Preprints/Roberts/Commentators/Halberg.html
2. Cornélissen G, Delmore P, Halberg F. Healthwatch 3: Why 7-day blood pressure monitoring: What everyone should know about blood pressure. Minneapolis. Halberg Chronobiology Center, University of Minnesota; 2003. 31 pp.

Scheme 2.

A neartransyear of ~1.05-year, presumably previously unknown to physicists, was also found by our chronomics in the changes of the speed of the solar wind and in its proton content and further in biologic variables [37, 38]. Most recent is a far-transyear found as yet in a very small sample of sudden cardiac deaths during the past 5 years in Minnesota and confirmed in Arkansas, Table 1, while a component corresponding to the calendar year is not detected. The transyears in Table 1 rest mostly on linear rhythmometry. Confirmation by the more conservative nonlinear approach awaits the availability of statistics on larger populations over a longer span with the same qualified diagnosis (ICD10 code I46.1). Far-transyears of about 1.3 and about 1.6 years found in human BP and HR are more prominent early and late in extrauterine human life than in young adults, as are about 7-day spectral components [39].

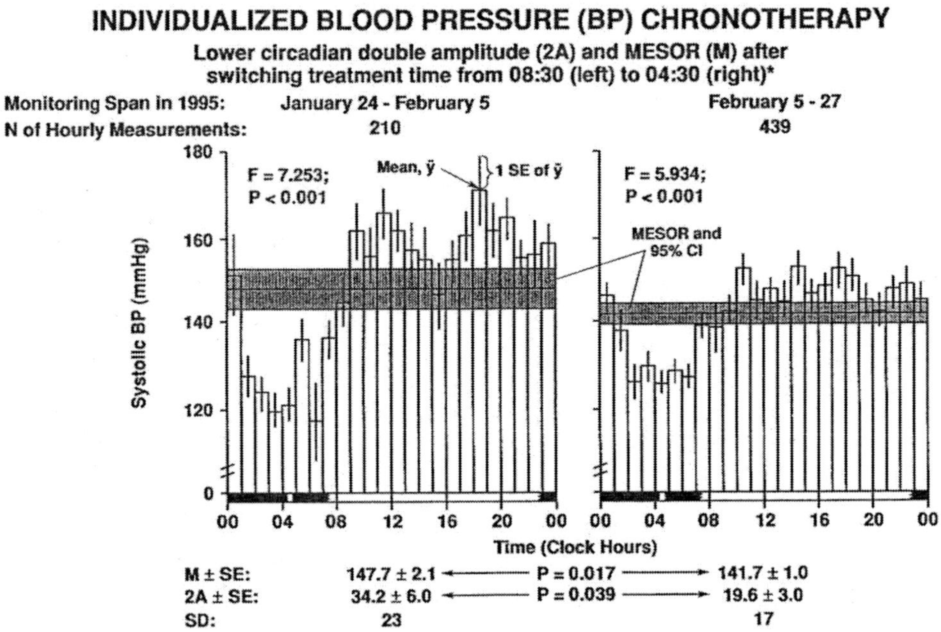

Figure 13a. Both the MESOR and the circadian amplitude of systolic blood pressure decreased when the same dose of the same medication was taken around 04:30 instead of around 08:30 by the same patient. The statistical significance of the effect is validated by parameter testing, an approach applicable to the individual patient for treatment optimization. © Halberg.

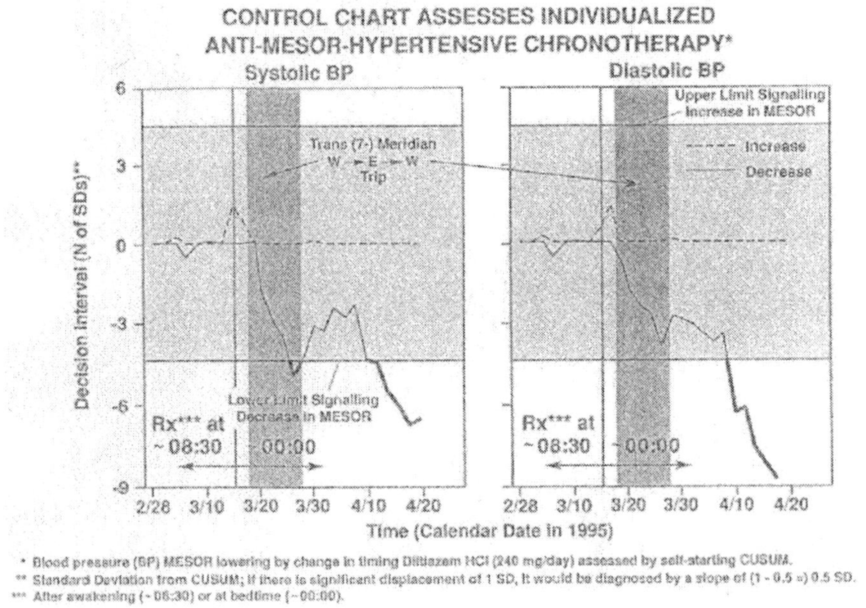

Figure 13b. The MESOR of systolic and diastolic blood pressure is further decreased when the same dose of the same medication is changed from awakening to bedtime in the same patient. The statistical significance of the effect is validated by a cumulative sum control chart. © Halberg.

Much remains to be done on much larger samples with rigorous attention to classification, notably since for myocardial infarction, a spectral component with a period of the calendar year is most prominent and a transyear very small in amplitude by comparison [40]. The winter's excessive cold is known to be a source of MI morbidity [41]. Mortality from MI has recently been investigated in relation to the duration of certain (Pc-1) geomagnetic pulsations, with a 10-100 pT and a 0.5-2.0 Hz frequency matching that of the cardiac cycle.

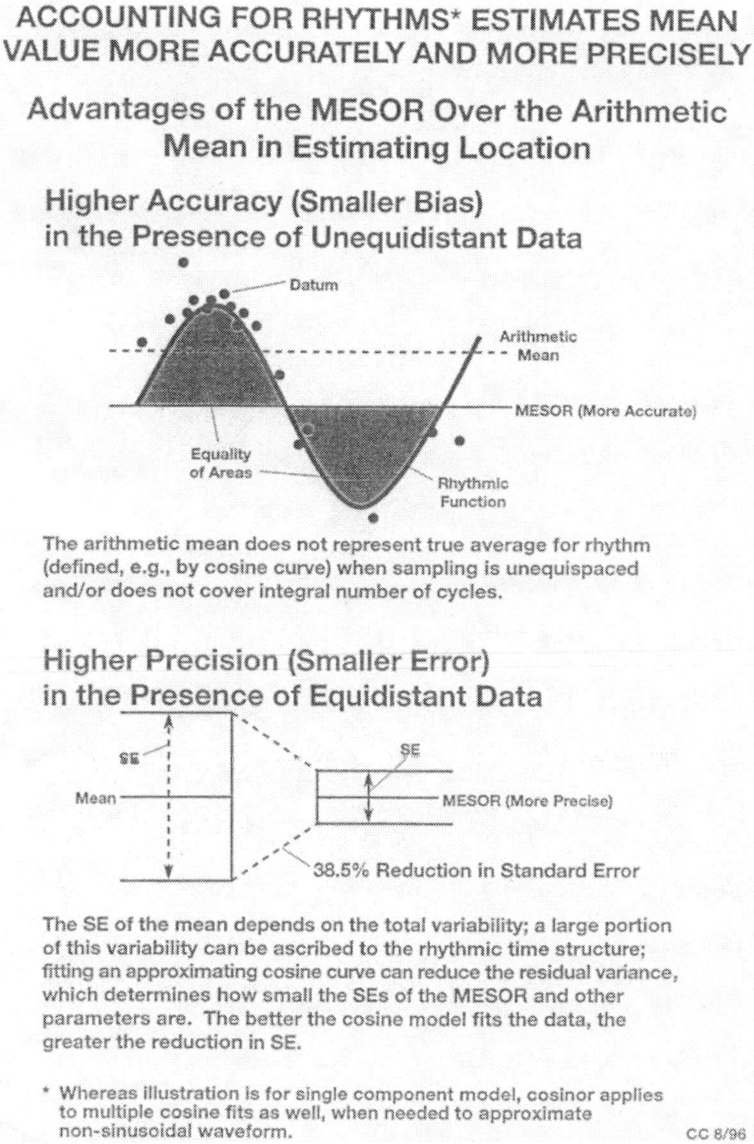

Figure 14. The MESOR, as compared to the arithmetic mean, is usually both more accurate and more precise since it is usually associated with a lesser bias when the data are non-equidistant and with a smaller standard error when the data are characterized by a prominent circadian variation. © Halberg.

Pc-1 pulsations are wave packages with durations of 0.3-1.0 minute at intervals of 1-4 minutes, with a maximal daily duration of about 6 hours [42]. "Pc-1 pulsation[s] are typical for the beginning phase and for the recovery phase of geomagnetic storms". A relation of MI morbidity to magnetic storms was found earlier by superposed epochs [43]. By contrast to a major about-yearly component in 85,819 MIs, it is the more noteworthy that in Table 1, a 1.39-year component constitutes a major spectral peak in a series of sudden cardiac deaths in Minnesota for the past 5 years, while a component corresponding to the calendar year is not detected, the change from warm summers to harsh winters notwithstanding.

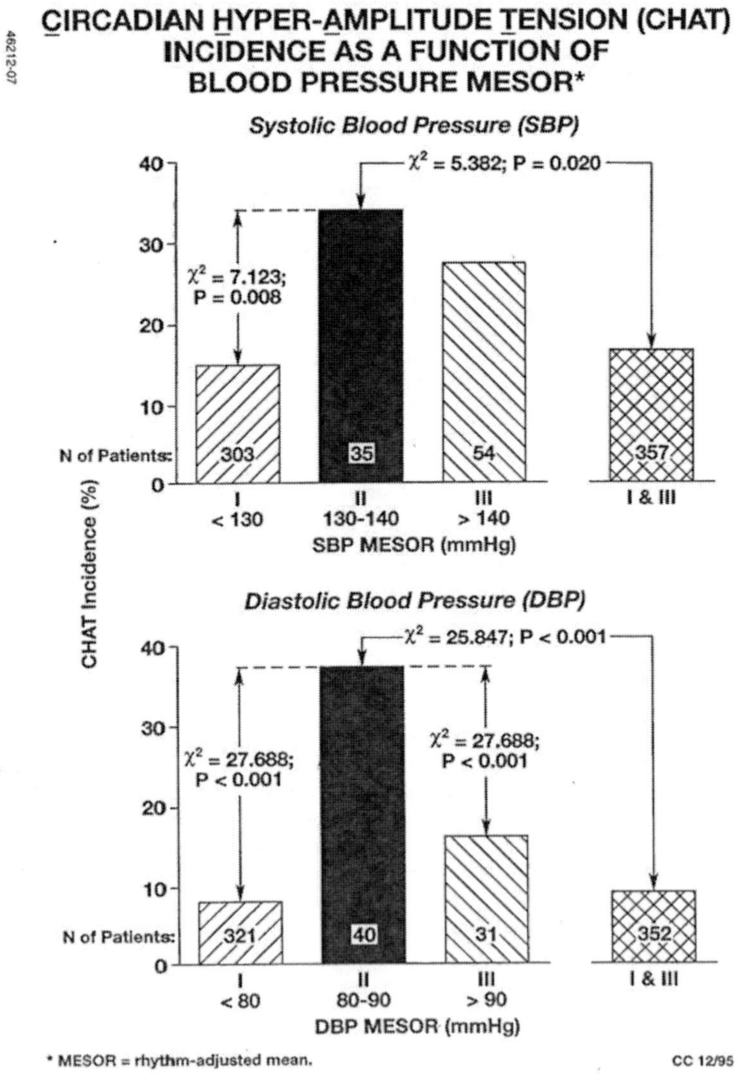

Figure 15a. CHAT (circadian hyper-amplitude-tension) occurs more often in patients with borderline hypertension than in patients with either MESOR-normotension or MESOR-hypertension. It may thus represent a warning sign for the development of later MESOR-hypertension. Judging from longitudinal studies on the SHR-SP rat, it is probably an intermediate, sometimes transient stage in the development of MESOR-hypertension. CHAT can also be observed as a transient stage at the start of anti-hypertensive therapy. © Halberg.

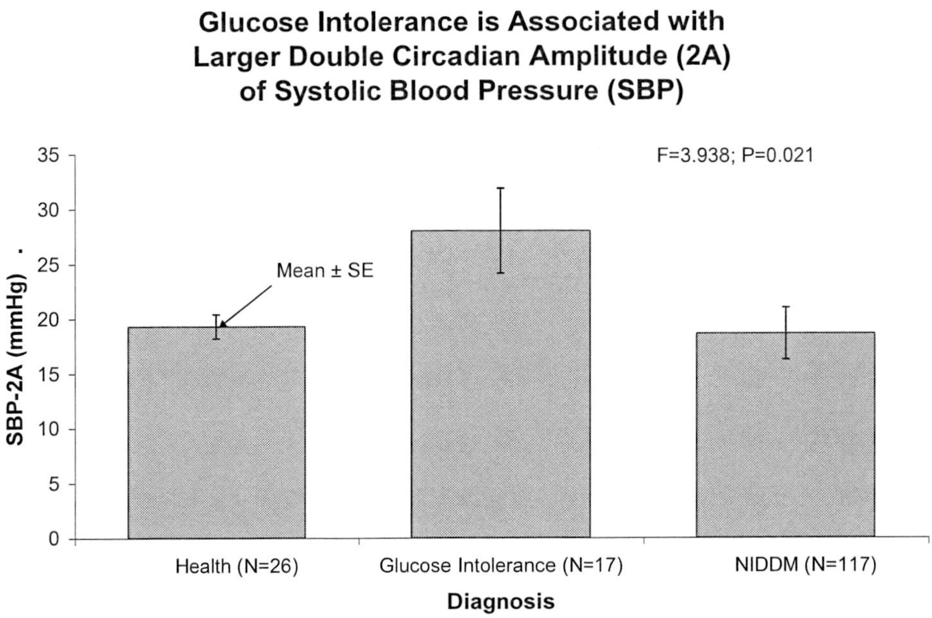

Figure 15b. CHAT occurs more often among patients with glucose intolerance than in healthy subjects or patients with non-insulin dependent diabetes mellitus. In conjunction with the evidence in Figure 15a, CHAT may be an early warning of a developing metabolic syndrome, a pre-metabolic syndrome, leading to MESOR-hypertension, non-insulin dependent diabetes mellitus, obesity and/or dyslipidemia. © Halberg.

Table 1. Fartransyears in Sudden Cardiac Death (SCD¶) in 2 North American Locations* (1999 - 2003)

Site (N data/N cases)	Variable	Linear Analysis		Nonlinear Analysis	
		τ (years)	P	τ (95% CI)	A (95% CI)
Sun (1826/NA)	Wind Speed	1.67	<0.001	1.70 (1.60, 1.80)	31.95 (22.13, 41.76)
Earth (1826/NA)	K_p	1.67	<0.001	1.67 (1.51, 1.83)	0.23 (0.11, 0.35)
Minnesota (MN) (1826/343)	SCD	1.39	0.014	1.39 (1.17, 1.61)	0.04 (0.00, 0.09)
Arkansas (AR) (1826/273)	SCD	1.67	0.043	1.68 (1.29, 2.08)	0.03 (0.00, 0.07)
"	"	1.09	0.045	1.095 (0.935, 1.255)	0.03 (0.00, 0.07)

From the International Classification of Diseases, ICD10 code I46.1 (residents in MN, cause of death in AR, excluding sudden deaths related to pulmonary embolism and cancer of the lung; when including the latter two categories, the about 1.67- and 1.09-year components are not statistically significant in AR).

*To be checked by nonlinear analyses on larger samples (these fail here, with the 95% CI of the A slightly overlapping zero, probably because of the very limited sample size and the brevity of the time series).

K_p: Planetary geomagnetic index; τ: Period; P: P-value (from zero-amplitude test); A: Amplitude (in km/s for the solar wind speed, in arbitrary units for K_p, in average N/day for SCD); 95% CI: 95% confidence interval, when anticipated from prior evidence and predicted by solar wind speed and K_p, to be found in a spectral region; each component fitted separately.

The methods for studying relations among time series have yet to be further developed. Figure 16 shows that phase synchronizations can be detected at multiple frequencies between several unseen environmental variables and a 29-year series of myocardial infarctions in Minnesota. These phase relations are time-varying in terms of their presence or absence and in terms of the frequencies involved. Whether we focus on sudden cardiac death, myocardial infarctions or stroke with a 50-year cycle [44], chronomics represents a method for investigations in the future, yet with immediate applicability in clinical practice.

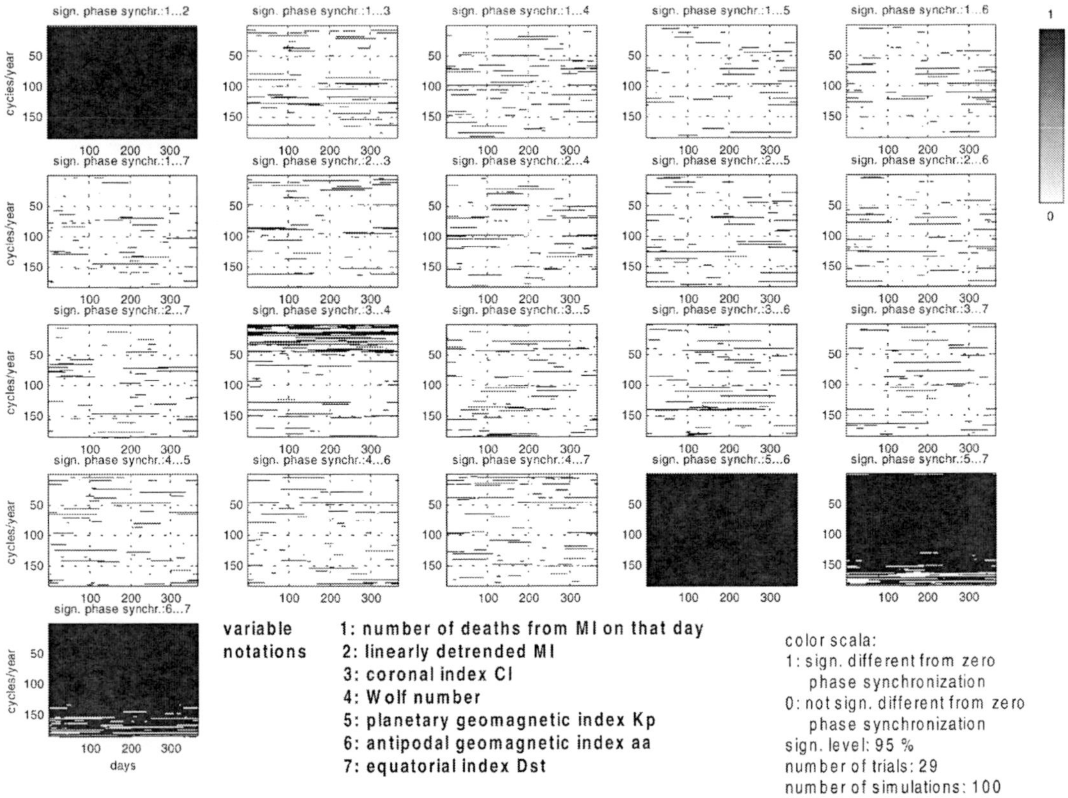

Figure 16. Non-zero time-varying phase synchronization between the daily incidence of mortality from myocardial infarction in Minnesota during 1968-1996 (29 years) and different physical environmental variables, reflecting, among others, the influence of the sun and/or that of geomagnetism, determine any mediating (such as resonating) frequencies at any given time, and assess the extent of consistency of any frequency-dependent effect over time. Black rectangle on top left shows phase synchronization between the original and detrended data on myocardial infarctions, whereas the last three, mostly black rectangles show the also anticipated phase synchronization at most if not all tested frequencies among three geomagnetic indices, anticipated to be closely related. These black rectangles thus constitute a replacement of the "standard" used in chemical determinations along with a series of other inferential statistical precautions (44). © Halberg.

Epilogue

In 1904, Theodore C. Janeway wrote:

> ... *it is essential* that a record of the pressure be made at frequent intervals *at some time previous* [presumably to an examination], to establish the *normal level* and the *extent of the periodic variations.* When this is done, it may be possible to demonstrate changes of small extent, which, lacking this standard for comparison, would be considered within the limits of normal variation (5).

And in 1974, Frederic C. Bartter wrote, in reference to his patient whose blood pressure was diagnosed differently by two physicians who saw him at different times of day [45]:

> By conventional standards, this patient is clearly normotensive every morning. But the blood pressure determined each day at 6 in the afternoon provides especially convincing evidence that this patient is a hypertensive. ...
>
> My plea today is that information contained in [data curves compiled under differing circumstances, such as 24 hours a day/7 days a week] become a *routine minimal amount* of information accepted for the description of a patient's blood pressure. *The analysis of this information by cosinor should become a routine.* It is essential that enough information be collected to allow objective characterization of a periodic phenomenon, to wit, an estimate of M [the time structure or chronome-adjusted mean, or MESOR] ... an estimate of [the amplitude] A itself, and finally an estimate of acrophase, ϕ [a measure of timing]. In this way, a patient can be compared with himself at another time, or under another treatment, and the patient can be compared with a normal or with another patient.

The clinician can now implement via BIOCOS today what was wanted 100 or 30 years ago, both in research and in practice, preferably with governmental support, since just as clean air and water and clean and safe streets are a public concern, so is a safe circulation.

References

[1] Sheps SG, Canzanello VJ. Current role of automated ambulatory blood pressure and self-measured blood pressure determinations in clinical practice. *Mayo Clin. Proc.* 1994; 69: 1000-1005.

[2] Halberg Franz, Cornélissen G, Katinas G, Syutkina EV, Sothern RB, Zaslavskaya R, Halberg Francine, Watanabe Y, Schwartzkopff O, Otsuka K, Tarquini R, Perfetto F, Siegelova J. Transdisciplinary unifying implications of circadian findings in the 1950s. J Circadian Rhythms 2003; 1: 2. 61 pp. www.JCircadianRhythms.com/content/pdf /1740-3391/1/2.pdf

[3] Halberg F, Cornélissen G, Stoynev A, Ikonomov O, Katinas G, Sampson M, Wang ZR, Wan CM, Singh RB, Otsuka K, Sothern RB, Sothern SB, Sothern MI, Syutkina EV, Masalov A, Perfetto F, Tarquini R, Maggioni C, Kumagai Y, Siegelova J, Fiser B, Homolka P, Dusek J, Uezono K, Watanabe Y, Wu JY, Sonkowsky R, Schwartzkopff O, Hellbrügge T, Spector NH, Baciu I, Hriscu M, Bakken E. Season's Appreciations 2002

and 2003. Imaging in time: The transyear (longer-than-the-calendar year) and the half-year. *Neuroendocrinol. Lett.* 2003; 24: 421-440.

[4] Hagen P (ed.) Mayo Clinic Guide to Self-Care: Answers for Everyday Health Problems. Rochester, MN/Jacksonville, FL/Scottsdale, AZ: *Mayo Clinic;* 2003. p. 180-181.

[5] Janeway TC. *The clinical study of blood pressure.* New York: D. Appleton and Co.; 1904. 300 pp.

[6] Günther R, Herold M, Halberg E, Halberg F. Circadian placebo and ACTH effects on urinary cortisol in arthritics. *Peptides* 1980; 1: 387-390.

[7] Halberg F, Bingham C, Cornélissen G. Clinical trials: the larger the better? *Chronobiologia* 1993; 20: 193-212.

[8] Cornélissen G, Halberg F, Prikryl P, Dankova E, Siegelova J, Dusek J, International Womb-to-Tomb Chronome Study Group: Prophylactic aspirin treatment: the merits of timing. *JAMA* 1991; 266: 3128-3129.

[9] Halberg F, Cornélissen G, Otsuka K, Schwartzkopff O, Halberg J, Bakken EE. Chronomics. *Biomedicine and Pharmacotherapy 2001*; 55 (Suppl 1): 153-190.

[10] Bittle CC Jr, Molina DJ, Bartter FC. Salt sensitivity in essential hypertension as determined by the cosinor method. *Hypertension* 1985; 7: 989-994.

[11] Itoh K, Kawasaki T, Cugini P. Effect of timing of salt intake to 24-hour blood pressure and its circadian rhythm. In: Portaluppi F, Smolensky MH (eds.) Time-dependent Structure and Control of Arterial Blood Pressure, *Ann. NY Acad. Sci.* 1996; 783: 324-325.

[12] Stinson SM, Cornélissen G, Scarpelli PT, Halberg F. Self-measurement and ambulatory monitoring of blood pressure: a subject's chronobiological perspective. *Biomed. Pharmacother* 2002; 56 (Suppl 2): 333s-338s.

[13] Halberg F, Cornélissen G, Schack B. Self-experimentation chronomics for health surveillance and science; also transdisciplinary civic duty? *Behavioral and Brain Sciences* 2004; 27 (2): 267-269.

[14] Verdecchia P, Schillaci G, Guerrieri M, Gatteschi C, Benemio G, Boldrini F, Porcellati C. Circadian blood pressure changes and left ventricular hypertrophy in essential hypertension. *Circulation* 1990; 81: 528-536.

[15] Otsuka K, Cornélissen G, Halberg F. Predictive value of blood pressure dipping and swinging with regard to vascular disease risk. *Clinical Drug Investigation* 1996; 11: 20-31.

[16] Calaprice A (ed.) *The Quotable Einstein.* Princeton, NJ: Princeton University Press, 1996, 269 pp.

[17] Halberg F, Cornélissen G, Wall D, Otsuka K, Halberg J, Katinas G, Watanabe Y, Halhuber M, Müller-Bohn T, Delmore P, Siegelova J, Homolka P, Fiser B, Dusek J, Sanchez de la Peña S, Maggioni C, Delyukov A, Gorgo Y, Gubin D, Carandente F, Schaffer E, Rhodus N, Borer K, Sonkowsky RP, Schwartzkopff O. Engineering and governmental challenge: 7-day/24-hour chronobiologic blood pressure and heart rate screening. *Biomedical Instrumentation and Technology* 2002; 36: Part I, 89-122; Part II, 183-197.

[18] Cornélissen G, Bakken E, Delmore P, Orth-Gomér K, Åkerstedt T, Carandente O, Carandente F, Halberg F. From various kinds of heart rate variability to chronocardiology. *Am. J. Cardiol.* 1990; 66: 863-868.

[19] Wood MA, Simpson PM, London WB, Stambler BS, Herre JM, Bernstein RC, Ellenbogen KA. Circadian pattern of ventricular tachyarrhythmias in patients with implantable cardioverter-defibrillators. *J. Am. Coll Cardiol.* 1995; 25: 901-907.

[20] Halberg F, Cornélissen G, Otsuka K, Watanabe Y, Wood MA, Lambert CR, Zaslavskaya R, Gubin D, Petukhova EY, Delmore P, Bakken E. Rewards in practice from recycling heart rate, ectopy, ischemia, and blood pressure information. *J. Medical Engineering and Technology* 1997; 21: 174-184.

[21] Halberg F, Cornélissen G, International Womb-to-Tomb Chronome Initiative Group: Resolution from a meeting of the International Society for Research on Civilization Diseases and the Environment (New SIRMCE Confederation), Brussels, Belgium, March 17-18, 1995: Fairy tale or reality? Medtronic Chronobiology Seminar #8, April 1995, 12 pp. text, 18 figures. http://www.msi.umn.edu/~halberg/

[22] Cornélissen G, Halberg F, Bakken EE, Singh RB, Otsuka K, Tomlinson B, Delcourt A, Toussaint G, Bathina S, Schwartzkopff O, Wang ZR, Tarquini R, Perfetto F, Pantaleoni GC, Jozsa R, Delmore PA, Nolley E. 100 or 30 years after Janeway or Bartter, Healthwatch helps avoid "flying blind". *Biomedicine and Pharmacotherapy* 2004; 58 (Suppl 1): S69-S86.

[23] Watanabe Y, Cornélissen G, Halberg F, Otsuka K, Kikuchi T. Long-acting carteolol lowers circadian and circaseptan blood pressure (BP) amplitude (A) as well as MESOR. Abstract, X National Symposium, Indian Society for Chronobiology, B.J. Medical College, Pune, India, August 21-22, 1995. p. 14-15.

[24] Shinagawa M, Kubo Y, Otsuka K, Ohkawa S, Cornélissen G, Halberg F. Impact of circadian amplitude and chronotherapy: relevance to prevention and treatment of stroke. *Biomedicine and Pharmacotherapy* 2001; 55 (Suppl 1): 125-132.

[25] JNC 7 Express: The Seventh Report of the Joint National Committee on Detection, Evaluation, and Treatment of High Blood Pressure. Bethesda, MD: US Department of Health and Human Services, National Institutes of Health, National Heart, Lung, and Blood Institute, National High Blood Pressure Education Program. NIH Publ. #03-5233, May 2003. 34 + xiii pp.

[26] Halberg F, Smith HN, Cornélissen G, Delmore P, Schwartzkopff O, International BIOCOS Group. Hurdles to asepsis, universal literacy, and chronobiology—all to be overcome. *Neuroendocrinol. Lett.* 2000; 21: 145-160.

[27] Cornélissen G, Halberg F, Hawkins D, Otsuka K, Henke W. Individual assessment of antihypertensive response by self-starting cumulative sums. *J. Medical Engineering and Technology* 1997; 21: 111-120.

[28] Bingham C, Arbogast B, Cornélissen Guillaume G, Lee JK, Halberg F. Inferential statistical methods for estimating and comparing cosinor parameters. *Chronobiologia* 1982; 9: 397-439.

[29] Halberg F, Cornélissen G, Regal P, Otsuka K, Wang ZR, Katinas GS, Siegelova J, Homolka P, Prikryl P, Chibisov SM, Holley DC, Wendt HW, Bingham C, Palm SL, Sonkowsky RP, Sothern RB, Pales E, Mikulecky M, Tarquini R, Perfetto F, Salti R, Maggioni C, Jozsa R, Konradov AA, Kharlitskaya EV, Revilla M, Wan CM, Herold M, Syutkina EV, Masalov AV, Faraone P, Singh RB, Singh RK, Kumar A, Singh R, Sundaram S, Sarabandi T, Pantaleoni GC, Watanabe Y, Kumagai Y, Gubin D, Uezono K, Olah A, Borer K, Kanabrocki EA, Bathina S, Haus E, Hillman D, Schwartzkopff O, Bakken EE, Zeman M. Chronoastrobiology: proposal, nine conferences,

heliogeomagnetics, transyears, near-weeks, near-decades, phylogenetic and ontogenetic memories. *Biomed. Pharmacother.* 2004; 58 (Suppl 1): S170-S186.

[30] Cornélissen G, Halberg F, Schwartzkopff O, Delmore P, Katinas G, Hunter D, Tarquini B, Tarquini R, Perfetto F, Watanabe Y, Otsuka K. Chronomes, time structures, for chronobioengineering for "a full life". *Biomed. Instrum. Technol.* 1999; 33: 152-187.

[31] Kumar A. Metabolic syndrome and CAD: a world overview. Abstract KS1, 3rd Int Congress on Cardiovascular Disease, Taipei, Taiwan, 26-28 Nov 2004. *Int. J. Cardiol.* 2004; 97 (Suppl 2): S3.

[32] Watanabe Y, Cornélissen G, Halberg F, Bingham C, Siegelova J, Otsuka K, Kikuchi T. Incidence pattern and treatment of a clinical entity, overswinging or circadian hyperamplitudetension (CHAT). *Scripta medica* (Brno) 1997; 70: 245-261.

[33] Sanchez de la Pena S, Gonzalez C, Cornélissen G, Halberg F. Blood pressure (BP), heart rate (HR) and non-insulin-dependent diabetes mellitus (NIDDM) chronobiology. Abstract S8-06, 3rd Int Congress on Cardiovascular Disease, Taipei, Taiwan, 26-28 Nov 2004. *Int. J. Cardiol.* 2004; 97 (Suppl 2): S14.

[34] Halberg F, Cornélissen G, Spector NH, Sonkowsky RP, Otsuka K, Baciu I, Hriscu M, Schwartzkopff O, Bakken EE. Stress/strain/life revisited. Quantification by blood pressure chronomics: benetensive, transtensive or maletensive chrono-vasculo-neuro-immuno-modulation. *Biomed. Pharmacother* 2003; 57 (Suppl 1): 136s-163s.

[35] Richardson JD, Paularena KI, Belcher JW, Lazarus AJ. Solar wind oscillations with a 1.3-year period. *Geophys. Res. Lett.* 1994; 21: 1559-1560.

[36] Mursula K, Zieger B. The 1.3-year variation in solar wind speed and geomagnetic activity. *Adv. Space Res.* 2000; 25: 1939-1942.

[37] Halberg F, Cornélissen G, Katinas G, Sampson M, Schwartzkopff O, members of the BIOCOS project, Spector NH, Faraone P, Tomescu S, Hriscu M. In memoriam: Ion Baciu. Mutually supporting neartransyears in solar and terrestrial magnetics, microbial and cell biology, physiology and pathology. In: Cornélissen G, Kenner R, Fiser B, Siegelova J (eds.) *Proceedings, Symposium: Chronobiology in Medicine.* Dedicated to the 85th Anniversary of Professor Franz Halberg. Brno: Masaryk University; 2004. p. 78-86.

[38] Cornélissen G, Masalov A, Halberg F, Richardson JD, Katinas GS, Sothern RB, Watanabe Y, Syutkina EV, Wendt HW, Bakken EE, Romanov Y. Multiple resonances among time structures, chronomes, around and in us. Is an about 1.3-year periodicity in solar wind built into the human cardiovascular chronome? *Human Physiology* 2004; 30 (2): 86-92.

[39] Gubin D, Cornélissen G, Halberg F, Gubin G, Uezono K, Kawasaki T. The human blood pressure chronome: a biological gauge of aging. *In vivo* 1997; 11: 485-494.

[40] Cornélissen G, Halberg F, Richardson JD, Katinas GS, Sothern RB, Watanabe Y, Otsuka K, Minne H, Bakken EE. About 1.3-year Richardson component of solar wind speed detected in human circulation and myocardial infarctions (MI). Abstract, *5th Japanese Annual Conference on Chronocardiology and Hypertension*, Sept. 12, 2003, Sapporo, Japan. Session (3) Ambulatory BP, 27.

[41] Danet S, Richard F, Montaye M, Beauchant S, Lemaire B, Graux C, Cottel D, Marécaux N, Amouyel P. Unhealthy effects of atmospheric temperature and pressure on the occurrence of myocardial infarction and coronary deaths. A 10-year survey: the

Lille-World Health Organization MONICA Project (Monitoring Trends and Determinants in Cardiovascular Disease). *Circulation* 1999; 100: e1-e7.

[42] Kleimenova NG, Obraztsova OI, Ivanova P, Breus TK, Rapoport S. Effects of Pc-1 geomagnetic pulsations on the cardiovascular system. *Presentation, Annual Conference on "Fundamental Sciences in Medicine*", Presidium, Russian Academy of Sciences, Moscow, December 2-3, 2004.

[43] Halberg F, Breus TK, Cornélissen G, Bingham C, Hillman DC, Rigatuso J, Delmore P, Bakken E, International Womb-to-Tomb Chronome Initiative Group. Chronobiology in space. Keynote, 37th Ann. Mtg. Japan Soc. For Aerospace and Environmental Medicine, Nagoya, Japan, November 8-9, 1991. University of Minnesota/Medtronic Chronobiology Seminar Series, #1, December 1991, 21 pp. of text, 70 figures.

[44] Halberg F, Cornélissen G, Otsuka K, Watanabe Y, Katinas GS, Burioka N, Delyukov A, Gorgo Y, Zhao ZY, Weydahl A, Sothern RB, Siegelova J, Fiser B, Dusek J, Syutkina EV, Perfetto F, Tarquini R, Singh RB, Rhees B, Lofstrom D, Lofstrom P, Johnson PWC, Schwartzkopff O, International BIOCOS Study Group. Cross-spectrally coherent ~10.5- and 21-year biological and physical cycles, magnetic storms and myocardial infarctions. *Neuroendocrinol. Lett.* 2000; 21: 233-258.

[45] Bartter FC. Periodicity and medicine. In: Scheving LE, Halberg F, Pauly JE (eds.) *Chronobiology*. Tokyo: Igaku Shoin Ltd., 1974: 6-13.

Support: U.S. National Institutes of Health (GM-13981) (FH), Supercomputing Institute (GC, FH).

"Dedicated, on the occasion of his birthday on June 22, 2008, to Prof. Miroslav Mikulecky, head emeritus of the Department of Internal Medicine and professor of statistics at Comenius University, Bratislava, who beyond extending the scope of cycles longer than a calendar year (transyears) to phenomena as diverse as natality in certain geographic locations, the incidence of stroke and of epilepsy, devoted a lifetime to rigorous inferential statistics in health care and the past decades to document the much neglected effects on human affairs of the moon, the sun and the cosmos."

In: World Heart Research Yearbook. Volume 1
Editors: Franz Halberg and R. B. Singh
ISBN: 978-1-60741-881-8

The Potential Benefits if Saponin from Canadian-Grown Fenugreek *(Trigonella Foenum-Graecum L.)* in Modifying Cholesterol Status

Debangshu Bhaumick[1], Surya Acharya[2] and Tapan K. Basu[1]*
[1]Department of Agricultural, Food and Nutritional Science, University of Alberta, Edmonton, Alberta, Canada
[2]Agriculture and Agri-Food Canada, Lethbridge, Alberta, Canada

Abstract

Background. Saponins are glycosidic steroidal compounds, which are composed of lipid-soluble aglycone (sapogenins) attached to a water soluble sugar molecule (s). There is now substantial body of evidence that dietary saponins can lower serum cholesterol levels. The hypocholesterolemic action is thought to be mediated by inhibiting absorption of cholesterol from the small intestine and reabsorption of bile acids. The present study was undertaken to examine *in vitro* cholesterol- and bile acid-binding capacities of the saponin-rich fraction, which was extracted from seeds of a Canadian-grown fenugreek line (*Trigonella foenum-graecum L.*). *Methods.* Saponin was extracted with ethanol (crude extract) followed by further purification through C-18 Sep-Pak column (purified extract). An *in vitro* binding capacity of either of the extracts to cholesterol and $[C^{14}]$-sodium taurocholic acid was examined. *Results.* The crude extract was found to contain a mixture of saponin, soluble fiber, simple sigar and proteins, while the purified extract contained essentially saponin. The formar contained 24.5 μg/mg and the latter contained 109.1 μg/mg of diosgenin, which is the predominant form of sapogenin in fenugreek seed. Both extracts displayed an appreciable amount of binding capacity to cholesterol, the crude extract having a greater capacity than the purified extract (41.8% vs. 35.4%; $p<0.001$). Unlike cholesterol, the capacity of taurocholic acid to bind crude extract was similar to that of the purified extract. Using the purified extract, however, the binding capacity was found to be the extract concentration-related. *Conclusion.* These results suggest that seeds from fenugreek, grown in Canada, have the ability to bind both cholesterol and bile acid, hence the potential to modify cholesterol metabolism. This is particularly important since a typical Western diet lacks in saponin.

Keywords: Fenugreek seeds; saponin, cholesterol-binding; bile acid-binding

---

* Correspondence should be addressed. Fax: (780) 492-4265; Tel. (780) 492-5338. Email: tapan.basu@ualberta.ca.

INTRODUCTION

Saponins are widely distributed secondary plant metabolites, consisting of steroidal or triterpenoid surface-active glycosides [1]. These compounds can also be produced by lower marine animals and some bacteria [2]. Saponins are composed of a lipid-soluble aglycone (sapogenins), which is usually either a tritepenoid or a steroid molecule. These molecules are glycosidically linked to water-soluble sugar molecule(s), which include glucose, glactose, glucuronic acid, xylose, rhamnose [3]. The complexity of saponin structures and properties arises from the variability of aglycone structure, the type of side chains, and the positions of attachment of sugar moieties on the aglycone. Saponis have the ability to form pores in membranes and that this property is thought to contribute to lytic action on erythrocytes [4-5]. Erythrocytes are thus disrupted in saponin solutions due to interactions with cholesterol in the erythrocyte membrane [6].

Many studies, involving humans and experimental animals, have shown that saponins from different sources lower serum cholesterol levels [7-9]. Diets containing foods rich in saponins (such as soya, chickpea and bean meal) have thus shown to reduce plasma cholesterol by 16-24% [10-11]. In rats, fed diets containing saponins from fenugreek [12], Soya [13] and chickpea [14] have all shown to modify lipid status. Such effects were observed both in the presence and absence of dietary cholesterol [15]. The hypercholesterolemic activity of dietary saponins is believed to form complex with dietary cholesterol, which is thereby unavailable for absorption [14]. According to an *in vitro* study saponins increase the permeability of intestinal mucosal cells, inhibit active mucosal transport, and facilitate uptake of substances that are normally not absorbed (J16).

The consumption of saponin rich foods increase the excretion of bile acid [17-18]. They form insoluble complexes with 3-ß-hydroxysteroids and thereby contribute to large mixed micelles with bile acids and cholesterol. The ability of saponins to prevent absorption of cholesterol via binding cholesterol and bile acids has made saponins to be of immense interest in relation to their potential to be hypocholesterolemic agents.

Fenugreek (*Trigonella foenum-graecum L.*) is an annual dicotyledon plant belonging to the family Papilionaceae Leguminasae and is thought to originate in Asia. In Indian sub-continent, the seeds are used in spice mixtures and as a condiment and hence constitute an important ingredient in chutney and spice blends [19]. The leaves are also commonly consumed as vegetables. In Egypt the seeds are either eaten as raw after sprouting or are used to make confection following roasting, grinding and cooking with triticale and sesame seeds [20]. The seeds of Asian fenugreek variety have been found to contain steroidal saponins mainly in the form of diosgenin, which comprised approximately 5-6% of the seed [20]. Hypocholesterolemic effects of the alcoholic extracts of Mediterranean and Asian fenugreek seeds and also of purified saponins derived from these seeds have been reported in both *in vitro* and *in vivo* studies [21-23]. In recent years, fenugreek has been adapted for cultivation in a Canadian province, Alberta. Unlike the Asian varieties and Asian-grown seed, the potential hypocholesterolemic effect of the Canadian adopted fenugreek seed has never been studied. The present study was undertaken to develop a simple and convenient method for the extraction of saponin from seeds of fenugreek, grown in Canada. Using this extract the study was further extended to examine its *in vitro* binding capacities with cholesterol and bile acids, indicating the hypocholesterolemic potential of the fenugreek saponin.

MATERIALS AND METHODS

Fenugreek Seed

The seed of Amber fenugreek (a cultivar grown for condimant market) was obtained from Agriculture and Agri-Canada Research Centre, Lethbridge, Alberta. They were ground, dried at room temperature for 72h, and then stored in polythene bags at -20^0C.

Extraction of Fenugreek Seeds

The ground seeds were best de-fatted with hexane and petroleum ether. It was found that for the extraction of saponins from the defatted seeds, 80% ethanol was the most suitable solvent when used with agitation at 60^0C. The C18 Sep-Pak column was found to be economical and easy way to use for the purification of the extract to obtain concentrated saponins. The schematic representation of the extraction and purification process of saponins is shown in Figure 1.

The filtered and dried ethanolic extract of fenugreek seeds containing saponin, soluble fibers, simple sugars and other polar compound like proteins, is referred to "crude extract", while the extract following its purification through C18 Sep-Pak column is referred to "purified extract".

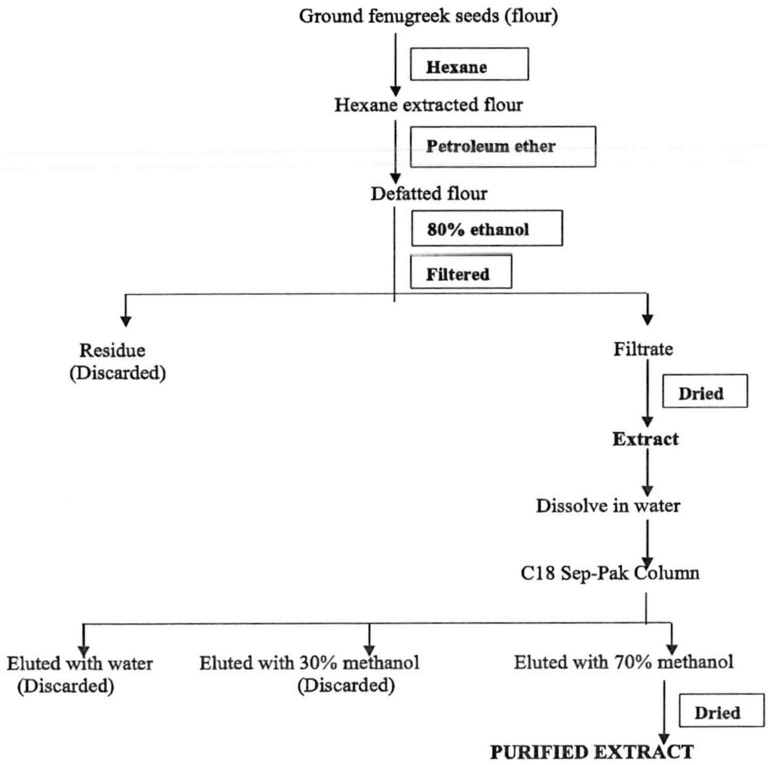

Figure 1. Extraction process of saponins from fenugreek seeds.

Cholesterol-Binding Capacity

The cholesterol-binding capacity of crude and purified extracts was determined by using the method described by Cayen and Dvornik [24]. A cholesterol solution (mg/ml) was prepared by dissolving cholesterol in ethanol-ether (1:1, v/v). Solutions (4 mg/ml) of either extract or purified extract were made by dissolving in ethanol-ether (1:1, v/v). The cholesterol and the extract solutions were mixed (1:1, v/v), incubated at room temp overnight, centrifuged, and subsequently the cholesterol content with and without the test compound was measured colorimetrically. The difference in cholesterol content with or without the binding agent indicated the amount of precipitated cholesterol.

Bile Acid-Binding Capacity

Different concentrations (1-8 mg/ml) of fenugreek extracts were prepared by dissolving in water. Labeled bile acid (^{14}C sodium taurocholic acid) solution was prepared in phosphate buffer (20uM, pH 6.5). A mixture of the labeled bile acid and the fenugreek extracts (1:1, v/v) was prepared, incubated at 37^{0}C for 1h, centrifuged, and subsequently the filtrate was used for scintillation count (Fisher Scientific, Canada). A control was also run maintaining the same experimental conditions without adding the extracts. The DPM counts were considered as the counts for the free bile acid.

RESULTS

The crude extract of fenugreek seeds displayed more binding capacity to cholesterol than the purified extract (44.83% vs. 35.38%), as shown in Figure 2. On the other hand, both the crude and the purified extracts showed an appreciable amount of binding capacity with labelled 14C Na-taurocholic acid (Figure 3).

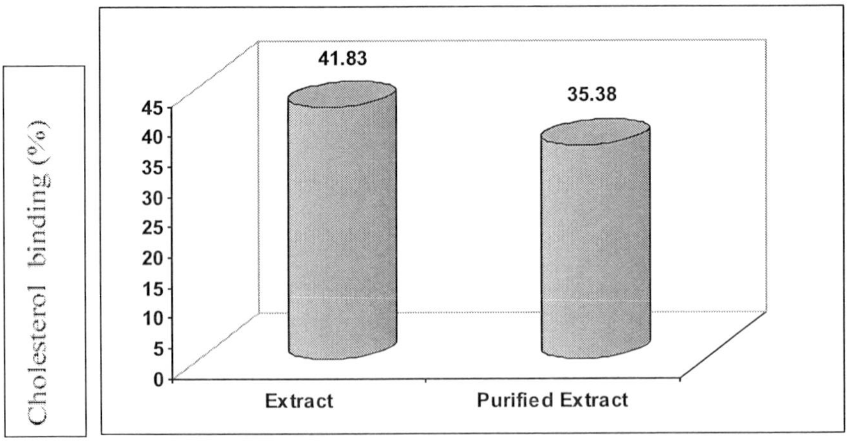

Figure 2. *In vitro* effects of fenugreek extracts on cholesterol-binding capacity.

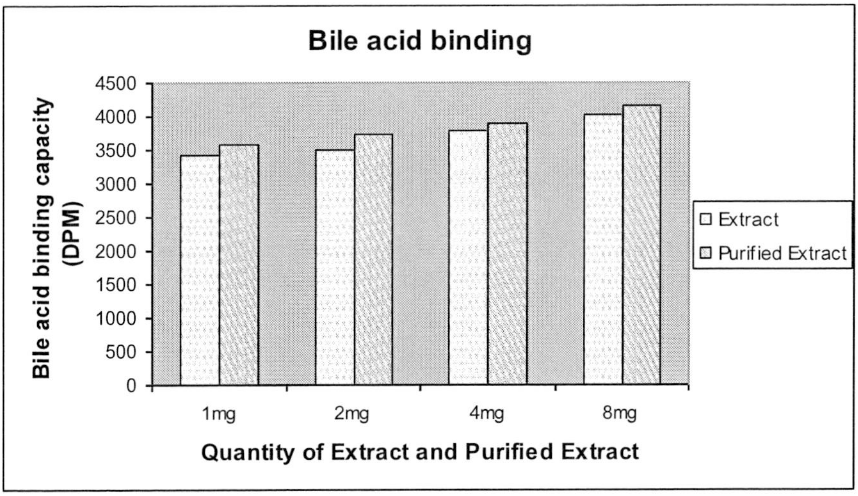

Figure 3. The dose-response effect of fenugreek extracts on the binding capacity (dpm) of ^{14}C sodium taurocholic acid *in vitro*.

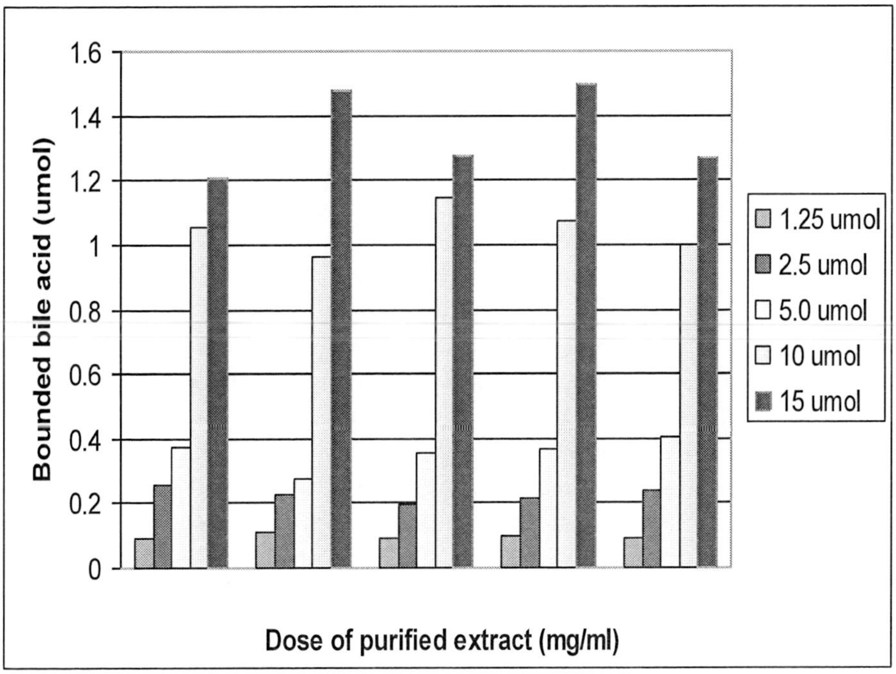

Figure 4. The *in vitro* binding capacity of 'purified extract' of fenugreek to different concentrations of taurocholic acid.

The latter was found to be related to the doses of the extracts (1 – 8 mg). Using the 'purified extract', the dose-response effect of the bile acid (1.25 – 15.0 μmol) was also examined. The magnitude of bile acid-binding to the fenugreek extract was increased with increasing concentrations of taurocholic acid (Figure 4).

DISCUSSION

The ability of fenugreek seed to modify cholesterol metabolism has been well recognized. It decreases total cholesterol, LDL-cholesterol and triglyceride levels without altering HDL –cholesterol concentrations [12]. Using an ethanol extract of fenugreek seeds containing saponin-rich isolate has been shown to have the cholesterol lowering property in hypercholesterolemic rats [21]. In the present study, saponin was, for the first time, extracted from Canadian-grown fenugreek seeds with ethanol, followed by further purification through C-18 Sep-Pak column. The dried ethanolic extract (crude extract) was found to contain a mixture of saponin, soluble fiber, simple sugar, and proteins, while the 'purified extract' contained essentially higher concentration of saponin (unpublished observation). The diosgenin (a predominant form of sapogenin in fenugreek seed) content in crude as well as in purified extracts was found to be 25 and 109 μg/mg, respectively. Both fractions of fenugreek displayed an appreciable amount of *in vitro* binding capacities to bile acid and cholesterol. Overall, the 'purified extract' had no added significance to the 'crude extract' fraction, which is relatively a simpler and economical process to be extracted. These results suggest that the dried ethanolic extract of Canadian-grown fenugreek seed has the ability to bind both cholesterol and bile acid, and hence the potential to modify cholesterol metabolism. The results also suggest that the binding capacity is not limited to saponin but to other components, which are present in the 'crude extract' fraction of fenugreek.

Based upon the *in vitro* evidence Based upon the in vitro evidence provided in this study, it is plausable that the underlying mechanism for cholesterol-lowering effect of saponins of Canadian-grown fenugreek seeds may be carried out via binding to dietary cholesterol and thereby preventing its absorption through binding to bile acids. The latter is supposed to interfere with the enterohepatic circulation of cholesterol and thereby increasing its fecal excretion [25]. Increased bile acid excretion by causing compensatory increase in bile acid synthesis from cholesterol in the liver can also, lower plasma cholesterol. Ginseng saponins have been shown to decrease cholesterol and triglycerides in rats and rabbits by sustaining lipoprotein lipase at a normal level or protecting LPL activity from being decreased by many factors, such as chemically induced hyperlipidemia or a high glycerol/fructose diet [26]. Saponins are anti-nutrient factors present in fenugreek. These factors appear to modify blood cholesterol status, and blood glucose, which might be even more beneficial in the context of high ω-3 and antioxidant diets [27].Singh et al [27], reported that fenugreek seeds may have antioxidant activity which poses the possibility that saponins may inhibit proinflammatory cytokines as well as protect beta cells of pancreas which are highly susceptible to damage due to free radical stress. Increased consumption of fenukgreek seeds or addition of saponins to diets rich in w-3 fatty acids, may provide a dietary regimen which may serve as wild food and protect against cardiovascular disease and diabetes [28].

ACKNOWLEDGMENT

This study was supported by grants received from the AVAC Ltd.

REFERENCES

[1] Yoshiki Y, Kudou S, and Okubo K. Relationship between chemical structures and biological activities of triterpenoid saponins from soybean (Review). *Biosci. Biotech. and Biochem.* 1998; 62: 2291 – 2299.

[2] Riguera R. Isolating bioactive compounds from marine organisms. *J. Marine Biotech* 1997; 5: 187-193.

[3] Fransis F, Kerem Z, Makkar HPS, et al. The biological action of saponins in animal systems: a review. *Br. J. Nutr.* 2002; 88: 587-605.

[4] Baumann E, Stoya G, Volkner A, et al. Hemolysis of human erythrocytes with saponin affects the membrane structure. *Acta Histochemica* 2000; 102: 21-35.

[5] Plock A, Sokolowska-Kohler W, Presber W. Application of flow cytometry and microscopical methods to characterize the effect of herbal drugs on *Lysimachia vulgaris* L. *Experimental Parasitology* 2001; 97: 141-153.

[6] Birk Y, Peri I . Saponins. In: *Toxic Constutuents of Plant Foodstuffs*, edited by Liener IE, Academic Press, New York, 1980; pp. 161-182.

[7] Harwood HJ Jr, Chandler CE, Pellarin LD, et al. Pharmacological consequences of cholesterol absorption inhibition: alteration in cholesterol metabolism and reduction in plasma cholesterol concentration induced by the synthetic saponin ß-tigogenin cellobioside (CP-88818; tiqueside). *J. Lipid Res.* 1993; 34: 377-395.

[8] Potter SM, Jimenez-Flores R, Pollack J, et al. Protein saponin interaction and its influence on blood lipids. *J. Agric Food Chem.* 1993; 41: 1287-1291.

[9] Matsuura M. Saponins in garlic as modifiers of the risk of cardiovascular disease. *J. Nutr.* 2001; 131: 1000S-1005S.

[10] Sharma RD. Effect of fenugreek seeds and leaves on blood glucose and serum insulin responses in human subjects. *Nutr. Res.* 1986; 6: 1353-1364.

[11] Thompson LU. Potential health benefits and problems associated with antinutrients in foods. *Food Res. International* 1993; 26: 131-149.

[12] Sharma RD, Raghuram TC. Hypoglycemic effect of fenugreek seeds in non-insulin dependent diabetic subjects. *Nutr. Res.* 1990; 10: 731-739.

[13] Oakenfull DG, Topping DL, Illman RJ, et al. Prevention of dietary hypercholesterolemia in the rat by soybean and quillaya saponins. *Nutr. Rep. Int.* 1884; 25: 1039-1046..

[14] Malinow MR, McLaughlin P, Papworth L, et al. Effect of alfalfa saponins on intestinal cholesterol absorption in rats. *Am. J. Clin. Nutr.* 1977; 30: 2061-2067).

[15] Rao AV, Kendall CW. Dietary saponins and serum lipids. *Food Chemistry and Toxicology* 1986; 24: 441-443.

[16] Johnson IT, Gee JM, Price K, et al. Influence of saponins on gut permeability and active nutrient transport in vitro. *J. Nutr.* 1986; 116: 2270-2277.

[17] Oakenfull DG. Aggregation of bile acids and saponins in aqueous solution. *Aust. J. Chem.* 1886; 39: 1671-1683.

[18] Oakenfull DG, Sidhu GS. Could saponin be useful treatment for hypercholesterolemia? *Euro J. Clin. Nutr.* 1990; 44: 79-88.

[19] Patil SP, Niphadkar PV, Bhat MM. Allergy to fenugreek (*Trigonella foenum graecum*). Ann Allergy *Asthma Immunol.* 1997; 78:297-300.

[20] Al-Habori M, Raman A. Antidiabetic and hypocholesterolemic effects of fenugreek. *Phytotherapy Res* 1998; 12: 233-242.

[21] Stark A, Madar Z. The effect of an ethanol extract derived from fenugreek (Trigonella foenum-graecum) on bile acid absorption and cholesterol levels in rats. *Br. J. Nutr.* 1993; 69: 277-287.

[22] Petit PR, Sauvaire YD, Hillaire-Buys DM, et al. Steroid saponins from fenugreek seeds: Extraction, purification and pharmacological investigation on feeding behavior and plasma cholesterol. *Steroids* 1995; 60: 674-680.

[23] Xue WL, Li XS, Zhang J, et al. Effect of Trigonella foenum-graecum (fenugreek) extract on blood glucose, blood lipid and hemorheological properties in streptozotocin-induced diabetic rats. *Asia Pac. J. Clin. Nutr.* 2007; 16(suppl 1): 422-426.

[24] Cayen MN, Dvornik D. Effect of diosgenin on lipid metabolism in rats. J Lip Res 1979; 20: 162-174.

[25] Sidhu GS, Oakenful DG. A mechanism for hypocholesterolemic activity of saponins. *Br. J. Nutr.* 1986; 55: 643-649.

[26] Inoue M, Wu CZ, Dou DQ, et al. Lipoprotein lipase activation by red ginseng saponins in hyperlipidemic model animals. *Phytomedicine* 1999; 6: 257-265.

[27] Singh RB, Niaz MA, Rastogi V, et al. Hypolipidemic and antioxidant effects of fenugreek seeds and triphala, as adjuncts to dietary therapy, in patients with mild to moderate hypercholesterolemia. *Perfusion* 1998; 11: 124-130.

[28] DeMeester F, Wild-type land based foods in health promotion and disease prevention: the LDL-CC:HDL-CC model. In *Wild Type Foods in Health Promotion and Disease Prevention*, editors Fabien DeMeester and RR Watson, Humana Press, NJ 2008,p 3-20.

In: World Heart Research Yearbook. Volume 1
Editors: Franz Halberg and R. B. Singh
ISBN: 978-1-60741-881-8

CAN WILD WHOLE SEEDS PROTECT AGAINST CARDIOVASCULAR DISEASE?

Viola Mechirova[1], Ram B. Singh[,2], Fabien DeMeester[3], Ronald R. Watson[4], Lekh Juneja[5], Jan Fedacko[1] and Daniel Pella[1]*

[1]Faculty of Medicine, Safaric University, Kosice, Slovakia
[2]Halberg Hospital and Research Institute, Moradabad, India
[3]Columbus Paradigm Institute, Waterloo, Belgium
[4] College of Public Health, University of Arizona, Tuscon, AZ, US
[5]Taiyo Kagaku, Yokkaichi, Japan

Katcher and co-workers' study on whole grains appears to be of great interest [1].

Whole-grain foods appear to be protective against cardiovascular disease (CVD) including acute coronary syndromes (ACS)[2]. However, no guidelines exist for administration of such foods in ACS patients. Katcher and co-workers have very nicely demonstrated that a whole grain-enriched hypocaloric diet may be superior to refined grain foods in decreasing risk of CVD in patients with metabolic syndrome [1]. However, no consideration has been given to w-6/w-3 fatty acid ratio of the two diets, which could have been the important factor in decreasing inflammation [2-5]. Wild whole seeds rich in w-3 fatty acids, antioxidants and magnesium may provide even better results compared to whole grain grown by modern farming.

Prior to the Agricultural Revolution, our diet was based on wild seeds, plants, eggs, fish and meat from wild animals, whereas today, the greatest percentage of food supply is contributed by refined cereal grains, refined carbohydrates and meat from supplemented farm sources. These foods are rich in w-6 fatty acids and low in w-3 fatty acids, fiber, phytoestrogens, minerals and antioxidants. CVD, diabetes mellitus, obesity, cancer, autoimmune diseases, rheumatoid arthritis, asthma and depression are associated with increased production of thromboxane A2(TXA2), leucotrienes, protacyclin, interleukins-1 and 6, tumor necrosis factor-alpha and C-reactive proteins. Increased dietary intake of w-6 fatty acids is known to enhance all these risk factors as well as atherogenicity of cholesterol which have adverse proinflammatry effects resulting into thrombosis and ACS [2-7].

ACS may be due to thrombosis in the unstable plaque, and may be associated with activation of neurohormones and proinflammatory cytokines, resulting into neuroendocrine dysfunction, which worsens the prognosis in these patients [8-10]. There also may be

* E-mail: drkk@dataone.in.

oxidative stress, hyperglycemia, hyperinsulinemia, hypertriglyceridemia, increased levels of catecholamines, free fatty acids and cortisol.

Recent studies [2-5, 8-10), indicate that eating high fat, refined carbohydrate rich fast foods (Western diet), can produce a similar proinflammatory state in our body. It increases oxidative stress, free fatty acids and triglycerides, resulting into endothelial dysfunction, which may have adverse effects in patients with ACS. It is therefore, logical to avoid Western diet in patients with ACS, and to administer Indo-Mediterranean foods, beneficial to vascular endothelium and myocardium [2-5, 8-10]. There is no precise and proven guideline for dietary advice for patients with ACS to protect against recurrent cardiac events. A Columbus soup (tomatoes, grapes, vegetables, walnuts, almonds + lin/chia seeds and olive oil) or yogurt containing, walnuts, almonds, raisins, could be prepared for nonpharmacological intervention among patients of ACS. These foods appear to be protective against metabolic syndrome [2]. Recipes have been commonly used in our studies and clinical practice [2-5, 8-10]. For prevention of metabolic syndrome, or ACS, we recommend eating 400g/day of fruits and vegetable and another 400g/day of legumes and other whole grains, and 50g/day of almonds and walnuts, in conjunction with 25-50g/day of Columbus oil(olive oil 88 %+ flax seed oil 12.0%) P:S = w-6:w-3 = 1:1 (Patent Application WO2005020698). Increased physical activity to control sedentary behavior is important in urban and affluent populations for prevention of metabolic syndrome and ACS as part of Columbus lifestyle [2]. Apart from designer foods and lifestyle changes, drug therapy with fibrates, statins, coenzyme Q10, w-3 fatty acids, ACE-inhibitors, beta blockers, metformin and glitozones may be useful for prevention and treatment of metabolic syndrome in w-6 fatty acid rich dietary environment.

In one study [11], among 54 patients with ACS, the control subjects (n=85) were randomly selected from the population. Increased consumption of trans fatty acids (TFA) (>5g/day) was significantly greater among ACS patients compared to controls (50.0 vs. 0.0%, n=27 vs. 0). Large meals (>1000 Kcal) (50.0 vs. 29.4%, n=27 vs. 25) and large breakfast (40.7% vs. 11.8%, n=22 vs. 10), rich in TFA, linoleic acid, saturated fat and refined carbohydrates and poor in whole grains intakes were also significantly ($p<0.02$) greater among patients, compared to control subjects. Metabolic syndrome was noted among half of the ACS patients.

Serum levels of nitrite (an indicator of nitric oxide, NO) were significantly lower in patients with ACS, compared to controls (mean+SD:0.36+1.42 vs. 0.96+1.48uM, CI difference 0.60,0.34-1.02,$p<0.03$).Serum levels of vitamins E, C and beta-carotene, coenzyme Q10,magnesium and potassium were significantly lower and insulin, glucose, triglycerides, and lipoprotein(a), TNF-alpha, and IL-6 were significantly higher in ACS, compared to their levels after 4 weeks of follow up. Nitrite deficiency as a risk factor for heart attack has been emphasized in recently [12].

In India ACS, diabetes and hypertension are more common among higher social classes compared to lower social classes, possibly due to lower fat intake and enormous occupational physical activity in lower social classes. *What are the social class differences in the western subjects? (delete).*

However, it would be very interesting to know the role of refined starches and sugar, large meals, decreased intake of fruits, vegetables, whole grains and nuts and serum nitrite levels as risk predictors of ACS. Fruits, vegetables, nuts, whole grains, animal foods rich in w-3 fatty acids are slowly absorbed and may prevent the increase in free fatty acids, and inflammation, which is a characteristic of Columbus foods (www.columbus-concept.com).

Therefore such foods may decrease the risk in ACS as well as metabolic syndrome [2,5,8].Omega-3 fatty acids can regulate leptin gene expression and the concentrations of anandamides in the brain, which in turn binds to endogenous cannabinoid receptors and regulate food intake and satiety and weight gain. International College of Cardiology is developing guidelines to include wild foods in the prevention of ACS.

REFERENCES

[1] Katcher HI, Legro RS, Kunselman AR et al. The effects of whole grain- enriched hypocaloric diet on cardiovascular disease risk factors in men and women with metabolic syndrome. *Am. J. Clin. Nutr.* 2008, 87:79-90.

[2] Singh RB, DeMeester F, Mechirova V, Pella D, Otsuka K. Fatty acids in the causation and therapy of metabolic syndrome. In *Wild Type Foods in Health Promotion and Disease Prevention*, editors Fabien DeMeester and RR Watson, Humana Press, NJ 2008,p 263-284.

[3] Harris WS, Reid KJ, Sands SA, et al. Blood omega-3 and trans fatty acids in middle aged acute coronary syndrome patients. *Am. J. Cardiol.* 2007;99:154–158.

[4] Singh RB,Dubnov G,Niaz MA,Ghosh S,Singh R,Rastogi SS,Manor O,Pella D,Berry EM. Effect of an Indo-Mediterranean diet on progression of coronary disease in high risk patients: a randomized single blind trial. *Lancet* 2002,360:1455-1461.

[5] Harper CR,Jacobson TA. Usefulness of omega-3 fatty acids and the prevention of coronary heart disease. *Amer. J. Cardiol.* 2005,96:1521-29.

[6] Ailhaud G, Massiéra F, Weill P, Legrand P, Alessandri JM, Guesnet P. Temporal changes in dietary fats: role of n-6 polyunsaturated fatty acids in excessive adipose tissue development and relationship to obesity. *Prog. Lip. Res.* 2006;45:203-236.

[7] Rolland-Cachera MF, Maillot M, Deheeger M, Bellisle F. Prediction of adult adiposity using two indicators: a 20 year follow-up study. *Int. J. Obes.* 2006;30:S12.

[8] Singh RB,Rastogi SS, Verma R et al. An Indian experiment with nutritional modulation in acute myocardial infarction. *Am. J. Cardiol. 1992, 69: 879-883.*

[9] Singh RB, Niaz MA, Kartik C.Can n-3 fatty acids provide myocardial protection be decreasing infarct size and inhibiting atherothrombosis? *Eur. Heart J.* 2001;3(Suppl. D)62-69.

[10] Singh RB,Pella D,DeMeester F..What to eat and chew in acute myocardial infarction. *Eur. Heart J.* 2006, 27:1628-29.

[11] Singh RB,Pella D,Sharma JP et al.Increased concentrations of lipoprotein(a), circadian rhythms and metabolic reactions, evoked by acute myocardial infarction in relation to large breakfast. *Biomed. Pharmacother.* 2004;58(Suppl.): 116-21.

[12] Maher AR, Milsom AB, Gunaruwan P, Abozguia K, Ahmad I,Weaver RA, Thomas P, Ashrafian H, Born GVR, James PE, Frenneaux MP. Hypoxic-modulation of exogenous nitrite-induced vasodilation in humans. *Circulation* 2008: 117: 670-677.

In: World Heart Research Yearbook. Volume 1
Editors: Franz Halberg and R. B. Singh

ISBN: 978-1-60741-881-8

Reducing Cardiovascular Disease Risk through Management of Hyperglycemia: Prospects and Pitfalls

*N. A. Abdella**
Departments of Medicine, Faculty of Medicine
Kuwait University, Kuwait

Abstract

A global epidemic of type 2 Diabetes exists and in the near future it may be closely associated with an epidemic of cardiovascular disease. Both diabetes mellitus and cardiovascular disease are major problems and among the diabetic population, the two problems taken together constitute a "double jeopardy".

Control of hyperglycaemia became an important target as proven by studies like the Diabetes Control Complications Study and the United Kingdom Prospective Diabetes Study (UKPDS).

At first review of some of the available oral antidiabetic agents with a focus on Sulphonylureas and the recently documented selectivity as regards their mechanism of action on the potassium ATP channels that completely mimicked the pre-conditioning phenomena, moreover, blocking these channels with some of the sulphonylurea compounds abolished this protective effect.

Metformin is currently, the most extensively used oral antidiabetic agent worldwide. Its use as monotherapy offers several advantages : improvement of insulin sensitivity and blood lipid profile. Based on UKPDS, metformin monotherapy in overweight diabetic subjects was the only arm of the study showing a significant reduction in cardiovascular events and overall mortality.

Thiazolidinediones are a relatively new class of agents that enhance insulin sensitivity in the liver, adipose tissue and muscles without affecting insulin secretion. There are still some controversial issues about the benefits of Thiazolidinediones on vascular function that might reduce cardiovascular risk.

There are on-going studies on the role of conventional and intensive insulin therapy in type 2 diabetes mellitus and its possible effect on cardiovascular disease and mortality. Recently the "Diabetes mellitus, Insulin Glucose Infusion in Acute Myocardial Infarction Study Group (DIGAMI-2)" in contrast to the DIGAMI-1 study showed no beneficial

* Corresponding Author: Dr. Nabila Abdella, Department of Medicine, Faculty of Medicine Kuwait University, Kuwait.Telephone: 965 531 9596 Fax : 965 533 8907Email : nabdella12@yahoo.com.

effect of insulin treatment in myocardial infarction patients. Patients on oral antidiabetic agents including Sulphonylureas had similar prognosis to those on insulin therapy.

There is some speculation on the role of intensive insulin therapy in stabilizing macrovascular disease or preventing progression in those already at risk.

The large-scale clinical trials in type 2 diabetes mellitus support the fact that lowering blood glucose significantly lowers the risk of diabetic complications. Quality of life studies performed as part of the UKPDS showed that allocation to different treatment did not in itself have an effect on quality of life.

The risks and benefits of a HbA1c goal of < 7% are currently being tested in an ongoing study Action to Control Cardiovascular Risk in Diabetes (ACCORD) which will show the efficacy of reducing cardiovascular risk factors in preventing or slowing cardiovascular disease. The American Diabetes Association recommends that targets of management should include blood pressure control, treatment of dyslipidaemia, aspirin therapy and cessation of smoking. Emphasis should be put on reducing cardiovascular risk factors as a main goal in addition to treating hyperglycaemia in subjects with type 2 diabetes mellitus.

INTRODUCTION

Type 2 Diabetes (DM) is a modern age epidemic that exists and in the near future it may be closely associated with an epidemic of cardiovascular disease (CVD). In the last decade the number of people with diabetes have risen sharply and a continued increase is projected, which will lead to a global prevalence of diabetes in excess of 220 million by 2010 [1]. Increases in both type 1 and type 2 DM have been observed in all societies studied in the last 30 years [2]. Type 2 DM accounts for most of the current and forecasted figures. In developing countries Type 2 DM is occurring with increasing frequency in younger people [3,4]. Of particular concern is the worldwide emergence of type 2 DM in the very young, including children and also adolescents [5]. This downward shift in the age at which DM develops has serious implications for the development of complications, in particular CVD which is more likely to develop at an earlier age. Both DM and CVD are major problems and among the diabetic population the two problems taken together constitute a "double jeopardy". The complex link between DM and CVD is based on a combination of insulin resistance state, hyperglycaemia and dyslipidaemia. Dysfunction of the endothelial cell monolayer leads to increased vascular tone and permeability and a prothrombotic environment. The poor outcome of CVD among diabetic compared to non-diabetic put an important focus on Type 2 DM treatment in relation to CVD and its outcome.

Control of hyperglycaemia became an important target as proven by studies like the Diabetic Control Complications study (DCCT) [6] and the United Kingdom Prospective Diabetes Study (UKPDS) [7]. The majority of studies that have evaluated the link between blood glucose levels and mortality among the population of people with DM find a positive, significant association [8].

Many prospective observational studies have found associations between hyperglycaemia and coronary artery disease [9]; stroke [10]; peripheral vascular disease [11] and lower extremity amputations [12]. Measures of glycaemia by fasting plasma glucose and HbA1C have been independently associated with death from macrovascular disease [13].

Having defined the magnitude of the problem of Type 2 DM and its close relationship to CVD disease there is definite evidence of the role of glycaemia control in prevention of diabetes – related macrovascular complications. It is clear that long term glycaemic control, best reflected by HbA1C levels, is an important factor in microvascular complications, as is already well established and also in myocardial infarction and cerebro vascular accident [6,7].

Therefore, antidiabetic treatment should be aimed at obtaining the best possible metabolic control.

- How then to achieve control of hyperglycaemia with groups of drugs with minimal effect on cardiovascular risks among the diabetic subjects?
- Does Sulphonylurea treatment of Type 2 DM contribute to the cardiovascular risk?

Historically, the concern about the safety of Sulphonylureas (SUs) dates back to 1970 when the UGDP [14] concluded that tolbutamide treatment caused increased cardiovascular mortality, a study which at the time led to curtailment of oral antidiabetic treatment in the USA, but was received with skepticism in Europe. Later criticism of its methodology reduced the impact of the study. However, the question of the safety of SUs in type 2 diabetic patients with CHD has been reopened because of new experimental data. SUs has been prescribed by three generations of diabetologists. SUs provided alternative therapy to insulin for type 2 diabetes. However, despite their relatively long use it is only recently that the mechanism of action of this therapeutic class of drugs at molecular level has been clearly understood. SUs stimulate insulin secretion in type 2 diabetic patients by blocking ATP-sensitive K^{+}_{ATP} channels in the pancreatic β-cell membrane by binding to the SU receptor (SUR1) subunit of the channel. K^{+}_{ATP} channels are also present in a range of extrapancreatic tissues, but may contain alternative types of SUR subunit (SUR2A in heart and SUR2B in smooth muscle) The SU sensitivity of K^{+}_{ATP} channels varies with the type of SUR subunit: thus, gliclazide and tolbutamide potently block the β-cell (SUR1), but not the cardiac (SUR2A) or smooth muscle (SUR2B) types of K^{+}_{ATP} channel. In contrast, glibenclamide and glimepiride block all three types of K^{+}_{ATP} channel with similar potency. Therefore, administration of SU compound such as glibenclamide that has a K^{+}_{ATP} -channel-blocking effect should be expected to increase ischaemic damage and abolish the protective action of channel openers.

It is known from, in vitro, as well as in vivo studies that activation of K^{+}_{ATP} channels constitutes an important cardioprotective mechanism against ischemic damage. Since the discovery of K^{+}_{ATP} channels in the heart, numerous investigators have evaluated their role in cardiac adaptation to ischaemic insults. The high levels of ATP in the normal cardiomyocyte probably keep most K^{+}_{ATP} channels in the closed state [15], but these are opened when the level is lowered thereby leading to multiple changes in cardiac metabolism, electrical activity and mechanical function, which results from ischemia. Soon after the onset of ischaemia, activation of outward flow of K+ currents through the K^{+}_{ATP} channels results in earlier repolarization of the myocyte and shortening of the action potential, which leads to a reduction of calcium influx through voltage-gated calcium channels [16-19]. The resulting decrease in contractility protects the ischaemic cardiomyocyte by reducing its oxygen demand. In addition, opened arterial wall K^{+}_{ATP} channels during ischaemia decrease the vascular resistance, thus increasing coronary blood flow [20,21]. Another consequence of ischaemia is intracellular accumulation of adenosine derived from the breakdown of ATP, which may leak out from cells and activate plasma membrane-A1 receptors in an autocrine manner, thus leading to opening of K^{+}_{ATP} channels [22, 23]. Adenosine has been suggested to be a major cardioprotective agent; it seems to mediate its effect through a variety of mechanisms, including direct vasodilatory and anti-arrhythmic actions, attenuation of the heart response to sympathetic stimuli, inhibition of platelet aggregation, and reduction of free radical formation [24-26]. The latter may be especially important in the protection against post-infarct reperfusion injury, believed to be caused by the burst of free radicals on reoxygenation.

Brief episodes of ischaemia render the heart more resistant to subsequent ischemic events, with marked reduction in infarct size and contractile dysfunction [27,28]. This phenomenon called ‘ischaemic preconditioning’, operates in most species including man [29, 30]. Activation of K^{+}_{ATP} channels completely mimicked the preconditioning, moreover, blocking the channels with antagonists such as glibenclamide abolished the protective effect of preconditioning [31, 32]. Adenosine also seems to be important for preconditioning: short-term infusion of adenosine reduced the extent of myocardial necrosis in dogs with the same efficiency as preconditioning, the effect being mediated through a K^{+}_{ATP} channel related mechanism, blocked by glibenclamide pretreatment [33,34]. Preconditioning is not limited to the heart, it is probably a major protective mechanism in many other tissues.

The other effects of SUs on cardiovascular risk factors should be taken into consideration, namely lowering lipid levels. It has been shown that SUs lowers plasma total cholesterol, total triglyceride, VLDL cholesterol, LDL cholesterol and apolipoprotein B [35]. In some [36] but not all studies [37] HDL cholesterol was lower in patients treated with insulin, despite comparable glycaemic control. Most of these investigations were conducted with gliclazide. In addition, gliclazide has been shown to inhibit thrombus formation, improve fibrinolysis and reduce platelet adherence and aggregation [38].

The UKPDS study [7] recruited 3,867 newly diagnosed type 2 diabetic patients into a multi-centre randomized controlled trial that sought to compare the effects of intensive blood glucose control (with SUs or insulin) with conventional treatment (diet) on risk of microvascular or macrovascular complications in diabetes. A total of 1,138 patients and 2,729 patients were, respectively, assigned conventional and intensive treatment in 23 centers in the UK. The study end-points were: diabetes-related death and all-cause mortality. The results suggested that intensive blood glucose control significantly decreased the risk of microvascular, but not macrovascular disease in patients with type 2 diabetes. There was no particular adverse cardiovascular risk with SUs or insulin. It would therefore appear that the potential advantage of SUs in modulating hyperglycaemia far outweighs any theoretical risk from a postulated increased liability to macrovascular disease.

Recently the GUIDE – Study (Glucose control in type 2 diabetes: Diamicron MR versus Glimepiride) [39] showed almost identical efficacy of both drugs in improving diabetes long term control, irrespective of the patients previous antidiabetic treatment (ie diet alone or metformin or α-glucosidase inhibitors). The safety of Diamicron MR (Gliclazide MR) was significantly better demonstrating about 50% less hypoglycaemic episodes in comparison with Glimepiride.

More recently the UKPDS investigators looked at case fatality in DM. Results clearly show that there is no difference in terms of myocardial infarction case fatality between those taking SUs (alone or in combination) and those not taking SUs.

This is a very important and reassuring finding, bearing in mind the millions of patients treated for years with SUs. Some previous publications [14] suggested that patients treated with SUs had a higher MI fatality than those not taking SUs, which created a number of difficulties in therapeutic decision making.

METFORMIN

This is currently the most extensively used oral agent for type 2 diabetes worldwide. Metformin has a variety of metabolic effects; it acts partly by improving insulin action and partly by effects that are not directly insulin dependent. Reduction of excessive hepatic glucose production is thought to be the principal mode of action. At the cellular level, metformin can improve insulin sensitivity by increasing the insulin stimulated tyrosine kinase signaling activity of the insulin receptor. Signaling is also increased through the enhanced activity of a range of post-receptor insulin-signaling pathways. Monotherapy with Metformin offers several advantages such as improvement of insulin sensitivity and blood lipid profile, thus plasma concentrations of triglycerides, free fatty acids and low density LDL-cholesterol tend to fall, while high density HDL– cholesterol tends to rise.

Based on the UKPDS [40] patients who started antidiabetic therapy with Metformin showed a reduced risk of myocardial infarction of 39% after 10 years. In addition to effects on body weight and lipid profile, several others potentially vasoprotective effects, including increased fibrinolysis and a reduced plasminogen activator inhibitor 1 (PAI-1) concentration has been reported. As monotherapy or in combination with other antidiabetic agents or insulin, Metformin, offers great benefits to diabetic subjects with CHD but precaution should be taken in gross congestive cardiac failure in addition to renal function impairment.

Metformin monotherapy in overweight diabetic subjects was the only arm of the UKPDS study [40] showing a significant reduction in CV events and overall mortality.

THIAZOLIDINEDIONES

Thiazolidinediones (TZD) are a relatively new class of agents that enhance insulin sensitivity in the liver, adipose tissue and muscles without affecting insulin secretion. Their site of action is believed to be mediated through selective activation of peroxisome proliferators-activated receptor gamma (PPAR Gamma), a nuclear receptor that plays an important role in adipogenesis [41]. The efficacy of TZD has been shown in multiple clinical trials [42, 43]. Obese and hyperinsulinaemic individuals are more likely to respond than those who have insufficient insulin. A significant disadvantage of the combination of TZDs and SUs is the associated weight gain that can be as high as 6.5 kg after one year of therapy. When TZDs are used as monotherapy a modest increase in body weight is observed [44].

As regards TZD effects related to CVD both LDL and HDL cholesterol tend to increase and serum triglyceride level may decrease with pioglitazone but not with rosiglitazone. While rosiglitazone has a pure PPAR gamma agonist activity, pioglitazone has in addition some PPAR alpha activity that may account for its effect on lowering serum triglyceride level.

TZDs are not recommended in patients with New York Heart Association (NYHA) class III or IV congestive heart failure as TZDs can lead to fluid retention and subsequent plasma volume expansion [45,46].

There are still some controversial issues about the benefits of TZDs on vascular function, which might reduce cardiovascular risk, as well as on the production of some inflammatory cytokines and its effects on transforming monocytes to macrophages in the vascular wall. The precautions related to heart disease, oedema, anemia and liver function include intermittent monitoring.

Exogenous Insulin Administration and Cardiovascular Risk in Type 2 Diabetes Mellitus

A progressive β-cell failure is a characteristic feature of type 2 DM based on the evidence in Type 1 DM treatment. Early epidemiological studies [8,9] reported insulin as an independent risk factor for cardiovascular disease. The 5-year follow-up analysis of the Helsinki Policemen Study [47] supported the hypothesis that high circulating level of insulin is related although probably indirectly to an increased incidence of complications of atherosclerosis such as myocardial infarction and angina pectoris. A current controversial issue is whether intensive insulin treatment of diabetes decreases the risk for cardiovascular complications by lowering glucose levels or increases the risk by postulated direct atherogenic effects of high circulating levels of exogenous insulin.

A growing number of investigators believe that the high circulating serum insulin level is simply a marker for the insulin-resistant state and therefore does not have a direct role in the pathogenesis of atherosclerosis. Although some in vitro experiments and animal models of atheroma formation have shown that high insulin level leads to accelerated plaque formation [48,49], clinical evidence does not exist as yet. A substantial amount of indirect data suggests that hyperglycaemia may have a causal role in atheroma formation [50,51] and may have a prothrombic effect on the coagulation cascade [52]. Improved glycaemic control has been shown to lower low-density lipoprotein cholesterol levels [53,54], which theoretically should lower the risk of developing CHD for patients with diabetes. Prospective epidemiologic studies [55] that had analyzed the relationship between the fasting blood glucose level or $HbA1_c$ level and the risk of CHD showed a linear association between worsening glycaemic control and an increased risk of CHD, although Singer et al. disagreed [13]. In the most compelling study, the Wisconsin Epidemiological Study of Diabetic Retinopathy, investigators analyzed cause-specific mortality over a 10-year period and found that death due to CHD was much more common in patients with worse glycaemic control (relative risk, 1.10 for each 1% increase in HbA1c; 95% confidence interval, 1.07-1.17) [56] than in others. In 3 randomized controlled trials of glycaemic control in type 2 diabetes, a sufficient number of cardiovascular events were recorded to make meaningful comparisons between treatment groups [57,58,59]. Too few events were recorded in the Kumamoto study [57] because of the exclusion of patients with hypertension, hypercholesterolemia and obesity. In the University Group Diabetes Program (UGDP) [58], no significant difference was found in the rate of myocardial infarction between the intensive and conventional treatment groups (20.6 vs. 20.2%, respectively, $p=1.00$), despite a much higher prevalence of cardiaovascular risk factors in the intensive treatment group. A shorter study, 'Diabetes mellitus, Insulin Glucose Infusion in Acute Myocardial Infarction Study Group (DIGAMI-1) [59], tested the hypothesis that intensive metabolic treatment with insulin glucose infusion followed by multidose insulin treatment in patients with diabetes mellitus and acute myocardial infarction improved the prognosis. The authors concluded that insulin treatment in diabetic patients with acute myocardial infarction improved long term survival by nearly a third, and the effect seemed to last for at least 3.5 years. Much more importantly, the absolute reduction in mortality was 11%, implying one saved life for 9 patients treated according to the insulin glucose infusion protocol. The reduction in mortality was most apparent in patients without previous insulin treatment and at a low cardiovascular risk. In contrast to the DIGAMI-1 study, in the DIGAMI-2 study, there was no beneficial effect of insulin treatment in myocardial infarction patients. Patients on oral antidiabetics, including SUs, had a similar prognosis to those on insulin treatment. But it was again confirmed that glucose level is a strong independent predictor of long-term mortality in patients with type 2 diabetes following myocardial infarction [60]

When all major CV and peripheral vascular events were combined in the DCCT, intensive therapy was found to reduce the risk of macrovascular disease by 41% (from 0.8 to 0.5 events per 100 patient-year), but the difference was not significant [61]. In addition, intensive therapy was associated with small but significant reductions in the development of hypercholesterolaemia and hypertriglyceridaemia [61]. Lawson et al [62] reviewed randomized controlled trials of intensive insulin therapy (IIT) in type 1 DM, the meta analysis demonstrated that IIT significantly decreased the total number of macrovascular events but had no significant effect on the number of subjects developing macrovascular disease or on macrovascular mortality. The authors speculate that IIT may stabilize macrovascular disease or prevent progression in those already already at risk. Although the authors conclude that long term prospective studies are needed to confirm these data and fully understand the effect of IIT on macrovascular disease in individuals with type 1 DM they also appropriately point out that future trials of IIT versus conventional therapy would seem to be unethical in patients with type 1 DM, given the positive effects of IIT on microvascular complications. Thus, the answer to this question may never to be more definitely answered.

CONCLUSION

The benefits of intensive glycaemic management do not come without risks. Essentially all of the studies of intensive therapy in type 1 DM for the prevention of microvascular and neuropathic complications demonstrated an increase of hypoglycaemia associated with intensive treatment.

The meta analysis by Egger et al [63] identified 26 deaths among patients with type 1 diabetes, 15 among those receiving intensive therapy and 11 among those receiving conventional therapy (OR 1.40, 95% CI 0.65-3.01). This analysis confirmed a non significant reduction in cardio-vascular mortality among intensive treated patients (OR 0.42, 95% CI 0.13-1.40).

Similar to the DCCT [64,65] results, the UKPDS [66] showed that intensive therapy included an increased risk of hypoglycaemia and increase in both weight, particularly among patients randomized to insulin. Weight gain was no greater in the metformin group than in the diet-controlled group. Quality of life studies performed as part of the UKPDS showed that allocation to different treatment did not in itself have an effect on quality of life.

A common problem in clinical practice is that monotherapy with oral agents either fails initially or fails over time. This important clinical observation was confirmed in the UKPDS. In order to achieve an optimal outcome, multiple drug therapy or a combination of oral agents and insulin is often needed. An important question that needs to be explored is whether triple oral therapy when used to avoid insulin use in particular in the elderly diabetic subject has any potential advantages over insulin therapy alone. When using such a regimen, one should consider the high cost of therapy and possible increased adverse events as a result of drug interactions.

This latter concern is very legitimate when dealing with a frail population with multiple coexisting medical conditions and where polypharmacy is common. Further studies are needed to evaluate the advantages and disadvantages of triple or quadruple oral therapy and its impact on the quality of life when compared with insulin monotherapy.

The large scale trials in type 2 DM, UKPDS [66],The Stockholm Diabetes Intervention Study (SDIS) [67], the Steno type 2 randomized study [68] support the fact that lowering blood glucose is an effective mean to lower the risk of diabetic complications. The UKPDS [66] and the Kumamoto study [57] show beyond doubt a significant risk reduction for microvascular complications with improved glycaemic control.

The UKPDS [66] results show that intensive blood glucose control was associated with a risk reduction of CVD but that the p value was 0.052. While this result is on the margin of statistical significance, the clinical significance is likely to be high; in part because the degree of risk reduction is so closely in line with what would have been expected from observational studies. The risk reduction associated with Metformin for CVD was very impressive possibly reflecting benefits from Metformin beyond those strictly related to glucose lowering.

The problem of defining the goals of glycaemic control is still under study as more stringent goals (i.e; a normal $HbA_1C<6\%$) can be considered in individual patients based on epidemiological analysis that suggest that there is no lower limit of Hb A_1C at which further lowering does not reduce risk of complications, at the risk of increased hypoglycaemia. The risks and benefits of a HbA_1C goal of <6% are currently being tested in an on going study ACCORD (Action to Control Cardiovascular Risk in Diabetes) [69].

Elevated post challenge (2-h OGTT) glucose has been associated with increased CV risk independent of fasting plasma glucose in some epidemiological studies. There are now pharmacological agents (for example Repaglinide) that primarily modify postprandial glucose and thereby reduce HbA_1C in parallel.

However, the effect of post prandial glycaemic control on micro or macrovascular complications has not been studied. Having discussed earlier the risks and benefits of therapy in its different form with particular re-assurance from the literature on prescribing SUs to type 2 diabetic subjects with CVD and the UKPDS results with Metformin in conclusion the focus should be on global management of cardiovascular risk factors among the diabetic population.

Studies have shown the efficacy of reducing cardiovascular risk factors in preventing or slowing CVD. Based on the American Diabetes Association recommendations management should also include blood pressure control [70], treatment of dyslipidaemia [71] aspirin therapy [72] and cessation of smoking [73].

Emphasis should be put on reducing cardiovascular risk factors as a main goal in addition to treating hyperglycaemia in subjects with type 2 DM.

REFERENCES

[1] Amos AF, McCarty DJ, Zimmet P: The rising global burden of diabetes and its complications: estimates and projections to the year 2010. *Diabet Med* 1997; 14(Suppl 5): S7-85.

[2] Gruber W, Leese B, Songer T, Williams R (eds): The economics of diabetes and diabetes care. *IDF and WHO*1997; Brussels, Belgium.

[3] King H, Aubert RE, Herman WH: Global burden of diabetes, 1995-2025: prevalence, numerical estimates and projections. *Diabetes Care* 1998; 21: 9.

[4] Onkano P, Vaananen S, Karvonen M, Tuomilehto J: Worldwide increase in incidence of type 1 diabetes – the analysis of the data on published incidence trends. *Diabetologia* 1999; 42: 1395-1403.

[5] Fagot-Campagna A : Emergence of type 2 diabetes mellitus in children: epidemiological evidence. *J. Paediatr. Endocrin. Metab.* 2000; 13: 1395-1402.

[6] The Diabetes Control and Complications: Trial Research Group: The effect of intensive treatment of diabetes on the development and progression of long term complications in insulin-dependent diabetes mellitus. *N. Engl. J. Med.* 1993; 329: 977-986.

[7] UK Prospective Diabetes Study (UKPDS) Group: Intensive blood glucose control with sulphonylurea or insulin compared with conventional treatment and risk of complications in patients with type 2 diabetes (UKPDS 33). *The Lancet* 1998; 352: 837-865.

[8] Eschwege E, Richard JL, Thibult N, et al: Coronary heart disease mortality in relation with diabetes blood glucose and plasma insulin levels: The Paris Prospective Study, ten years later. *Horm. Metab. Res.* (Suppl) 1985; 41-46.

[9] Welborne TA, Wearne K: Coronary heart disease and Cardiovascular mortality in Busselton with reference to glucose and insulin concentrations. *Diabetes Care* 1979; 2: 154-160.

[10] Nielsen NV, Ditzel J: Prevalence of macro- and Microvascular disease as related to glycosylated hemoglobin in type 1 and 2 diabetic subjects: an epidemiologic study in Denmark.. *Horm. Metab. Res.* (Suppl.)1985; 15:19-23.

[11] Adler A, Stevens R, Neil H, Holman R, Turner R: Hyperglycaemia and other potentially modificable risk factors for peripheral vascular disease in type 2 diabetes. *Diabetic Medicine* 1999; 16:16.

[12] Lehto S, Ronnemaa T, Pyörälä K, Laakso M: Risk factors predicting lower extremity amputations in patients with NIDDM. *Diabetes Care* 1996; 19:607-612.

[13] Singer DE, Nathan DM, Anderson KM, Wilson PW, Evans JC : Association of HbA1c with prevalent cardiovascular disease in the original cohort of the Framingham Heart Study. *Diabetes* 1992; 41: 202-208.

[14] University Group Diabetes Program: A study of the effects of hypoglycemic agents on vascular complications in patients with adult- onset diabetes. V1. Supplementary report on non fatal events treated with tolbutamide. *Diabetes* 1976; 25:1129-1152.

[15] Noma A: ATP-regulated K^+_{ATP} channels in cardiac muscle. *Nature* 1983; 305: 147-148.

[16] McPherson C, Pierce G, Cole W: Ischemic cardioprotection by ATP-sensitive K^+ channels involves high energy phosphate preservation. *Am. J. Physiol.* 1993; 265: H1809-H1818.

[17] Lee C : Gating mechanisms of ATP sensitive potassium channels:implication in reperfusion injury and preconditioning. *Cardiovasc. Res.* 1994; 28: 729-734.

[18] Gross GJ, Yao Z, Pieper GM, Auchampach JA: The ATP-regulated potassium channel in ischemia-reperfusion injury. *Ann. N. Y. Acad. Sci.* 1994; 723: 71-81.

[19] Sanguinetti MC : Modulation of potassium channels by antiarrhythmic and hypertensive drugs. *Hypertension.* 1992; 19:228-236.

[20] Brayden JE : Hyperpolarization and relaxation of resistance arteries in response to adenosine diphosphate. *Circ. Res.* 1991;69:1415-1420.

[21] Daut J, Maier-Rudolph W, von Beckerath N, Mehrke G, Gunther K, Goedel-Meinen L: Hypoxic dilatation of coronary arteries is mediated by ATP-sensitive potassium channels. *Science* 1990; 247:1341-1344.

[22] Auchampach JA, Gross GJ: Adenosine A1 receptors, K_{ATP} channels and ischemic preconditioning in dogs. *Am. J. Physiol.* 1993; 264: H1327-H1336.

[23] Kirsch GE, Codina J, Birnbaumer L, Brown AM : Coupling of ATP-Sensitive K^+ channels to A1 receptors by G proteins in rat ventricular myocytes. *Am. J. Phsiol.* 1990; 259:H820-H826.

[24] Wainwright CL, Parrat JR: An antiarrhythmic effect of adenosine during myocardial ischemia and reperfusion. *Eur. J. Pharmacol.* 1988 ; 145: 183-194.

[25] Belardinelli L, Linden J, Berne RM: The cardiac effects of adenosine. *Prog.Cardiovasc. Dis.* 1989; 32: 73-97.

[26] Smits P, Lenders JWM, Willemsen JJ, Thien T: Adenosine attenuates the response to sympathetic stimuli in man. *Hypertension* 1991; 18: 216-223.

[27] Murray CE, Jennings RB, Reimer KA : Preconditioning with ischemia : a delay of lethal cell injury in ischemic myocardium. *Circulation* 1986; 74:1124-1136.

[28] Fralix TA, Steenbergen C, London RE, Murphy E: Glibenclamide does not abolish the protective effect of preconditioning on stunning in the isolated perfused rat heart. *Cardiovasc. Res.* 1993; 27: 630-637.

[29] Schulz R, Rose J, Heusch G : Involvement of activation of ATP-dependent potassium channels in ischemic preconditioning in swine. *Am. J. Physiol.* 1994; 267:H1341-H1352.

[30] Tomai F, Crea F, Gaspardone A, et al : Ischemic preconditioning during coronary angioplasty is prevented by glibenclamide, a selective ATP-sensitive K+ channel blocker. *Circulation* 1994; 90: 700-705.

[31] Gross G, Auchampach J: Blockade of ATP- sensitive potassium channels prevents myocardial preconditioning in dogs. *Circ. Res.* 1992; 70:223-233.

[32] Kubota I, Yamaki M, Shibata T, Ikeno E, Hosoya Y, Tomoike H: Role of ATP-sensitive K^+ channels on ECG ST segment elevation during a bout of myocardial ischemia. A study on epicardial mapping in dogs. *Circulation* 1993; 88: 1845-1851.

[33] Downey JM, Liu GS, Thornton JD: Adenosine and anti-infarct effects of preconditioning. *Cardiovasc. Res.* 1993; 27:3-8.

[34] Yao Z, Gross GJ: A comparison of adenosine-induced cardioprotection and ischemic preconditioning in dogs. Efficacy, time course, and role of K_{ATP} channels. *Circulation* 1994 ; 89:1229-1236.

[35] Taskinen MR, Beltz WF, Harper I, et al: Effects of NIDDM on very low-density lipoprotein triglyceride and apolipoprotein B metabolism : studies before and after sulfonylurea therapy. *Diabetes* 1986; 35:1268-1277.

[36] Calvert GD, Graham JJ, Mannik T, Wise PH, Yeates RA : Effects of therapy on plasma high-density-lipoprotein-cholesterol concentration in diabetes mellitus. *Lancet* 1978;2:66-68.

[37] Huupponen RK, Viikari JS, Saarimaa H : Correlation of serum lipids with diabetes control in sulfonylurea-treated diabetic patients. *Diabetes Care* 1984; 7:575-578.

[38] Colwell JA : Pathophysiology of vascular disease in diabetes: effects of gliclazide. *Am. J. Med* .1991;90 (suppl 6A): 505-545.

[39] Schernthaner G, Grimaldi A, Di Mario U, Drzewoski J, Kempler P, Kvapil M, Novials A, Rottiers R, Rutten GE, Shaw KM: GUIDE study: double-blind comparison of once-daily gliclazide MR and glimepiride in type 2 diabetic patients. *Eur. J. Clin. Invest.* 2004;34(8):535-542.

[40] UKPDS Group: Effect of intensive blood glucose control with metformin on complications in overweight patients with type 2 diabetes (UKPDS 34). *Lancet* 1998; 352: 854-865.

[41] Day C : Thiazolidinediones: a new class of antidiabetic drug. *Diabetic Med* 1999; 16:1-14.

[42] Evans AJ, Krentz AJ: Recent developments and emerging therapies for type 2 diabetes mellitus. In: Krentz AJ, Ed. Drug treatment of type 2 diabetes. *Auckland: Adis International*, 2000; 1-22.

[43] Howlett HCS, Bailey CJ: A risk-benefit assessment of metformin in type 2 diabetes mellitus. In: Krentz AJ, Ed. Drug treatment of type 2 diabetes. *Auckland: Adis International*, 2000; 61-76.

[44] Murphy E, Nolan JJ: Insulin sensitizer drugs. *Exp. Opin. Invest. Drugs* 2000; 9:1347-1361.

[45] Schoonjans K, Auwerx J: Thiazolidinediones: an update. *Lancet* 2000; 355:1008-1010.

[46] Spiegelman BM : PPARγ: adipogenic regulator and Thiazolidinedione receptor. *Diabetes* 1998; 47:507-514.

[47] Pyörälä K, Savolainen E, Kaukola S, Haapakoski J: Plasma insulin as coronary heart disease risk factor: relationship to other risk factors and predictive value over 9.5 year follow up of the Helsinki Policeman Study population. *Acta Med. Scand.* 1985;(Suppl): 38-52.

[48] Sato Y, Shiraishi S, Oshida Y, Ishiguro T, Sakamoto N: Experimental atherosclerosis-like lesions induced by hyperinsulinism in Wistar rats. *Diabetes* 1989; 38: 91-96.

[49] Stout RW, Bierman EL, Ross R : Effect of insulin on the proliferation of cultured primate arterial smooth muscle cells. *Circ. Res.*1975; 36: 319-327.

[50] Bruno G, Cavallo-Perin P, Bargero G, Borra M, D'Errico N, Pagano G : Association of fibrinogen and glycemic control and albumin excretion rate in patients with non-insulin-dependent diabetes mellitus. *Ann. Intern. Med.* 1996;125: 653-657.

[51] Yegin A, Ozben T, Yegin H : Glycation of lipoproteins and accelerated atherosclerosis in non-insulin-dependent diabetes mellitus. *Int. J. Clin. Lab. Res.* 1995; 25: 157-161.

[52] Colwell JA: Vascular thrombosis in type 2 diabetes mellitus. *Diabetes* 1993; 42:8-11.

[53] Taskinen MR, Kuusi T, Helve E, Nikkila EA, Yki JH: Insulin therapy induces antiatherogenic changes of serum lipoproteins in non-insulin-dependent diabetes. *Arteriosclerosis* 1988; 8: 168-177.

[54] Agardh CD, Nilsson EP, Schersten B: Improvement of the plasma lipoprotein pattern after institution of insulin treatment in diabetes mellitus. *Diabetes Care* 1982; 5: 322-325.

[55] Gall MA, Borch-Jonhnsen K, Hougaard P, Nielsen FS, Parving HH: Albuminuria and poor glycemic control predict mortality in NIDDM. *Diabetes* 1995; 44: 1303-1309.

[56] Moss SE, Klein R, Klein BE, Meuer SM: The association of glycemia and cause-specific mortality in a diabetic population. *Arch. Intern. Med.* 1994; 154: 2473-2479.

[57] Ohkubo Y, Kishikawa H, Araki E, et al: Intensive insulin therapy prevents the progression of diabetic microvascular complications in Japanese patients with non-insulin –dependent diabetes mellitus: a randomized prospective 6-year study. *Diabetes Res. Clin. Pract.* 1995; 28: 103-117.

[58] Kilo C, Miller JP, Williamson JR: The Achilles heel of the University Group Diabetes Program. *JAMA* 1980; 243: 450-457.

[59] Malmberg K: Prospective randomized study of intensive insulin treatment on long term survival after acute myocardial infarction in patients with diabetes mellitus. *BMJ* 1997; 314: 1512-1515.

[60] Mogensen CE : Interesting positive news about Sulfonylureas, especially gliclazide, from the EASD congress in Munich (2004). *Int. J. Metab.* 2004;7:29.

[61] The Diabetes Control and Complications Trial Research Group: The effect of intensive treatment of diabetes on the development and progression of long term complications in insulin-dependent diabetes mellitus. *N. Engl. J. Med.* 1993; 329:977-986.

[62] Lawson ML, Tsui E, Gerstein HC, Zinman B: Effect of intensive therapy on early macrovascular disease in young individuals with type 1 diabetes – a systematic review and meta-analysis. *Diabetes Care* 1999; 22(2): B35-B39.

[63] Egger M, Smith GD, Stettler C, Diem P: Risk of adverse effects of intensified treatment in insulin-dependent diabetes mellitus: a meta-analysis. *Diabetic Med.* 1997;14: 919-928.

[64] The Diabetes Control and Complications Trial Research Group: Influence of intensive diabetes treatment on quality-of-life outcomes in the The Diabetes Control and Complications Trial. *Diabetes Care* 1996; 19: 195-203.

[65] The Diabetes Control and Complications Trial Research Group: The absence of a glycemic threshold for the development of long-term complications: the perspective of the The Diabetes Control and Complications Trial . *Diabetes* 1996; 45: 1289-1298.

[66] American Diabetes Association: Implications of the United Kingdom Prospective Diabetes Study. *Diabetes Care* 2002; (Suppl 1): 28-32.

[67] Reichard P, Berglund B, Britz A, Cars I, Nilsson BY, Rosenqvist U: Intensified conventional insulin treatment retards the microvascular complications of insulin-dependent diabetes mellitus (IDDM): the Stockholm Diabetes Intervention Study (SDIS) after five years. *J. Intern. Med* .1991; 230: 101-108.

[68] Gaede P, Vedel P, Parving HH, Pedersen O: Intensified multifactorial intervention in patients with type 2 diabetes mellitus and microalbuminuria: the Steno type 2 randomised study. *Lancet* 1999; 353(9153): 617-622.

[69] Halimi S, Charpentier G, Grimaldi A, Grenier JL, Baut F, Germain B, MagnetteJ: Effect on compliance, acceptability of blood glucose self-monitoring and (1c) of a self-monitoring system developed according to patients wishes ACCORD study. *Diabetes Metab.* 2001; 6: 681-687.

[70] American Diabetes Association: Hypertension management in adults with Diabetes. *Diabetes Care* (Middle East edn.) 2004; (Suppl 1): 65-67.

[71] American Diabetes Association: Dyslipidemia management in adults with Diabetes. *Diabetes Care* (Middle East edn.) 2004; (Suppl 1): 68-71.

[72] American Diabetes Association: Aspirin Therapy in Diabetes. *Diabetes Care* (Middle East edn.) 2004; (Suppl 1): 72-73.

[73] American Diabetes Association: Smoking and Diabetes. *Diabetes Care*(Middle East edn.) 2004; (Suppl 1): 74-75.

In: World Heart Research Yearbook. Volume 1
Editors: Franz Halberg and R. B. Singh
ISBN: 978-1-60741-881-8

PREVENTION OF ISCHEMIC HEART DISEASE IN PATIENTS WITH DIABETES MELLITUS

Hector Bueno *

Hospital General Universitario "Gregorio Marañón",
Department of Cardiology, Madrid, Spain

ABSTRACT

Cardiovascular disease (CVD) is the most prevalent and detrimental complication of diabetes mellitus, accounting for aproximately 80% of chronic complication hospitalizations suffered by this patients.

The incidence of CVD among diabetic patients is so high that diabetes mellitus is currently defined as a cardiovascular disease equivalent. Furthermore, the prognosis of diabetic patients after a cardiac event is significantly worse than that observed in non-diabetics. Therefore, primary and secondary preventive measures have a critical importance in this population subgroup.

There is substantial evidence that the efficacy of pharmacological therapies for primary and secondary cardiovascular prevention is much higher in diabetic patients than in nondiabetics. This chapter reviews the evidences of the efficacy of pharmacological prevention therapies in diabetic patients to support an aggressive pharmacological preventive strategy for them. An intesified multifactorial treatment aproach involving multiple risk factors like hypertension or dyslipidemia should be recommended. Every diabetic patient without known cardiovascular disease should receive treatment with angiotensina-converting enzyme inhibitors and statins, and in high-risk individuals, with low-dose aspirin.

There is consistent evidence that the benefits of secondary cardiovascular prevention with β-blockers, angiotensin converting enzyme inhibitors and statins is higher among diabetic patients than in non-diabetics. In our view, unless formal contraindications are present, diabetic patients with ischemic heart disease, particularly those with previous myocardial infarction, should receive always treatment with aspirin, β-blockers, angiotensin converting enzyme inhibitors and statins, regardless of lipid levels, left ventricular systolic function or the presence of congestive heart failure.

Despite the strong evidence that supports an aggressive pharmacological cardiovascular prevention treatment for diabetic patients, a number of registries throughout the world consistently reveal a significant underuse of these therapies. There is a need to develop strategies aimed to expand the degree of education about the importance of cardiovascular prevention in diabetics, to increase the use of proven useful

* Correspondence: Dr. Hector Bueno , Hospital General Universitario "Gregorio Marañón", Department of Cardiology, Dr Esquerdo, 46, 28007, Madrid, Spain; E-mail: hecbueno@jet.es.

preventive interventions, and to narrow the gap between clinical practice and the recommendations of guidelines among physicians involved in the management of these patients, particularly primary care physicians.

Keywords: Diabetes. Ischemic heart disease. Myocardial infarction. Primary prevention. Secondary prevention

Diabetic patients have a markedly increased risk of cardiovascular disease compared with non diabetic individuals, particularly of ischemic heart disease.

Approximately 50 to 75% of deaths in patients with diabetes are attributable to cardiovascular disease.

In fact, the prognosis of diabetic patients without established ischemic heart disease is similar to that of non-diabetics with previous myocardial infarction. [1]

This significant effect of diabetes on morbidity and mortality has resulted in diabetes being described as a coronary heart disease risk equivalent.[2-5]

Furthermore, diabetic patients who develop clinical ischemic heart disease have a significantly lower survival rate than do patients without diabetes.

This implies that preventive interventions for asymptomatic diabetic individuals are especially important, particularly measures to control the metabolic syndrome and those focused in other cardiovascular risk factors that are frequently associated.

Table 1. Therapeutic Goals For Preventive Treatment in Diabetic Patients without Cardiovascular Disease

Glycemic control	Hb $A_{1C} \leq 6.1\%$ Pre-prandial glycemia < 110 mg/dl Post-prandial glycemia < 135 mg/dl
Stop smoking all forms of tobacco	
Avoiding overweight	
Blood pressure control	BP < 130/80 mmHg
Plasma lipids	Total cholesterol < 175 mg/dl LDL-cholesterol < 100 mg/dl Triglycerides < 150 mg/dl

Primary prevention measures must include lifestyle changes (healthy diet, avoidance of overweight, increase in physical activity, and the absolute cessation of smoking) [6-9].

Once non-pharmacological measures have been introduced, pharmacological treatment for the prevention of the development of cardiovascular diseases must be considered (Table 1).

Several recommendations for the control of all these risk factors in diabetic patients have been released by scientific societies, although its implementation is still far away from optimal.

PHARMACOLOGICAL TREATMENT OF DIABETIC PATIENTS WITHOUT CARDIOVASCULAR DISEASE (PRIMARY PREVENTION)

Glycemic Control

The pathophysiology of type 2 diabetes is characterized by metabolic abnormalities beginning several years before the onset of overt hyperglycemia. Insulin resistance and compensatory hyperinsulinemia are the main causes of this process. Furthermore, insulin resistance not only produces hyperglycemia but is associated to a series of abnormalities that have been called the metabolic syndrome (central obesity, hypertriglyceridemia, low levels of HDL-cholesterol, hypertension and abnormal fibrinolysis), which is responsible at least in part of the increased incidence of cardiovascular diseases in diabetic patients.

There is convincing evidence from randomized controlled trials that good metabolic control prevents microvascular complications in patients with type 1 and type 2 diabetes. Glycemic control, evaluated by glycosylated hemoglobin levels, has been shown to predict cardiac events and mortality in patients with diabetes [10] and even in those without diabetes who have levels at the upper end of the normal range.[11] Although it is clear that strict glycemic control improves microvascular disease, its effect on macrovascular disease is not so obvious. An analysis of the UKPDS data by glycemic control showed a significantly lower incidence of cardiovascular events in patients whose levels of glycosylated hemoglobin were below 7%. A recent meta-analysis estimated in 13% (95% CI, 1% to 26%) the risk reduction in cardiovascular events (total mortality, cardiovascular mortality, non-lethal myocardial infarction, and stroke) associated with pharmacological interventions to strictly control glycemia in diabetic patients.[12] However, several pharmacological interventions directed to improve glycemic control have failed to demonstrate a reduction in the risk of cardiovascular events.[13,14] In one of the most important of these studies, UKPDS (*UK Prospective Diabetes Study*), the intensive treatment of hyperglycemia with a sulfonylurea or insulin in 2,729 patients with recently diagnosed type 2 diabetes mellitus only produced a non-significant reduction in the incidence of acute myocardial infarction (16%; $p = 0.052$), which was more marked among the 342 obese diabetics treated with metformin (39%; $p = 0.01$).[13] So, metformin is one of the few drugs that has been shown to decrease cardiovascular events in patients in patients with type 2 diabetes to date. Although metformin has a small effect as a peripheral insulin sensitizer, its main mechanism is inhibiting hepatic gluconeogenesis. It has been suggested that the use of drugs that directly improve insulin sensitivity, such as thiazolidinediones, may have direct vascular effects beyond glycemic control. Ongoing clinical trials such as ACCORD (*Action to Cardiovascular Control Risk in Diabetes*), DREAM (*Diabetes Reduction Approaches with Ramipril and Rosiglitazone Medications*) or ADOPT (*A Diabetes Outcome Progression Trial*) will evaluate their cardiovascular protective effect in diabetic patients. A recent multicenter study, the STOP-NIDDM trial, randomized 1,429 patients with impaired glucose tolerance to receive acarbose 100 mg three times a day or placebo. After a three year follow-up, treatment with acarbose was associated with a 49% relative risk reduction in the incidence of cardiovascular events (a combined end-point including coronary heart disease, cardiovascular death, congestive heart failure, cerebrovascular events and peripheral vascular disease). Acarbose was also associated with a

34% relative risk reduction in the incidence of new cases of hypertension, even after adjustment for major risk factors [15].

Therefore, multifactorial interventions directed to obtain a strict control of glycemia are essential in the prevention of diabetic microvascular complications, however they will not completely prevent the development of macrovascular disease.

Lipid Lowering Therapy

Dyslipidemia is a typical feature in diabetic patients. Among individuals with diabetes mellitus, 97% have at least one lipid abnormality and, as demonstrated the MRFIT (*Multiple Risk Factor Intervention Trial*) study, a two to threefold increase in cardiovascular risk for each lipid level (Figure 1) [16] The most common pattern of dyslipidemia in diabetics is hypertriglyceridemia and low HDL cholesterol levels. LDL concentrations do not usually differ in diabetics and non-diabetics, but non-HDL cholesterol (VLDL + LDL) levels are usually high in diabetics. In addition, type 2 diabetic patients typically have a preponderance of smaller, oxidized and denser LDL particles, which possibly increases atherogenicity even if the absolute concentration of LDL cholesterol is not significantly increased. Finally, it has to be considered that glycemic control usually improves lipid levels in the diabetic patient, but it does not always optimize the lipid profile.

Most of the information we have regarding primary pharmacological prevention in patients with diabetes mellitus comes from *post hoc* analyses of small subgroups of diabetic patients enrolled in some of the large primary prevention clinical trials. The AFCAPS/TexCAPS (*Air Force/Texas Coronary Atherosclerosis Prevention Study*) was designed to assess whether treatment with lovastatin for at least 5 years could reduce the incidence of first major coronary events (non-lethal acute myocardial infarction, unstable angina, or sudden death) in individuals without known cardiovascular disease, intermediate levels of total and LDL-cholesterol, and low HDL-cholesterol. Six percent of the patients were diabetic (n= 394). They showed a greater reduction in the incidence of coronary events (43%) compared with the whole group (37%), although the difference did not reach statistical significance.[17] In the Helsinki Heart Study, treatment with gemfibrozil was also associated with a non-significant reduction in the incidence of ischemic heart disease in diabetics [18].

The first study that prospectively demonstrated the efficacy of a lipid lowering drug in reducing morbidity and mortality in diabetics was HPS (*Heart Protection Study*). In this trial, 20,536 patients at high risk of coronary artery disease and no clear indication for cholesterol-lowering therapy were randomized to receive simvastatin 40 mg, antioxidant vitamins, both or placebo. Simvastatin therapy was associated with a significant 12% overall mortality reduction (12.9% versus 14.6%) and a 17% reduction in cardiovascular mortality (7.7% versus 9.2%). A 24% reduction (19.9% versus 25.4%) in the incidence of acute cardiovascular events (coronary events, stroke, and coronary revascularization) was also observed. This study recruited 5,963 patients with type 1 or type 2 diabetes, approximately 4,000 of them without known cardiac or peripheral arterial disease. The relative reduction in the risk of cardiovascular events in this subgroup was similar to that observed in high-risk patients, regardless of patient's age, sex or cholesterol level.[19]

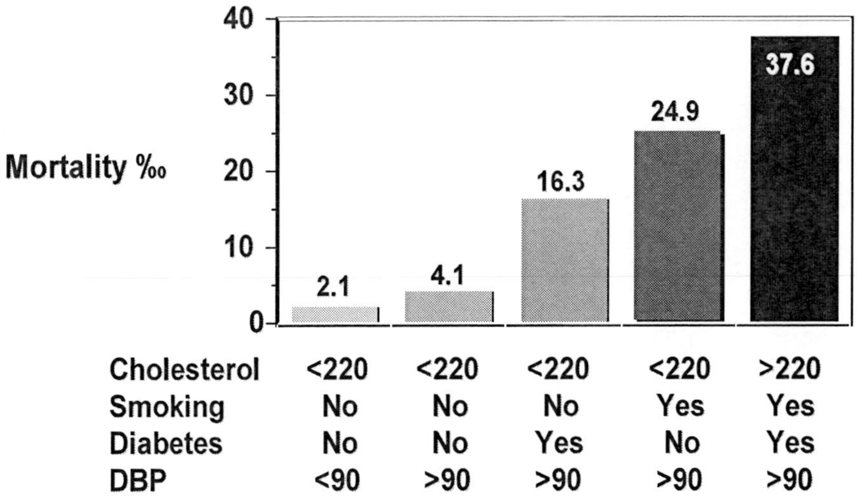

Figure 1. Cardiovascular risk assesment according to the number of risk factors. (adapted from the Multiple Risk Factor Intervention Trial). DBP: dyastolic blood pressure.

The Steno-2 trial, compared the effect of a targeted, intensified, multifactorial intervention with that of conventional treatment on modifiable risk factors for cardiovascular disease (hyperglycemia, hypertension, and dyslipidemia) in patients with type 2 diabetes and microalbuminuria, which included treatment with atorvastatin. This study showed a significant reduction not only in the risk of microvascular events but also in cardiovascular risk.[20] Currently, there is a number of ongoing trials designed to confirm the benefit on cardiovascular risk of different lipid lowering agents in diabetic patients without evidence of ischemic heart disease, such as ASPEN (*Atorvastatin Study for the Prevention of coronary heart disease End-points in NIDDM*) and FIELD (*Fenofibrate Intervention and Event Lowering in Diabetes*) study.

Although the published evidence is scarce, there is a high degree of consensus in the recommendations of the main scientific societies clinical guidelines. The current recommendations for the treatment of hyperlipidemia of the American Diabetes Association, American Heart Association and the third report of the National Cholesterol Education Program (NCEP III) establish a common therapeutic goal of LDL-cholesterol <100 mg/dl for all diabetics, recommending non-pharmacological measures such as behavioral counseling, physical activity, weight control and dietary measures for patients with values beyond that level.[3-5] The undisputed LDL-cholesterol threshold to begin pharmacological treatment in diabetic patients without known cardiovascular disease is 130 mg/dl,[3,4] whereas in patients with c-LDL values between 100 and 129 mg/dl, the decision should be based on a global cardiovascular risk assessment (Table 2).[3,5]

No specific treatment goals are defined for HDL-cholesterol or triglycerides, but their concentrations are used as markers of increased risk. HDL-cholesterol >40 mg/dl in men, >46 mg/dl in women, or triglycerides >150 mg/dl are markers of an increased cardiovascular risk and can be used to guide the choice of drug therapy.

The priorities in the treatment of dyslipidemias in diabetics must be: *a)* to reduce high LDL levels; *b)* to raise HDL levels, and *c)* to reduce triglyceride levels.[4] Pharmacological treatment should begin with moderate doses of statins as the first choice. The use of fibrates or bile acid sequestrants in combined treatment is recommended only when monotherapy fails to control dyslipidemia.[3-5] The benefit of treating hypertriglyceridemia is not well known. However, drug therapy is recommended for severe hypertriglyceridemia (>400 mg/dl) in the absence of other risk factors and for moderate hypertriglyceridemia (>200 mg/dl) in patients with other risk factors. Statins are the drugs of choice when high LDL-cholesterol levels are associated, and fibrates when only triglyceride levels are elevated (Table 2) [4]

Table 2. Current Indications of Pharmacological Treatment in DIABETIC Patients without Cardiovascular Disease

	Condition	Indication	Drugs	Observations
Antihypertensive therapy				
	BP > 135 / 80 mmHg	Always	ACEI, ARB Diuretic, BB, ACEI, ARB or CCB	If + Proteinuria If – Proteinuria
Lipid-lowering therapy				
	c-LDL ≥130 mg/dl	Always	Statin	
	c-LDL 100 to 129 mg/dl	10-year risk > 5%	Statin	
	Triglycerides >400 mg/dl	Always	Statin Fibrate	If c-LDL >100 mg/dl If c-LDL normal
	Triglycerides 200-400 mg/dl	>1 CVRF	Statin Fibrate	If c-LDL >100 mg/dl If c-LDL normal
Antithrombotic therapy				
	Age >55	>1 CVRF	Aspirin 75-150 mg/day	Class IIA

ACEI: angiotensin-converting enzyme inhibitors. ARB: angiotensin II receptor blockers. BB: beta-blockers. CCB: calcium channel blockers. c-LDL: cholesterol low density lipoproteins. CVRF: cardiovascular risk factor.

Blood Pressure Control

Hypertension is an extremely common comorbid condition in diabetes. The incidence of hypertension is approximately twice as frequent in patients with diabetes than in normal individuals.[21] A recent registry performed in Spain revealed that 75% of diabetic patients are also hypertensive.[22] On the other hand, metabolic abnormalities are more frequent in hypertensive patients. These data suggest that there is an association between hypertension and diabetes mellitus, a pernicious coexistence strongly linked to cardiovascular disease, stroke, progression of renal disease and diabetic retinopathy [23-25].

Pharmacological treatment of hypertension prevents the development of cardiovascular disease in the general population. The decrease in blood pressure in hypertensive individuals is associated with a reduction in mortality and cardiovascular events. Several studies have shown a superior benefit of treating hypertension in diabetic patients compared with non-diabetics. This advantage is observed regardless of the drugs and doses used.[26-28] The question of which agent class is superior for lowering blood pressure is not so important if we consider that the majority of diabetic patients will require two or more drugs to achieve blood pressure control. Randomized controlled trials that have included large diabetic populations, including UKPDS, HOT (*Hypertension Optimal Treatment*), Syst-EUR (*Systolic Hypertension in Europe*), HOPE (*Heart Outcomes Prevention Evaluation Study Investigators*), LIFE (*Losartan Intervention For Endpoint Reduction in Hypertension Study*), SHEP (*Systolic Hypertension in the Elderly Program*), and ALLHAT (*Antihypertensive and Lipid-Lowering treatment to prevent Heart Attack Trial*), have demonstrated that adequate blood pressure control improves cardiovascular outcomes, especially stroke, when aggressive targets are achieved [29-35].

The studies that compared strategies of different intensity in blood pressure control demonstrated that the maximal benefit is obtained achieving the lowest levels of blood pressure.[27-29] Therefore, regimes directed to obtain tight a blood pressure control are desirable. The HOT study randomly allocated 18,790 hypertensive patients to three progressive strategies of control, based on diastolic blood pressure (<90, <85 and <80 mm Hg, respectively). Among the 1,501 diabetic patients included, a progressive reduction in major cardiovascular episodes was observed as a more accurate control of diastolic blood pressure was reached. In addition, diabetics assigned to the group of more strict control of blood pressure (diastolic pressure <80 mm Hg) had a cardiovascular mortality rate three times lower than that observed in the other two groups.[28] The hypertension control arm of the UKPDS showed a 15% reduction in diabetes-related mortality, 11% in myocardial infarction and 13% in microvascular complications such as retinopathy and nephropathy for each 10 mm Hg decrease in systolic blood pressure. This benefit was obtained even in ranges of blood pressure considered normal [30].

These findings suggest that blood pressure reduction *per se* improves cardiovascular prognosis in diabetic patients. The benefit is greater as control of blood pressure is tightest. This is the rationale on which the recommendation to set a lower threshold of blood pressure to initiate pharmacological treatment in diabetic patients stands. The current recommendations of the seventh report of the Joint National Committee (JNC-VII) are concordant with the American Diabetes Association guidelines, which recommend a blood pressure level lower than 130/80 mmHg for diabetic patients [31].

However, it is not clear if the beneficial effect of lowering blood pressure in patients with diabetes mellitus is independent of the antihypertensive agent used. In the ALLHAT study the doxazosine treatment arm was discontinued because it was associated with more than two-fold increase in the incidence of heart failure and a 24% increase in cardiovascular episodes in comparison with the chlorthalidone-treated group, both in diabetic and non-diabetic patients [32]. Chlorthalidone reduced the incidence of myocardial infarction and cardiovascular mortality similarly to lisinopril or amlodipine.

In the ABCD (*Appropriate Blood Pressure Control in Diabetes*) study, in which 470 non-insulin-dependent diabetics with hypertension were randomized to receive treatment with nisoldipine or enalapril, the nisoldipine arm was prematurely discontinued because of the higher incidence of lethal and non-lethal acute myocardial infarction in this group of patients (adjusted RR, 4.2; 95% CI, 1.8%-10.1%).[33,34] A recent meta-analysis suggests that, compared with other antihypertensive drugs, the use of calcium-channel blockers in diabetic patients is associated with a significant increase of 55% in the incidence of myocardial infarction and 44% in major cardiovascular events.[35] However, the ABCD-2 study, published later, showed that in diabetic patients with normal blood pressure levels, nisoldipine is similar to lisinopril in the prevention of stroke or development of albuminuria.[36] The CAPP (*Captopril Prevention Project*) study compared captopril with conventional therapy in 10,985 patients, 572 of them diabetics. Captopril showed no benefit in non-diabetic individuals, but was associated with a 46% reduction in total mortality (95% CI, 4-54%) and 66% in the incidence of acute myocardial infarction (95% CI, 33%-83%) in diabetic patients.[37] The LIFE study compared the treatment with losartan and atenolol during an average of 4.7 years in hypertensive patients with electrocardiographic signs of left ventricular hypertrophy. Among the 1,195 diabetic patients enrolled losartan showed a 27% reduction (95% CI, 5%-43%) in the primary endpoint (cardiovascular death, acute myocardial infarction or stroke) compared with atenolol, mainly due to a 38% reduction (95%CI, 8%-59%) in cardiovascular mortality. In addition, a 40% reduction in total mortality and 43% in the incidence of heart failure was found.[38]

In the Micro-HOPE study,[39] a predefined substudy of the HOPE trial, 3,577 diabetic patients without clinical proteinuria, heart failure, or left ventricular systolic dysfunction were randomly distributed to receive placebo or ramipril 10 mg daily. The treatment group showed a significantly lower incidence of the combined endpoint (25% risk reduction) and of each of its components: myocardial infarction (22%), stroke (33%), and cardiovascular death (37%). A significant reduction in total mortality (24%), heart failure of any degree (20%), and overt nephropathy (24%) was also found. This beneficial effect was observed with a reduction in systolic blood pressure at the end of the study of only 1.9 mm Hg, and 3.3 mm Hg in diastolic pressure. All subgroups of diabetic patients showed some degree of risk reduction, although it was more evident in patients with dietetic control of hyperglycemia, in those with microalbuminuria at the beginning of the study, and in those with previous cardiovascular disease (secondary prevention). The maximal benefit was observed in patients with type 1 diabetes, although the differences did not reach statistical significance because this patient subgroup was very small.[39]

Regarding microvascular complications, a recent meta-analysis confirmed that treatment with ACE inhibitors in type 1 normotensive diabetics with microalbuminuria reduces the progression to macroalbuminuria and increases the probability of regression to normoalbuminuria regardless blood pressure control.[40] More recently, angiotensin receptor blockers such as irbesartan (IRMA II: *Irbesartan in Patients with type II Diabetes and Microalbuminuria Study*, or IDNT: *Irbesartan Diabetic Nephropathy Trial*),[41,42] and losartan (RENAAL: *Reduction of Endpoints in NIDDM with the Angiotensin II Antagonist Losartan*)[43] have demonstrated their ability to reduce the progression of diabetic nefropathy but with no significant effect in terms of mortality or macrovascular complications. The American Diabetes Association recommends ACE inhibitors or angiotensin receptor blockers for diabetic patients with chronic kidney disease, in order to prevent deterioration of glomerular filtration or worsening of albuminuria.

All these findings suggest that drugs that block the renin-angiotensin-aldosterone system may be superior to other antihypertensives for the prevention of renal dysfunction as well as for cardiovascular risk reduction in patients with diabetes mellitus. Therefore, ACE inhibitors must be considered the treatment of choice in all diabetics with a blood pressure above the threshold value (130/80 mm Hg), regardless of the presence of proteinuria. Nevertheless, in the light of the results of the Micro-HOPE study, the indication of ACE inhibitors may be extended to all diabetic patients with other risk factors, regardless of blood pressure levels.

Antithrombotic Therapy

There are several evidences supporting the beneficial effect of aspirin for cardiovascular prevention in diabetics. In primary prevention, the *Physicians' Health Study* investigated the effect of 325 mg of aspirin every other day to reduce cardiovascular mortality in a placebo-controlled randomized trial that studied 22,071 USA male physicians. After a 5 year follow-up period, aspirin did not prove any significant effect on cardiovascular mortality but reduced the risk of myocardial infarction by 44% (95% CI: 30% to 65%). The risk reduction was 61% among the 533 diabetic participants (4.0% versus 10.1%) compared with 40% among non-diabetics (1.2% versus 2.0%). The difference in risk reductions between both groups was not statistically significant, suggesting that the efficacy is at least similar in diabetics as in non-diabetics.[44] The *Early Treatment Diabetic Reninopathy Study* (ETDRS) enrrolled 3,711 diabetics with diabetic retinopathy —30% type 1 diabetes mellitus, and 48% with known cardiovascular disease—, that were randomized to receive a relatively high dose of aspirin (650 mg daily) or placebo. After 5 years of follow-up, the incidence of myocardial infarction decreased by 28% (99% CI: 5% to 45%), from 12.3% in the placebo group to 9.1% in the treated group.[45] The HOT (*Hypertension Optimal Treatment*) trial randomized 18,790 patients with hipertension —less than 10% of them with cardiovascular disease— to receive antihypertensive therapies with three different intensities in the degree of diastolic blood pressure to address the optimal blood pressure therapeutic target. In addition, the HOT trial investigated the benefit of adding 75 mg of aspirin daily, through a parallel placebo-controlled randomization. Aspirin therapy decreased by 36% the incidence of myocardial infarction, but did not influence cardiovascular mortality or the risk of stroke. Quantitatively analyzed, it was estimated that aspirin could prevent 15 myocardial infarctions per 10,000 patients/year in the whole group, with a reduction of 25 myocardial infarctions per 10,000 diabetic patients/year.[28] The results of the 4,961 diabetics without cardiovascular disease included in the placebo-controlled trials investigating antiplatelet therapies performed until 1997 were pooled in the *Antithrombotic Trialists' Collaboration* metanalysis, which confirms the beneficial effect of aspirin therapy, with a 1% absolute and 7% relative reduction (8% standard deviation) in the incidence of major vascular events.[46] The authors pointed out that the lack of statistical significance must not be interpreted as a lack of efficacy but as a lack of difference in effect with that observed in other high risk subgroups, such as those with previous myocardial infarction or stroke, because the 99% confidence interval includes the 25% risk reduction, that observed in the whole population included in the analysis.

The main limitation of chronic aspirin therapy is the increase in bleeding risk. According to the findings of ETDRS and HOT trials, aspirin does not increase the incidence of lethal hemorrhages, stroke, or cerebral or retinal hemorrhage, but it does increase by 80% the rate of major non-lethal hemorrhages and minor bleedings [28,47].

Based on these evidences, the use of aspirin is recommended in all diabetic patients with concomitant cardiovascular disease and in those without disease but at a high risk. Provided that low doses of aspirin (75-150 mg daily) are associated with a similar or greater efficacy than higher doses [46] and that they should be associated with a lower incidence of bleeding, particularly of a gastric origin, the generalized recommendation is to use low doses of aspirin for cardiovascular prevention therapy. The *Antithrombotic Trialists' Collaboration* metanalysis concludes that "it may be appropriate to consider antiplatelet therapy in diabetic patients who are at substantial risk of a first vascular event (such as those with proteinuria)".[46] The sixth *American College of Chest Physicians* guideline on antithrombotic therapy, establishes a 2A type recommendation for the use of aspirin for primary prevention in men and women over 50 years of age with diabetes mellitus that have no contraindications to its use [48].

The *American Diabetes Association* recommends to consider treatment with aspirin at a dose of 75-325 mg/day in type I or type II diabetics older than 30 years of age at a high cardiovascular risk (with family history of coronary artery disease, any other risk factor, micro o macroalbuminuria or obesity) that do not show contraindications.[49,50] More generically, the *American Heart Association* recommend to use 75–160 mg of aspirin daily for individuals without cardiovascular disease at a high risk of developing it (particularly in those with an estimated risk ≥10% in 10 years) [51].

Finally, the *American Diabetes Association* recommends considering clopidogrel as an alternative to aspirin in non-tolerant patients and as a combined therapy in very high-risk patients [50].

Pharmacological Treatment of Diabetics with Coronary Artery Disease (Secondary Prevention)

Diabetics who survive an acute coronary event have a much higher incidence of short- and long-term complications and mortality compared with non-diabetics. Consequently, diabetic patients with ischemic heart disease deserve an aggressive strategy of secondary cardiovascular prevention.

Beta-Blocker Therapy

Early oral beta-blocker treatment.[51,53-54] is associated with a better outcome in patients with acute myocardial infarction. However, there is not much information from randomized trials regarding the specific efficacy of long-term beta-blocker therapy in diabetic patients surviving an acute myocardial infarction compared with non-diabetics. On the contrary, several observational studies suggest a much greater benefit in patients with diabetes mellitus, particularly in older patients.[55]

Lipid Lowering Therapy

There is a robust evidence demonstrating the efficacy of lipid lowering therapies for secondary cardiovascular prevention in diabetic patients with known cardiovascular disease. In the LIPID study (*Long-Term Intervention with Pravastatin in Ischaemic Disease*), pravastatin showed a favorable effect on the incidence of death due to coronary artery disease and non-lethal acute myocardial infarction both in diabetic and non-diabetic patients with ischemic heart disease and cholesterol concentrations of 155 to 271 mg/dl.[57] The 4S (*Scandinavian Simvastatin Survival Study*) trial, in which only 202 of 4,444 patients were diabetics (4.5%), the reduction in 5-year death rate was much greater in absolute terms (10.4%) among the diabetic patients than in non-diabetics (3%).

The reduction of both non-lethal coronary and other cardiovascular events showed a parallel pattern to that observed for mortality, with the exception of stroke, the only event not significantly reduced in diabetics.[58] The CARE (*Cholesterol and Recurrent Events Trial*) evaluated the effect of pravastatin in 4,159 patients <76 years old with previous myocardial infarction, total cholesterol <240 mg/dl, and LDL-cholesterol <175 mg/dl, 14% of them diabetics. The relative reduction in the cumulative incidence of coronary events (death due to coronary artery disease, non lethal acute myocardial infarction, coronary artery bypass grafting and coronary angioplasty) was similar in diabetics (25%) and non-diabetics (23%). Nevertheless, since the number of events was approximately two times greater in diabetics, the benefit was also greater in absolute terms. Of note, the divergence in the survivals curves in diabetics began to be apparent in the fourth year of treatment.[58]

A recent analysis of the *Pravastatin Pooling Project*, focused on the 20% of patients with LDL-cholesterol values <125 mg/dl included in the CARE and LIPID trials, has shown that while 5.5 years of pravastatin therapy was not associated with any beneficial effect in non-diabetic patients, the incidence of coronary events was reduced by 44% (95% CI, 17% to 63%) in diabetics (an absolute reduction of 12%, from 34% to 22%).[59] This analysis showed no significant differences the incidence of cancer in patients treated with pravastatin or placebo.

A reduction in the incidence of adverse episodes in patients with diabetes mellitus has been demonstrated not only with statins. The VA-HIT study (*Veteran Affairs High-Density Lipoprotein Cholesterol Intervention Trial*), which enrolled patients with known coronary artery disease, intermediate LDL-cholesterol levels (<140 mg/dl), and low HDL-cholesterol concentrations (<40 mg/dl), treatment with gemfibrozil 1,200 mg daily produced a 24% relative reduction in the primary endpoint (death due to coronary artery disease, non lethal acute myocardial infarction or confirmed stroke) in both groups, but the absolute reduction in events was greater in diabetics (8%) than in non diabetics (5%).[60] In a similar way, the Helsinki Heart Study confirmed that gemfibrozil reduces the incidence of coronary events in type 2 diabetic patients [18].

Current guidelines recommend beginning pharmacological therapy with moderate doses of statins in diabetic patients with macrovascular disease (ischemic heart disease, cerebrovascular disease or peripheral arterial disease) and LDL-cholesterol levels over 100 mg/dl. [4,5] Pharmacological treatment is recommended for triglyceride levels above 150 mg/dl in patients with known cardiovascular disease (Table 2). Statins are recommended as the first choice, particularly when cholesterol levels are elevated. If an adequate control is not obtained, a fibrate should be added, although potential side effects such as hepatic toxicity and rhabdomyolysis must be ruled out during follow up.

Treatment with ACE Inhibitors

One of the most consistently documented beneficial effects in secondary cardiovascular prevention in diabetes mellitus is the reduction in mortality observed with ACE inhibitors in diabetic patients with previous myocardial infarction.[8,61-63] All placebo-controlled randomized trials that have analyzed the influence of diabetes on the efficacy of ACE inhibitors in this context have shown comparable results: a significant mortality reduction in the whole group, based mainly on the reduction in mortality in diabetic patients (Table 3). In addition, long-term therapy with ACE inhibitors decreases the incidence of heart failure [39,61,63] and acute myocardial infarction.[39]

Antithrombotic Therapy

The efficacy of aspirin for secondary cardiovascular prevention is very clearly established, with an effect that seems to be maximal at doses of 75-150 mg daily (absolute reduction of 4.3 major vascular events per 100 patients treated) [46].

There is no evidence that the clinical efficacy of aspirin may be less in diabetics with cardiovascular disease, therefore as these patients do have a much higher risk of subsequent vascular events than non-diabetics, it seems that the benefit of secondary cardiovascular prevention with aspirin in absolute terms is superior in diabetics than in non-diabetic patients. Regarding the efficacy of other antiplatelet agents, the CAPRIE (*Clopidogrel versus Aspirin in Patients at Risk of Ischemic Events*) trial evaluated the effect of clopidogrel on the incidence of ischemic (cardiovascular death, myocardial infarction, stroke and rehospitalization due to ischemic events) and hemorrhagic events (rehospitalization due to hemorrhage) in patients with known cardiovascular disease, compared with aspirin.

Table 3. Efficacy of Angiotensin-Converting Enzyme Inhibitors for Cardiovascular Secondary Prevention in Diabetic and Non-Diabetic Patients

Study Drug	Group	Follow-up	Mortality Placebo	Mortality ACEI	Absolute reduction	Relative reduction	95% CI
GISSI-3		6 weeks					
Lisinopril	DM		12.4	8.7	3.7	32	14 – 47
	Non-DM		5.9	5.6	0.3	5	-9 – 17
TRACE		26 months					
Trandolapril	DM		61	45	16	36	9 – 55
	Non-DM		39	33	6	18	3 – 31
SMILE*		6 weeks					
Zofenopril	DM		16.5	7.2	9.3	61	16 – 82
	Non-DM		9.0	7.1	1.9	23	-17 – 50
HOPE		5 years					
Ramipril	DM		14.0	10.8	3.2	24	8 – 37
	Total		12.2	10.4	1.8	16	5 – 25

ACEI: angiotensin-converting enzyme inhibitors. CI: confidence interval. DM: diabetic patients. Non-DM: non-diabetic patients. * Death + severe CHF.

A *post-hoc* analysis of this trial estimated that among 3,866 diabetic patients enrolled, treatment with clopidogrel could prevent 21 ischemic or hemorrhagic events a year compared with the treatment with aspirin. This benefit was greater in insulin-treated diabetics (38 events prevented a year). A multivariate analysis adjusting for baseline clinical features selected treatment with clopidogrel as an independent predictor of a lower rate of ischemic-hemorrhagic events compared with aspirin (risk reduction: 13.1%; 95% CI: 1.2% to 23.7%, p=0.032).[64]

PHARMACOLOGICAL CARDIOVASCULAR PREVENTION AND DIAGNOSIS OF NEW ONSET DIABETES

An interesting aspect of the relation between cardiovascular prevention and diabetes is the finding that several preventive pharmacological interventions used in a non-diabetic population may reduce the incidence of new onset type 2 diabetes mellitus (Figure 2). The ARIC (*Atherosclerosis Risk In Communities*), carried out on 12,550 individuals without diabetes, evaluated the relation between antihypertensive therapy and risk of developing diabetes mellitus in a 6-year follow-up cohort study. It was observed that among all antihypertensive therapies, beta-blockers were the only ones associated with an increased risk of new diagnosis of diabetes mellitus during follow-up (probably due to their ability to reduce insulin sensitivity). However, the main determinant of the risk of developing diabetes was the presence of hypertension, regardless of the treatment received [65]. In the LIFE trial, treatment with losartan was associated with a 25% lower incidence of newly diagnosed diabetes mellitus compared with atenolol, although both groups showed a similar reduction in blood pressure.[66] In the CAPPP study, hypertensive patients who received treatment with captopril had an 14% lower incidence (95% CI, 1% to 26%) of newly diagnosed diabetes mellitus than those individuals who received conventional therapy [37].

In the HOPE study the incidence of development of new onset diabetes mellitus (diagnosed after the study began) was 30% lower in the patients who received ramipril than in those in the placebo arm [67]. These studies suggest an ethiologic and pathophysiological relationship between hypertension and type 2 diabetes mellitus. Moreover, pharmacological treatment of hypertension may influence the rate of diabetes incidence.

While drugs that block the renin-angiotensin-aldosterone system seem to prevent or delay the development of type 2 diabetes mellitus, beta-blockers may accelerate it. The mechanisms by which ACE inhibitors and angiotensin II receptor antagonists may exert their protective are unknown, but it has been hypothesized that their ability to improve insulin resistance in hypertensive patients may play a role [68].

Not only antihypertensive agents but also statins have been shown to prevent the appearance of type 2 diabetes mellitus. Thus, in the WOSCOPS (*West Of Scotland Coronary Prevention Study*) trial, the incidence of new onset diabetes mellitus was 32% lower in patients treated with pravastatin than in those who received placebo.[69] The mechanism of this protective effect are not known. It has been speculated that it might be due their anti-inflammatory effect [70]. Insulin resistance has been related to the concentrations of C reactive protein, a mediator of inflammation [71]. The mechanism by which the statins can reduce reactive protein C values [72,73] could be similar to that associated with the reduction of insulin resistance, although other mechanisms have been proposed, such as the improvement in physical activity capacity of patients treated with statins due to the reduction in the incidence of angina associated with their use [74,75].

These findings open new research pathways about the pathophysiological relationship between cardiovascular risk factors, their prevention and treatment, but also strengthen the evidences supporting an aggressive treatment strategy with these drugs in diabetic patients, regardless of the presence of known cardiovascular disease.

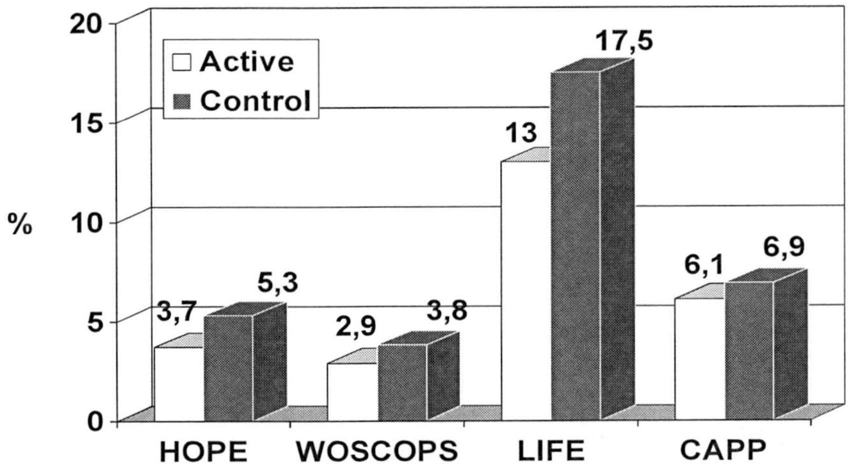

Figure 2. Incidence of new-onset type 2 diabetes mellitus in clinical trials testing pharmacological cardiovascular preventive therapies according to allocated treatment. HOPE (Heart Outcomes Prevention Evaluation): ramipril versus placebo.WOSCOPS (West Of Scotland Coronary Prevention Study): pravastatin versus placebo.LIFE (Losartan Intervention For Endpoint Reduction in Hypertension Study): losartan versus atenolol.CAPP (Captopril Prevention Project): captopril versus conventional antihypertensive treatment (diuretics or beta blockers).

Use of Cardiovascular Prevention Interventions in Diabetic Patients in the Real World

In spite of the strong evidences supporting the fact that a number of pharmacological interventions may improve prognosis in high-risk populations through a reduction in cardiovascular risk, these therapies are frequently underused in diabetic patients. Several registries have evaluated the patterns of use and appropriateness of pharmacological treatment in diabetic patients. All them show that the adherence to evidence-based medicine is generally poor in the community.[76-80]

The RISK-HIA *(Register of Information and Knowledge about Swedish Heart Intensive care Admissions*) registry collected data from 25,633 patients with acute coronary syndromes admitted to 58 coronary care units in Sweden, 5,193 of them (20%) diabetics. During hospitalization, patients with diabetes mellitus received significantly less reperfusion therapy (41% versus 31%, $p<0.001$) or intravenous beta blockers. Thrombolytic therapy was less utilized even after multiple regression analyses. Serious events were, however, more common among the diabetic patients. In parallel, a similar pattern of underutilization of several evidence-based therapies at hospital discharge was found. The use of β-blockers was high in both groups (75% in diabetics, 80% in non-diabetics), but only 25% of diabetic patients were discharged on statin therapy. There was an exception, the use of ACE inhibitors was more common in diabetics [76].

Underuse of effective therapies is not the only problem observed in diabetics, but lack of achievement of therapeutic goals is also relevant in diabetic patients receiving pharmacological treatment. The EUROASPIRE survey, focused on patients with established coronary artery disease, found that only 54% of diabetic patients were receiving beta blockers and 30% ACE inhibitors. In addition, 49% of patients who were on lipid-lowering therapy still had their cholesterol above 5.5 mmol/l.[77] The L-TAP (*Lipid Treatment Assesment Project*) study showed similar results in patients with diabetes: less than 10% were taking lipid lowering drugs and, among treated patients, almost none of them achieved recommended cholesterol values (only 1% had levels of LDL-cholesterol below 100 mg/dl).[78] These limitations have been found also in primary care. The TranSTAR, a prospective study that recorded blood pressure, lipid levels and pharmacological therapy in 388 consecutive type 2 diabetes patients visited in 326 primary care centers in Spain during October 2001, found that underutilization of preventive measures is common in general practice. The prevalence of hypertension and dyslipidemia in these patients was 58% and 52%, respectively and 10% had known cardiovascular disease. The rate of use of lipid lowering therapies, ACE inhibitors and β-blockers was 57%, 27% and 4%, respectively. During the visits, 86% of hypertensives showed blood pressure values above the current recommendations. Only 8% of the patients who were receiving lipid-lowering agents showed a fully appropriate lipid profile. Among diabetics with cardiovascular disease, the proportion of patients on statins was 36%, 50% on ACE inhibitors and 11% on β-blockers.[79,80]

Despite the fact that aspirin is very efficient for cardiovascular prevention, particularly in very high risk patients such as those with diabetes and cardiovascular disease, and that it is an inexpensive therapy, its use is far from common. A recently published study based on 1,718 answers to an interview sent to the 4,707 adult members of a local diabetic association in Spain found that the rate of regular aspirin use was 21% in this population, ranging from 53% among those with known cardiovascular disease and 14% in those without. [81] These results are very similar to those obtained in the third *National Health and Nutrition Examination Survey* (NHANES III) [82] and concordant with other studies suggesting that the use of aspirin in diabetic patients with ischemic heart disease is still low (between 37% and 63%) [83,84]. It is important to realize that the main determinant of aspirin use for cardiovascular prevention in diabetic patients is being counseled about aspirin use by a physician,[85] so even in groups with low aspirin prescription rates, as much as 80% of patients who received counseling were on aspirin regardless the presence of cardiovascular disease.[81]

CONCLUSION

Diabetic patients are at a high-risk of future cardiovascular disease, particularly coronary artery disease. Whereas lifestyle and pharmacological interventions directed to optimize glycemic control reduce the incidence of microvascular disease (nephropathy, retinopathy...), their effect on macrovascular disease is limited. Therefore, the use of other proven therapies to reduce cardiovascular risl is warranted in these patients. At the present moment, there is a robust evidence to recommend treatment with statins and ACE inhibitors in all diabetic patients, regardless of their lipid profile and blood pressure levels. Hypertensive diabetics must have strict blood pressure control that should always include an ACE inhibitor (or an angiotensin II receptor blocker when proteinuria is present). In diabetic patients with other risk factors or at a high cardiovascular risk, the association of low dose aspirin should also be weighed.

The risk of new cardiovascular events in diabetic patients with coronary artery disease is very high, but the potential benefit of secondary prevention interventions is also higher than that obtained in the general population. All diabetics with known coronary artery disease —and probably those with carotid artery disease or peripheral artery disease— must receive treatment with aspirin (75-150 mg daily), beta-blockers, ACE inhibitors and statins regardless of their clinical characteristics (lipid profile, blood pressure, left ventricular systolic function, presence of congestive hear failure...) unless formal contraindications are present.

In spite of the magnitude of the benefits achieved in diabetic patients with primary and secondary pharmacological cardiovascular prevention interventions, registries of clinical practice consistently reveal a large gap with guidelines recommendations and a significant underuse of these therapies. This adverse scenario must be viewed as an opportunity for improvement, in which strategies aimed to expand the degree of education about the importance of cardiovascular prevention in diabetics, to increase the use of proven useful preventive interventions, and to narrow the gap between clinical practice and the recommendations of guidelines must be developed. These interventions should be directed to all physicians involved in the management of diabetic patients: endocrinologists, diabetologists, cardiologists, internal medicine physicians, geriatricians, and specially to primary care physicians.

REFERENCES

[1] Haffner SM, Lehto S, Rönnemaa T, Pyörälä K, Laakso M. Mortality from coronary heart disease in subjects with type 2 diabetes and in nondiabetic subjects with and without prior myocardial infarction. *N. Engl. J. Med.* 1998; 339:229-34.

[2] Grundy SM, Benjamin IJ, Burke GL, Chait A, Eckel RH, Howard BV, et al. Diabetes and cardiovascular disease: A statement for health professionals from the American Heart Association. *Circulation* 1999;100: 1134 –1146.

[3] A Joint Editorial Statement by the American Diabetes Association; the National Heart, Lung, and Blood Institute; the Juvenile Diabetes Foundation International; the National Institute of Diabetes and Digestive and Kidney Diseases; and the American Heart Association. Diabetes Mellitus: A Major Risk Factor for Cardiovascular Disease. *Circulation* 1999;100: 1132-1133.

[4] American Diabetes Association Management of dyslipidemia in adults with diabetes. *Diabetes Care* 2002; 25 (Suppl. 1): S74-S77.

[5] Expert Panel on Detection, Evaluation, and Treatment of High Blood Cholesterol in Adults. Executive Summary of the Third Report of the National Cholesterol Education

Program (NCEP) Expert Panel on Detection, Evaluation, and Treatment of High Blood Cholesterol in Adults (Adult Treatment Panel III). *JAMA* 2001; 285:2486-2497.

[6] American Diabetes Association Position Statement: Evidence-based nutrition principles and recommendations for the treatment and prevention of diabetes and related complications. *J. Am. Diet. Assoc.* 2002; 102:109-118.

[7] Tuomilehto J, Lindstrom J, Eriksson JG, Valle TT, Hämäläinen H, Ilanne-Parikka P, et al. Prevention of type 2 diabetes mellitus by changes in lifestyle among subjects with impaired glucose tolerance. *N. Engl. J. Med.* 2001; 344:1343–1350.

[8] Eriksson KF, Lindgarde F. Prevention of type 2 (non-insulin-dependent) diabetes mellitus by diet and physical exercise: the 6-year Malmö feasibility study. *Diabetologia* 1991; 34: 891-8.

[9] American Diabetes Association. Smoking and Diabetes. *Diabetes Care* 2002; 25 (Suppl. 1):S80-S81.

[10] Kuusisto J, Mykkänen L, Pyörälä K, Laakso M. NIDDM and its metabolic control predict coronary heart disease in elderly subjects. *Diabetes* 1994; 43:960–967.

[11] Khaw KT, Wareham N, Luben R, Bingham S, Oakes S, Welch A, Day N. Glycated haemoglobin, diabetes, and mortality in men in Norfolk cohort of European Prospective Investigation of Cancer and Nutrition (EPIC-Norfolk). *BMJ* 2001; 322:15–18.

[12] Huang ES, Meigs JB, Singer DE. The effect of interventions to prevent cardiovascular disease in patients with type 2 diabetes mellitus. *Am. J. Med.* 2001;111: 633– 642.

[13] UK Prospective Diabetes Study (UKPDS) Group. Intensive blood-glucose control with sulphonylureas or insulin compared with conventional treatment and risk of complications in patients with type 2 diabetes (UKPDS 33). *Lancet* 1998; 352:837-53.

[14] Diabetes Control and Complications Trial Research Group. The effect of intensive treatment of diabetes on the development and progression of long-term complications in insulin-dependent diabetes mellitus. *N. Engl. J. Med.* 1993;329: 977–986.

[15] Chiasson JL, Josse RG, Gomis R, Hanefeld M, Karasik A, Laakso M. Acarbose treatment and the risk of cardiovascular disease and hypertension in patients with impaired glucose tolerance. The STOP-NIDDM trial. *JAMA* 2003;290:486-94.

[16] Multiple Risk Factor Intervention Trial Research Group. Multiple Risk Factor Intervention Trial: risk factor changes and mortality. *JAMA* 1982; 248:1465–77.

[17] Downs JR, Clearfield M, Weis S, Whitney E, Shapiro DR, Beere PA, et al. Primary prevention of acute coronary events with lovastatin in men and women with average cholesterol levels. *JAMA* 1998;279:1615–1622.

[18] Koskinen P, Manttari M, Manninen V, Huttunen JK, Heinonen OP, Frick MH. Coronary heart disease incidence in NIDDM patients in the Helsinki Heart Study. *Diabetes Care* 1992;15:820–825.

[19] MRC/BHF Protection Study of cholesterol-lowering with simvastatin in 5963 people with diabetes: a randomised placebo-controlled trial. Heart Protection Study Collaborative Group. *Lancet* 2003; 361:2005-16.

[20] Gaede P., Pernillo V., Larsen N., et al. Multifactorial intervention and cardiovascular disease in patients with type 2 diabetes. *N. Engl. J. Med.* 2003; 348:383-93.

[21] Simonson DC. Etiology and prevalence of hypertension in diabetic patients. *Diabetes Care* 1998; 11: 821-27.

[22] González Juanatey JR, Alegría E, García Acuña JM, et al. Impacto de la diabetes en las enfermedades cardíacas en España. Estudio Cardiotens 1999. *Med. Clin. (Barc)* 2001; 116: 686-91.

[23] Hinderliter AL, Runge MS. Who´s on first? Does hypertension in type 1 diabetes result from nephropathy or metabolic alterations? *Circulation* 2001; 104: 508-510.

[24] Mogensen CE, Osterby R, Hansen KW, et al. Blood pressure elevation versus abnormal albuminuria in the genesis and prediction of renal disease in diabetes. *Diabetes Care* 1992;15:1192–1204.

[25] La Rocca E, Gobbi C, Ciurlino D, et al. Improvement of glucose/insulin metabolism reduces hypertension in insulin-dependent diabetes mellitus recipients of kidney-pancreas transplantation. *Transplantation*. 1998;65: 390–393.

[26] Curb JD, Pressel SL, Cutler JA, Savage PJ, Applegate WB, Black H, et al. Effect of diuretic-based anti-hypertensive treatment on cardiovascular risk in older diabetic patients with systolic hypertension. *JAMA* 1996;276: 1886-92.

[27] Tuomilehto J, Rastenyte D, Birkenhäger WH, Thijs L, Antikainen R, Bulpitt CJ, et al. Effects of calcium-channel blockade in older patients with diabetes and systolic hypertension. *N. Engl. J. Med.* 1999;340:677-684.

[28] Hansson L, Zanchetti A, Carruthers SG, Dahlof B, Elmfeldt D, Julius S, et al. Effects of intensive blood-pressure lowering and low-dose aspirin in patients with hypertension: principal results of the Hypertension Optimal Treatment (HOT) randomised trial. HOT Study Group. *Lancet* 1998; 351:1755-62.

[29] Hansson L, Lindholm LH, Ekborn T, Dahlof B, Lanke J, Scherstén B, et al. Randomised trials of old and new antihypertensive drugs in elderly patients: cardiovascular mortality and morbidity. The Swedish Trial in Old Patients with Hypertension-2 study. *Lancet* 1999;354:1751-1756.

[30] UK Prospective Diabetes Study Group. Tight blood pressure control and risk of macrovascular and microvascular complications in type 2 diabetes: UKPDS 38. *Br. Med. J.* 1998; 317:703-713.

[31] The Seventh Report of the Joint National Committee on Prevention, Detection, Evaluation, and Treatment of High Blood Pressure. Bethesda, Md: National Institutes of Health, National Heart, Lung, and Blood Institute, National High Blood Pressure Education Program. *Hypertension* 2003; 42: 1206-1252.

[32] The ALLHAT Officers and Coordinators for the ALLHAT Collaborative Research Group. Major cardiovascular events in hypertensive patients randomized to doxazosine vs chlortalidone. The Antihypertensive and Lipid-Lowering treatment to prevent Heart Attack Trial (ALLHAT). *JAMA* 2000; 283;1967-75.

[33] Estacio RO, Jeffers BW, Hiatt WR, Biggerstaff SL, Gifford N, Schrier RW. The effect of nisoldipine as compared with enalapril on cardiovascular outcomes in patients with non-insulin-dependent diabetes and hypertension. *N. Engl. J. Med.* 1998;338:645-52.

[34] Schrier RW, Estacio RO. Additional follow-up from the ABCD Trial in patients with type 2 diabetes and hypertension. *N. Engl. J. Med.* 2000;342:1969.

[35] Pahor M, Psaty BM, Alderman MH, Applegate WB, Williamson JD, Cavazzini C, et al. Health outcomes associated with calcium antagonists compared with other first-line antihypertensive therapies: a meta-analysis of randomised controlled trials. *Lancet* 2000; 356:1949–54.

[36] Schrier RW, Estacio RO, Esler A, Mehler P. Effects of aggressive blood pressure control in normotensive type 2 diabetic patients on albuminuria, retinopathy and strokes. *Kidney Int.* 2002;61:1086–1097.
[37] Hansson L, Lindholm LH, Niskanen L, Lanke J, Hedner T, Niklason A, et al. Effect of angiotensin-converting-enzyme inhibition compared with conventional therapy on cardiovascular morbidity and mortality in hypertension: the Captopril Prevention Project (CAPPP) randomised trial. *Lancet* 1999;353:611-6.
[38] Lindholm LH, Ibsen H, Dahlöf B, Devereux RB, Beevers G, de Faire U, et al. Cardiovascular morbidity and mortality in patients with diabetes in the Losartan Intervention For Endpoint reduction in hypertension study (LIFE): a randomised trial against atenolol. *Lancet* 2002;359: 1004–10.
[39] Heart Outcomes Prevention Evaluation (HOPE) Study Investigators. Effects of ramipril on cardiovascular and microvascular outcomes in people with diabetes mellitus: results of the HOPE study and MICRO-HOPE substudy. *Lancet* 2000;355:253–59.
[40] The ACE Inhibitors in Diabetic Nephropathy Trialist Group. Should all patients with type 1 diabetes mellitus and microalbuminuria receive angiotensin-converting enzyme inhibitors? A meta-analysis of individual patient data. *Ann. Intern. Med.* 2001;134:370-379.
[41] Parving H-H, Lehnert H, Brochner-Mortensen J, Gomis R, Andersen S, Arner P. The effect of irbesartan on the development of diabetic nephropathy in patients with type 2 diabetes. *N. Engl. J. Med.* 2001;345:870-878.
[42] Lewis EJ, Hunsicker LG, Clarke WR, Berl T, Pohl MA, Lewis JB, et al. Renoprotective effect of the angiotensin-receptor antagonist irbesartan in patients with nephropathy due to type 2 diabetes. *N. Engl. J. Med.* 2001;345:851-60.
[43] Brenner BM, Cooper ME, de Zeeuw D, Keane WF, Mitch WE, Parving H-H, et al. Effects of losartan on renal and cardiovascular outcomes in patients with type 2 diabetes and nephropathy. *N. Engl. J. Med.* 2001;345:861-869.
[44] Steering Committee of the Physicians' Health Study Research Group. Final report on the aspirin component of the ongoing Physicians' Health Study. *N. Engl. J. Med.* 1989; 321:129-135.
[45] ETDRS Investigators. Aspirin effects on mortality and morbidity in patients with diabetes mellitus. *JAMA* 1992; 268:1292-1300.
[46] Antithrombotic Trialists' Collaboration. Collaborative meta-analysis of randomised trials of antiplatelet therapy for prevention of death, myocardial infarction, and stroke in high risk patients. *Br. Med. J.* 2002;324:71-86.
[47] Chew EY, Klein ML, Murphy RP, Remaley NA, Ferris FL. Early Treatment Diabetic Retinopathy Study Research Group. Effects of aspirin on vitreous/preretinal hemorrhage in patients with diabetes mellitus. *Arch. Ophthalmol.* 1995;113:52-55.
[48] Cairns JA, Théroux P, Lewis HD Jr., Ezekowitz M, Meade TW. Antithrombotic Agents in Coronary Artery Disease. *Chest.* 2001;119: 228S–252S.
[49] American Diabetes Association. Aspirin Therapy in Diabetes. *Diabetes Care* 2003;25 (suppl.1): S87-S88.
[50] American Diabetes Association. Standards of medical care for patients with diabetes mellitus. *Diabetes Care* 2003; 26 (Suppl. 1): S33-S50.
[51] Pearson TA, Blair SN, Daniels SR, Eckel RH, Fair JM, Fortmann SP, et al. AHA Guidelines for primary prevention of cardiovascular disease and stroke: 2002 Update.

Consensus panel guide to comprehensive risk reduction for adult patients without coronary or other atherosclerotic vascular diseases. *Circulation* 2002; 106:388-91

[52] ISIS-2 (Second International Study of Infarct Survival) Collaborative Group. Randomised trial of intravenous streptokinase, oral aspirin, both, or neither among 17,187 cases of suspected acute myocardial infarction: ISIS-2. *Lancet* 1988; 2:349-60.

[53] Malmberg K, Herlitz J, Hjalmarson A, Rydén L. Effects of metoprolol on mortality and late infarction in diabetics with suspected acute myocardial infarction. Retrospective data from two large studies. *Eur. Heart J.* 1989;10: 423– 8.

[54] Gundersen T, Kjekshus J. Timolol treatment after myocardial infarction in diabetic patients. *Diabetes Care* 1983;6:285–90.

[55] Chen J, Marciniak TA, Radford M, Wang Y, Krumholz HM. Beta-Blocker Therapy for Secondary Prevention of Myocardial Infarction in Elderly Diabetic Patients. Results From the National Cooperative Cardiovascular Project. *J. Am. Coll. Cardiol.* 1999; 34: 388-94.

[56] The Long-Term Intervention with Pravastatin in Ischaemic Disease (LIPID) Study Group. Prevention of cardiovascular events and death with pravastatin in patients with coronary heart disease and a broad range of initial cholesterol levels. *N. Engl. J. Med.* 1998;339:1349-1357

[57] Pyörälä K, Pedersen TR, Kjekshus J, Faergeman O, Olsson AG, Thorgeirsson G, for the Scandinavian Simvastatin Survival Study (4S) Group. Cholesterol lowering with simvastatin improves prognosis of diabetic patients with coronary heart disease: a subgroup analysis of the Scandinavian Simvastatin Survival Study (4S). *Diabetes Care* 1997;20:614 –620.

[58] Goldberg RB, Mellies MJ, Sacks FM, Moyé LA, Howard BV, Howard WJ, el al. Cardiovascular events and their reduction with pravastatin in diabetic and glucose-intolerant myocardial infarction survivors with average cholesterol levels subgroup analyses in the cholesterol and recurrent events (CARE) Trial. *Circulation* 1998; 98:2513-19.

[59] Sacks FM, Tonkin AM, Craven T, Pfeffer MA, Shepherd J, Keech A, et al. Coronary heart disease in patients with low LDL-cholesterol benefit of pravastatin in diabetics and enhanced role for HDL-cholesterol and triglycerides as risk factors. *Circulation* 2002;105:1424-1428.

[60] Rubins HB, Obins SJ, Collins D, Fye CL, Anderson JW, Elam MB, et al. Gemfibrozil for the secondary prevention of coronary heart disease in men with low levels of high-density lipoprotein cholesterol. *N. Engl. J. Med.* 1999;341:410-8.

[61] Zuanetti G, Latini R, Maggioni AP, Franzosi MG, Santoro L, Tognoni G, for the GISSI 3 Investigators. Effect of the ACE inhibitor lisinopril on mortality in diabetic patients with acute myocardial infarction. Data from the GISSI-3 Study. *Circulation* 1997;96:4239-4245.

[62] Gustafsson I, Torp-Pedersen C, Køber L, Gustafsson F, Hildebrandt P. Effect of the angiotensin-converting enzyme inhibitor trandolapril on mortality and morbidity in diabetic patients with left ventricular dysfunction after acute myocardial infarction. Trace Study Group. *J. Am. Coll. Cardiol.* 1999;34:83-89. Ambrosioni E, Borghi C, Magnani B, for the Survival of Myocardial Infarction Long-Term Evaluation (SMILE) Study Investigators. The effect of the angiotensin-converting–enzyme inhibitor

zofenopril on mortality and morbidity after anterior myocardial infarction. *N. Engl. J. Med.* 1995;332:80-85.

[64] Bhatt DL, Marso SP, Hirsch AT, Ringleb PA, Hacke W, Topol EJ. Amplified benefit of clopidogrel versus aspirin in patients with diabetes mellitus. *Am. J. Cardiol.* 2002; 90: 625– 628.

[65] Gress TW, Nieto FJ, Hahar E, Wofford MR, Brancati FL, for the Atherosclerosis Risk In Communities Study. Hypertension and antihypertensive therapy as risk factors for type 2 diabetes mellitus. *N. Engl. J. Med* 2000;342:905-12.

[66] Lindholm LH, Ibsen H, Borch-Jonsen K, Hetch Olsen M, Wachtell K, Dahlöf B et al. The LIFE study group. Risk of new-onset diabetes in the Losartan Intervention For Endpoint reduction in hypertension study. *J. Hypertens.* 2002; 20: 1879-1886.

[67] The Heart Outcomes Prevention Evaluation Study Investigators. Effects of an angiotensin-converting-enzyme inhibitor, ramipril, on cardiovascular events in high-risk patients. *N. Engl. J. Med.* 2000;342:145-153.

[68] Mykkänen L, Kuusisto J, Pyörälä K, Laakso M, Haffner SM. Increased risk of non-insulin-dependent diabetes mellitus in elderly hypertensive subjects. *J. Hypertens.* 1994;12:1425–1432.

[69] Freeman DJ, Norrie J, Sattar N, Neely DG, Cobbe SM, Ford I, et al. Pravastatin and the development of diabetes mellitus: evidence for a protective treatment effect in the West of Scotland Coronary Prevention Study. *Circulation* 2001;103:357–362.

[70] Haffner SM. Do interventions to reduce coronary heart disease reduce the incidence of type 2 diabetes? A possible role for inflammatory factors. *Circulation* 2001;103:346-7.

[71] Schmidt MI, Duncan BB, Sharrett AR, Lindberg G, Savage PJ, Offenbacher S, et al. Markers of inflammation and prediction of diabetes mellitus in adults (Atherosclerosis Risk in Communities study): a cohort study. *Lance*t 1999;353:1649 –1652.

[72] Ridker PM, Hennekens CH, Buring JE, Rifai N. C-reactive proteins and other markers of inflammation in the prediction of cardiovascular disease in women. *N. Engl. J. Med.* 2000;342:836 –843.

[73] Ridker PM, Rifai N, Pfeffer MA, Sacks F, Braunwald E. Long-term effects of pravastatin on plasma concentrations of C-reactive protein: the Cholesterol and Recurrent Events (CARE) Investigators. *Circulation* 1999;100:230 –235.

[74] Ur E, Shlossberg A. Do statins reduce the risk for diabetes by improving exercise capacity? *Circulation* 2001;104:E104-E105.

[75] Ross SD, Allen IE, Connelly JE, Korenblat BM, Smith ME, Bishop D, et al. Clinical outcomes in statin treatment trials: a meta-analysis. *Arch. Intern. Med.* 1999;159:1793–1802.

[76] Norhammar A, Malmberg K, Rydén L. Underutilisation of evidence-based treatment partially explains for the unfavourable prognosis in diabetic patients with acute myocardial infarction. *Eur. Heart. J.* 2003;24:838-44.

[77] Pearson TA, Laurora I, Chu H, Kafonek S. The lipid treatment assessment project (L-TAP): a multicenter survey to evaluate the percentages of dyslipemic patients receiving lipid-lowering therapy and achieving low-density lipoprotein cholesterol goals. *Arch. Intern. Med.* 2000; 160:459-67.

[78] EUROASPIRE Study Group. A European Society of Cardiology survey of secondary prevention of coronary heart disease: principal results. *Eur. Heart. J.* 1997; 18: 1569±82.

[79] Sarnago Cebada F, Bueno H, Gambús G. Grupo TranSTAR. ¿Cómo se utilizan las medidas de prevención cardiovascular basadas en el control lipídico en la población diabética española? *Rev. Esp. Cardiol.* 2003; 56 (Suppl 2): 160-161 (Abstr).

[80] Sarnago Cebada F, Bueno H, Gambús G. Grupo TranSTAR. Inadecuado control de la tensión arterial en la población diabética española. Resultados del estudio TranSTAR. *Rev. Esp. Cardiol.* 2003; 56 (Suppl 2): 163-164 (Abstr).

[81] Esmatjes E, Castell C, Franch J, Puigoriol E, Hernáez R. Consumo de ácido acetil salicílico en pacientes con diabetes mellitus. *Med. Clin (Barc)* 2004;122: 96-98.

[82] Rolka DB, Fagot-Campagna A, Narayan V. Aspirin Use Among Adults With Diabetes. Estimates from the Third National Health and Nutrition Examination Survey. *Diabetes Care* 2001;24:197-201.

[83] Wood DM, Plehwe WE, Colman PG. Aspirin usage in a large teaching hospital diabetes clinic setting. *Diabet Med.* 1999:16:605–608.

[84] Krumholz HM, Chen YT, Wang Y, Radford MJ. Aspirin and angiotensin-converting enzyme inhibitors among elderly survivors of hospitalization for an acute myocardial infarction. *Arch. Intern. Med.* 2001;161:538–544.

[85] Krein Sl, Vijan S, Pogach LM, Hogan MM, Kerr EA. Aspirin use and counseling about aspirin among patients with diabetes. *Diabetes Care.* 2002;25:965–970.

In: World Heart Research Yearbook. Volume 1
Editors: Franz Halberg and R. B. Singh
ISBN: 978-1-60741-881-8

ETHNIC DIFFERENCES IN DIET AND LIFESTYLE FACTORS AND AMBULATORY BLOOD PRESSURE AND HEART RATE IN ASIAN INDIANS LIVING IN UNITED STATES

Viola Vargoa[1], *Viola Mechirova*[2], *Daniel Pella*[*1], *Fabien De Meester*[2], *Lekh Juneja*[3] *and Taiyo Kagaku*[3]
[1] Faculty of Medicine, PJ Safaric University, Kosice, Slovakia
[2] Columbus Paradigm Institute, Waterloo, Belgium
[3] Yokkaichi, Mie, Japan

Recent evidence on ethnic differences in ambulatory blood pressure (ABP) in African Americans compared to people of European origin appears to be quite interesting [1]. Data on ABP and heart rate (HR) on American Indians and Asian Indians could have made this study even more interesting [2]. Details on diet and lifestyle factors also appear to be important for mapping circadian changes in blood pressure in populations studied by the BIOCOS group [3]. Circadian changes in blood pressure are synchronized by the daily routine of living via plasma concentrations of neurotransmitters, released by the pineal, pituitary and adrenal cortices, coordinated by clock genes situated in the brain's suprachiasmatic nucleus [2], and elsewhere [4,5].The role of ABP monitoring [6] should include detection of abnormal BP variability such as circadian hyper-amplitude-tension (CHAT) [7] and their correlation with diet and lifestyle factors,to find out preventive measures [2-7].

Many studies focusing on this issue have relied mostly on single measurements of blood pressure (BP) and heart rate (HR) rather than on week-long profiles obtained with an AMBP, interpreted with a view of their time structure (chronome) [3]. It is now accepted that ABPM is superior to clinical spot-checks in terms of diagnosis and prognosis [6]. Our study involved 209 subjects (142 men and 67 women) 42.4 ± 18.0 years of age living in Moradabad, India.

Anticipated relationships were found. Namely, the MESOR of SBP, DBP and HR increased with age (SBP: $r= 0.260$, $P<0.001$; DBP: $r=0.269$, $P<0.001$; HR: $r=0.242$; $P<0.005$), as well as with BMI (SBP: $r=0.232$, $P<0.005$; DBP: $r=0.257$, $P<0.001$). The MESOR of HR also decreased with increased activity ($F=5.558$, $P=0.001$). The MESOR of SBP also decreased slightly with increased activity, yet the relationship is not statistically significant.

* E-mail: pellad@hotmail.com.

Additional relations were uncovered. The SD of DBP increased as a function of BMI (r=0.248, P=0.002), whereas the SD of HR slightly decreased with age (r=-0.177, P=0.015). The percentage time DBP was elevated above time-specified reference values was elevated in subjects who reported consuming alcohol (17.2% vs. 7.1% in subjects who did not report consuming alcohol, Student t=2.367, P=0.020). Both the MESOR and the circadian double amplitude of both SBP and DBP, as well as the SD of DBP decreased as a function of social class. Of particular importance is the effect of consumption of fruits, vegetables and legumes (FVL) on the MESOR of HR (r=-0.192, P=0.011). The circadian double amplitude of HR was also found to be higher among Hindus who prayed (11.7 beats/min) as compared to Hindus who did not pray (8.1 beats/min) (Student t=2.137, P=0.035).

High BP is a serious public health problem in developing as well as developed countries, to the point that the World Health Organization (WHO) is considering using affordable ABPM around the world, a project now underway by a group of volunteering engineers in Minnesota (http://www.phoenix.tc-ieee.org/). Immigration of Asian Indians has been shown to influence BP, partly related to effects of urbanization [7].

High BP and altered BP variability can be treated [6]. The effect treatment on BP variability can be very different from one agent to another and from one treatment schedule to another . Because CHAT, that is too large a circadian variation in BP has been associated with an increase of 720% in the risk of adverse cerebral events [3], it is important to determine a given treatment's effect not only on the MESOR but also on the circadian amplitude of BP.

Drugs such as ACE-inhibitors,and coenzyme Q10 which is rich in the mitochondria of the arterial smooth muscle and is being tried for treatment of BP variability by our group. Wild type and functional foods rich in ω-3 fatty acids, which are rich in neurons and cell membrane phospholipids, may also have a beneficial effect as these fatty acids, can influence the brain-heart connection [2,8].

REFERENCES

[1] Wang X, Poole JC, Treiber FA et al. Ethnic and gender differences in ambulatory blood pressure trajectories. Results from a 15-year longitudinal study in youth and young adults. *Circulation* 2006 doi:10.1161/CIRCULATIONAHA.106.643940.

[2] Singh RB, Weydahl A, Otsuka K et al. Can nutrition influence circadian rhythm and heart rate variability? *Biomed. Pharmacother* 2001,55(Suppl1):115-24.

[3] Cornélissen G, Delcourt A, Toussaint G et al. Opportunity of detecting prehypertension: worldwide data on blood pressure overswinging. *Biomed. Pharmacother.* 2005,59 (Suppl1):152-7.

[4] Pickering TG, Shimbo D, Haas D. Ambulatory blood pressure monitoring. *N. Engl. J. Med.* 2006;354:2368-74.

[5] Cornélissen G, Chen CH, Halberg F. Predictive value of blood pressure variability: relative merits of circadian parameters versus dipping patterns. *N. Engl. J. Med.* 2006;355:850-1.

[6] Otsuka K, Cornélissen G, Halberg F. Predictive value of blood pressure dipping and swinging with regard to vascular disease risk. *Clin. Drug Invest.* 1996;11:20-31.

[7] Sundaram B, Holley DC, Cornélissen G et al. Circadian and circaseptan (about-weekly) aspects of immigrant Indians' blood pressure and heart rate in California, USA. *Biomed. Pharmacother* 2005;59 (Suppl1):S76-85.

[8] DeMeester F, Wild-type land based foods in health promotion and disease prevention: the LDL-CC:HDL-CC model. In *Wild Type Foods in Health Promotion and Disease Prevention,* editors Fabien DeMeester and RR Watson, *Humana Press, NJ* 2008,p 3-20.

In: World Heart Research Yearbook. Volume 1
Editors: Franz Halberg and R. B. Singh
ISBN: 978-1-60741-881-8

ACUTE CORONARY SYNDROME: A PROGRESSION OF PRE-METABOLIC SYNDROME

R. B. Singh*[*,1], Viola Vargoa[2], Viola Mechirova[2] and Daniel Pella[2]
[1]Halberg Hospital and Research Institute, Civil Lines, Moradabad, India
[2]Faculty of Medicine, PJ Safaric University, Kosice, Slovakia

Acute coronary syndromes(ACS) and coronary risk factors; hypertension, hyperlipidemia,obesity and type 2 diabetes have become a major health problem in Asia with economic development, due to interaction of gene and environmental factors.[1,2] Overswinging,that is an excessive circadian variation in blood pressure (BP) has been associated with a large increase in cardiovascular risk, present even in absence of hypertension and prehypertension itself.The prevalence of obesity varies between 5-7%, in the Asian urban population.The paradox is that despite low rates of obesity, the prevalence of central obesity (40-60%), prediabetes(10-15%), overswinging of BP(10-15%), type 2 diabetes(6-15%), and ACS (9-14%) are higher, in urban areas, which are much higher among Asian immigrants to developed countries [2].The prevalence of metabolic syndrome is 5% in rural and 15%in urban south India whereas in north and western India, the prevalences appear to be slightly lower.

In a cross-sectional survey, in five Indian cities,among 6940 subjects aged 25years and above, the prevalence of obesity was approximately 7% but more than half of the subjects had central obesity and one third had prehypertension, one quarter hypertension and one fifth prediabetes. About three quarters of hypertensives had central obesity in both sexes.

In a subsample,(n=1633), the prevalence of metabolic syndrome comprising of central obesity, hypertension and hypertriglyceridemia and low HDL was approximately 13% and premetabolic syndrome comprising of prehypertension, prediabetes and central obesity in 19.5%. The emerging typical South Asian, urban or immigrant has phenotype of higher percentage of body fat at a lower value of BMI,high WHR at a relatively low waist circumference and less lean body mass compared to other ethnic groups. A similar genotype is present among Chinese and other Asians.However,in case control studies, the mean age in south Asia varies between 48 to 51 years, which is againt the finding of 61 years mean age among Asians,(3) in the study by Teo and co-workers[1,3].

---

* icn2005@sancharnet.com.

In one study among 54 patients with acute coronary syndromes(ACS), 41 patients had acute myocardial infarction(AMI), 5 possible MI, 4 cases unstable angina and rest 4 angina pectoris.The control subjects(n=85) were randomly selected from the population from the city of Moradabad, drawn from a similar age and sex of the subjects.Serum level of nitrite(a indicator of nitric oxide,NO) was significantly lower in patients with ACS compared to controls(mean+SD:0.36+1.42 vs 0.96+1.48uM,CI difference 0.60,0.34-1.02,P<0.03). After 4 weeks of follow up,serum nitrite level recovered showing significant increase without such changes in the control group.(0.88 vs 1.09uM;CI 0.21,0.67-1.12,P<0.05)

The incidence of lipoprotein(a) excess(>30mg/dl) and mean levels of lipoprotein(a) (difference 6.4mg/dl,95% confidence interval 2.8-10.5,P<0.05) was significantly greater in the acute ACS group compared to control subjects.Serum levels of vitamins E, C and beta-carotine, coenzyme Q10, magnesium and potassium were significantly lower and insulin, glucose, triglycerides, and lipoprotein(a) were significantly higher in ACS compared to their levels after 4 weeks of follow up.There was a significantly greater occurrence of acute ACS events in the second quarter of the day compared to other quarters.A circadian rhythm was also noted for serum level of NO showing significantly lower nitrite in 6.00-12.00 AM period compared to afternoon,12.00-18.00hours period (0.27+1.12 vs 0.42+1.44 uM,P<0.04).

The differences in the nitrite levels in the two groups indicate that low levels of nitrite appears to be a risk factor of ACS. Lower levels of nitrite during acute stage of AMI and its recovery after 4 weeks of follow up indicate that transient hyperglycemia and hyperinsulinemia may also be responsible for its increase, (apart from low arginine intake and sedentary behaviour,) by inhibiting the expression of NO receptors caused by metabolic reactions evoked by ACS. Reduction in antioxidants vitamins may be due to increased oxidative stress which is common in AMI due to enhanced free radical generation which may also influence NO levels and cause endothelial dysfunction.More studies would be necessary to demonstrate that NO deficiency is a risk factor of ACS.There is a need to compare association of protective factors; physical activity, fruit and vegetable intake, n-6/n-3 ratio in the diet, moderate alcohol intakes and stress to find out their roles in the pathogenesis of ACS among Asians and Caucasians [1-5].

In rural population of India and China, there is low plasma insulin, low glucose, triglycerides and angiotensin.There is low prevalence of central obesity and obesity is uncommon in rural areas of Asia.When these populations migrate to urban slums or to industrialized countries, they substitute whole grain based diet from ready prepared fast foods containing more linoleic acid, saturated fat, trans fatty acids, sugar, and flesh foods and dairy products in conjunction with sedentary behaviour and increased mental stress.It seems that rapid changes in diet and lifestyle due to modest but unsustainable, economic development, without learning of methods of prevention, result into maladaptations, that are important in the pathogenesis of acute coronary syndromes among Asians and in newly industrialized countries such as Hong Kong ,Singapore, Slovakia etc.Wild type foods, due to their slow absorption and higher content of w-3 fatty acids and other micronutrients may modulate cardiovascular risk among ACS patients [6].

REFERENCES

[1] Teo M, Lalondrel S, Roughton M, Mason RG, Dubrey SW.Acute coronary syndromes and their presentation in Asian and Caucasian patients in Britain. *Heart* 2007, 93: 183-188.

[2] Singh RB, Suh IL, Singh VP et al. Hypertension and stroke in Asia ;prevalence, control, and strategies in developing countries for prevention. *J. Human Hyper* 2000 ,14:740-763.

[3] Singh RB,Rastogi SS, Verma R et al. An Indian experiment with nutritional modulation in acute myocardial infarction. *Am. J. Cardiol* 1992, 69: 879-885.

[4] Singh RB, Pella D, De Meester F.What to eat and chew in acute myocardial infarction. *Eur. Heart J.* 2006,27: 1628-29.

[5] Janus ED,Postiglion E,Singh RB, lewis B. Coronary heart disease in Asia. *Circulation* 1996,94: 2671-73.

[6] DeMeester F, Wild-type land based foods in health promotion and disease prevention: the LDL-CC:HDL-CC model. In *Wild Type Foods in Health Promotion and Disease Prevention*, editors Fabien DeMeester and RR Watson, *Humana Press, NJ* 2008,p 3-20.

In: World Heart Research Yearbook. Volume 1
Editors: Franz Halberg and R. B. Singh

ISBN: 978-1-60741-881-8

Continued 7-Day/24-Hour Monitoring Required in (MESOR-) Hypertension and Other VVDs (Vascular Variability Disorders)

***Ranjana Singh*[*1], *N. S. Verma*[2], *R. K. Singh*[1], *S. Singh*[1], *R. B. Singh*[3], *Rajesh K. Singh*[1], *O. Schwartzkopff*[4], *G. Cornelissen*[4] *and F. Halberg*[4]**

[1, 2]Departments of Biochemistry and Physiology, Chhatrapati Shahuji Maharaj Medical University (Formerly King George's Medical University), Lucknow, India
[3]Halberg Hospital and Research Institute, Moradabad, India
[4]Halberg Chronobiology Center, University of Minnesota, Minneapolis, MN, US

Abstract

Background: The diagnosis of hypertension by the time-unqualified conventional measurement of blood pressure (BP) in a health care office is associated with many false positive and false negative diagnoses, since a single measurement session can render the diagnosis dependent upon time of day, and even in around-the-clock profiles limited to a few days, normotensives can be hypertensive and vice-versa. Ambulatory blood pressure monitoring (ABPM) is now an available tool. Its results can be evaluated chronobiologically (C-ABPM) based on an initial record of at least 7 days while monitoring continues. It should be stopped only if no abnormality is found; if abnormality is found, monitoring continues, notably if the second 7-day record is also abnormal. There is an organismic time structure (chronome) and components of the spectral element in the chronome have physical as well as sociological environmental counterparts, in the chronomes, among others, of both societal and physical environments, including geomagnetics and the solar wind.

The chronomic interpretation of the circadian and very much broader spectral element of the time structure of BP and heart rate (HR) (variability) and of its clinical relevance has now resulted in the recognition of vascular variability disorders, VVDs, including MESOR-hypertension, that is a reliably diagnosed high BP based on C-ABPM. An overswing of the within-day change, dubbed CHAT (circadian hyper-amplitude-tension), is another VVD, as is circadian ecphasia, i.e., an odd timing of the high BPs, while the HR acrophases are acceptable (to distinguish this condition from a shift in work-rest schedule such as that in shiftwork or after transmeridian flights).

* Corresponding author: Senior Professor and Head, Department of Biochemistry, *King George's Medical University, Lucknow 226003 (India).* E-mail: singhrk23a@hotmail.com; Tel: +91-522-2257449, Fax: +91-522-2257539.

Further VVDs are an above-threshold pulse pressure and a below-threshold variability in HR, gauged in the standard deviation. All VVDs should be based on replication of at least a 7-day/24-hour record interpreted by C-ABPM.

Design: We examined whether monitoring sessions planned to be each of 7 days, at varying intervals corresponding to sometimes casual contacts with the patient, may suffice. They do not. There is a need for much longer monitoring and for not discontinuing the completed 7-day monitoring until the record shows no longer abnormality for at least 7 days.

Aim: To detect and treat VVDs based on the 7-day/24-hour C-ABPM with focus upon the diagnosis of CHAT -- a higher risk of cardiovascular complications than a high blood pressure in itself.

Method: The present study involves planned about (~) 7-day BP/HR monitoring of a 40-year-old man with known type 2 diabetes mellitus and MESOR-hypertension coexisting with ischaemic heart disease. He had dyslipidemia and angiographically documented triple vessel disease. He was purely vegetarian. His BP/HR were recorded through an ambulatory BP monitor (TM-2430 from A and D, Tokyo, Japan) on five different occasions between October 2004 and November 2007 with changes in the schedule of drug therapy given by reference to awakening time.

Results: The diagnosis of systolic CHAT in 3 profiles and, on one occasion, of complicating diastolic CHAT, and on still another occasion of systolic MESOR-hypertension, was made on the basis of a chronobiologic interpretation of circadian characteristics by sphygmochron, a summary of BP and HR variation with time. The patient received (at the time of the first monitoring) Metoprolol 100mg twice a day, on getting up and retiring for sleep; Ramipril 5mg in the morning, and other drugs for diabetes and heart disease.

During the second recording, Ramipril 5 mg was prescribed in the evening, 12-14 hours after awakening (presumably by misunderstanding advice to the contrary from The Biosphere and the Cosmos [BIOCOS] project), while all other drugs were continued with the same timing at the 3rd, 4th and 5th monitoring. Starting during the third record, two antihypertensive drugs were added to the treatment plan in the morning.

Conclusion: This case study indicates the need for continued surveillance, notably in case of CHAT complicating MESOR-hypertension. When a 7/24 profile is done, the monitoring is to be continued until the results of analysis (promptly provided by BIOCOS) are in hand. When these results are negative, BP and HR surveillance can be discontinued, but not when abnormality is found.

This was not done in the case reported herein. Had this patient been monitored until the diagnosis was in hand, and then had the switching of medication, such as a beta-blocker, from a twice-a-day schedule to a full dose in the morning-only, been implemented with continued surveillance, perhaps his VVD could have been eliminated several years earlier. Whether (and, if so, how much) peripheral end organ damage occurred in the interim will have to be assessed by outcomes in clinical trials with more than single patients.

But the single case suffices to emphasize the need for monitoring while 1. waiting for analyses, and if these show abnormalities, 2. further monitoring follows after changing treatment. The addition of diuretics in this case may have (possibly!) with a delay, contributed to eliminating both CHAT and MESOR-hypertension, but for how long it worked is unknown. Further monitoring is indicated.

Keywords: Chronomics, ABPM, CHAT, chronotherapy, Ramipril

INTRODUCTION

The diagnosis of hypertension in an office by the conventional time-unqualified measurement of HR and BP is associated with false positive and false negative diagnoses, due to the influence of various environmental and organismic factors [1-5]. It is known that in single measurement sessions, normotensives can have hypertensive values and vice-versa (6; cf. 1-5). It has been shown that a 7-day/24-hour ABPM, while appropriate to rule out a VVD, is not enough to rule one in; 14 or more days of chronobiologically interpreted ambulatory BP monitoring (C-ABPM) are required to consider a tentative diagnosis and treatment [7-9] unless a hypertensive crisis requires prompt intervention.

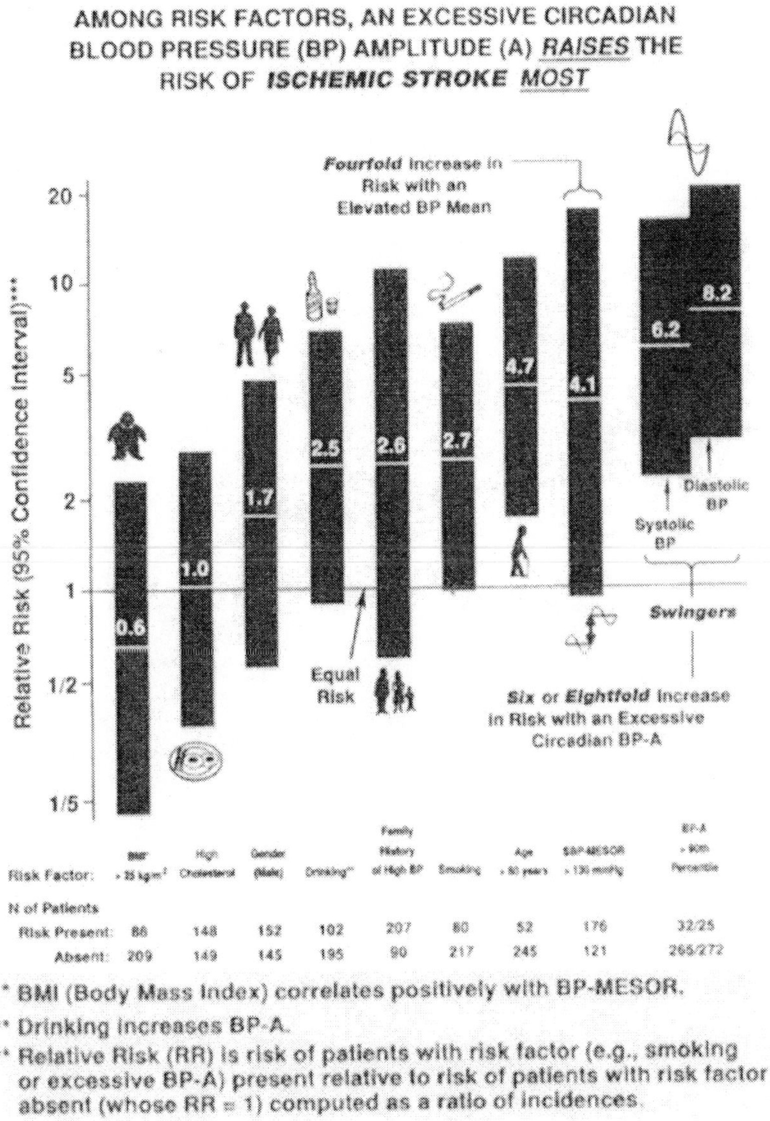

Figure 1. A systolic or diastolic overswing of blood pressure carries a risk of ischemic stroke greater than hypertension as shown by a comparison of the last two columns with the preceding column. © Halberg.

If a VVD is found the C-ABPM is to be continued to assess changes along the scale of a year, to assess not only circadians but also any infradian, e.g., seasonal overswinging or other infradian changes in BP or HR [10-13]. The 7-day C-ABPM gives an opportunity for the tentative diagnosis, among other VVDs, of Circadian Hyper-Amplitude-Tension (CHAT), but cannot (yet) rule out transient CHAT. In laboratory experiments and in a series of clinical studies, CHAT has been associated with the largest risks of stroke and nephropathy among the factors tested concomitantly [3, 4]. By comparison to the diagnosis of MESOR-hypertension, CHAT is a better predictor of target organ damage and clinical hard events, Figure 1 [1-4].

Circadian changes in BP as well as in various biochemical predictors of hypertension can influence response to drug therapy [14, 15]. Usually, in subjects active by day and retiring at night, BP starts rising about midsleep [16] and rises even more after awakening in the morning and remains high in the afternoon, then declines at night. Studies have focused on the increased frequency of cardiovascular events occurring in the morning [17]. When antihypertensive drugs administered once daily are typically taken upon awakening and arising, the end of their action, the trough effect tends to coincide with the rapid increase in BP early in the morning. On the other hand, treatment in the evening has been associated with an increase rather than decrease in the circadian amplitude of BP. Adjusting the timing of administration of the same dose of the same drug can play a major role in decreasing the BP-MESOR and reducing the circadian amplitude of BP as well as its MESOR, Figure 2 (18; cf. 19). Herein, we illustrate the need for continuous surveillance of patients taking multiple medications after changes of timing these medications.

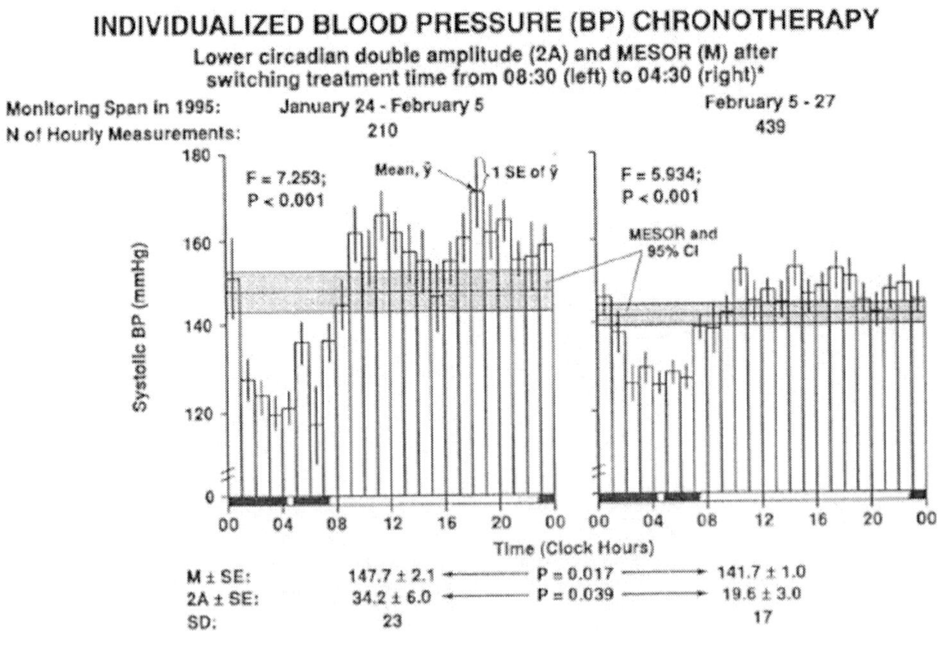

Figure 2. Chronotherapy achieves normalization, i.e., acceptability of MESOR and circadian amplitude by changing only the timing of medication (18). © Halberg.

SPHYGMOCHRON-TM

Monitoring Profile over Time;
Computer Comparison with Peer Group Limits

Blood Pressure (BP) and Related Cardiovascular Summary.

Name:——————
Age: 43
Monitoring From: 12/7/2004 11:00
Comments:

Patient #: RKSin066
Sex: M
To: 12/12/2004 16:31

CHRONOBIOLOGIC CHARACTERISTICS

	SYSTOLIC BP (mmHg) Patient Value	SYSTOLIC BP (mmHg) Peer Group Reference Limits	DIASTOLIC BP (mmHg) Patient Value	DIASTOLIC BP (mmHg) Peer Group Reference Limits	HEART RATE (bpm) Patient Value	HEART RATE (bpm) Peer Group Reference Limits
ADJUSTED 24-h MEAN (MESOR)	130.6	98.4-135.1 Range	82.4	60.3-87.2 Range	69.3	56.4-91.2 Range
PREDICTABLE CHANGE (DOUBLE AMPLITUDE)	**43.72**	6.4-39.40 Range	**30.08**	4.84-29.80 Range	18.31	5.26-36.20 Range
TIMING OF OVERALL HIGH VALUES (ACROPHASE) (hr:min)	16:12	11:48-17:40 Range	15:24	11:08-16:48 Range	16:00	11:44-17:20 Range

	STD (MIN; MAX)*	STD (MIN; MAX)*	STD (MIN; MAX)*
PERCENT TIME OF ELEVATION	19.5%	13.2%	0.0%
TIMING OF EXCESS	15:13 (hr:min)	14:26 (hr:min)	0:00 (hr:min)
EXTENT OF EXCESS DURING 24 HOURS HBI*	30 (mmHg x hour)	11 (mmHg x hour)	0 (mmHg x hour)
10-YEAR CUMULATIVE EXCESS	111 (mmHg x hour)(in 1,000's units)	41 (mmHg x hour)(in 1,000's units)	0 (mmHg x hour)(in 1,000's units)

Individualized bounded indices: (STD = Standard)(Min = Minimum)(Max = Maximum)(HBI = Hyperbaric Index)

INTERVENTION NEEDED
No
Yes Drug Non-Drug

MORE MONITORING NEEDED
Annually
As soon as possible
Other specify________________

CHAT (2 tpts slightly changed to enable prg to run)

Prepared By_____Germaine Cornelissen_______________ Date_24_/_Jun_/_2008____

1) Unusually long standing or lying down during waking: unusual activity, such as exercise, emotional loads, or schedule changes, e.g. shiftwork; etc.; 2) Salt, calories, kind and amount, other, etc.

Copyright, Halberg Chronobiology Center, University of Minnesota, Mayo Hospital, Rooms 715, 733-5 (7th floor), Minneapolis Campus, Del Code 8609, 420 Delaware Street SE, Minneapolis, MN 55455, USA. Fax 612-624-9989.
For questions, call F. Halberg or G. Cornelissen at 612-624-6976.

Figure 3. Sphygmochron showing CHAT by systolic BP amplitude (in bold). © Halberg.

a

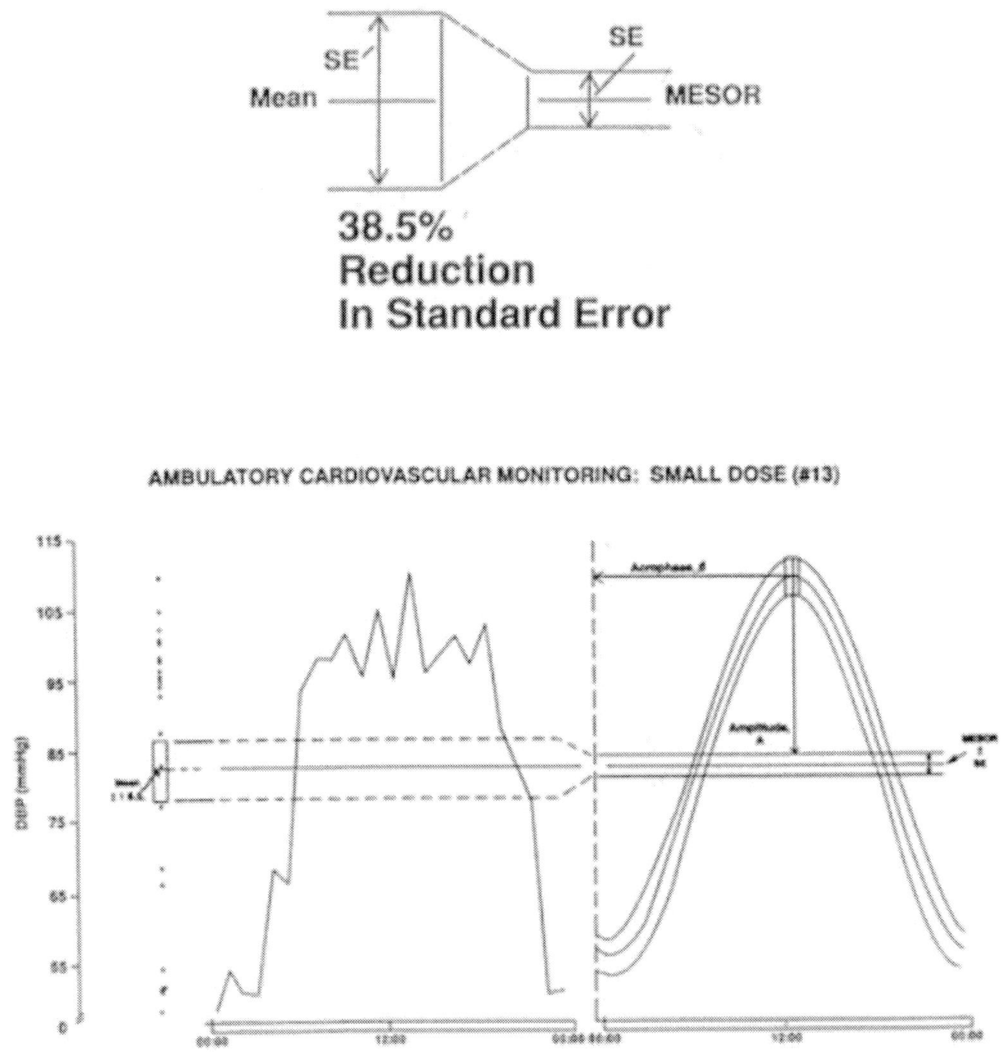

Figure 4. Merits of MESOR over arithmetic average. *4a, Top:* A merit of chronobiologic MESOR, M, vs. arithmetic mean, $\overline{y}$. When data characterized by rhythms are equidistant and dense (available at intervals, $\Delta \ll$ period, τ) and cover an integral number of τs, the M (though identical to the arithmetic mean) has a smaller standard error (SE). This is because the SE of the mean depends on the total variability in the data. But if a large portion of the variability can be ascribed to the rhythmic time structure in the data, fitting an approximating cosine curve can considerably reduce the residual variance, which in turn determines how large (or rather how small) the SEs on the MESOR and on the other parameters of the fitted model are. Thus, the better the cosine model fits the data, the greater the reduction in SE on the (rhythm-adjusted) mean. *4a, Bottom:* While the residual error is reduced around the cosine model fitted to the data, new parameters can also be defined, such as the amplitude and acrophase which provide valuable information in their own right.

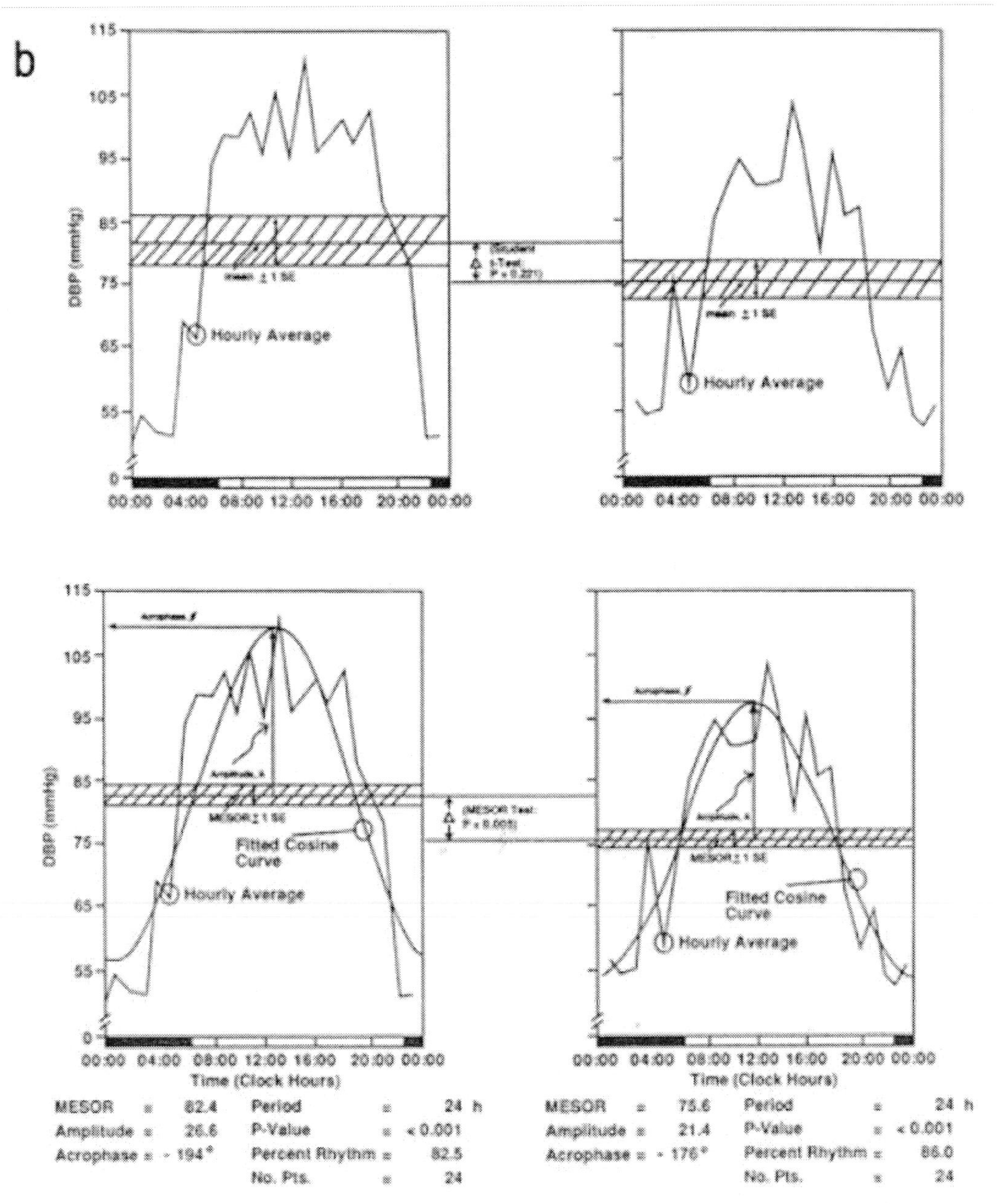

Figure 4b. *Top*: When the data are plotted as a function of time, it is readily seen that they do not present a random pattern of change (as the use of the Student t-test, comparing the data without accounting for their timing, would assume), but rather a circadian variation of large amplitude already apparent to the naked eye. It is inefficient and inappropriate to apply the Student t-test in this case. *4b, Bottom:* When the circadian variation is taken into consideration and the Student t-test is replaced by a MESOR-test, the same decrease of 6.8 mm Hg in diastolic blood pressure after institution of treatment with a beta-blocker is highly significant (P=0.005). The chronobiologic approach is thus more powerful at detecting changes in blood pressure for the individual patient, apart from also providing new endpoints. © Halberg.

Case Report and Methods

The study was to involve a target monitoring span of 7 days/24 hours of BP and HR (which was not consistently reached) of a 40-year-old subject with known type 2 diabetes mellitus, hypertension and ischaemic heart disease. He had dyslipidemia and angiography-documented triple vessel disease. His BP and HR were recorded on five different occasions from 11-10-2004 to 18-10-2004, 07-12-2004 to 12-12-2004, 08-01-2005 to 14-01-2005, 20-01-2006 to 25-01-2006 and 26-10-2007 to 01-11-2007 with changed schedules of drug therapy by reference to the time of awakening in the morning, Table 1. The patient was advised to take antihypertensive drugs either 1-2 hours (morning) or 12-14 hours (evening) after awakening.

Table 1. Medication kind, dose and time of subject investigated

Period	Name	Desired effect	Dosage	Timing
10.12.2004 to 10.18.2004 (N=226; T= 7 days)	Mononitrate	Antianginal	30 mg	BD
	Metoprolol	Beta-blocking	100 mg	BD
	Ramipril	ACE inhibition	5 mg	Morning
	Ecosprin	Antiplatelet activity	75 mg-	-evening
	Clopidogrel	Antiplatelet activity	75 mg	Morning
	Glimipride	Oral hypoglycemic	2 mg	Morning
	Atorvastatin	Lipid lowering	10 mg	Evening
12.07.2004 to 12.12.2004 (N=292; T= 6 days, 6 hours)	Mononitrate	antianginal	30 mg	BD
	Metoprolol	antihypertensive	100 mg	BD
	Ramipril	antihypertensive	5 mg	Evening
	Ecosprin	antiplatlet	75 mg	evening
	Clopidogrel	antiplatlet	75 mg	Morning
	Glimipride	antidiabetic	2 mg	Morning
	Atorvastatin	lipid lowering	10 mg	Evening
01.08.2005 to 01.14.2005 (N=215; T= 6 days, 2 hours)	Mononitrate	antianginal	30 mg	BD
	Metoprolol	antihypertensive	100 mg	BD
	Ramipril	antihypertensive	5 mg	Evening
	Ecosprin	antiplatlet	75 mg	evening
	Clopidogrel	antiplatlet	75 mg	Morning
	Glimipride	antidiabetic	2 mg	Morning
	Atorvastatin	lipid lowering	10 mg	Evening
	Furosemide	Diuretic	40 mg	Morning
	Amiloride	Diuretic	12.5 mg	Morning
01.20.2006 to 01.25.2006 (N=190; T= 5 days, 1 hour)	Same as above			
10.26.2007 to 11.01.2007 (N=332; T= 6 days)	Same as above			

N: N of measurements.

T: Time in days and fractions of a day covered by record.

Table 2. Circadian vascular rhythm parameters for systolic and diastolic blood presure (BP) and heart rate in a male subject, 40 years of age at start of monitoring span, on antihypertensive medication

Monitoring span		Systolic BP (mm Hg)			Diastolic BP (mm Hg)			Heart Rate (bpm)		
From	To	MESOR	2A	ϕ	MESOR	2A	ϕ	MESOR	2A	ϕ
10.12.2004 (19:30)	10.18.2004 (19.00)	128.6	42.86	15:40	79.5	27.14	14:55	69.6	19.98	15.42
12.07.2004 (11:00)	12.12.2004 (16:30)	130.7	43.46	16:12	82.4	29.93	15:22	69.3	18.19	16.01
01.08.2005 (11:00)	01.14.2005 (10:00)	126.6	49.06	16:31	78.8	28.31	16:42	69.3	16.28	15:16
01.20.2006 (11:30)	01.25.2006 (11:30)	136.0	30.56	14:09	85.3	18.40	13:31	70.5	14.15	14:57
10.26.2007 (07:00)	11.01.2007 (00:00)	124.7	20.99	15:32	74.9	13.56	16:01	72.5	11.41	14:24

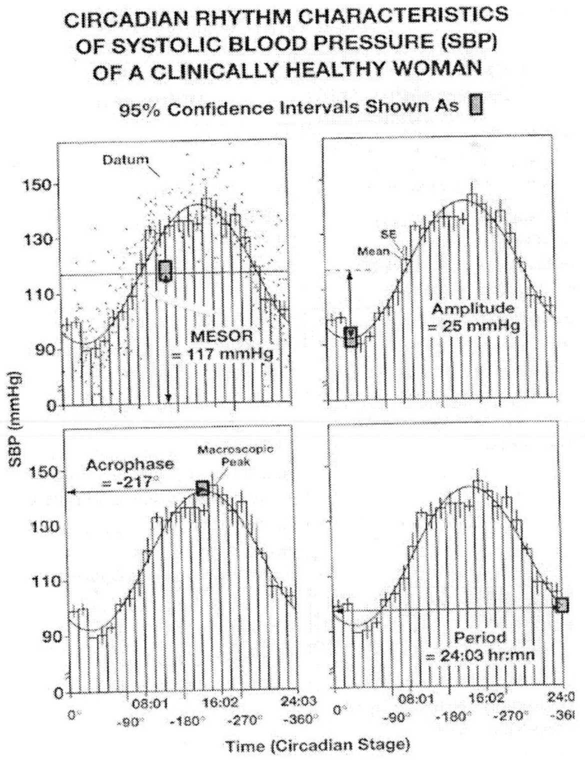

Figure 5. Illustration of circadian rhythm characteristics for the case of a series of systolic blood pressures collected over several weeks by a clinically healthy woman. Data are shown as dots (top left), plotted after stacking over an idealized circadian cycle. The data have been analyzed by linear-nonlinear rhythmometry, consisting of the linear least squares fit of cosine curves with different trial periods, followed by the nonlinear analysis. The latter allows the period to be estimated as a parameter in the model, together with other parameters, each with a measure of uncertainty, the 95% confidence interval (shown as a dark rectangle). The four parameters are illustrated separately for the same data series: 1. The MESOR (midline estimating statistic of rhythm), a time structure (chronome)-adjusted mean value (top left). 2. The circadian amplitude, half the extent of predictable change within a day (top right). 3. The circadian acrophase, a measure of the timing of overall high values recurring in each cycle (bottom left). 4. The period, the duration of one cycle (bottom right). © Halberg.

The patient wore an ambulatory BP monitor (TM-2430 from A and D, Tokyo, Japan), programmed to automatically measure BP and HR at 30-minute intervals while awake and at 1-hourly intervals during hours of habitual sleep. The data were downloaded after every monitoring span to a local PC via an interface (TM-2421), also obtained from A and D, Japan. Each BP and HR profile was analyzed by a sphygmochron [18], utilizing both a parametric and a non-parametric approach, Figure 3.

The parametric approach consists of fitting cosine curves with periods of 24 and 12 hours to the data to estimate the MESOR (M, chronome-[time-structure] adjusted mean), Figure 4; the double circadian amplitude (2A), a measure of the extent of predictable change within a day; the circadian acrophase (ϕ), a measure of the timing of overall high values recurring each day, Figure 5; and the double amplitude and acrophase of the 12-hour component aimed at assessing any non-sinusoidality of the circadian waveform. C-ABPMs were done each time on records sent to the University of Minnesota for analysis. The diagnosis of systolic CHAT was made in this patient on data from the first 3 records and was accompanied by diastolic CHAT during the second record. Systolic MESOR-hypertension was diagnosed during the 4th record. On all occasions, different drugs were given by the treating physician, as summarized in Table 1. Results from the five profiles are given in Table 2.

The patient received Metoprolol 100 mg twice a day, Ramipril 5 mg in the morning hours, Mononitrate 30 mg twice a day, Ecosprin 150 mg evening hours, Glimipride 2 mg morning hours, Clopidogril 75 mg morning hours and Atorvastatin 10 mg in the evening hours during first span of monitoring. He continued the same drugs at the time of second and third recordings where Ramipril 5mg antihypertensive drug was changed to evening hours, 12-14 hours after awakening.

The same medication and timing schedule was followed in the fourth and fifth monitoring that included additional medication, namely the diuretic Furosemide (40mg) and Amiloride (12.5mg) in the morning.

COMMENTS

The change of Ramipril from morning to evening was contrary to suggestions from a project on The BIOsphere and the COSmos (BIOCOS). The project advice, verbatim, was:

> ...there is a real chance that you can eliminate CHAT (a great risk of stroke) simply by changing medication time. If and only if the treating physician agrees (and he could be part of the study), case 60 should monitor for the next several weeks or until CHAT is removed, whichever occurs earlier. After one week's data have accumulated, we shall analyze them again, and if CHAT is confirmed, he would take one of his evening medications in the morning. After another week's data have accumulated on the new regime, we would analyze again and then decide on the next step ... [FH, personal communication to RKS, 3 Dec 2004]

The advice was misunderstood, and the opposite was done. Instead of switching, e.g., the beta blocker's evening dose to morning, Ramipril was switched from the morning to the evening, where it likely contributed more to CHAT. The next monitoring, as Table 2 shows, occurred only after 2 weeks, as were follow-up recordings of 6 or 5 days at arbitrary times.

About 9 months later, following the addition of two diuretic drugs, MESOR-hypertension was noted, and only another year later could normalization be ascertained.

The chronomic interpretation of the circadian and very much broader spectral element of the time structure of BP and HR variability and of its clinical relevance has resulted in the discovery of disease risk syndromes [20]. This case report illustrates the need for continued surveillance of BP and HR, notably when multiple medications are taken and the patient presents with one or several VVDs. Whether the addition of two diuretics in the morning helped reduce the circadian amplitude of BP and eliminated CHAT cannot be answered with any certainty in view of the long time spans between consecutive recordings. Ramipril was administered in the evening, in view of the results from the HOPE study of high-risk patients with cardiovascular disease, resulting in a marked reduction in cardiac events when Ramipril was taken in the evening [21; cf. 22].

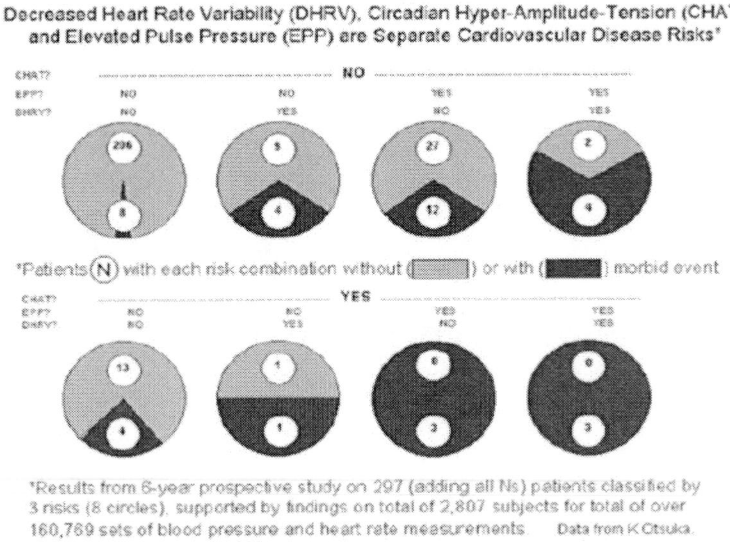

Figure 6. Decreased heart rate variability (DHRV), circadian hyper-amplitude-tension (CHAT) and elevated pulse pressure (EPP) are separate cardiovascular disease risks. CHAT is one of several conditions related to the variability in blood pressure (BP) and/or heart rate (HR) that is associated with an increase in vascular disease risk. The circadian (or preferably circaseptan profile) with too large a pulse pressure (the difference between systolic [S] BP and diastolic [D] BP, i.e., between the heart's contraction or relaxation, or the extent of change in pressure during a cardiac cycle) and a decreased HR variability (gauged by the standard deviation of HR) in relation to a threshold, preferably eventually all in gender- and age-matched peers are two other risk conditions (as is an abnormal circadian timing of BP but not of HR, not shown). Vascular disease risk is elevated in the presence of any one of these risk factors, and is elevated further when more than a single risk factor is present, suggesting that these abnormalities in variability of BP and HR are mostly independent and additive. Abnormalities in the variability of blood pressure and heart rate, impossible to find in a conventional office visit (the latter aiming at the fiction of a "true" blood pressure), can raise cardiovascular disease risk (gauged by the occurrence of a morbid event like a stroke in the next six years) from 4% to 100%. By comparison to subjects with acceptable blood pressure and heart rate variability, the relative cardiovascular disease risk associated with a **d**ecreased **h**eart **r**ate **v**ariability (DHRV), an **e**levated **p**ulse **p**ressure (EPP) and/or **c**ircadian **h**yper-**a**mplitude-**t**ension (CHAT) is greatly and statistically significantly increased. These risks, silent to the person involved and to the care provider, notably the risk of CHAT, can usually be reversed by chronobiologic self-help, also with a non-pharmacologic approach in the absence of MESOR-hypertension. © Halberg.

The day-night changes in BP result from an interplay of circadian rhythms in neurohumoral mechanisms responding to temporally patterned physical activity and mental loads, so that blood pressure monitoring becomes in itself revealing of the extent of known and, what is equally important, of unknown loads, if a good diary is maintained [1-6].

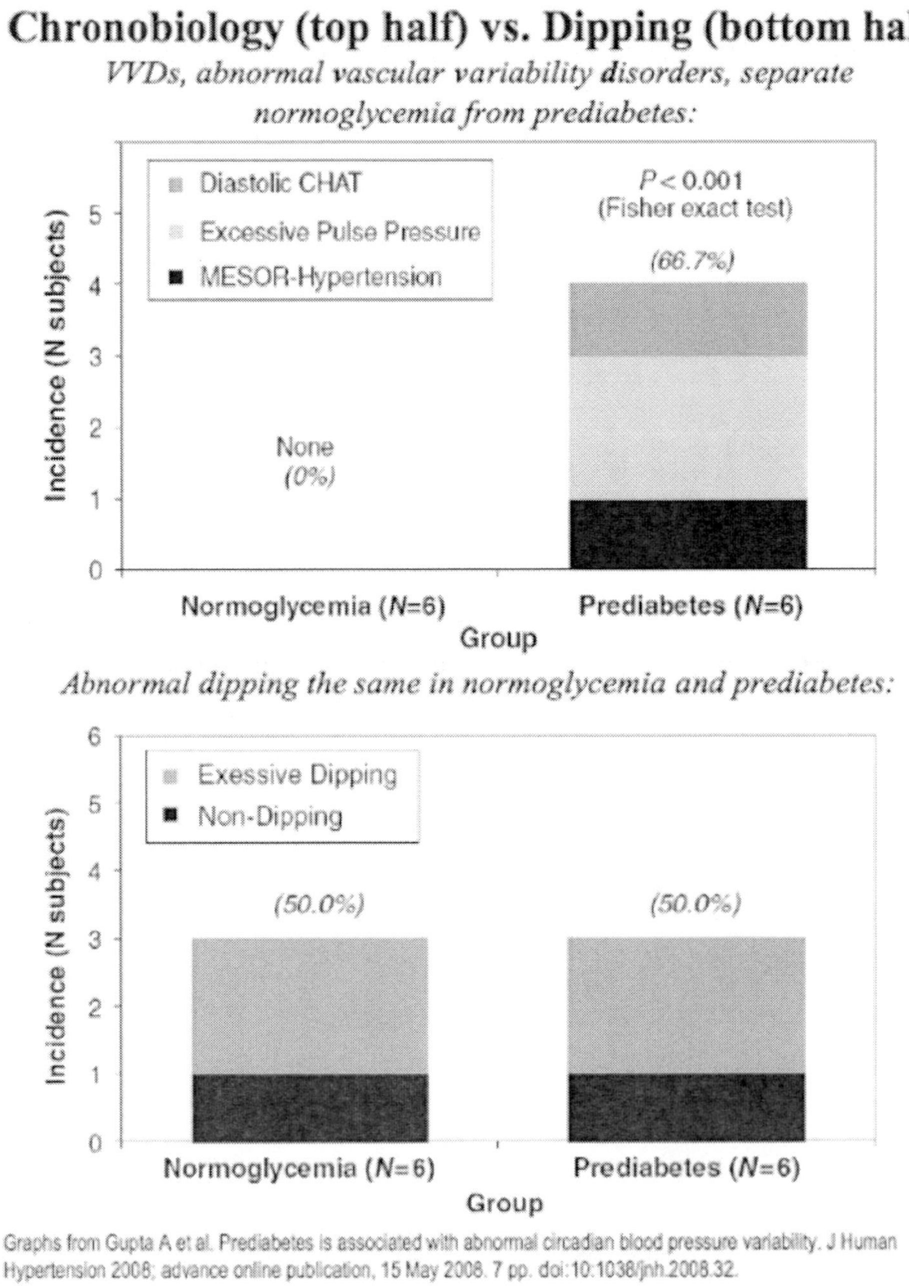

Figure 7. Chronobiology vs. dipping. Top: abnormal circadian blood pressure variability in normoglycemia and prediabetes. Bottom: Incidence of abnormal dipping in normoglycemics and prediabetics. From Alok Gupta et al. (8; cf. 23, 24).

The composite effects of endogenous and exogenous factors, including seen and unseen cyclic phenomena, among other conditions, can give rise to elevated BP, usually but not invariably, during diurnal activity. BP is usually reduced at night in both normotension and uncomplicated so-called "essential" MESOR-hypertension. C-ABPM also reveals the efficacy of antihypertensive medication throughout the 24 hours and as a function of drug administration. 24-hour/7-day BP/HR monitoring is not enough once VVDs are diagnosed; one needs continued monitoring, whenever the day-to-day variability in circadian parameters is present on some days but absent on other days. Other VVDs associated with increased cardiovascular disease risk in addition to MESOR-hypertension and CHAT include an above-threshold pulse pressure, an odd timing of the circadian rhythm in BP but not in that of HR, and/or a reduced infradian HR variability, Figure 6; all these risk syndromes are best treated [17, 18]. The importance of ABPM and of the indices derived from its chronomic application are just beginning to be documented and need greater appreciation and exploration, Figure 7 [8, 23, 24].

EPILOGUE

In the Lucknow, India, segment of BIOCOS, it was planned to examine chronobiologically analyzed records (C-ABPM), also to detect and correct VVDs. Eventually, the aim is to construct time-specified reference intervals for Indians as a function of gender and age and to identify problems in so doing. We do so with this case report, which documents CHAT in toto, as it was also documented in Indian immigrants to Silicon Valley [25]. Sometimes switching treatment timing leads to elimination of high risk of severe vascular disease, Figure 1. This opportunity was missed in the case here reported and there are other cases of incomplete compliance [26].

It could be argued that automatic monitors are expensive even via the BIOCOS project (corne001@umn.edu) with an 80% cost reduction in exchange for the data. Hard events and their treatment are much more costly, not only financially but in suffering, including incapacitation. Health planners can use C-ABPM to detect earliest changes by BP/HR monitoring in a premetabolic syndrome, including prediabetes and prehypertension. Here lies the challenge, which is the greater, the weaker the economy, and the greater one's concern for the proverbial ounce of prevention vs. pound of cure. Education of the population in the need to help itself, preferably in earliest schooling, remains the task on hand [27].

REFERENCES

[1] Cornelissen G, Chen CH, Halberg F. Predictive value of blood pressure variability. *N. Engl. J. Med.* 2006; 355: 850-851. Cf. Cornélissen G, Halberg F, Otsuka K, Singh RB, Chen CH. Chronobiology predicts actual and proxy outcomes when dipping fails. *Hypertension* 2007; 49: 237-239. doi:10.1161/01.HYP.0000250392.51418.64.

[2] Singh RB, Cornelissen G, Weydahl A et al. Carcadian heart rate and blood pressure variability considered for research and patient care. *Int. J. Cardiol.* 2003; 87: 9-28.

[3] Otsuka K, Cornelissen G, Halberg F, Oehlert G. Excessive circadian amplitude of blood pressure increases risk of ischaemic stroke and nephropathy. *J. Med. Engin. Tech.* 1997; 21: 23-30.

[4] Otsuka K, Cornelissen G, Halberg F. Predictive value of blood pressure dipping and swinging with regard to vascular disease risk. *Clin. Drug Invest* 1996; 11: 20-31.

[5] Scarpelli PT, Gallo M, Chiari G. Chronobiology of blood pressure. *J. Nephrol.* 2000; 13: 197-204.

[6] Pickering TG, Shimbo D, Haas D. Ambulatory blood pressure monitoring. *N. Engl. J. Med.* 2006; 354: 2368-74.

[7] Halberg F, Cornélissen G, Otsuka K, Katinas GS, Schwartzkopff O, Halpin C, Mikulecky M, Revilla M, Siegelova J, Homolka P, Dusek J, Fiser B, Singh RB. Chronomics* (*the study of time structures, chronomes) detects altered vascular variabilities constituting risks greater than hypertension: with an illustrative case report. In: Mitro P, Pella D, Rybar R, Valocik G, editors. *Proceedings, 2nd Congress on Cardiovascular Diseases,* Kosice, Slovakia, 25-27 April 2002. Bologna: Monduzzi Editore; 2002. p. 223-258.

[8] Gupta AK, Greenway FL, Cornélissen G, Pan W, Halberg F. Prediabetes is associated with abnormal circadian blood pressure variability. *J. Human Hypertension* 2008; advance online publication, 15 May 2008. 7 pp. doi:10:1038/jnh.2008.32.

[9] Schaffer E, Cornélissen G, Rhodus N, Halhuber M, Watanabe Y, Halberg F. Outcomes of chronobiologically normotensive dental patients: a 7-year follow-up. *JADA* 2001; 132: 891-899.

[10] Halberg F, Cornélissen G, Haus E, Northrup G, Portela A, Wendt H, Otsuka K, Kumagai Y, Watanabe Y, Zaslavskaya R. Clinical relevance of about-yearly changes in blood pressure and the environment. *Int. J. Biometeorol.* 1996; 39: 161-175.

[11] Singh RB, Cornelissen G, Siegelova J, Homolka P, Halberg F. About half weekly circasemiseptan pattern in blood pressure and heart rate in men and women of India. *Scripta Medica* (Brno) 2002; 75: 125-28.

[12] Halberg F, Cornélissen G, Katinas G, Tvildiani L, Gigolashvili M, Janashia K, Toba T, Revilla M, Regal P, Sothern RB, Wendt HW, Wang ZR, Zeman M, Jozsa R, Singh RB, Mitsutake G, Chibisov SM, Lee J, Holley D, Holte JE, Sonkowsky RP, Schwartzkopff O, Delmore P, Otsuka K, Bakken EE, Czaplicki J, International BIOCOS Group. Chronobiology's progress: season's appreciations 2004-2005. Time-, frequency-, phase-, variable-, individual-, age- and site-specific chronomics. *J. Applied Biomedicine* 2006; 4: 1-38. http://www.zsf.jcu.cz/vyzkum/jab/4_1/halberg.pdf.

[13] Cornélissen G, Masalov A, Halberg F, Richardson JD, Katinas GS, Sothern RB, Watanabe Y, Syutkina EV, Wendt HW, Bakken EE, Romanov Y. Multiple resonances among time structures, chronomes, around and in us. Is an about 1.3-year periodicity in solar wind built into the human cardiovascular chronome? *Human Physiology* 2004; 30 (2): 86-92.

[14] Cugini P, Letizia C, Scarvo D. The circadian rhythmicity of serum angiotensin converting enzyme: its phasic relation with circadian cycle of plasma rennin and aldosterone. *Chronobiologia* 1988; 15:229-32.

[15] Neutal JL, Smith DHG, Venkatram C, Kaplan NM, et al. Application of ambulatory blood pressure monitoring in differentiating between antihypertensive agents. *Amer. J. Med.* 1993; 94: 181-187.

[16] Halberg E, Halberg F, Shankaraiah K. Plexo-serial linear-nonlinear rhythmometry of blood pressure, pulse and motor activity by a couple in their sixties. *Chronobiologia* 1981; 8: 351-366.

[17] Smolensky M, Halberg F, Sargent F II. Chronobiology of the life sequence. In: Itoh S, Ogata K, Yoshimura H, editors. *Advances in Climatic Physiology*. Tokyo: Igaku Shoin Ltd.; 1972. p. 281-318.

[18] Halberg F, Cornélissen G, International Womb-to-Tomb Chronome Initiative Group: Resolution from a meeting of the International Society for Research on Civilization Diseases and the Environment (New SIRMCE Confederation), Brussels, Belgium, March 17-18, 1995: Fairy tale or reality? *Medtronic Chronobiology* Seminar #8, April 1995, 12 pp. text, 18 figures. URL http://www.msi.umn.edu/~halberg/

[19] Shinagawa M, Kubo Y, Otsuka K, Ohkawa S, Cornélissen G, Halberg F. Impact of circadian amplitude and chronotherapy: relevance to prevention and treatment of stroke. *Biomedicine and Pharmacotherapy* 2001; 55 (Suppl 1): 125s-132s.

[20] Halberg F, Cornelissen GG, Wall D, Ostuka K, Halberg J, Katinas G, Watanabe Y, Halhuber M, Muller- Bohn T, Delmore P, Siegelova J, Homolka P, Fiser B, Dusek J, Sanchez de la Pena S, Maggioni C, Delyokov A, Gorgo Y, Gubin D, Carandente F, Schaffer E, Rhodus N, Borer K, Sonkowsky RP, Schwarrtzkopff O. Engineering and governmental challenge: 7-day/24-hour chronobiologic blood pressure and heart rate screening. *Biomedical Instrumentation and technology* 2002; Part I, 36: 89-122; Part II, 36: 183-197.

[21] The HOPE investigators. Effects of an angiotensin-converting-enzyme inhibitor, ramipril, on cardiovascular events in high risk patients. *N. Engl. J. Med.* 2000; 342: 145-53.

[22] Svensson P, de Faire U, Sleight P, Yusuf S, Östergren J. Comparative effects of ramipril on ambulatory and office blood pressures: a HOPE substudy. *Hypertension* 2001; 38: e28-e32.

[23] Cornélissen G, Halberg F, Otsuka K, Singh RB, Chen CH. Chronobiology predicts actual and proxy outcomes when dipping fails. *Hypertension* 2007; 49: 237-239. doi:10.1161/01.HYP.0000250392.51418.64.

[24] Halberg F, Cornélissen G, Halberg J, Schwartzkopff O. Pre-hypertensive and other variabilities also await treatment. *Am. J. Medicine* 2007; 120: e19-e20. doi:10.1016/j.amjmed.2006.02.045.

[25] Sundaram B, Holley DC, Cornélissen G, Naik D, Hanumansetty R, Singh RB, Otsuka K, Halberg F. Circadian and circaseptan (about-weekly) aspects of immigrant Indians' blood pressure and heart rate in California, USA. *Biomedicine and Pharmacotherapy* 2005; 59 (Suppl 1): S76-S85.

[26] Pati AK, Parganiha A, Pradhan RK, Agrawal A, Cornélissen G, Halberg F. Compliance with monitoring needed after switching treatment timing to eliminate vascular disease risks. *Proceedings, International Conference on the Frontiers of Biomedical Science: Chronobiology*, Chengdu, China, September 24-26, 2006, p. 55-57.

[27] Halberg F, Smith HN, Cornélissen G, Delmore P, Schwartzkopff O, International BIOCOS Group. Hurdles to asepsis, universal literacy, and chronobiology—all to be overcome. *Neuroendocrinol. Lett.* 2000; 21: 145-160.

In: World Heart Research Yearbook. Volume 1
Editors: Franz Halberg and R. B. Singh
ISBN: 978-1-60741-881-8

MODIFYING EFFECT OF *PUNICA GRANATUM* FLOWERS ON LIPIDS AND LIPIDS-METABOLIZING ENZYMES STATUS IN STREPTOZOTOCIN INDUCED DIABETIC RATS

S. Manoharan**, *P. Ranezab Anishkumar*, *K. Panjamurthy*, *L. Vellaichamy* and *A. Linsa Mary

Department of Biochemistry and Biotechnology,
Faculty of Science
Annamalai University,
Tamil Nadu, India

ABSTRACT

Our aim was to investigate the anti-hyperglycemic and anti-hyperlipidemic effects of ethanolic extract of *Punica granatum* flowers (PgFEet) in streptozotocin induced diabetic rats. Diabetes mellitus was induced in Wistar rats by single intraperitoneal injection of streptozotocin (50mg/kg b.w.) dissolved in 0.1M-citrate buffer (pH 4.5), after overnight fasting for 12 h.

Hyperglycemia associated with significant alterations in lipids and lipoproteins pattern and activities of lipids-metabolizing enzymes were noticed in streptozotocin induced diabetic rats.

Oral administration of ethanolic extract of *Punica granatum* flowers (400 mg/kg b.w.) to diabetic rats brought back the status of blood glucose, lipids and lipoproteins pattern and the activities of lipids-metabolizing enzymes to near normal concentrations. Our study thus demonstrated the significant anti-hyperglycemic and anti-hyperlipidemic effects of *Punica granatum* flowers in streptozotocin induced diabetic rats.

Keywords: Diabetes mellitus, lipids, lipids- metabolizing enzymes, Punica granatum

---

* Corresponding author: Dr. S. Manoharan, Reader, Department of Biochemistry and Biotechnology, Faculty of Science, Annamalai University, Annamalainagar – 608 002, Tamil Nadu, India. Tel: +91 - 4144 – 238343. Fax: +91 - 4144 – 238080. e-mail: manshisak@yahoo.com.

INTRODUCTION

Diabetes mellitus is a metabolic disorder characterized by hyperglycemia due to disturbances in carbohydrate, fat and protein metabolism, resulting from defects in insulin secretion, insulin action, and or both.

Diabetes mellitus if not controlled and properly managed, leads to acute metabolic complications (diabetic ketoacidosis, hyperosmolar non–ketotic coma and hypoglycemia) and long-term complications (retinopathy, nephropathy and neuropathy). People with diabetes are also at increased risk of cardiovascular, peripheral vascular and cerebrovascular diseases.

According to World Health Organization, approximately 171 million people worldwide are affected by diabetes mellitus and assumed that by the year 2030 this number will double. In India, approximately 30 million people are affected by diabetes mellitus and this figure will double by the year 2030, due to its vast population [1, 2].

Streptozotocin, a glucosamine nitrosourea compound, shows selective cytotoxicity to pancreatic β-cells and therefore used as an agent to induce diabetes mellitus in experimental animals. Streptozotocin induce diabetes mellitus in experimental animals through overproduction of reactive oxygen species, such as superoxide, hydrogen peroxide, hydroxyl radical and singlet oxygen, which cause DNA strand breaks and damages in β-cells of pancreatic islets [3].

Lipids are a group of heterogeneous metabolically active substances that play an important role in determining a number of properties and functions of normal cells. Liver, an important metabolic organ, plays a pivotal role in glucose and lipid homeostasis and is severely affected during diabetes [4].

The liver participates in oxidation and metabolic conversion of free fatty acids, synthesis of cholesterol and phospholipids and in the secretion of specific classes of plasma lipoproteins. Diabetes affects large number of metabolic pathways including lipid metabolism by altering the activities of various enzymes involved in these pathways.

As insulin is an important regulator of many enzymes involved in lipolysis and lipogenesis, its deficiency causes major changes in the activity of these enzymes and thereby affects overall lipid metabolism in various tissues.

In recent years, considerable interest has been directed towards the investigation of plasma lipids in diabetes mellitus due to the fact that abnormal lipid levels lead to the development of coronary artery disease in diabetic patients. Altered pattern of lipids were reported in both experimental and human diabetes mellitus [5, 6].

Medicinal plants and herbs have been used for the treatment and prevention of diabetes mellitus and its complications in Ayurvedha and other indigenous systems of medicine. Most of these medicinal plants are not scientifically validated for their antidiabetic efficacy. Scientific studies on theses plants may therefore provide invaluable antidiabetic drugs. *Punica granatum*, a fruit-bearing deciduous shrub or small tree, is popularly known as "Pomegranate" in English and occurs throughout India.

Different parts of *Punica granatum* are used in Indian traditional medicine for treating several disorders including diabetes mellitus [7]. To the best of our knowledge, there were no scientific report on modifying effect of *Punica granatum* flowers on lipids and lipid metabolizing enzymes status in streptozotocin induced diabetic rats.

The present study was thus designed to focus the effect of *Punica granatum* flowers on lipids and lipids- metabolizing enzymes status in streptozotocin induced diabetic rats.

MATERIALS AND METHODS

Chemicals

Streptozotocin was purchased from Sigma Aldrich Chemicals, Pvt., Ltd., Bangalore. All other chemicals and reagents used were of analytical grade.

Animals

Albino Wistar male rats 7-8 weeks old and weighing180-200g were used for the present study. The animals were obtained from Central animal house, Rajah Muthiah Institute of Health Sciences, Annamalai University, India and were maintained under controlled conditions of temperature and humidity with a 12 h light/dark cycle. The animals were randomized into control and experimental groups and were housed four or five in polypropylene cages. Standard pellets obtained from Kamadenu agency, Agro Corporation Private Limited, Bangalore, India, were used as a basal diet during the experiment. The control and experimental animals were provided food and drinking water *ad libitum*.

Preparation of Ethanolic Extract of Punica Granatum Flowers

Five hundred grams of fresh flowers of *Punica granatum* were dried powdered and then soaked in 1500ml of 95% of ethanol overnight. After filtration, the residue obtained was again resuspended in equal volume of 95% ethanol for 48 h and filtered again. The above two filtrates were mixed and the solvent was evaporated in a rotavapor at 40°-$50^{o}C$ under reduced pressure. A 12% semisolid dark brown material obtained was stored at 0-$4^{o}C$ until used. A known volume of the ethanolic residual extract is suspended in distilled water and was orally administered to the animals by gastric intubation using a force-feeding needle during the experimental period.

Induction of Diabetes Mellitus

Diabetes mellitus was induced in Wistar rats by single intraperitoneal injection of freshly prepared solution of streptozotocin (50mg/kg bw) in 0.1M-citrate buffer (pH 4.5) after overnight fasting for 12h [8]. The diabetes mellitus was assessed in streptozotocin-induced rats by determining the blood glucose concentration, 48 hours after the injection of streptozotocin. The rats with blood glucose level above 250 mg/dl were selected for the experimental studies.

Experimental Design

Group I animals: Served as untreated control

Group II animals: Received oral administration of PgFEet (400mg/kg b.w.) alone for 45 days

Group III animals: Treated with single intraperitoneal injection of streptozotocin (50 mg/kg. b.w.) after overnight fast for 12h. (Diabetic control)

Group IV animals: Received oral administration of PgFEet (400mg/kg b.w.) for 45 days after diabetes mellitus was confirmed

Group V animals: Received oral administration of glibenclamide (600 μg/kg. b.w.) for 45 days after diabetes mellitus was confirmed

Biochemical Estimations

Blood glucose was determined by the method of Sasaki *et al* [9] using O-toluidine reagent. Total haemoglobin was measured by the method of Drabkin and Austin [10] and glycosylated haemoglobin was determined by the method of Sudhakar Nayak and Pattabiraman [11]. Plasma insulin was estimated by ELISA method using Boehinger Mannheim GmbH Kit [12]. Total cholesterol and phospholipids were assayed according to the methods of Parekh and Jung [13] and Zilversmlt and Davis [14] respectively. Free fatty acids and triglycerides were estimated by the methods of Falholf ef al. [15] and Foster and Dunn [16] respectively. HDL cholesterol was estimated by the method of Gidez and Webb (17). LDL cholesterol was calculated using the formula,

$$\text{LDL cholesterol} = \text{Total cholesterol} - \text{HDL} + \left(\frac{TG}{5}\right)$$

Lecithin cholesterol acyl transferase (LCAT) activity was assayed by the method of Hitz et al. [18]. Lipoprotein lipase (LPL) activity was assayed by the method of Korn [19].

Statistical Analysis

The data are expressed as mean ± SD. Statistical comparisons were performed by one-way analysis of variance (ANOVA) followed by Duncan's multiple comparisons test (DMRT). The results were considered statistically significant if the p values were 0.05 or less.

Results

The status of blood glucose, urinary sugar, total haemoglobin, glycosylated haemoglobin, and plasma insulin content in control and experimental animals in each group are shown in table 1. Blood glucose and glycosylated haemoglobin levels were significantly increased whereas plasma insulin and total haemoglobin were decreased in diabetic animals as compared to control animals. The urinary sugar was (+++) in diabetic animals. Oral administration of PgFEet to diabetic animals brought back the status of blood glucose, urinary sugar, glycosylated haemoglobin, total hemoglobin and plasma insulin to near normal range. The antihyperglycemic effect of PgFEet was much comparable to that of glibenclamide. Wistar rats treated with PgFEet alone showed no significant difference in the above mentioned biochemical parameters as compared to control rats.

The status of lipids (total cholesterol, triglycerides, phospholipids, and free fatty acids) and lipoproteins pattern (HDL-cholesterol and LDL-cholesterol) in plasma and liver of control and experimental animals in each group is shown in table 2 and 3 respectively. Lipids pattern were significantly increased in plasma and liver of streptozotocin induced diabetic animals as compared to control animals. LDL-cholesterol was increased whereas HDL-cholesterol was significantly decreased in plasma of diabetic animals compared to control animals. However, oral administration of PgFEet to diabetic animals brought back all the biochemical variables to near normal range. The modifying effect of PgFEet on lipids and lipoproteins pattern was much comparable to that of glibenclamide. Wistar rats treated with PgFEet alone showed no significant difference in the above mentioned biochemical parameters as compared to control rats.

Table 4 shows the activities of lipoprotein lipase (LPL) and lecithin cholesterol acyl transferase (LCAT) in plasma of control and experimental animals in each group.

Table 1. Blood glucose, urine sugar, plasma insulin, total hemoglobin and glycosylated hemoglobin concentrations in control and experimental animals in each group

Groups/Parameters	Control	Control+ PgFEet (400mg/kg bw)	Diabetic control	Diabetic+ PgFEet (400mg/kg bw)	Diabetic+ glibenclamide (600μg/kg bw)
Fasting blood glucose (mg/dl)	91.6±5.64^{a}	88.5±4.82^{a}	286.3±12.9^{b}	103.83±6.88^{c}	105.8±9.30^{c}
Urine Sugar*	Nil	Nil	+++	Nil	Nil
Plasma Insulin (μU/ml)	15.1±0.78^{a}	15.6±0.96^{a}	10.5±0.86^{b}	13.1±1.00^{c}	13.7±1.02^{c}
Total hemoglobin (g/dl)	14.0±0.86^{a}	14.2±1.12^{a}	9.12±0.94^{b}	12.6±0.98^{c}	12.4±1.02^{c}
Glycosylated hemoglobin (HbA1%)	3.92±0.30^{a}	3.84±0.38^{a}	6.98±0.73^{b}	4.62±0.45^{c}	4.84±0.49^{c}

Values are expressed as mean ± SD (n=6).
Values not sharing a common superscript letter in the same row differ significantly at $p< 0.05$ (DMRT)
PgFEet – *Punica granatum* flowers ethanolic extract
* - (+++) Indicates more than 1% Sugar.

The activities of LPL and LCAT were significantly decreased in diabetic animals as compared to control animals. However, oral administration of PgFEet to diabetic animals significantly increased the activities of LPL and LCAT. The effect of PgFEet and was much comparable to that of glibenclamide. Wistar rats treated with PgFEet alone showed no significant difference in the activities of LPL and LCAT as compared to control rats.

Table 2. Plasma lipids and lipoprotein patterns in control and experimental animals in each group

Groups/Parameters	Total cholesterol (mg/dl)	Phospholipids (mg/dl)	Triglycerides (mg/dl)	Free fatty acids (mg/dl)	HDL-C (mg/dl)	LDL-C (mg/dl)
Control	82.1±7.1 [a]	95.2±7.82 [a]	78.5±6.5 [a]	10.5±0.68 [a]	25.20±1.62 [a]	58.4.4±6.25 [a]
Control+PgFEet (400mg/kg bw)	80.5±6.1 [a]	92.5±7.65 [a]	75.3±7.9 [a]	10.02±0.72 [a]	26.30±1.45 [a]	58.41±6.82 [a]
Diabetic control	156.43±9.2 [b]	152.1±10.4 [b]	147.6±8.25 [b]	18.6±0.88 [b]	17.44±0.82 [b]	124.1±8.92 [b]
Diabetic+PgFEet (400mg/kg bw)	100.22±8.2 [c]	114.6±8.20 [c]	99.14±9.8 [c]	12.44±1.16 [c]	22.03±1.28 [c]	79.15±7.98 [c]
Diabetic+glibenclamide (600µg/kg bw)	103.2±8.5 [c]	115.2±9.46 [c]	102.4±9.5 [c]	13.12±0.84 [c]	22.30±0.98 [c]	82.0±6.60 [c]

Values are expressed as mean ± SD (n=6).
Values not sharing a common superscript letter in the same column differ significantly at $p < 0.05$ (DMRT).
PgFEet – *Punica granatum* dried flowers ethanolic extract.

Table 3. Activities of lecithin cholesterol acyltransferase (LCAT) and lipoprotein lipase (LPL) in plasma of control and experimental animals in each group

Groups/Parameters	LCAT (U^A/I)	LPL (U^B/I)
Control	62.35±4.15 [a]	6.82±0.9 [a]
Control+PgFEet (400mg/kg bw)	62.36±4.4 [a]	6.96±0.8 [a]
Diabetic control	42.62±2.10 [b]	4.52±0.67 [b]
Diabetic+PgFEet (400mg/kg bw)	52.15±3.9 [c]	3.90±0.32 [c]
Diabetic+glibenclamide (600µg/kg bw)	53.25±3.62 [c]	4.1±0.39 [c]

Values are expressed as mean ± SD (n=6 rats).
Values not sharing a common superscript letter in the same column differ significantly at $p < 0.05$ (DMRT)
PgFEet – *Punica granatum* dried flowers ethanolic extract.
A = µmolholesterol liberated/hr., B = µmol glycerol liberated/hr.

Table 4. Lipid profile in the liver of control and experimental animals in each group

Groups/Parameters	Total cholesterol (mg/g tissue)	Triglycerides (mg/g tissue)	Phospholipids (mg/g tissue)	Free fatty acids (mg/g tissue)
Control	4.42±0.44 [a]	3.96±0.28 [a]	20.4±1.8 [a]	7.68±0.9 [a]
Control+PgFEet (400mg/kg bw)	4.08±0.41 [a]	3.93±0.30 [a]	19.4±1.85 [a]	7.35±0.86 [a]
Diabetic control	8.60±0.69 [b]	6.74±0.50 [b]	42.3±2.92 [b]	14.60±2.26 [b]
Diabetic+PgFEet (400mg/kg bw)	5.47±0.40 [c]	4.41±0.24 [c]	32.1±1.74 [c]	8.48±0.90 [c]
Diabetic+glibenclamide (600µg/kg bw)	5.65±0.52 [c]	4.63±0.25 [c]	32.5±1.58 [c]	8.62±0.81 [c]

Values are expressed as mean ± SD (n=6 rats).
Values not sharing a common superscript letter in the same column differ significantly at $p < 0.05$ (DMRT).
PgFEet – *Punica granatum* dried flowers ethanolic extract.

DISCUSSION

In the present study, an increase in blood glucose was accompanied by a decrease in plasma insulin, total hemoglobin and increase in glycosylated hemoglobin was noticed in diabetic rats as compared to control rats. Oral administration of ethanolic extract of *Punica granatum* flowers to diabetic rats brought back the levels to near normal concentrations. The antidiabetic efficacy of *Punica granatum* flowers suggests its ability to stimulate insulin secretion from surviving pancreatic β-cells. Several authors reported flavonoids, sterols, alkaloids and phenolics as bioactive antidiabetic principles [20]. The phytochemical examination of *Punica granatum* flowers revealed the presence of polyphenols such as pomegranatate, ellagic acid, 3,3',4'-tri-o-methyl ellagic acid, gallic acid, urolic and maslinic acids [20]. The antihyperglycemic effect of *Punica granatum* flowers is probably due to the presence of these bioactive antidiabetic principles and their synergistic properties. Oral administration of ethanolic extract of *Punica granatum* flowers to diabetic rats for 45 days decreased the levels of glycosylated hemoglobin and increased the content of total hemoglobin. Our results suggest that *Punica granatum* flowers improved the glycemic control mechanism in diabetic rats. In the present study, the antidiabetic effect of *Punica granatum* flowers was also compared with glibenclamide, the standard reference drug. The effect of *Punica granatum* flowers in diabetic rats was much comparable to that of the reference drug.

In the present study we observed an altered lipid, lipoprotein and lipoprotein metabolizing enzymes pattern in streptozotocin induced diabetic rats. A positive association between diabetes mellitus and lipid abnormalities has been shown [21]. Altered lipids and lipoprotein profile in diabetic patients contribute to the development of atherosclerosis [22, 23]. Elevated plasma and tissue cholesterol and phospholipids have been reported in diabetic rats [5, 24]. Hyperglycemia associated plasma triglycerides and LDL levels and decrease in HDL levels in diabetic patients are often associated with development of premature atherosclerosis. Elevated total cholesterol in plasma is probably due to increased mobilization of free fatty acids from peripheral fat depots. Hypertriglyceridaemia associated with increased VLDL are the common dyslipidemia in Indian diabetic subjects [6]. High concentration of fatty acids in plasma promotes the liver in the conversion of some fatty acids into phospholipids and cholesterol. Reduction in HDL cholosterol and increased VLDL and LDL cholesterol has been well documented in diabetes mellitus [24]. Our results corroborate these observations. Liver has a crucial role in the metabolism of lipids and lipoproteins. Increase in total cholesterol in the liver of diabetic rats is probably due to defect in insulin secretion and function. Elevated triglycerides in the liver of diabetic rats are probably due to increased synthesis or decreased output from liver as VLDL or combination of both [24, 25].

Lipoprotein lipase (LPL) plays a central role in the catabolism of triglyceride rich lipoprotein. Lipoprotein lipase has a role in the production of high density lipoprotein (HDL) and anti- atherogenic lipoproteins [26]. Decreased LPL activity observed in the present study is therefore due to hypertriglyceridaemia and hypo-HDL cholesterolemia. Lopes-Virella et al [27] reported that treatment of diabetes with insulin lowered the plasma triglycerides levels, by returning LPL activity to normal status.

Lecithin cholesterol acyltransferase (LCAT) is the plasma enzyme responsible for formation of most of the cholesterol ester (EC) found in circulation. It has been reported that

LCAT and LPL are suppressed when insulin levels are lowered in circulation, which in turn adversely affects HDL metabolism [28]. Fielding et al [29] and Dirican et al [30] have reported decrease in LCAT activities in diabetic patients. HDL helps to scavenge cholesterol from extra-hepatic tissues in the presence of LCAT and brings it to the liver. Decreased HDL observed in the present study therefore responsible for diminished LCAT activity, which in turn contribute to elevated plasma cholesterol levels.

Oral administration of ethanolic extract of *Punica granatum* flowers to diabetic rats brought back the levels of lipids and lipoproteins and the activities of lipid metabolizing enzymes to near normal concentrations. The protective effect of *Punica granatum* flowers on lipids status is probably due to its role in the inhibition of endogenous synthesis of lipids and antagonizing the aberrations of lipids and lipoproteins metabolism. The antihyperlpidemic effect of *Punica granatum* flowers is also due to presence of polyphenols such as ellagic acid and gallic acid, which are shown to have antihyperlipidemic effect in experimental animal models [31,32]. The effect of *Punica granatum* flowers on status of lipids, lipoproteins and the activities of lipid metabolizing enzymes was much comparable to that of glibenclamide. The present study thus demonstrated that *Punica granatum* flowers maintained the status of lipids, lipoproteins and the activities of lipid metabolizing enzymes in streptozotocin induced diabetic rats. Our study thus concludes that *Punica granatum* flowers have shown protective effect on diabetes-induced dyslipidemia in streptozotocin induced diabetic rats. Further studies are needed to test the efficacy of *Punica granatum* flowers on lipids-related metabolic disorders such as coronary artery diseases.

REFERENCES

[1] Vasudevan AR, Burns A, Fonseca VA. The effectiveness of intensive glycemic control for the prevention of vascular complications in diabetes mellitus. *Treat Endocrinol* 2006, 5: 273-286.

[2] Mohan V. Why are Indians more prone to diabetes? *Journal Association Physicians India* 2004, 54: 468-474.

[3] Weis RB. Streptozotocin: a review of its pharmacology, efficacy and toxicity. Cancer. *Teat.Rep* 1982, 66:427-438.

[4] Umesh, CS. Yadav, KM, Najma ZB. Efeect of sodium- orthovanadate and *Trigonella foenum-graecum* seeds on hepatic and renal lipogenic enzymes and lipid profile during alloxan diabetes. *J. Biosci* 2004, 29: 81-91.

[5] Pavana P. Manoharan S. Renju GL, Sethupathy S. Antihyperglycemic and antihyperlipidemic effect of *Tephrosia purpurea* leaf extract in streptozotocin induced diabetic rats. *J. Enviorn. Biol.* 2007, 28: 833-837.

[6] Das S. Presidential Oration - 2003. Lipids, Diabetes and Coronary Artery Disease in Indians. *Int. J. Diab. Dev. Countries* 2004, 24: 87-95.

[7] Satyavati GV, Gupta AK, Tandon N. *Medicinal plants of India,* vol. 2. Indian Council of Medical Research, New Delhi, 1978, p539-544.

[8] Torrico F, Cepeda M, Guerrero G, et al. Hypoglycaemic effect of *Croton cuneatus* in streptozotocin-induced diabetic rats. *Braz. J. Pharmacogn* 2007, 17: 166-169.

[9] Sasaki T, Matsy S, Sonac A. Effect of acetic and concentration on the colour reaction in the O-toluidine boric acid method for blood glucose estimation. *Rinsho Kagaku* 1972, 1: 346-353.

[10] Drabkin DL, Austin JM. Spectophotometric constants for common haemoglobin derivatives in human, dog and rabbit blood. *J. Biol. Chem* 1932, 98: 719-733.

[11] Sudhakar Nayak S, Pattabiraman TN. A new colourimetric method forms the estimation of glycosylated haemoglobin. *Clin. Chem. Acta* 1981, 109: 267-274.

[12] Anderson L, Dinesen B, Jorgesen PN, Poulsen F, Roder MF. Enzyme Immunoassay for intact human insulin in serum or plasma. *Clin. Chem. Acta* 1993, 38: 578-585.

[13] Parkeh AC, Jung DH. Cholesterol determination with ferric acetate uranium acetate reagent and sulfuric acid-ferrous sulfate reagents. *Anal. Chem.* 1970, 1423-1427.

[14] Zilversmit DB, Davis. Micro determination of phospholipids by trichloro acetic acid precipitation. J *Lab Clin. Med.* 1950, 35, 155-159.

[15] Falholf K, Falholf W, Lund B. An assay colorimetric method for routine determination of free fatty acids in plasma. *Clin. Chim. Acta* 1973, 46,105-111.

[16] Foster LB, Dunn RT. Stable reagents for determination of serum triglycerides by colorimetric hantzsch condensation method. *Clin. Chim. Acta* 1973, 19,338-340.

[17] Gidez WM, Webb M. revision of cholesterol determination. *J. Biochem.* 1950, 187, 97-106.

[18] Hitz J, Steormetry J, Siest G. Plasma LCAT reference values and effects of xenobiotics. *Clin. Chim. Acta.* 1983,133, 85-86.

[19] Korn ED. A heparin activated lipoprotein lipase isolation and characterization of enzyme from normal rats. *J. Biol. Chem.* 1955, 215, 1-26.

[20] Wang R, Wang W, Wang L et al. Constituents of the flowers of *Punica grantum. Fitoterapia* 2006, 77: 534-537.

[21] Goldberg RB, Lipid disorders in diabetes. *Diabetes Care* 1981; 4: 561-572.

[22] Orchard TJ. Dyslipoproteinemia and diabetes. *Endocrinol. Metab. Clin. North Am.* 1990, 19: 361-380.

[23] Betteridge DJ. Diabetic dyslipidemia. *Am. J. Med.* 1994, 96: 25-31.

[24] Ruzaidi A, IN Amin, AG Awalvah, M Hamid, HA Faizul. The effect of *Malaysian cocoa* extract on glucose levels and lipid profiles in diabetic rats. *J. Ethanopharmcol.* 2005, 98: 55-60.

[25] Bhandaru R, Srinivasan SR, Radhakrishna murthy B, Berenson GS. Effects of diabetes and high fat–high cholesterol diet on plasma lipid levels and on erythrocyte membrane composition. *Atherosclerosis* 1982, 42, 263-272.

[26] Takeshi T, Kenji U, Toshiki S et al. Cilostazol, a selective type III phosphodiesterase inhibitor, decreases triglyceride and increases HDL cholesterol levels by increasing lipoprotein lipase activity in rats. *Atherosclerosis* 2000, 152: 299-305.

[27] Lopes-Virella MF, Wohltmann HJ, Mayfield RK, Loadholt CB, Colwell JA. Effect of metabolic control on lipid, lipoprotein, and apolipoprotein levels in 55 insulin-dependent diabetic patients. A longitudinal study. *Diabetes* 1983, 32: 20-25.

[28] Fossati P, Romon-Rousseaux M. Insulin and HDL-cholesterol metabolism. *Diabetes Metab.* 1987, 13:390-394.

[29] Fielding CJ, Shore VG, Fielding PE. A protein cofactor of lecithin cholesterol acyl transferase. *Biochem. Biophys. Res. Commun.* 1972, 46:1493–1498.

[30] Dirican M, Serdar Z, Sarndol E, Surmen-gur E. Lecthin cholesterol acyltransferase activity and cholesterol ester transfer rate in patients with diabetes mellitus. *Turk. J. Med. Sci.* 2003,. 33: 95-101.

[31] Devipriya N, Sudheer AR, Vishwanathan P, Menon VP. Modulatory potential of ellagic acid, a natural plant polyphenol on altered lipid profile and lipid peroxidation status during alcohol-induced toxicity: a pathohistological study. *J. Biochem. Mol. Toxicol.* 2008, 22: 101-112.

[32] Hsu CL, Yen GC. Effect of gallic acid on high fat diet-induced dyslipidaemia, hepatosteatosis and oxidative stress in rats. *Br. J. Nutr.* 2007;98:727-735.

In: World Heart Research Yearbook. Volume 1
Editors: Franz Halberg and R. B. Singh
ISBN: 978-1-60741-881-8

BODY COMPOSITION AND CARDIO-VASCULAR STATUS OF INDIAN SCHOOL GOING GIRLS

*Anindita Mandal (Majee)**
Raja Peary Mohan College
Dist: Hooghly
West Bengal, India

ABSTRACT

While the growth and development of an individual is dependant upon multiple factors, body composition and cardio-vascular fitness play a prominent role in indicating the body fitness level including the power to combat the cardio-vascular diseases .Again the benefit of modern civilization vis-à-vis industrialization and technical innovations allow to curb the physical labour thereby reducing the cardio-vascular fitness of an individual.

In order to deal with problem specially the body composition and cardio-vascular fitness pattern, a cross sectional study was conducted on 490 Bengalee school going girls (9-18yrs) of middle class families in semi-urban area of Hooghly district of West Bengal, India.

The study revealed that maximum gain in body height and body weight attained in the range of 11-15 yrs but triceps and subscapular skinfold thickness and % body fat showed peak values having age ranging of 14-16 years. Systolic blood pressure values showed maximum gain in between 12-13 years and 14-16 years but Diastolic blood pressure values showed maximum gain within 12-13 years. Maximum oxygen uptake was measured indirectly by QCT and when it was compared with vo_2 max values of Indian (Bengalee) girls from Kolkata ,West Bengal ,India by direct method ,it was found that Vo_2max (lit/min) values of these two studies were not significantly different but significant difference was observed in Vo_2max(ml/Kg/min) values.

There was high correlation between Vo_2max(lit/min) with physical parameters of these population .Thus on the basis of age, body height and body weight ,simple regression equations were reproduced ,which are as follows:

Vo_2max(lit/min)= 0.087 Age + 0.037 (r = 0.65,P< 0.001, SEE = 0.25)
Vo_2max(lit/min)= 0.025 body weight + 0.228 (r = 0.88, P<0.001,SEE= 0.16)
Vo_2max(lit/min)= 0.024 body height – 2.31(r = 0.73, P< 0.001, SEE= 0.22)

* Address for correspondence: 27, Mohanlal Mukherjee street, p.o-uttarpara, dist- hooghly, pin-712258. West Bengal (india); permanent address—do; e-mail-anindita11us@rediffmail.com; tel no.-o33-26636745®; o33-26634155(o); 9433910161.

Among these prediction equations , Vo_2 max(lit/min) from body weight was considered as most reliable one because of highest correlation coefficient between Vo_2max and body weight as well as minimum SEE.

On the basis of body composition and predicted Vo_2max value, the young adolescent girls should take care of their food habits and physical activities to avoid excess body fat and cardio-vascular complications right from their early age.

Keywords: Body composition, Vo2max, Cardio-vascular fitness, % body fat

INTRODUCTION

Maximum aerobic power is a well defined indicator of cardio-vascular fitness and it has, therefore, been widely studied in both adults and children. Maximum O_2 uptake of a children starts to develop during elementary school ages between 10 – 12 years and continues to develop during puberty. Peak maximum O_2 uptake of a children is useful in determining the growth and development of cardio-respiratory and musculo energetic system (Dey and Debray, 2003). Civilization and industrialization make our life pleasant, jubilant and luxuriant. But automation and technological upliftment reduce our physical labour both at home and outside which inturn increases the incidence of cardio-vascular disease (Sadhan et al, 2007). So the assessment of blood pressure, percentage of body fat, blood lipids and cardio vascular fitness in children and adolescent has been applied widely because atherosclerotic process is initiated early in life (Rowland and Green, 1988) and on the basis of this study proper dietary and exercise habits are implemented at young age. The regional variation of morphological characteristics of Indian Children occurs due to socio-economic, climatic and genetic variation. Swaminathan et al (1997) concluded that nutritional and socio-cultural factors may play an important role in determining peak O_2 uptake (Vo_{2max}) of children from different population rather than ethnic difference alone.

In India, physical growth and maximum aerobic power of girls (eastern region) have been studied only by chatterjee et al (1979). But the relationship among cardio-respiratory fitness, body composition and blood pressure in school children specially school going girls are scanty (Guerra et al, 2002) So the *purpose* of the present project is:

1) To establish growth pattern, body composition and cardio-vascular fitness pattern of Indian Bengalee girls.
2) To determine the relationship between cardio-vascular fitness, percentage of body fat and blood pressure.
3) To establish prediction equations for maximum O_2 uptake on the basis of age, body height and body weight.

MATERIALS AND METHODS

Subjects: This study was carried out on four hundred ninety (490) Indian Bengalee school going girls of age range 9-18 yrs. During the year 2006-07. The subjects were randomly sampled from different schools of Semi urban area of West Bengal, eastern India and all the subjects were considered to be normal and healthy according to the criteria stated by Gill et al (1969). The subjects were chosen mainly from middle class families. 40% of the total population of each age was randomly selected. A total of 490 out of 1225 girl students were investigated having age range of 9-18 years.

Age of the subject was determined from their date of birth from school register and it is rounded off to their nearest whole members. The distribution of subjects with respect to different ages is shown in Table I.

The test item administered and the method used are given below:

(1) *Body weight (Kg.)*:- By standard weighting machine with light clothing without putting on shoes.

(2) *Body height (cm.)*:- By anthropometric rod without putting on shoes.

(3) *BMI*:- From height and weight body mass index (BMI) was calculated by the equations of Meltzer et al (1988)

$$\text{BMI (Kg/m}^2) = \frac{\text{Body weight in Kg.}}{(\text{Body height in m})^2}$$

(4) *Skin fold measurements*: The Skin fold measurements were taken by Holtain Skinfold caliper (Holtain Ltd. UK) with constant tension by following the guideline of Johnson and Nelson (1982).Triceps and subscapular skinfolds were measured on the right side of the body with the subject standing in proper posture (Chatterjee and Mandal, 1993; Johnson and Nelson, 1982)

(5) *Percentage of body fat* (% body fat): It was calculated by using the formulae of Parizkova et al (1961)

9-12 year girls:-Body density = 1.088 – 0.014 log X 4 – 0.036 log X 5
13-16 years girls:-Body density = 1.114 – 0.031 log X 4 – 0.041 log X 5
X_4 – triceps skinfold thickness, X_5 – Subscapular skinfold thickness
% of body fat = (4.950/BD – 4.50) 100
BD= Body density

(6) *Resting heart rate and blood pressure* were measured with the subject in a seated position. Resting HR was measured from carotid artery. Resting blood Pr. was measured using a sphygmomanometer (Mercury type) and stethoscope by the auscultatory method (Guyton, 1991).

(7) *Cardio-respiratory fitness by Queen's college step test (QCT):* Queen's college step test (McArdle et al, 2001) was used to predict max: aerobic capacity. It is a standard method to measure one's max. O_2 uptake using bench stepping sub maximal exercise, suitable for both sexes of adults. It is a good indirect method for predicting cardio respiratory fitness in terms of Vo_2 max among Indian females (Chatterjee et al, 2005) to avoid the hazardous, laborious, exhaustive, time consuming and expensive protocol of direct Vo_2 max measurement. QCT was performed on a stool of 16.25 inches height for a total duration of 3 min. at the rate of 22 cycles/min. The cadens of the steps was maintained by the rhythm set on a metronome.

Table I. Mean and SD values of physique,body fat pattern and cardio-vascular parameters of Bengalee girls (9-18years) from West Bengal, India

Parameters Age Group	n	Body Height (cm)	Body Weight (Kg)	BMI (Kg/m2)	Systolic Blood Pressure (mmHg)	Diastolic Blood Pressure (mmHg)	Triceps Skinfold Thickness (mm)	Subscapular Skinfold Thickness (mm)	%Body fat	Vo2max ml/Kg/min	Vo2max Lit/min
mean ±SD	70	133.53 7.5	27.53 6.28	15.22 2.57	95.99 8.35	62.13 8.59	8.74 3.2	8.06 2.76	24.31 3.30	33.13 3.5	0.90 0.21
11 mean ±SD	58	136.60 7.44	29.21 6.36	15.49 2.22	96.21 7.39	61.55 7.84	8.17 3.39	7.6 2.68	23.83 2.88	32.58 4.50	0.95 0.22
12 mean ±SD	57	141.42 6.71	31.43 6.23	15.66 2.27	98.68 10.33	62.72 8.30	7.82 2.99	8.03 3.11	24.02 3.21	31.85 3.43	0.99 0.21
13 mean ±SD	58	148.05 6.63	38.10 6.37	17.35 2.51	104.48 11.11	68.62 10.83	8.67 2.83	10.13 3.77	23.17 4.24	31.54 2.93	1.2 0.20
14 mean ±SD	50	151.54 5.59	42.01 9.62	18.43 2.87	106.7 11.98	69.8 8.39	8.68 3.11	10.70 2.56	23.95 4.02	31.03 3.14	1.31 0.20
15 mean ±SD	68	152.3 5.10	46.93 10.13	20.17 3.89	110.74 11.79	70.29 9.1	13.15 5.45	12.32 4.13	27.59 5.52	29.74 5.0	1.39 0.28
16 mean ±SD	63	153.03 5.89	49.38 10.50	21.05 4.03	114.37 13.36	72.84 9.43	17.01 7.09	12.51 4.56	25.55 8.50	30.22 3.47	1.48 0.33
17-18 mean ±SD	66	154.51 5.39	48.48 6.92	20.17 2.76	116.97 7.84	73.78 7.79	17.56 7.23	13.56 4.74	24.69 8.71	29.62 3.53	1.43 0.26

Table II. Correlation coefficients between Physique, Body fat Pattern and Cardio-vascular parameters of Bengalee girls

BMI	1	0.66***	0.50***	0.68***	0.82***	0.57***	0.35***	0.80***
SBP		1	0.82***	0.56***	0.59***	0.32***	0.37***	0.55***
DBP			1	0.44***	0.46***	0.20***	0.28***	0.46***
Triceps skinfold				1	0.61***	0.22***	0.33***	0.55***
Subscaular skinfold					1	0.69***	0.33***	0.55***
% Body fat						1	0.2***	0.39***
Vo2max ml/kg/min							1	0.02
Vo2max l/min								1

(9-18 yrs) from West Bengal ,India
(*** = P< 0.001. ** = P< 0.01).

The step test began after a brief demonstration and practice period. The subjects were asked to perform each stepping cycle to a 4 step cadens continuously for 3 minutes. After completion of test, subjects remained standing while pulse rate was measured for 15 secs, 5-20 secs. into recovery. Recovery HR was converted to beats/min. (15 Sec. HR X 4).

Following *equation* was used for estimation of Vo_2max (ml/kg/min)

Vo_2max = 65.81 – [0.1847 X step test pulse rate (b/min)]

The preclicted Vo_2max (ml/kg/min) was converted to lit/min by multiplying predicted Vo_2max value (ml/kg/min) X body weight/1000.

Statistical Analysis

Two tail t-test was performed to test the significant variation between the mean values and Pearson's product moment correlation was computed to test the relationship between two variables with level of significance. Linear Regression analysis was made for Vo_2max, on the basis of age, body height, body weight.

RESULTS

The mean values and standard deviations of different physical and cardio-vascular fitness parameters for each age group are shown in table I. Mean values for body height and body weight gradually increased from 9 to 18 years of age but significant changes in different ages were observed ($P<0.01-0.001$) uto 14 years in case of body height and 11-15years in case of body weight($P<0.1-0.001$).BMI values increased significantly ($P<0.05-0.001$) from 12 to 15 years of age.

The study also revealed that there is steady progression in SBP and DBP values with age having significant increase ($P<0.01$) in between 12-13 years and in between 14-16 years ($P<0.05-0.1$) in case of SBP but only in between 12-13 years ($P<0.001$) in case of DBP. Triceps skinfold thickness shows significant increase ($P<0.001$) in between 14-16 years but 12-13 and 14-15 years incase of subscapular thickness ($P<0.001$) and 14-16 years in case of % of BF ($P<0.1-0.001$).

Regarding max O_2 uptake capacity, girls of this study show significant increase in Vo_2max (lit/min) in between 12-16 years ($P<0.01-0.001$), but no significant increase is noted when Vo_2max is expressed in ml/kg/min.

Table II, represents the correlation coefficients between variables and it is indicated that all the correlation coefficients are highly significant ($P<0.001$) and positive except the correlation between Vo_2max (lit/min) and Vo_2max (ml/kg/min).

Figure 1 represents the comparison of the Vo_2max values of Bengalee girls from West Bengal with a previous study in which Vo_2max was measured directly (Chatterjee et al 1979). It is found that Vo_2max (lit/min) values of Bengalee girls of present study are not significantly different with the previous one of same age group. But significant difference ($P<0.01-0.001$) is observed when Vo_2max is expressed in ml/kg/min in each age group.

Table III represents the prediction equations of Vo_2max (lit/min) on the basis of age, height and weight. Among these prediction equations, body weight was considered as the most reliable one because of highest correlation value between Vo_2max and body weight as well as minimum SEE.

Table III. Linear Regression Equations of Vo_2max(L/min) based on Age, Body height, Body Weight

Linear regression equations	Multiple R	R^2	SEE
VO2max(l/min) = 0.087 Age + 0.037	0.65	0.42*	0.25
VO2 max (l/min)= 0.025 Weight + 0.228	0.88	0.77*	0.16
VO2 max(l/min) = 0.024 Height - 2.31	0.73	0.52*	0.23

* = P< 0.001.

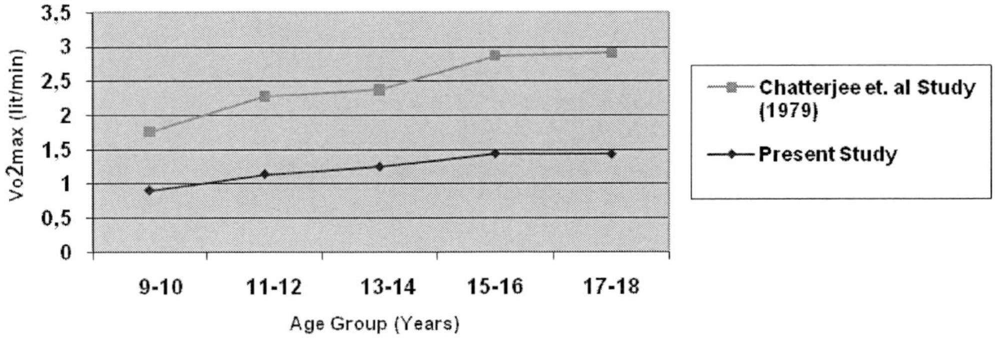

Figure 1. Comparison of Vo2max (lit./min.) value of girls of present study to Indian (Bangalee) girls of Kolkata.

DISCUSSION

We have measured aerobic capacity and cardio respiratory status of Indian Bengalee girls (9-18 yrs.) of West Bengal and also studied body height, body weight, BMI, skinfold thickness and % of body fat of school going girls of this population. Body height and body weight values when compared with the Indian (Bengalee) girls studied by Mandal (2005), reveal that girls of the present study have significantly (P<0.01-0.001) lower body height and body weight values upto 15 yrs of age. BMI values of semi-urban Bengalee girls (Mandal,2005) also show higher value in comparison to the girls of present study. This is probably due to girls of the present study having been taken from lower middle class families whereas semiurban Bengalee girls of West Bengal (Mandal,2005) were taken from upper middle class families. But young girls of West Bengal (Chatterjee et al, 1979) had significantly lower (P<0.05-0.001) values in body weight in comparison to the girls of the present study but body height values were not significantly different in these two groups of girls. The differences are probably due to variation in population, young girls of West Bengal were taken from different schools of Kolkata and no. of subject of that study was much lower in comparison to the present study.

In our study systolic blood Pr. has positively significant correlation ($P<0.001$) with diastolic blood Pr. in Bengalee girls which corroborates with the findings of Sadhan et al (2007) on Punjabi Collegiate population. They also stated that body mass is the most important determinant of SBP and DBP. As regards SBP and DBP values of girls of the present study when compared with the girls of Pondichery (average age 14.8-15.5 yrs) studied by Ravisankar et al (2005) it is observed that SBP and DBP values of these two studies are comparable only with their overweight group of girls although BMI value of girls of present study is in normal range in the respective age group. This is probably due to the interferences of other variables like genetic (Malina et al, 1991), socio-economic status (Reddy,1998) and other metabolic risk factors (Blair et al, 1988).

In the present study, effect of puberty on the aerobic capacity is found to occur at 12-16 yrs. which coincides with the peak body height and body weight. But Vo_2max when expressed in ml/kg/min (relative Vo_2max), decreases insignificantly with age which is different from the finding of aerobic capacity of girls of Kolkata, eastern India (Chatterjee et al, 1979) where Vo_2max /kg body wt. reduced very significantly at the onset of puberty. This variation is probably due to variation in sample size in these two population and body weight of young adolescent girls (n varies from 10-16 in each age group) of Kolkata, West Bengal where it has been found to be significantly high in comparison to the girls of the present study due to the method of Vo_2max determination. (Figure 1).

In case of Vo_2max of Bengalee girls of West Bengal when compared with the South Indian girls (Swaminathan et al, 1997) of comparable age, it is found that both Vo_2max (lit/min) and Vo_2max (ml/kg/min) of South Indian girls are significantly ($P<0.1$-0.001) higher in comparison to the Bengalee girls of the present study at their age of 11 and 12 which coincides with their growth spurt. This is probably due to more active life style, environmental factors and method of Vo_2max determination (swaminathan et al, 1997).

Besides, aerobic capacity of black adolescent girls studied by pivarnik et al,(1993) (age range 11.4 – 15.8 yrs.) had Vo_2max value of 37.3 + 6.2 ml/kg/min and was significantly correlated with height, body mass index and % Body fat. Black adolescent girls when compared with the Bengalee girls of present study, it is observed that adolescent black girls have significantly ($P<0.001$) higher values of Vo_2max in comparison to the girls of present study. This is probably due to diversity in genetic, racial, climatic, geographical and nutritional factors (Dey and Debray, 2002).

In the present study correlation values of relative Vo_2max (ml/kg/min) with age, height, weight and BMI are low but significant ($P<0.01$-0.001) in comparison to the absolute Vo_2max (lit/min) values ($P<0.001$).Thus linear regression equations of absolute Vo_2max value are reproduced to predict the Vo_2max on the basis of age, body height, body weight.

CONCLUSION

Thus, it may be concluded that a correlation exists for various parameters between cardio-respiratory fitness, body composition and blood Pressure specially with age, body heightand body weight . So on the basis of these above parameters linear regression equations of Vo_2max (max O_2 uptake) was reproduced which can be applied to predict max O_2 uptake of school going Bengalee girls when survey and screening of large no. of subjects are deemed necessary.

This study also gives valuable information regarding growth pattern, body composition and cardio-vascular fitness pattern of Bengalee girls which will help them to monitor the fitness profile, cardio vascular complication and obesity.

On the basis of this report young girls should take care of their food habits and physical activity to avoid excess body weight and cardio vascular complication from their early life.

Acknowledgment

Author is very much thankful to University grant commission for their financial assistance to conduct this project.

References

Blair SN, Ludwig DA and Goodyear NN. A canonical analysis of central and peripheral subcutaneous fat distribution and coronary heart disease risk factors in men and women aged 18-65 year. *Hum. Biol.* 1988; 60: 111-122.

Chatterjee S, Banerjee PK, Chatterjee P and Maitra SR, Aerobic capacity of young girls. *Indian J. Med. Res.* 1979; 69: 327-333.

Chatterjee S, Chatterjee P and Bandyopadhyay A. Validity of Queen's college step test for estimation of maximum oxygen uptake in female students. *Indian J. Med. Res.* 2005; 121: 32-35.

Chatterjee S, Mandal A and Das NK. Physical and motor fitness level of Indian School going boys. *J. Sports Med. Phys. fitness,*1993; 33, 268-77.

Dey SK and Debray PS. A comparative study of Maximal aerobic power of school boys of East and North East Regions of India. *Indian pediatries* 2003; 40: 105-11.

Gill PS, Prasad BG and Shrivastava RN. Natritional status of primary school children in a rural area of Lucknow. 1968; *Indian J. Pediat*: 35, 314.

Guerra S, Rebero JC, Costa R, Durato J and Mota J. Relationship between cardiorespiratory fitness body composition and blood pressure in school children. *J. Sports Med. Phys. Fitness*. 2002; 42(2): 207-213.

Guyton AC. *Textbook of medical physiology*, Philadelphia: W.B. Saunders Company, 1991.

Johnson BL and Nelson JK. Practical Measurements for evaluation in physical education. Third Edition, New Delhi (India) Surjeet Publication P.180.

MacArdle WD, Katch FI, Katch VL. *Exercise physiology, energy, nutrition and human performance*. 5th edition Lippincott Willium and Wilkins. 2001, P-244.

Malina RM and Bouchard C: Genetic regulation of growth maturation and performance. In *growth, Maturation and physical activity*. R.M. Malina,C.Bouchard and Bar-or-ored (Eds) Human kinetics publishers Inc; Champaign Illinosis, 1991, P 303-327.

Mandal A. Anthropometric studies in adolescent Bengalee girls from semiurban area of Hooghly district of West Bengal. *Journal of Medical Sciences*. 2005; 8(1): 62-67.

Meltzer A, Mueller W, Annegers J, Grines B and Albright D. Weight history and hypertension. *Clinical Epidermiology*. 1988; 41: 867-874.

Parikova J. Total body fat and skinfold thickness in children. *Metabolism*. 1961; 10: 794-807.

Pivarnik JM, Fulton JE, Taylor WC, Snider SA. Aerobic capacity in black adolescent girls. *Res. Q Excrc. Sport.* 1993; 64(2): 202-207.

Ravisankar P,Madanmohan, Kaviraja U and Sankaranarayanan Prakash. Correlation between body mass index and blood pressure indices, handgrip strength and handgrip endurance in underweight, normal weight and overweight adolescents. *Indian J. physiol. Pharmacol.* 2005; 49(4): 455-461.

Reddy BN. Blood Pressure and Adiposity: a comparative study of socio-economically diverse groups of Andhra Pradesh, India. *Am J Hum Biol.* 1998; 10: 5-21.

Rowland TW, Green GM. Physiological responses to treadmill exercise in females: Adult-child differences. *Med. Sci. .sports exercs* 1988; 20: 474-478.

Sadhan B, koley S and Sandhu JS, Relationship between Cardio-respiratory fitness, body composition and blood pressure in Punjabi collegiate population. *J. Hum. Ecol.* 2007; 22(3): 215-219.

Swaminathan S, Vijayan VK, Venkatesan P and Kuppurao KV. Aerobic capacity and cardiopulmonary response to exercise is healthy South Indian children. *Indian Pediatrics*, 1997; 34 : 112-118.

In: World Heart Research Yearbook. Volume 1 ISBN: 978-1-60741-881-8
Editors: Franz Halberg and R. B. Singh

Association of Increased Mortality with Underweight, Overweight and Obesity among Urban Decendents in North India, Dying Due to Various Causes

Ram B. Singh*[*,1], *Surendra Singh*[1], *Vijendra Singh*[1], *Shelendra K. Kulshresth*[1], *Viola Michirova*[2] and *Daniel Pella*[2]

[1]Halberg Hospital and Research Institute,Moradabad,
Hindu College, Moradabad, India
[2]Safaric University, Kosice, Slovakia

Abstract

Introduction: While overweight and obesity are important risk factors of death due to cardiovascular disease CVD) and diabetes, underweight predisposes deaths due to infections. In the present study, we examine the association of body mass index(BMI) with causes of deaths among urban decendents in a middle income country.

Methods: For the period 1999-2001, we studied the randomly selected records of death of 2222 (1385 men and 837 women) decedents, aged 25-64 years, out of 3034 death records overall from the records at Municipal Corporation, Moradabad. All the families of these decendents could be contacted individually to find out the causes of death, by scientist/doctor administered, informed consented, verbal autopsy questionnaire, completed with the help of the spouse and local treating doctor practicing in the appropriate health care region. Clinical data and causes of death were assessed by a questionnaire based on available hospital record and verbal autopsy questionnaire, suggested by WHO. Decendents were classified in to underweight, normal weight, overweight and obese based on new criteria of WHO and International College of Nutrition. The association of BMI with causes of death was calculated by Mantel-Haesnzel Chi square test.

Results: Majority of the decendents (n=792,35.6%) (men 31.1%,n=431; and women 43.1%,n=361) had normal BMI of 18.5-22.9Kg/m2.The prevalence of underweight victims was 14.2%(n=315),overweight 29.4%(n=654)and obese 20.8%(n=461).There was an overall increase in risk factors;diabetes mellitus, hypertension, and CAD among overweight and obese victims based on BMI criteria, and the trend was significant. However, tobacco intake showed nonsignificant trend, highest in the underweight

* Correspondence: Dr. R.B. Singh,MD Former Professor of Medicine,Subharti Medical College, Halberg Hospital and Research Institute, Civil Lines, Moradabad-10(UP) 244001, India; Email: icn2008@mickyonline.com , icn2005@sancharnet.in.

victims, without significant differences in the other categories of BMI.BMI was positively associated with significant rising trend in the prevalence of circulatory causes of death, both among men and women. Infections and cancers as the cause of death were inversely associated with increase in BMI among both men and women. Injury and miscellaneous causes of death showed no association with BMI among men whereas among women, miscellaneous causes of death were positively and significantly associated with BMI. No such association was noted for injury with BMI among women. Among circulatory causes of death, 25.0%(n=108) of the victims had normal BMI (18.5-22.9Kg/m2),which was because of victims dying due to rheumatic heart diseases and heart failure, where lower BMI may be the result of these diseases.

Conclusions: Overweight (>23Kg/m 2) and obesity(>25Kg/m 2) are important determinant of mortality due to circulatory diseases and underweight due to infections. Those decendents dying of heart failure, rheumatic heart disease and cancers, may have underweight during the deaths, similar to those dying of infections, as a result of the complication of the disease rather than cause of the deaths. Larger studies would be necessary to demonstrate the association of BMI with causes of death in India.

Keywords: Mortality, coronary heart disease, sudden death, stroke, infections, cancer

Responsibilities: Study design, questionnaire, writing of manuscript by RBS, collection of data by VS, SKK, RBS. Others experts; DP, SS helped in the writing of manuscript, calculations and review of references

INTRODUCTION

There is evidence that those who suffer from excessive body weight and body fat have an increased prevalence of cardiovascular disease (CVD) ,diabetes and cancer [1-4]. Dietary fat intake, increased consumption of energy, physical inactivity and family history are important risk factors of obesity [3-12]. Excessive weight gain is not only a cause of several of cardiovascular risk factors but is in itself a risk factor for coronary artery disease (CAD), sudden cardiac death (SCD) diabetes, insulin resistance, and stroke [3-5]. There is increased risk of death from CVD, CAD, and diabetes when obese people become older [3]. The elevated risk associated with excess weight occurred even in the absence of other cardiovascular risk factors such as smoking, hypertension, and hypercholesterolemia [3]. While modest increase in body mass index (BMI) have adverse effects, small downward shifts in the distribution of BMI levels could have tremendous societal impact on public health [1-4]. International agencies, consider overweight in presence of a body mass index (BMI) of 25.0-29.9 kg/m^2 and obesity, 30.0-39.9 kg/m^2 [2,4,10,11] . Since Asians [10-12], particularly south Asians have a smaller body frame size and increased susceptibility for central obesity; these guidelines appear to be inappropriate for these populations [6-9]. Therefore, Indian Consensus group in 1996 and later on WHO in 2000, have suggested that BMI of 25 kg/m^2 and above should be considered obesity and above 23Kg/m2 overweight, among Asians [10, 11].In the present study,we examine the association of BMI with causes of death among urban decendents,in which data have been collected based on verbal autopsy questionnaire.

MATERIAL AND METHODS

Moradabad is situated in north India and is an urban area with the population of 0.641 million residing in 306 streets or 60 wards of the city. Based on 2001 census, all the deaths that occurred in the city of Moradabad may be verified in the birth and death record section of municipal board, office. Since autopsy is not possible, due to religious considerations, causes of death recorded at Municipal Board might not be correct. These records are based on certificates issued by the doctors based on clinical diagnosis and laboratory examinations. We studied the records of randomly selected,2842 adult victims, aged 25-64years, of which 2222 victim's relatives, could respond for this study, during the last two years,July1999 to July 2001.Of 2222 victims, 1385 were males and 837 were females. All the families of these 2222 victims were contacted, individually to find out the causes of deaths by verbal autopsy questionnaire [4]. In developing countries due to religious considerations, WHO has suggested to investigate the causes of death by detailed questionnaires administered to spouse and concerned doctors. The head of every family was personally called after communication with the help of the local accessible doctor in the lane. At least three calls, via letter/telephone and personal contact via lane doctor were made before any subject or family was declared non- contact or non-replier, one in the morning, one in the evening, around 17.00 hrs., and last one at the weekend.

Our team included a scientist; a health worker and a doctor, who were trained and briefed regarding the details of questionnaires before starting the survey. The case record form was pre-tested by the concerned committee in roughly 30 to 60 families. It was found that 10% of the families who came within reach of survey were declared non-contact or non-responder as observed in other survey [5].Detailed interviews were possible among 90% of the families approached. Clinical data on age, sex, height, weight, marital status, occupation, education, past and family history, history of hypertension, diabetes, stroke, heart attack, alcohol intake, drug intake, tobacco intake, lung tuberculosis, bronchitis, asthma, cancer, mental diseases, diarrhea and dysentery, and renal, liver, brain, CVD, infectious diseases, and accidents etc, were recorded based on medical record of the victim, death certificate issued by the doctor, interview of the doctor and the family doctor, interview of the spouse and other family members, with the help of a pretested questionnaire, to know the cause of death. Lane doctor or spouse of the victim were asked to suggest a person with identical age, sex, height and weight as that of the victim. In those victims records, data on height and weight were not available, we collected. These data from these subjects. Body weights were measured by the trained scientist independently, in light under-clothes, to the nearest of 0.5Kg.Height was measured in standing position. BMI was calculated by deviding the body weight in Kg, with height in meter square(weight in Kg/height in Meter 2).Subjects were classified according to BMI into underweight (BMI >18.5), normal weight(18.5-22.9Kg/m2), overweight(23-24.9kg/m3), and obese (25-29.9Kg/m2) and >30Kg/m2. The socio- economic status (SES) of the family was classified based on attributes of housing condition, education, occupation, per capita income and ownership of consumer durables like car, television, auto etc in the household [13]. Per capita income was calculated by dividing the total income of the family, by the number of family members. The diagnosis of risk factors was based on available records, inquiry from the spouse and concerned doctors and the criteria of diagnosis were based on our earlier studies [13].

Statistical Analysis

We used chi square test for the comparison of two groups. Only P values <0.05 and two tailed t-test, were considered significant among both sexes. A relation was determined between BMI and prevalence of risk factors as well as causes of deaths and the significance of any trend was calculated with the Mantel-Haenszel X 2test.

RESULTS

The results indicating clinical data based on the records and by questionnaire, and measurement in identical subjects (approximately in 10% of victims where height and weight were not recorded or not known to spouse or doctor), among 2222 victims, aged 25-64 years, dying due to various causes, are given in the table 1.The mean age, body mass index and body weight were significantly higher among men compared to women victims. There was a high prevalence of obesity, and tobacco intake among men compared to women (table 1). Table 2 shows the BMI in relation to age groups. Approximately, half(49.8%,n=1107) of the decendents with overweight and obesity died prematurely by the age of 64 years. Majority of the men(31.1%,n=431) and women(43.1%,n=361) had normal BMI of 18.5-22.9Kg/m2.Obese subjects(n=461) were mainly from social classes 1-3(82.8%,n=382).The prevalence of underweight victims was 14.2%(n=315),overweight 29.4%(n=654)and obese 20.8%(n=461).

Table 1. Clinical data and risk factors among victims studied, based on records and assessment by questionnaire

Clinical Data	Male (n=1385)	Female (n=837)
	Mean (Standard deviation)	
Mean age	42.12** (13.02)	40.05 (11.60)
Body weight	60.12** (6.24)	53.10 (6.95)
Body mass index (kg/m)	23.18* (2.18)	23.65 (2.46)

Prevalence of risk factors,n(%).
Obesity (BMI>25Kg/m2) 277(20.0) 184(22.0).
Overweight (23-24.9Kg/m2) 470(33.9)* 184(22.0).
Underweight (<18.5Kg/m2) 207(14.9) 108(12.9).
Hypertension (>140/90mmHg)457(33.0) 251(30.0).
Diabetes mellitus (known) 110(8.0) 58(7.0).
Tobacco intake 623(45.0)* 125(15.0).
*=P <0.05,**=P <0.001, P value were obtained by Analysis of variance and chi square test.

We found an overall increase in risk factors; diabetes mellitus, hypertension, and CAD among overweight and obese victims based on BMI criteria for Asia Pacific region [10,11], and the trend was significant as shown in table 3. However, tobacco intake showed non-significant trend, highest in the underweight victims, without significant differences in the other categories of BMI. Table 4 shows the prevalence of causes of mortality among victims dying due to various causes. An increasing level of BMI was associated with significant rising trend in the prevalence of circulatory causes of death, both among men and women. Infections and cancers as the cause of death showed an decreasing trend with increase in BMI among both men and women (table 4).Injury and miscellaneous cause of death showed no association with BMI among men whereas among women miscellaneous causes of death showed significant increasing trend with increase in BMI.

Table 2. Body mass index (%) in relation to age groups based on records and questionnaires

BMI (Kg./M2)	No.	<18.5	18.5-22.9	23.0-24.9	25.0-29.9	>30.0
Age Groups	Men					
25-34	715	105(14.7)	210(29.4)	283(39.6)	116(16.2)	1(0.1)
35-44	420	74(17.6)	121(28.8)	126(30.0)	98(23.3)	1(0.2)
45-54	189	18(9.5)	86(45.5)	40(21.2)	40(21.2)	5(2.6)
55-64	61	10(16.4)	14(22.9)	21(34.4)	12(19.6)	4(6.5)
Total	1385	207(14.9)	431(31.1)	470(33.9)	266(19.2)	11(0.8)
	Women					
25-34	462	42(9.1)	212(45.9)	104(22.5)	104(22.5)	-
35-44	247	28(11.3)	115(46.5)	56(22.6)	47(19.0)	1(0.4)
45-54	98	30(30.6)	22(22.4)	21(21.4)	20(20.4)	5(5.1)
55-64	30	8(26.6)	12(39.9)	3(10.0)	3(10.0)	4(13.3)
Total	837	108(12.9)	361(43.1)	184(21.9)	174(20.8)	10(1.2)
G.Total	2222	315(14.2)	792(35.6)	654(29.4)	440(19.8)	21(0.9)

Values are number (%).

Table 3. Risk factors in relation to body mass index, based on available records and questionnaires

Body Mass Index (Kg/m^2)	n	Diabetes mellitus	Hypertension >140/90 mmHg	CAD	Tobacco intake
Men					
BMI <18.5	207	6 (2.9)	4 (1.9)	-	110 (53.1)
BMI 18.5-22.9	431	31 (7.2)	66 (15.3)	9 (2.1)	187 (43.4)
BMI 23-24.9	470	42 (8.9)	202 (42.9)	51 (10.8)	200 (42.5)
BMI 25-29.9	266	28 (10.5)	180 (67.6)	69 (25.9)	125 (46.9)
BMI >=30	11	3 (27.2)	6 (54.5)	3 (27.2)	1 (9.0)
Total	1385	110 (7.9)	458(33.1)	132 (9.5)	623 (45.0)
Mantel-Haenszel X^2		13.3	21.8	12.2	8.1
P Value		<0.001	<0.001	<0.02	>0.05
Body Mass Index (Kg/m^2)	n	Diabetes mellitus	Hypertension >140/90 mmHg	CAD	Tobacco intake
Women					
BMI <18.5	108	-	2 (1.8)	-	22 (20.3)
BMI 18.5-22.9	361	9 (2.5)	43 (11.9)	2 (0.5)	56 (15.5)
BMI 23-24.9	184	20 (10.8)	95 (51.6)	12 (6.5)	26 (14.1)
BMI 25-29.9	174	26 (14.9)	105 (60.3)	26 (14.9)	20 (11.5)
BMI >=30	10	3 (30.0)	6 (60.0)	2 (20.0)	1 (10.0)
Total	837	58 (6.9)	251 (30.0)	42 (5.0)	125 (14.9)
Mantel-Haenszel X^2		16.6	22.8	10.9	7.5
P Value		<0.001	<0.001	<0.05	>0.05
Values are number and %,BMI=body mass index,CAD=Coronary artery disease.					

Table 4. Causes of death in relation to body mass index based on records and assessed by questionnaires

Body Mass Index (Kg/m^2)	Infections	Circulatory	Malignant	Injury	Miscellaneous
Men(%)					
BMI (<18.5) (n=207)	180 (86.9)	2 (0.9)	14 (6.7)	6 (2.9)	5 (2.4)
BMI (18.5-22.9) (n=431)	248 (57.5)	108 (25.0)	28 (6.5)	25 (5.8)	22 (5.1)
BMI (23-24.9) (n=470)	146 (31.0)	135 (28.7)	25 (5.3)	114 (24.2)	50 (10.6)
BMI (25-29.9) (n=266)	35 (13.1)	155 (58.3)	10 (3.7)	52 (19.5)	14 (5.2)
BMI (<30) (n=11)	-	6 (54.5)	-	2 (1.8)	3 (27.2)
Total (n=1385)	609(43.9)	406(29.3)	77(5.5)	199(14.3)	94(6.8)
Mantel-Haenszel X 2	23.7	18.8	8.7	7.6	6.1
P value	<0.001	<0.001	<0.05	<0.05	>0.05
Women(%)					
BMI (<18.5) (n=108)	75 (69.4)	5 (4.6)	16 (14.8)	10 (9.2)	2 (1.8)
BMI (18.5-22.9) (n=361)	180(49.8)	64 (17.7)	27 (7.5)	58 (16.0)	32 (8.8)
BMI (23-24.9) (n=184)	40 (21.7)	70 (38.0)	10 (5.4)	24 (13.0)	40 (21.7)
BMI (25-29.9) (n=174)	11 (6.3)	97 (55.7)	1 (0.6)	18 (10.3)	47 (27.0)
BMI (>30) (n=10)	-	4 (40.0)	-	4 (40.0)	2 (20.0)
Total (n=837)	306(36.5)	240(28.6)	54(6.4)	114(13.6)	123(14.7)
Mantel-Haenszel X2	22.5	18.5	8.8	6.2	9.2
P value	<0.001	<0.001	<0.05	>0.05	<0.05

Values are number (%).BMI=body mass index.

No such association was noted for injury with BMI among women. Among circulatory causes of death, 25.0%(n=108) of the victims had normal BMI (18.5-22.9Kg/m2),which was because of victims dying due to rheumatic heart diseases and heart failure.

Discussion

This study shows that infections were the major cause of death among decendents with underweight, which showed a decreasing trend with increase in BMI among both sexes (table 4).Similar association was observed for cancer deaths, however underweight among cancer deaths, may be due to the effect of cancer cachexia rather than underweight causing cancers. We also found that BMI was positively associated with significant rising trend in the prevalence of deaths due to circulatory diseases among both men and women. Among deaths due to circulatory causes, 25.7%(n=110) men and 27.1%(n=69) women decendents were associated with BMI <23 Kg/m 2,and the causes of death were rheumatic heart disease and heart failure. Rest of the men and women decendents were associated with BMI of 23Kg/m 2 and above and causes of death were mainly CAD,SCD and stroke (table 4).These findings indicate that BMI was an important determinant of deaths due to various causes; underweight causing more deaths due to infections and overweight and obesity due to diseases of affluence.

We can not compare our results with other studies because such studies are rare from India. There is increased mortality due to cardiovascular disease and diabetes among migrants of Indian origin living in developed countries [15] as well as in South India compared to North India(15,16).In a 6 year, follow up study [16] in South India, among 1262 subjects, aged 20years and above, the causes of deaths were ; cardiovascular disease (34%, n=17),renal diseases (12%,n=6), gastrointestinal diseases (8%, n=4), infections(4%,n=2), respiratory and cancers each in 6%(n=3). Mean BMI was greater among survivors compared to dead subjects(22.6 vs 21.7 Kg/m 2).In another recent study from India [17],lower BMI cut point of 21.5 for men and 19.0Kg/m 2 for women have been suggested, although this study included subjects from slums.

CAD and coronary risk factors were two or three times higher among urban compared to rural subjects of India, which may be due to more sedentary behavior and greater alchohol intake, and obesity among urban people [18]. In both sexes, central obesity was four times more common in the urban than in the rural population .There was a significant association between CAD and age, hypercholesterolemia, hypertension and central obesity [18]. Energy expenditure during routine and spare-time physical activity was significantly higher in rural than in urban subjects. A West London cohort study [19], comparing migrants from the Indian subcontinent of Punjabi origin with their siblings in Punjab found that the West London cohort had a greater mean BMI and higher serum cholesterol and apolipoprotein B levels, lower HDL cholesterol levels and higher fasting blood glucose levels than their counterparts in India. Insulin sensitivity was lower in men in West London and beta-cell function was lower in Indians in West London compared with their siblings in the Punjab. The Indian Women's Health Study [20], comprising of 3257 women, aged 25-64 years, showed that 5.0%(n=164) were underweight,54.0% had BMI> 23 Kg/m 2, and rest BMI >25Kg/m 2.Hypertension,hyperlipidemia and glucose intolerance were significantly associated with BMI.

In developed countries, obesity has been recognized as a risk factor of deaths due to CAD, SCD, stroke, diabetes and cancers [2, 14, 21-25]. The elevated risk associated with excess weight occures even in the absence of other cardiovascular risk factors such as smoking, hypertension and hyperlipidemia. The Chicago Heart Association Detection Project in Industry study(2),comprising of 17,643 subjects, aged 31 to 64 years, who were free of CAD, diabetes were studied up to the age of 65 years. The adds ratio for CAD death for obese subjects compared with those of normal weight in the same risk category was 1.43 for those at low risk and 2.07 for those at moderate risk after adjustment for systolic blood pressure and serum total cholesterol levels. The risk for CAD hospitalization was 4.25 times higher in obese subjects at low risk, compared with those of normal weight, and 2.04 times higher for those at moderate risk. The association was stronger for diabetes with obesity conferring a 11 fold greater mortality among low risk subjects and a 7.84 fold increased risk of hospitalization. In the Framingham Study [24],among 3457 subjects , aged 30 to 49 years, overweight and obesity were associated with large decreases in life expectancy and increases in early mortality. BMI at ages 30 to 49 years, predicted mortality after ages 50 to 69 years, even after adjustment for BMI at age 50 to 69 years. In a further recent study [25], among 527,265 subjects, excess body weight during midlife, including overweight, was associated with an increased risk of death, among both sexes, in all ethnic groups. However, the risk of death among underweight persons was attenuated in this study but not among study in Indians [26].

There is experimental and physiological evidence that dietary fat is particularly conducive to weight gain [1-3]. Excess dietary fat is more readily stored than dietary carbohydrate. However, changes in body fat depend mainly, on an imbalance between energy intake and energy expenditure. Thus obesity develops when energy intake is in excess of expenditure for a sustained period of time. Social and environmental factors that either increase energy intake or reduce physical activity place a greater demand on the normal mechanisms of appetite control and metabolic regulation. Therefore changes in the environmental factors which influence the level of energy expenditure may result in the development of obesity.

Recently, abdominal obesity has been suggested to be a better predictor of death than BMI [2,14,17]. The distribution of obesity may be dependent on genetic, environmental and hormonal factors which are important predictor of obesity-associated comorbidities and mortality [1-3].However, genetic do not mean nonnutritional or nonmetabolic because several genetic expressions related to obesity are under influence of nutrients. Omental adipose tissue contains more number of glucocorticoid receptors (GR) compared to subcutaneous adipose tissue with similar Kd values whereas lipoprotein lipase activity (LPL) activity in subcutaneous adipose tissue is lower compared to omental adipose tissue. A positive correlation between LPL activity and glucocorticoid binding exists. Human adipose tissue glucocorticoid binding is higher in omental than in subcutaneous adipose tissue, whereas LPL activity is higher in omental than in subcutaneous adipose tissue. Leptin mRNA expression is higher in abdominal subcutaneous adipocytes compared with omental adipocytes. An inverse relationship exists between adipocytes. An inverse relationship exists between adipocytes, PPAR-γ expression and body mass index (BMI) [27].

In brief,the findings in our study indicate that BMI indicating overweight and obesity, are significant predictors of deaths due to circulatory diseases and underweight for deaths due to infections.Larger studies are necessary to confirm our findings.

Acknowledgments

We are grateful to Centre of Nutrition Research, International College of Nutrition for the financial support for conducting this study.

References

[1] Flegal KM, Graubard BI, Williamson DF,Gail MH.Excess deaths associated with underweight,overweight and obesity. *JAMA* 2005, 293:1861-67.

[2] Weight control and physical activity, Lyon, International Agency for research on cancer, 2002 (*IARC Hand looks on cancer prevention*, Vol. 6)

[3] Yan LL and Chicago Heart Association Detection Project in Industry Study Group.Midlife body mass index and hospitalization and mortality in older age. *JAMA* 2006,295:192-198.

[4] Sachs JD Commission on Macroeconomics and Health. A Race against Time: The Challenge of Cardiovascular Disease in Developing Economies. The Earth Institute of Columbia University, New York, 2004.

[5] Singh RB, Ghosh S, Beegum R, Chibo H, Shoumin Z. Epidemiologic study of diet and coronary risk factors in relation to central obesity and insulin levels in rural and urban populations of north India. *Int. J. Cardiol.* 1995, 47:245-255.

[6] Singh RB, Suh IL,Singh VP, Chaithiraphan S. Hypertension and stroke in Asia: prevalence, control and strategies in developing countries for prevention. *J. Human Hyperten.* 2000, 14: 749-763.

[7] INCLEN Multicentre Collaborative Group. Body mass index and cardiovascular disease risk factors in seven Asian and five Latin American centres. Data from the International Clinical Epidemiology Network (INCLEN).*Obesity Res.* 1996, 4:221-228.

[8] Singh RB, and Five City Study Group. Prevalence and determinants of central obesity and age-specific waist-hip ratio of people in five cities, the Indian Womens Health Study. *J. Cardiovasc. Risk* 1998, 5:73-77.

[9] Gopinath N, Chadha SL, Jain P, Shekhawat S, Tandon R. An epidemiologic study of obesity in adults in the urban population of Delhi. *J. Assoc Physicians India* 1994, 421:212-215.

[10] Indian Consensus Group.Indian Consensus for prevention of hypertension and coronary artery disease. *J. Nutr. Environ. Med.* 1996,6:309-18.

[11] World Health Organization Regional office for the western pacific / International Association for the study of obesity, International obesity task force: The Asia –pacific perspective: redefining obesity and its treatment Sydney, Health communications, Australia, 2000.

[12] Singh RB,Niaz MA,Beegum R,Wander GS,Thakur AS,Rissam HS.Body fat percent by bioelectrical impedence analysis and risk of coronary artery disease among urban men,with low rates of obesity:The Indian paradox. *J. Am. Coll. Nutr.* 1999,18:268-73.

[13] Singh V.Chemical Analysis of Inorganic Metal Ions in the Diets of Victims in Relation to Cause of Death. PhD Thesis Accepted by MJP Rohilkhand University, 2002.

[14] Romero-Coral A,Montori VM, Somers VK,Korinek. J. Thomas RJ, Allison AG, Mookadam A,Lopez-Jimenez , F:Association of body weight with total mortality and with cardiovascular events in coronary artery disease: a systemic review of cohort studies. *Lancet* 2006,368:666-678.

[15] Ma S,Cutter J,Tan CE ,Chew SK, Tai ES Associations of diabetes mellitus and ethnicity with mortality in a multiethnic Asian population;data from the 1992 Singhapore National health Survey. *Am J. Epidemiol.* 2003,158:543 52.

[16] .Mohan V,Shanthirani CS,Deepa M,Deepa R,Unnikrishnan RI,Datta M.Mortality rates due to diabetes in a selected urban south Indian population-the Chennai Urban Population Study(CUPS-16). *J. Asso. Phys. India* 2006,54:113-117.

[17] Dudeja V,Misra A,Pandey RM,Devina G,kumar G,Vikram NK. Body mass index does not accurately predict overweight in Asian Indians in north India. *Br. J. Nutr.* 2001,86:105-112.

[18] Singh RB,Sharma JP,Rastogi V,Rastogi SS,Raghuvanshi R.Prevalence of coronary artery disease and coronary risk factors in rural and urban populations of north India. *Eur. Heart J,* 1997,18:1728-35.

[19] Bhatanagar D,Anand IS,Durrington PN et al.Coronary risk factors from the people from the Indian subcontinent living in west London and their siblings in Indias. *Lancet* 1995,345:405-409.

[20] Singh RB,Beegum R,Mehta AS,Niaz MA,De AK,Mitra RK,Haque M,Verma SP,Dube GK,Siddiqui HM,Wander GS,Janus ED,Postiglione A,Haque MS.Social class,coronary risk factors and undernutrition,a double burden of diseases during transition,in five Indian cities. *Int. J. Cardiol.* 1999,69:139-147.

[21] Kiselbah A.H, Freednan D.S. and Peris A.M. Health risks of obesity. *Med. Clin. North Am.*, 1998., 73 (1), 111-38.

[22] Bray G.A. Overweight is risking fate: Obesity a modern day epidemic. *J. Clin. Endo. Metab*, 1999;84:7-10.

[23] Gerber Y, Jacobsen J, Frye RL, Weston SA, Killian JM, Roger VL. Secular trends in deaths from cardiovascular diseases . A 25year community study. *Circulation* 2006, 113: 2285-92.

[24] Peeters A, Barendregt JJ, Willekens F, Mackenbach JP, Mamun AA, Bonneux L. Obesity in adulthood and its consequences for life expectancy: A life table analysis. *Ann. Intern. Med.* 2003,138:24-32.

[25] Adams KF, Schatzkin A, Harris TB, Kipnis V, Mouw T, Ballard-Barbash R, Hollenbeck A, Leitzmann MF. Overweight, obesity,and mortality in a lage prospective cohort of persons 50 to 71 years old. *N. Engl. J. Med.* 2006;355:763-778.

[26] Singh RB, Singh V, Kulshrestha SK, Singh S, Gupta P, Kumar R, Krishna A, Srivastav SSL, Gupta SB, Pella D, Cornelissen G. Social class and all cause mortality in an urban population of north India. *Acta Cardiol.* 2005,60:611-617.

[27] Orel M, Lichnovska R, Gwozdziewiczova S, Zlamalova N, Klementa I, Merkunova A, Hrebicek J. Gender differences in tumor necrosis factor-alpha and leptin secretion from subcutaneous and visceral fat tissue. *Physiol. Res.* 2004;53:501-505.

In: World Heart Research Yearbook. Volume 1
Editors: Franz Halberg and R. B. Singh
ISBN: 978-1-60741-881-8

Plasma Brain Natriuretic Peptide – An Independent Predictor of Mortality and Rehospitalization in Congestive Heart Failure – A Meta-Analysis

Dragos Vesbianu, Carmen Vesbianu, Paul Bernstein and Ruth Kouides

Abstract

Background: CHF is one of the most important cardiac disorders in the US with a high incidence and prevalence as well as increased number of hospitalizations, deaths and, subsequently, increased health care costs.

Design: Meta-analysis of studies assessing BNP as a prognostic indicator.

Methods: Our objective is to determine if discharge BNP is an independent predictor of mortality and rehospitalization in patients admitted with CHF exacerbation. Our personal archives, MEDLINE, and reference lists of retrieved articles were searched. Two reviewers checked the list of abstracts and then the full papers for eligible studies and extracted data independently. We have started our search with 954 articles out of which 82 were selected for more detailed review. Only five studies met the eligibility criteria for the final meta-analysis. Our inclusion criteria were: age more than 18 years, CHF diagnosed by Framingham or echo criteria, BNP assessment in the 24 hour period prior to discharge and a minimum follow up period of one month. The outcomes assessed were all cause mortality and rehospitalization. Only observational, prospective cohort studies published in English language were included. We excluded all randomized control trials (as different treatment of different groups will introduce an additional bias), case series, case reports, case control studies, as well as studies that did not indicate clear clinical end points. The quality of the studies was assessed using the QUADAS (Quality Assessment of Diagnostic Accuracy Studies) score. Statistical analyses were performed using the fixed effects model calculated with Stats Direct and results were expressed as relative risks (RR). Receiver Operating Characteristics (ROC) curves were prepared using Dr. ROC software. We have used the I square test to appreciate the heterogeneity of the combined studies.

Results: The RR of death or rehospitalization for the three BNP cutoffs used 250, 350 and 500 pg/ml were 3.87, 4.66 and 5.73 respectively. For the 250 and 350 BNP cutoffs the Area Under the Curve (AUC) was 0.82 and 0.80.

Conclusion: BNP level at discharge is a strong independent predictor of early readmission or death in patients hospitalized with CHF exacerbation. Prior to discharging those patients health care providers should not only assess for clinical stability but also for circulatory stability by checking discharge BNP.

INTRODUCTION

The clinical assessment of congestive heart failure (CHF) is notoriously difficult. It is hard to determine which patients have heart failure and, once the diagnosis is established, to predict which patients are at risk of death or rehospitalization [1].

If we believe in one of the axioms of epidemiology, that disease and death are not chance-determined events, then there must be as yet unidentified characteristics of the patients or interventions that determine the differences in outcome [2].

Brain Natriuretic Peptide (BNP) is a member of the natriuretic peptide family synthesized mainly in the ventricles and secreted in response to myocardial tension or increased intravascular volume. BNP and the amino-terminal fragment of its molecule, N-terminal proBNP (NT-proBNP) have been shown to be independent predictors for mortality and cardiac composite endpoints for populations at risk for coronary artery disease (CAD), diagnosed CAD, and diagnosed HF [3].

Despite many assessments in the literature, the exact relationship between BNP and the prognosis in CHF remains ambiguous. This ambiguity results mainly from the broad range of studies and study designs addressing this topic.

It is well known that heart failure is a syndrome that carries a bad prognosis. Hospitalization is common and rehospitalization rate is high, factors which influence the cost of care [4].

We anticipate that finding a good prognostic indicator for these outcomes will have a major impact on heath care costs of this disease. Hence the objective of this review is to determine if discharge BNP at the time of CHF exacerbation is an independent prognostic factor for mortality or short term rehospitalization.

MATERIAL AND METHODS

Design

We conducted a literature review to estimate the prognostic value of BNP in patients admitted with CHF exacerbation. Only studies that looked at adult patients hospitalized for CHF exacerbation, diagnosed using Framingham [5] or echo criteria were included in the final meta-analysis. Other inclusion criteria were assessing BNP in the 24 hour period prior to discharge and a minimum follow up period of one month. The outcomes assessed were all cause mortality and rehospitalization. Only observational, prospective cohort studies published in English language were included. We excluded all randomized control trials, case series, case reports, case control studies, as well as studies that did not indicate clear clinical end points.

Literature Search

The search for the relevant articles was conducted by three people (the two reviewers and the librarian) using Medline. References from review articles as well as our personal archives were used to find more articles. The time frame was 1989, first year a BNP assay was reported to 2008. We used 5 MeSH terms for BNP and 8 MeSH terms for heart failure. Two different reviewers (DV and CV) evaluated the studies. Conflicts regarding inclusion of the studies were solved by consensus or by the intervention of a third reviewer (RK).

Validity Assessment

The two reviewers independently assessed the methodological quality of prognostic accuracy of each study included in the final analysis using the QUADAS criteria [6]. A quality score based on those criteria was given to each of the studies. We looked at the inclusion criteria, study design, length and completeness of follow up, as well as the blinding of the investigators to the index test or reference standard results.

Data Abstraction

We extracted data on BNP cutoff, the method of measuring BNP, the outcomes assessed, number of events, length of follow up, the number of patients, mean ejection fraction, clinical setting, and study type. The reviewers extracted data independently.

Analysis

Statistical analyses were performed using the fixed effects model calculated with Stats Direct and the results were expressed as relative risks. For the summary ROC curves, AUC as well as for calculating I square to estimate the heterogeneity, we used dr.-ROC software.

RESULTS

We found 926 studies after the MEDLINE search, and we added 28 studies from our personal files and reference lists. After careful evaluation of the titles and abstracts we identified 82 articles for more detailed review. The main reasons for exclusion of the studies were, BNP used to evaluate the response to therapy, the use of NT-proBNP, or usage of BNP as a diagnostic tool. After reviewing the full text of the 82 articles, 77 were excluded mainly for assessing different outcomes, following outpatients only, or no mention of the discharge BNP (Figure 1).

The 5 studies that were included [7, 8, 9, 10, 11] in the final analysis had a total of 607 patients with sample sizes ranging from 50 to 202. The follow up was between 1 and 18 months. The BNP cutoffs used were from 200 to 1170 (Table 1).

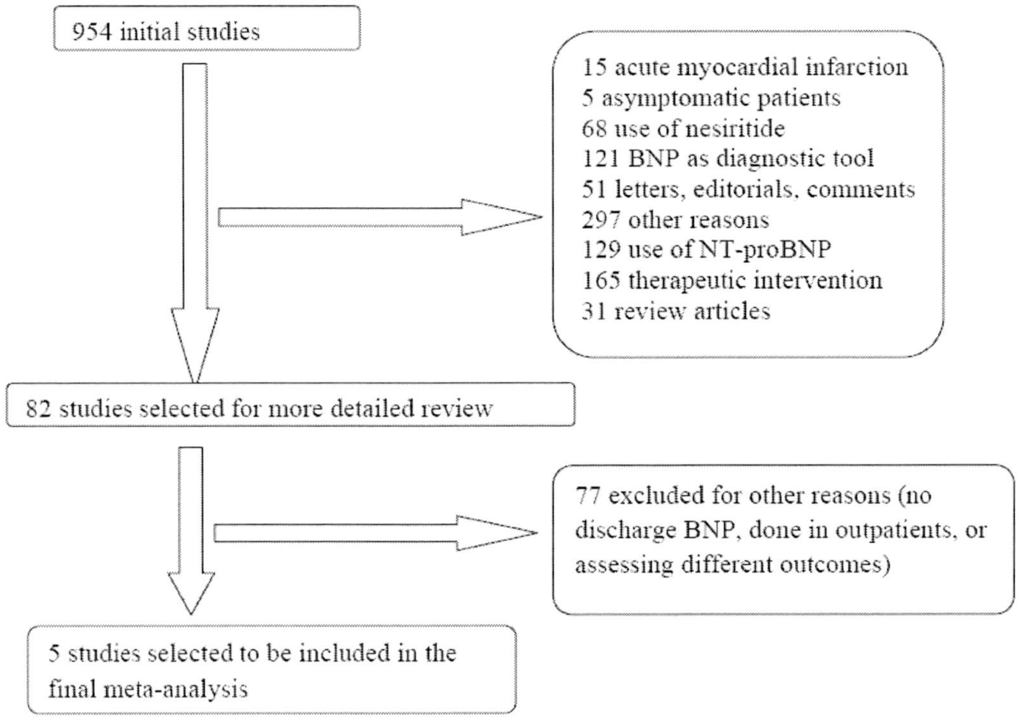

Figure 1. Search strategy.

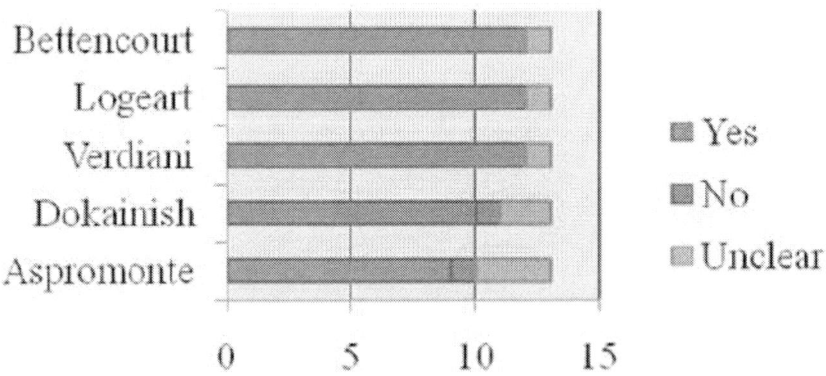

Figure 2. QUADAS criteria per each study.

The QUADAS score was calculated for each study. Each study receives one point for each quality criterion met. If a study does not satisfy a criterion or if this is not reported it receives zero points. By adding all the points together each study can have a maximum score of 13 points that would denote an ideal study from a methodological quality standpoint. (Figure 2).

We combined the studies depending on their BNP cutoffs. To show the amount of variation between studies and to estimate the overall result (relative risk) we have done a forest plot (Figure 3). Our outcome was death or rehospitalization during the follow up.

All 5 studies showed a consistently increased relative risk for death or rehospitalization during follow up for higher BNP. It is also very evident that the relative risks were steadily increasing as the BNP cutoff used increases.

To appreciate the accuracy we calculated summary ROC curves and the AUC for each BNP cutoff (Figure 4). The ROC curves for the three BNP cutoffs used (225, 350, 500) were relatively similar with AUCs of 0.82, 0.81 and 0.84. I square was used to estimate the heterogeneity. We found a moderate to high heterogeneity.

Table 1. Baseline characteristics

Study name	No of patients	BNP cutoffs	Follow up (months)	Mean age	Mean EF %	Outcome	No of events
Aspromonte	145	200,250,350 500	6	72	42	Death or readmission	41
Dokainish	110	250	18	59	40	Death or readmission	54
Bettencourt	50	321	6	71	NR	Death or readmission	20
Logeart	202	350, 700	6	70	34	Death or readmission	86
Verdiani	100	506, 696, 789, 1170	1	78	38	Death or readmission	17

DISCUSSION

The cost of CHF hospitalization is very high and numerous attempts were done to determine which factors can increase hospital readmission or mortality.

Our meta-analysis of the various published data showed that discharge BNP is an excellent prognostic indicator for hospital readmission or death in patients hospitalized for heart failure exacerbation.

There are several factors that seemed to be fair predictors of mortality. Older age, comorbidities such as diabetes mellitus or renal dysfunction, higher NYHA class, lower ejection fraction, hyponatremia, lower body mass index, lower blood pressure, and lower quality life scores. However none of these is a strong predictor [11].

It is difficult to point to the exact BNP cutoff that we should aim for. Health care providers should not only assess the patients' clinical stability but also their circulatory stability by checking BNP prior to discharge. Doing so we may be able to identify those patients who have a high risk of rehospitalization or death and either postpone their discharge or arrange for a closer follow up as outpatients.

We have conducted a high-quality and reproducible review there are a few limitations. Although we have started with a large number of trials we had to limit our final analysis to only five. Because the BNP cutoffs used were so heterogeneous we had to split them in more subgroups. Taking into consideration only studies that were published in English, there is a potential for publication bias. It is possible that small studies or studies that did not come up with positive results were never published.

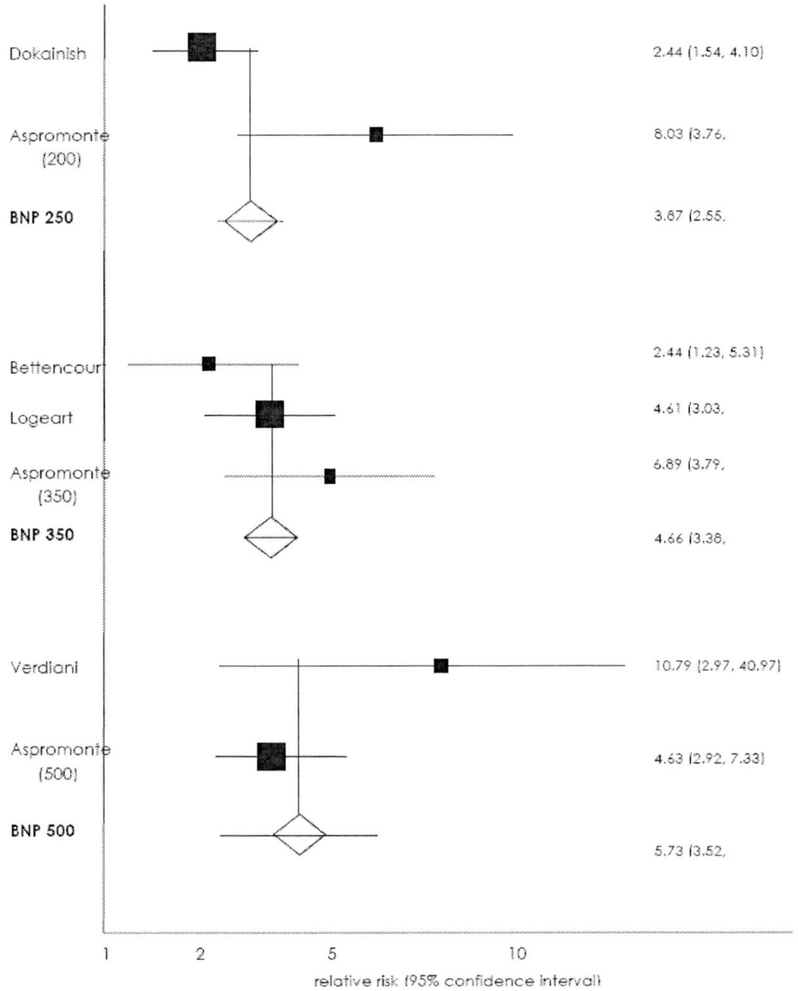

Figure 3. Relative risk meta-analysis plot (fixed effect) for all three BNP cutoffs.

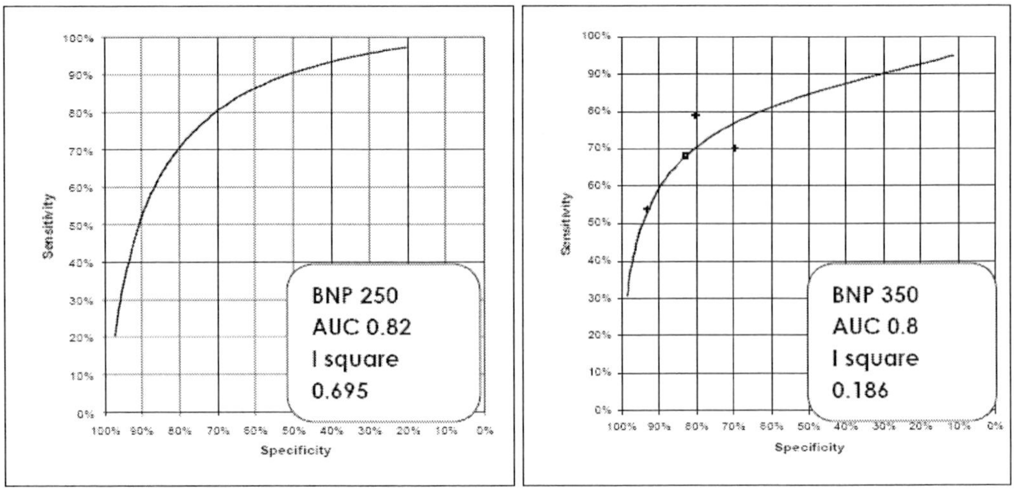

Figure 4. ROC curves, AUCs and I square for two of the BNP cutoffs.

References

[1] Doust JA, Pietrzak E. How well does B-type natriuretic peptide predict death and cardiac events in patients with heart failure: systematic review. *BMJ* 2005; 330.

[2] Bettencourt P, Frioes F, Azevedo A. Prognostic information provided by serial measurements of brain natriuretic peptide in heart failure. *International Journal of Cardiology* 2004; 93:45-48.

[3] Testing for BNP and NT-proBNP in the diagnosis and prognosis of heart failure. AHRQ (Agency for Healthcare Research and Quality). Publication No. 06-E014, Sept. 2006.

[4] Linee A. Health care costs of heart failure: results from a randomized study of patient education. *European Journal of Heart Failure* 2000; 2:291-297.

[5] McKee PA, Castelli WP, McNamara PM, Kannel WB. The natural history of CHF. The Framingham study. *N Engl J Med* 1971; 285:1442-1446.

[6] Hatjimihail A. Quality of diagnostic accuracy studies: the development, use and evaluation of QUADAS. *Evid. Based Med.* 2006; 11:189.

[7] Aspromonte N, Feola M, Milli M. prognostic role of B-type natriuretic peptide in patients with diabetes and acute decompensated heart failure. *Diabetic Medicine* 2007; 24:124-130.

[8] Dokainish H, Zoghbi WA, Ambriz E. Comparative cost-effectiveness of B-type natriuretic peptide and echocardiography for predicting outcome in patients with congestive heart failure. *Am. J. Cardiol* 2005; 97:400-403.

[9] Bettencourt P, Ferreira S, Azevedo A. Preliminary data on the potential usefulness of B-type natriuretic petide levels in predicting outcome after hospital discharge in patients with heart failure. *Am J Med.* 2002; 113:215-219.

[10] Logeart D, Thabut G, Jourdain P. Pre-discharge B-type natriuretic peptide assay for identifying patients at risk of re-admission after decompensated heart failure. *J. Am. Coll Cardiol.* 2004; 43:635-41.

[11] Verdiani V, Nozzoli C, Bacci F. Pre-discharge B-type natriuretic peptide predicts early reccurence of decompensated heart failure in patients admitted to a general medical unit. *Eur J. Heart Failure* 2005; 7:566-571.

In: World Heart Research Yearbook. Volume 1
Editors: Franz Halberg and R. B. Singh
ISBN: 978-1-60741-881-8

FALSE TENDON INDUCED SUBAORTIC HYPERTROPHY — A NEW VARIANT OF HYPERTROPHIC CARDIOMYOPATHY?

James Ker*
Department of Physiology, University of Pretoria
Gesina, Pretoria, South Africa

ABSTRACT

Left ventricular false tendons are a common echocardiographic finding and consist of thin fibrous or fibromuccular structures traversing the left ventricular cavity. They have no connection to any valvular cusps and may be single or multiple. Histologic examination has shown that they can be composed of any combination of cardiac muscle, fibrous tissue, blood vessels and Purkinje cells.

At present the clinical significance of the false tendons is uncertain, with some studies showing a possible causal role for ventricular arrhythmias. These tendons have been divided into five categories, based on the site of implantation.

In this study a sixth category of left ventricular false tendon is identified, with implantation into the ventricular septum in a subaortic position. These subaortic false tendons is associated with localized subaortic hypertrophy and it is suggested that they play a causale role in the genesis of localized subaortic hypertrophy with a possible new variant of hypertrophic cardiomyopathy—false tendon induced subaortic hypertrophy.

Keywords*:* False tendons, hypertrophy, cardiomyopathy

INTRODUCTION

Left ventricular false tendons are thin, fibrous or fibromuscular structures that traverse the left ventricular cavity [1]. They may be single or multiple and have no connection to the valvular cusps [1].

False tendons can be an isolated finding or can be associated with cardiac abnormalities [2]. These tendons are usually of no clinical significance but has been associated with rate-

* Address for correspondence: Department of Physiology, University of Pretoria, Gesina, Pretoria, South Africa. MRCP, PhD, FESC, FACC. PO Box 24318. 0031; E-mail: jker@wol.co.za; Tel: +2712-3414341; Fax: +2712-3414342.

dependent ventricular arrhythmias and has also been shown to be a cause of musical murmurs when pulled taut by ventricular dilatation [2].

Loukas et al [3] examined 200 formalin fixed, adult hearts and divided false tendons into five categories: In type I the false tendon is located between the posteromedial papillary muscle and the ventricular septum. In type II the false tendon is located between the two papillary muscles. In type III the false tendon is located between the anterolateral papillary muscle and the ventricular septum. In type IV the false tendon is located between the ventricular septum and the free wall. In type V the false tendons appear weblike and have three or more points of insertion. After careful histological examination Abdulla et al [2] suggested that false tendons may be intracavitary radiations of the bundle of His and that their clinical significance may be more relevant than previously believed and merits further study.

METHODS

This study was a retrospective analysis.A total of 3000 adult echocardiograms, performed between 2004 and 2008 for various clinical indications, were reviewed and analyzed for the presence of a left ventricular false tendon in the subaortic position.

RESULTS

A total of 6 adult echocardiograms clearly demonstrated the presence of a false tendon located between the left ventricular lateral wall and the subaortic interventricular septum (see figure 1-6). In all 6 of these cases a striking local ventricular hypertrophic response was present at the site of septal implantation of the false tendon (see figure 1-6).

No systolic and/or diastolic dysfunction, valvular disease or pericardial disease were present in any of these patients. All 6 echocardiograms were from men, aged from 35 years to 64 years.

DISCUSSION

A sixth type of left ventricular false tendon is identified—with the specific location between the subaortic portion of the interventricular septum and the left ventricular free wall. In each of the six cases presented, a striking localized ventricular hypertrophic response is present at the site of subaortic implantation of the false tendons.

Hypertrophic growth is the primary mechanism by which the heart reduces stress on the ventricular wall [4]. Mechanical stress on the ventricular wall elicits auto-and paracrine signaling by inducing the synthesis and secretion of growth factors, such as angiotensin II, insulin like growth factor I and endothelin 1 and furthermore, mechanical stretch is also capable of activating angiotensin II receptors directly, without the involvement of angiotensin II [4, 5]. The predominant feature of the hypertrophic cardiomyopathy phenotype is increased thickness of the left ventricular wall [6]. However, hypertrophic cardiomyopathy is both genotypically and phenotypically a highly heterogenous disorder with more than 150 mutations, scattered throughout 10 genes, encoding various proteins of the cardiac sarcomere, as known genetic causes for the condition [7, 8, 9].

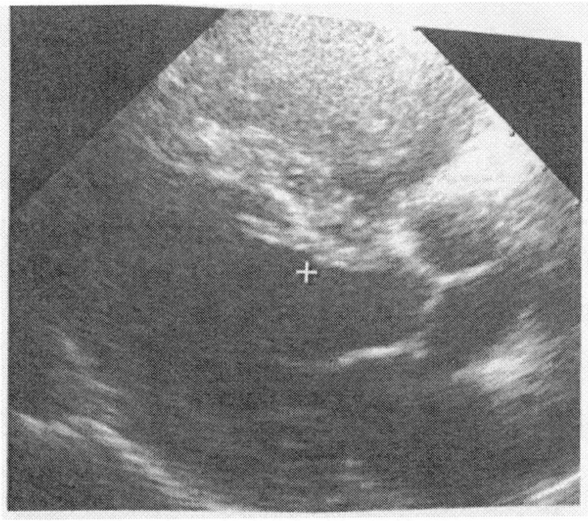

Figure 1. Parasternal long-axis view on transthoracic echocardiogram of patient 1. Note the subaortic implantation of a false tendon, with a prominent localized hypertrophic response.

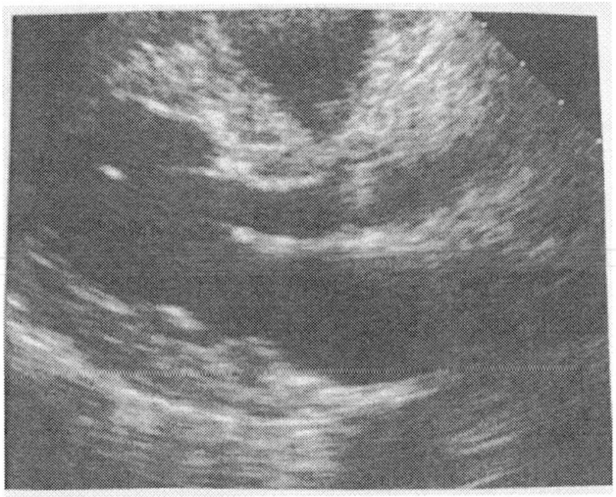

Figure 2. Parasternal long-axis view of transthoracic echocardiogram of patient 2, demonstrating the same subaortic false tendon as in patient 1, also with a localized hypertrophic response.

Phenotypically, there can be marked regional differences in ventricular wall thickness [10], with the hypertrophic process affecting either the left and/or right ventricle [7], being symmetrical or asymmetrical [7]. Septal hypertrophy is the most common phenotype, with midventricular and apical hypertrophy less common [7]. Even in patients with identical mutations striking inter-and intra-family variations have been noticed in the presence and severity of left ventricular hypertrophy [11]. So-called modifier genes may contribute to this phenotypic diversity and indeed the rs2106809 and rs6632677 polymorphisms of the angiotensin-converting enzyme 2 gene have been shown to increase the risk for expressing greater magnitude of ventricular hypertrophy in hypertrophic cardiomyopathy [11].

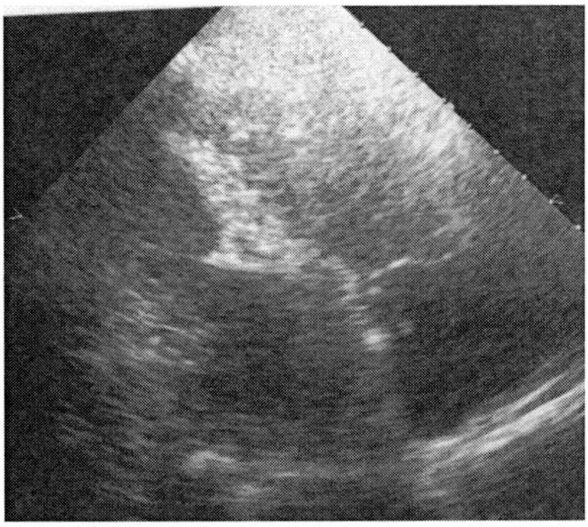

Figure 3. Parasternal long-axis view of patient 3. The presence of the same type of subaortic false tendon with localized hypertrophy is shown.

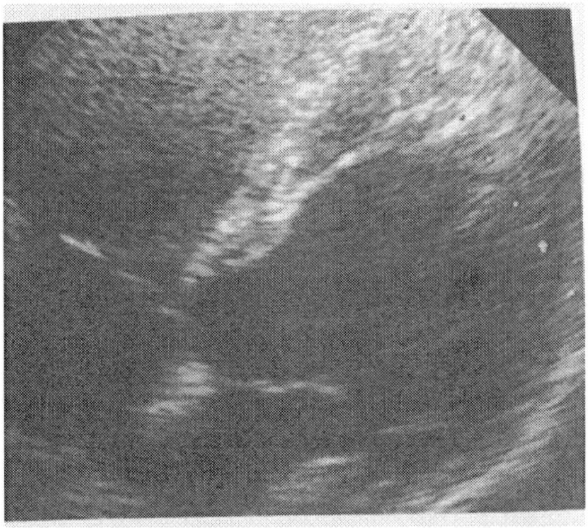

Figure 4. Apical two-chamber view of patient 4. The presence of a subaortic false tendon with a striking localized hypertrophic response is shown.

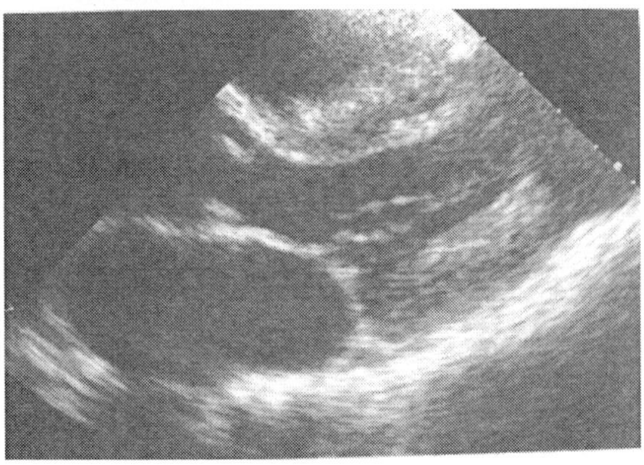

Figure 5. Apical two-chamber view of patient 5.

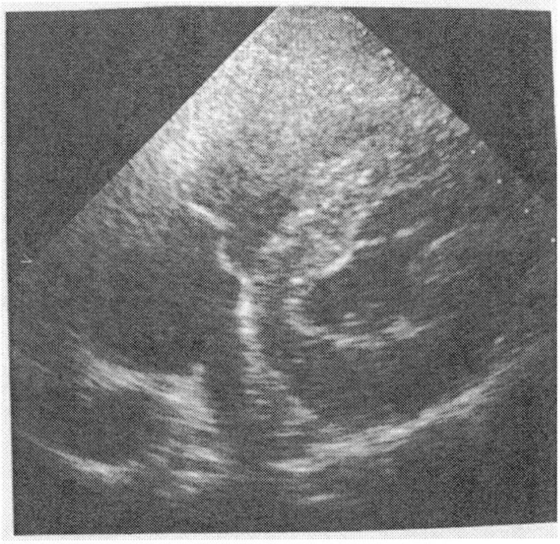

Figure 6. Parasternal short-axis view of patient 6. The localized hypertrophic response is clearly shown.

Kobashi *et al* [12] noted that patients can present with isolated papillary muscle hypertrophy and suggested that this is a newly identified subtype of hypertrophic cardiomyopathy.

Harrigan *et al* [6] have shown on the other hand, that in patients with established hypertrophic cardiomyopathy, both the number and the mass index of the papillary muscles may be increased and that in these patients accessory papillary muscles can even contribute to ventricular outflow obstruction.

Adult-onset hypertrophic cardiomyopathy is a prevalent condition [13] and is caused by either inherited or new mutations in cardiac sarcomere protein genes, such as: cardiac beta-myosin heavy chain (MYH7), cardiac myosin-binding protein C (MYBPC3), cardiac troponin T (TNNT2), cardiac troponin I (TNNI3), essential myosin light chain (MYL3), regulatory myosin light chain (MYL2), alpha-tropomyosin (TPM1), cardiac actin (ACTC) and titin (TTN). The age range at clinical diagnosis of hypertrophic cardiomyopathy is broad, however, clinical manifestation before the age of 14 years are atypical [13].

In view of the above background of hypertrophic cardiomyopathy three issues are relevant to this study: First, it is possible that the local hypertrophic response is due to local mechanical stretch, induced by the false tendon attachment. Second, the involvement of the papillary muscles in hypertrophic cardiomyopathy has been clearly shown—an increase in their mass index and number with accessory papillary muscles—has been documented. It is perhaps time to focus on false tendons in hypertrophic cardiomyopathy—will there be an increase in their mass index and number the same as for the papillary muscles? Thirdly, the striking local hypertrophic response at the site of septal implantation of these false tendons may be caused by the false tendon itself in a manner other than a local stretch induced response—a true false tendon-induced hypertrophic cardiomyopathy. Lastly, an important clinical question is whether these localized hypertrophic responses will remain static or will progress with generalized ventricular involvement over time?

A sixth type of ventricular false tendon is proposed—the subaortic false tendon, giving rise to false tendon-induced subaortic hypertrophy. Whether this is due to a local stretch response or a true hypertrophic cardiomyopathy will need to be determined by further studies, also performing genetic analyses for possible mutations in genes encoding proteins of the cardiac sarcomere.

REFERENCES

[1] Kervancioglu M, Ozbag D, Kervancioglu P, Hatipoglu ES, Kiliuc M, Yilmaz F, Deniz M. Echocardiographic and morphologic examination of left ventricular false tendons in human and animal hearts. *Clinical Anatomy* 2003; 16(5): 389-395.

[2] Abdulla AK, Frustaci A, Martinez JE, Florio RA, Somerville J, Olsen EGJ. Echocardiography and pathology of left ventricular false tendons. *Chest* 1990; 98: 129-132.

[3] Loukas M, Louis RG, Black B, Pham D, Fudalej M, Sharkees M. False tendons: An endoscopic cadaveric approach. *Clinical Anatomy* 2007; 20(2): 163-169.

[4] Hill JA, Olson EN. Cardiac plasticity. New *England Journal of Medicine* 2008; 358: 1370-1380.

[5] Sadoshima J, Izumo S. The cellular and molecular response of cardiac myocytes to mechanical stress. *Annu. Rev. Physiol.* 1997; 59: 551-571.

[6] Harrigan CJ, Appelbaum E, Maron BJ, Buros JL, Gibson M, Lesser JR, Udelson JE, Manning WJ, Maron MS. Significance of papillary muscle abnormalities identified by cardiovascular magnetic resonance in hypertrophic cardiomyopathy. *The American Journal of Medicine* 2008; 101(5): 668-673.

[7] Wigle ED, Rakowski H, Kimball BP, Williams W. Hypertrophic cardiomyopathy: clinical spectrum and treatment. *Circulation* 1995; 92: 1680-1692.

[8] Runge MS, Stouffer GA, Sheahan RG, Lerakis S. Hypertrophic cardiomyopathy: presentation and pathophysiology. *Circulation* 1997; 314: 324-329.

[9] Van Driest SL, Ackerman MJ, Ommen SR. Prevalence and severity of benign mutations in the beta-myosin heavy chain cardiac troponin T and alpha-tropomyosin genes in hypertrophic cardiomyopathy. *Circulation* 2002; 106: 3085-3090.

[10] Ganame J, Mertens L, Eiden BW, Claus P, D`hooge J, Havemann LM, McMahon CJ, Elayda MA, Vaughn WK, Towbin JA, Ayres NA, Pignatelli RH. Regional myocardial deformation in children with hypertrophic cardiomyopathy: morphological and clinical correlates. *European Heart Journal* 2007; 28(23): 2886-2894.

[11] Wang SX, Fu CY, Zou YB, Wang H, Shi Y, Xu XQ, Chen JZ, Song XD, Huan TJ, Hui RT. Polymorphisms of angiotensin-converting enzyme 2 gene associated with magnitude of left ventricular hypertrophy in male patients with hypertrophic cardiomyopathy. *Chinese Medical Journal* 2008; 121(1): 27-31.

[12] Kobashi A, Suwa M, Ito T, Otake Y, Hirota Y, Kawamura K. Solitary papillary muscle hypertrophy as a possible form of hypertrophic cardiomyopathy. *Japanese Circ. J.* 1998; 62: 811-816.

[13] Hiroyuki M, Rehm HL, Menesses A, McDonough B, Roberts AE, Kucherlapati R, Towbin JA, Seidman JG, Seidman CE. Shared genetic causes of cardiac hypertrophy in children and adults. *New England Journal of Medicine* 2008; 358: 1899-1908.

In: World Heart Research Yearbook. Volume 1
Editors: Franz Halberg and R. B. Singh
ISBN: 978-1-60741-881-8

CARDIOVASCULAR DISEASE AND ERECTILE DYSFUNCTION: THE EVOLVING ROLE OF PHOSPHODIESTERASE-5-INHIBITORS

Ujjaini Khanderia* and Randolph E. Regal
University of Michigan Health Systems, Ann Arbor, US

INTRODUCTION

The exact prevalence of erectile dysfunction (ED) is difficult to determine due to under-reporting of this condition. This is because of patient reluctance to talk about personal problems related to sexual functioning. One of the most frequently cited studies on the epidemiology of ED is the Massachusetts Male Aging Study.[1] This landmark study interviewed 1,290 men with a self-administered questionnaire regarding sexual activity. The findings showed that 52% of men age 40 to 70 years had some degree of ED, and that about 10% of these men experienced a total absence of erectile function. With increased age, the prevalence of ED also increased, such that 68% of men aged 60 to 70 years experienced ED of some magnitude. After adjusting for age, ED directly correlated with the presence of coronary artery disease (CAD), hypertension, diabetes mellitus, low serum levels of high-density lipoprotein cholesterol (HDL-C), depression, and cigarette smoking.

There is compelling evidence that ED precedes the formation of atherosclerotic plaques and may serve as an early marker of coronary atherosclerosis. The manifestation of ED may therefore, serve as a useful clinical tool for identifying men at high risk for cardiovascular disease (CVD). [2,3] ED and CVD share many conventional risk factors including hypertension, [1,4] dyslipidemia, [5,6] type 2 diabetes mellitus [7,8], cigarette smoking [l,9] and obesity [10] The severity of ED appears to correlate with the presence of an increasing number of risk factors, all of which are associated with endothelial dysfunction. It is now well established that the endothelium plays a key role in the pathogenesis of all systemic vascular diseases, including ED [11]

In this chapter, we review the association between ED and underlying CVD. The pharmacology, clinical efficacy and safety of the available phosphodiesterase -5 inhibitors (PDEIs) will be discussed. Clinical trials that have investigated the use of PDEIs in men with ED and concomitant cardiovascular conditions such as heart failure (HF), hypertension, pulmonary hypertension, diabetes mellitus, and coronary artery disease will be addressed.

* Ujjaini Khanderia: shamo@med.umich.edu.

Endothelial Dysfunction

The link between ED and atherosclerosis is endothelial dysfunction. The endothelium is present throughout the arterial vasculature and consequently, symptoms of endothelial dysfunction manifested as ED, may also indicate problems in the coronary arteries. Indeed, the pathogenesis of ED is closely related to the atherosclerotic process, [12-14] with both conditions being characterized by disturbed endothelial function [2,15]. Endothelial dysfunction results from the inability of arterial smooth muscle to relax in a process regulated by the nitric oxide-cyclic guanosine-3'5'-monophosphate (NO-cGMP) system [14,16,17,18]. Nitric oxide (NO), synthesized by nitric oxide synthase (NOS) from the amino acid L-arginine, regulates vasomotor tone and plays a major role in mediating smooth muscle relaxation in normal penile erection. Oxidative stress, which interferes with the NO pathway and is directly toxic to the endothelium, causes vascular damage associated with both preclinical as well as clinically evident CVD. A deficiency in NO, brought about by impaired production or increased degradation by reactive oxidant species (i.e., superoxides), prevents normal vasodilation in the penile arteries [19,20].

ED resulting from insufficient NO-mediated dilatation of relatively small penile arteries may occur at a stage when atherosclerosis in the larger coronary, carotid or femoral arteries is not yet clinically manifested [21]. In one study using flow mediated brachial artery vasodilation, systemic endothelial function was examined in 30 men with ED compared with 27 age-matched controls [17]. Men with ED had impaired endothelium-dependent flow-mediated vasodilation ($p \leq 0.05$) as well as endothelium-independent vasodilation, defined as a blunted response to sublingual nitroglycerin, compared with the control group ($p=0.02$) [17]. The abnormalities preceded any evidence of coronary or vascular disease.

Erectile Dysfunction as a Surrogate Marker for Cardiovascular Disease

The prevalence of ED in patients with CVD is higher than that seen in the general population, ranging from 60% in men with previous myocardial infarction (MI) or who had undergone coronary artery bypass surgery [22] to 75% of men with chronic CAD [23]. Infact, one study found that men with ED had a twofold increased risk for acute MI compared to their cohorts without ED [24].

Until recently, ED was generally regarded as a late consequence of generalized atherosclerosis. This view has been contradicted in recent times, and questions have arisen as to whether ED could be a marker predating the development of future cardiac events. The Prostate Cancer Prevention Trial [25] was a landmark study that used data from 9457 men to determine whether ED was associated with the subsequent development of CVD. Around 15% of the men (1394 of 9457) had CVD at study entry. All patients were evaluated every three months over a 9-year period for evidence of ED and CVD. Of the 4247 men who did not have ED at study entry, 2420 (57%) developed ED (incident ED) in the subsequent 5 years. After adjusting for other CVD risk factors, incident ED was associated with a hazard ratio of 1.25 for the development of new CV events ($p=0.04$). Thus, ED had significant prognostic value for the subsequent development of CVD. For men who either had ED at the start of the study or developed it during the course of the study, the hazard ratio for developing CVD during the course of the study was 1.45 ($p<0.001$).

ED may already be present prior to the clinical manifestations of coronary artery or peripheral vascular disease [3,26,27]. A large study of 25, 650 men found a 75% increased risk of peripheral vascular disease in men with pre-existing ED [28] Pritzker [29] studied 50 men who had ED but no history or symptoms of CVD, yet 80% of these men had multiple risk factors for CAD as assessed by questionnaire analysis. Furthermore, 56% failed a treadmill stress test and had an abnormal exercise electrocardiogram (ECG). When 20 of these 28 men had coronary angiography, all were found to have one- to three- vessel disease. Vlachopoulos et al. [30] documented that up to 19% of patients with ED have documented silent CAD.

ED is now considered to be a surrogate marker for occult vascular or coronary artery disease (CAD). The diameter of penile arteries is around 1-2 mm, which is a much smaller compared with that of the coronary artery (3-4 mm) or carotid artery (5-7 mm). Consequently, the amount of plaque sufficient to block blood flow through the penile artery, and therefore cause ED, produces only a 30-40% stenosis and no apparent symptoms in arteries with a larger diameter [21]. Thus, compared to penile arteries, the larger coronary arteries can better tolerate the same amount of atherosclerotic plaque without inducing obstructive flow-limiting stenosis. It follows then that damage to the penile vascular bed precedes the development of atherosclerotic lesions, and may serve as an early marker of systemic atherosclerosis. Thus, ED may be the first clinical manifestation of coronary atherosclerosis, and patients presenting with ED should be investigated for CVD. Early detection could facilitate prompt intervention and aggressive management of CV risk factors to prevent future cardiovascular events.

PHOSPHODIESTERASE INHIBITORS

At the time of this writing, three phosphodiesterase inhibitors (PDEIs), sildenafil (Viagra®), vardenafil (Levitra®), and tadalafil (Cialis®) are available in the US market for treating ED of organic, psychogenic, or mixed etiology. Sildenafil has also been recently labeled under a different strength and trade name (Revatio®) for treating pulmonary hypertension. Ironically, before these agents became widely marketed and aggressively publicized as the drugs of choice for ED, the PDEIs were studied as a potential pharmaceutical panacea for a gamut of cardiovascular-related diseases such as chronic heart failure, essential hypertension, and diabetes mellitus. However, further long-term studies are necessary to measure their true overall utility for these conditions.

Mechanism of Action: Thus far, eleven discrete phosphodiesterase (PDE) families have been identified within the human body, and at least 40 different isoforms have been described. The enzyme families are similar in structure, but differ in terms of tissue distribution, selectivity for cyclic nucleotides, and sensitivity for inhibitors and activators. Because of these differences, each family occupies a unique niche in terms of its ultimate physiological role. As will be further addressed in this section, the currently marketed PDEIs are relatively specific to the family known as PDE 5 [31-33].

PDE enzymes catalyze the degradation of both cyclic adenosine monophosphate (cAMP) and cyclic guanosine monophosphate (cGMP). It is established that cAMP and cGMP play pivotal roles in a plethora of intracellular signaling pathways. In the case of cGMP, this compound acts as a vital messenger that initiates complex signaling cascades which regulate such diverse functions as vascular smooth muscle tone , homeostasis of interstitial fluid and electrolytes, and induction of phototransduction within the retina. In terms of its function on vascular smooth muscle within the penis, specifically, cGMP is the second messenger in the enzymatic cascade that elicits relaxation of the smooth muscle in the penile vascular spaces and penile vessels, including the corpus cavernosa.. Of course, potentiation of these processes then facilitates the effect of penile erection. [32]. Once introduced into the systemic circulation, PDEIs penetrate into smooth muscle cells to inhibit tissue-local PDE. Obviously, when PDEIs prevent the degradation of cGMP, they subsequently induce vasodilation leading to an increase in penile blood flow; and ultimately potentiate the achievement of penile erection [31-34].

It is important to understand the synergistic physiologic process which PDEIs exact with nitric oxide (NO). NO is a potent activator of guanylate cyclases, a group of enzymes which catalyze the synthesis from guanosine triphosphate to cGMP. One can recall that these compounds make up part of the NO-cGMP system which was alluded to earlier in the article. As a result of their ability to activate guanylate cyclases, NO and related nitrates directly elevate cGMP levels. This NO effect of elevating cGMP levels acts in consort with PDEIs, since PDEIs prevent cGMP degradation. Understanding the synergy between PDEIs and NO/nitrates helps to practically explain two important clinical pearls that clinicians must remember about PDEI therapy. First, this helps explain why the concomitant use of nitrates and PDEIs can cause a profound and prolonged drop in blood pressure; the hypotension results from vasodilation caused by excessive cGMP buildup. Second, this helps explain why in order to facilitate optimal erectile responses, PDEIs still need the concomitant presence of endogenous nitric oxide from neuronal or endothelial cells, a process initiated by normal sexual stimulation, in order to be optimally effective [31,33,35,36]

History of Pharmaceutical Development: Of the eleven PDE families, much research initially focused on the subtype known as PDE5. This is because in the mid -1980s, the PDE5 family was found to be present in high concentrations in vascular smooth muscle as well as within platelets. Of course, both of these effects were already recognized as being of benefit in treating various cardiovascular conditions, such as angina [31]. Thus, in hopes of synthesizing an agent that elicited vasodilator effects as well as platelet anti-aggregation, a selective PDE5 inhibitor was sought after for research and development. Although the PDE5 enzyme is especially plentiful in the corpus cavernosum of the penis, it was recognized earlier that the PDE5 family was ubiquitous, and could be found in vascular smooth muscles throughout the body [31,32].

In 1989, sildenafil citrate was synthesized as a potent and selective inhibitor of PDE5. Though initially studied for angina, this aspiration was countermanded by the emergence of self-limiting and transient visual side effects. Vision changes were observed at high doses of 150mg and 200mg daily. It was later realized that these side effects were due to sildenafil's weak inhibitory effect on PDE6, an enzyme concentrated in the photoreceptor cells within the retina. Serendipitously, another side effect reported in clinical trials was penile erections. Shortly thereafter, the somewhat parallel and complementary role of NO in sexual stimulation and erectile production was also discovered. With the added knowledge of PDE5's presence in the smooth muscle of the corpus cavernosum, sildenafil's first pilot study in men with ED was started in 1993 [31]. The drug was eventually approved for the treatment of ED in 1998.

Since then, two more PDE inhibitors under the generic names of vardenafil and tadalafil, were approved in or around 2004.

In terms of PDE5 potency, sildenafil and tadalafil appear to have equal potency, whereas vadalafil has greater potency [32]. Vardenafil appears to share the same cross-affinity for PDE6 receptors as does sidenafil, whereas tadalfil apparently cross-reacts with PDE 11 enzymes, which happen to be located in cardiac tissue, the pituitary gland, and the testes [32]. In addition, sildenafil, but not vardenafil or tadalafil, shows relatively high affinity for PDE1c, a subtype PDE enzyme which has been found to distribute in high concentrations in lung tissue. This last observation regarding sildenafil's PDE1c selectivity may explain its emergence as the first PDEI to be studied and approved to treat pulmonary hypertension [37].

Table 1. PDE5 -Inhibitor Comparison: Dosing and Pharmacokinetics

Parameter	Sildenafil(Viagra)	Vardenafil(Levitra)	Tadalafil(Cialis)
Dosage Availability (mg)	25, 50, 100	2.5, 5, 10, 20	5, 10, 20
Dosing	50mg orally 1hr (usally 0.5-4hr) prior to sexual intercourse (may decrease to 25mg or increase to 100mg per day as tolerated)	10mg orally 1hr prior to sexual intercourse (max 20mg/day)	10mg orally prior to sexual intercourse (may decrease to 5mg or increase to 20mg per day as tolerated)
Onset of Action (min)	30-60	30-120	16-30
Duration of Action (hr)	3-5	4-5	24-36
Half-life (hr)	4	4-5	17.5
Metabolism	Hepatic	Hepatic	Hepatic
P-450 Isozyme Pathways	3A4 (major) 2C9 (minor)	3A4 3A5, 2C	3A4
Plasma Protein Binding	96%	95%	94%
Mean Volume of Distribution (L)	105	208	63
Absorption	F= 0.40 Time to peak prolonged and Cmax reduced with high-fat foods. No change in AUC	F=0.15 Time to peak prolonged and Cmax reduced with high-fat foods. No change in AUC.	F=0.36 Unchanged with food; decreased with antacids
Dose Adjustments for Renal or Hepatic Impairment	Dose reduction for patients > 65yr, hepatic impairment, severe renal impairment (CrCl < 30ml/min)	Dose reduction for patients > 65yr, hepatic impairment, moderate to severe renal impairment (CrCl < 50ml/min)	No dosage adjustment for age; not recommended for use with severe hepatic impairment; decrease dose for moderate to severe renal impairment (CrCl < 50ml/min)

Pharmacokinetics and Dosing: The pharmacokinetics of PDEIs is summarized in Table 1. [38] The most clinically important difference between the three agents is that tadalafil possesses a much longer half-life than either sildenafil or vardenafil [39-41] In this class of drugs, the durations of action appear commensurate with the elimination half-lives, thus owing tadalafil to nicknames such as "*Le weekender*" in France.

The PDEIs share many similarities. All are primarily hepatically eliminated, with CYP 3A4 as the major CYP pathway for metabolism. Thus, caveats exist for use and dosing of PDEIs in patients with liver disease, as well at those taking concomitant drugs which have been identified as potent CYP 3A4 inhibitors (see Table 2 and Drug Interactions).

Conversely, drugs that may induce the CYP 3A4 system could reduce PDEI effectiveness.[33,37] Both sildenafil and vardenafil have 2C isozymes listed as secondary pathways, but no warnings exist as to drug interactions with important 2C inhibitor drugs for either one of these drugs [38-41].

In addition to hepatic elimination, the PDE inhibitors also have sufficient renal elimination such that dose reductions are recommended for patients with creatinine clearances between 30 and 50 ml/min and below, depending on the drug [39-41].

Table 2. PDE5 Inhibitor Comparison of Side Effects, Drug Interactions

Parameter	Sildenafil(Viagra)	Vardenafil(Levitra)	Tadalafil(Cialis)
Side Effects	Headache, flushing, dyspepsia, nasal congestion, abnormal vision, priapism	Headache, flushing, dyspepsia, rhinitis, abnormal color vision, priapism	Headache, flushing, nasal congestion, dyspepsia, back pain, myalgia 12-24hr after dose, rare color vision changes, priapism
Collateral PDE Family Inhibition	PDE 6, PDE 1c	PDE 6	PDE 11
Precautions/ Contraindications	Hypersensitivity; concurrent use of nitrates; not for use in children	Hypersensitivity; concurrent use of nitrates; not for use in children	Hypersensitivity; concurrent use of nitrates; not for use in children
Drug Interactions	Non-specific interactions w/ strong CYP3A4 inhibitors (e.g., ritonavir, indinavir, ketoconazole, itraconazole) & moderate CYP3A4 inhibitors (e.g., erythromycin); increased plasma levels w/ CYP450 inhibitor cimetidine; potential hypotension w/ nitrates and α-adrenergic blockers	Increased plasma levels w/ strong CYP3A4 inhibitors (e.g., ritonavir, indinavir, ketoconazole, itraconazole); potential hypotension w/ nitrates and α-adrenergic blockers	Increased plasma levels w/ strong CYP3A4 inhibitors (e.g., ritonavir, indinavir, ketoconazole, itraconazole); potential hypotension w/ nitrates and α-adrenergic blockers
Additional Information	None	May prolong QT interval	Nitrates given no sooner than 48hr after dose; substantial consumption of EtOH increases orthostatic hypotension; no BP drop w/ tamsulosin

For example, in the case of tadalafil's active catechol metabolite, its half-life increases from 36 hours in healthy individuals to 54-77 hours in patients with end stage renal disease [37].

In terms of systemic oral absorption, bioavailability tends to be low for the PDEIs, at 40, 36, and 15% for sildenafil, tadalafil, and vardenafil, respectively [37]. In the case of at least sildenafil, the low systemic bioavailability is attributed to a high first pass effect [37]. All three agents bypass absorption in the stomach, and are rapidly absorbed in the small intestine. Thus, delays in drug onset can result from conditions or activities that delay gastric emptying [32]. The absorption of both sildenafil and vardenafil are slowed by high fat meals, such that the time to peak is increased and maximum drug concentration in the serum is decreased, but the AUC is apparently not changed [33]. Tadalafil's absorption is not affected significantly by food consumption, but the concomitant use of antacids may reduce its absorption [38-41].

All three agents are highly lipophilic and highly protein bound at approximately 95% [32,38-41]. High protein binding may limit the dialyzability of PDEIs, as reported with sildenafil [39].

Clinical Efficacy for ED: Sildenafil, the prototype PDEI, appears to be effective in about 50-80% of men with ED. Response rates in men with primarily psychogenic disease is reported to be as high as 84% compared to 68% in those thought to have primarily organic disease [33]. Response rates to sildenafil appear to be slightly lower (about 59%) in men who have diabetes mellitus, and even lower (around 31%) in those who have undergone radical retropubic prostectomy, especially when the local nerve fibers were not spared. In patients with ED secondary to radiotherapy, response rates to sildenafil have been around 70% [36].

Nitric oxide deficiency has been identified as one of the underlying causes of ED.[32] PDEIs have been less effective in various disease states associated with deficiencies in neuronal or endothelial nitric oxide synthetase, leading to low local levels of NO. As previously discussed in the "Mechanism of Action" section earlier in this text, both stimulation of cGMP production from endogenous NO and inhibition of cGMP breakdown from PDEIs are important features in inducing cGMP mediated vasodilation in the corpus cavernosum and surrounding tissues. The presence of endogenous nitric acid is necessary for PDEIs to work effectively, and men with underlying organic disorders appear to be relatively deficient in endogenous NO production and/or secretion [36].

There is a paucity of head-to-head clinical trials comparing response rates to sildenafil with that of the two newer agents, vardenafil and tadafadil. Despite differences in terms of pharmacokinetics, the clinical efficacy for treating ED appears to be comparable between the three agents [31,32,36]. Response rates of 80% have been reported with vardenafil [36,42]. One study with tadalafil showed an 81% improvement rate compared to 17% in the placebo group [43].

Tolerability and Side Effects: Table 2 provides a summary of the various side effects reported with each of the three agents. The preponderance of side effects attributed to the PDEIs are usually related to either their PDE5-mediated vasodilatory effects or "collateral damage" from affected PDE enzymes outside of the PDE5 isozyme.

Headache, a classic vasodilator-related effect, is the most common side effect reported with all three PDE inhibitors (11-16%) [39-41]. Other side effects include flushing, reported in 11% of patients on vardenafil, 4-14% on sildenafil, and only 2-3% with tadalafil. Direct comparison data are lacking, however. It is possible that the longer half-life and more gradual time-to-peak effect of tadalafil might somewhat ameliorate the flushing. Nasal congestion has been reported with sildenafil (4%) as well as vardenafil (3-9%) and tadalafil (2-3%); and dizziness may occur with all three agents (around 2%) [39-41].

Gastrointesinal (GI) side effects including indigestion and diarrhea have been reported with all three PDEIs, with an incidence of around 4% [39-41]. The "dyspeptic" GI side effects are of interest, because they are though to be primarily due to relaxation of the lower esophageal sphincter muscle. In other words, PDEIs may cause or potentiate gastroesphageal reflux disease (GERD), a malady that already afflicts a large percentage of the male population taking these medications [33]. In one study with sildenafil that used a direct question and answer design to assess each side effect associated with the medication, patient response to "heartburn" was positive 10.5% of the time. When side effects are specifically elicited in this manner, the reported numbers are generally higher than open-end volunteering of complaints. For instance, in the same study using self-referred males in a university-based practice, all side effects, including flushing (30.8%), headache (25.4%), nasal congestion (18.7%), and visual changes (5.8%) were higher than the rates reported in clinical trials [33,44].

For reasons related to the aforementioned collateral PDEI inhibition of PDE6 which subsequently leads to an effect on retinal transduction, visual changes have been reported with all three agents [39-41]. However, the incidence has been lowest with tadalafil, probably because, unlike sidenafil and vardenafil, tadalafil has very little affinity for PDE 6 receptors [32]. While the visual changes are often mild and transient, PDEIs have been associated with non-arteritic anterior ischemic optic neuropathies (NAAION) with attendant permanent vision loss [45]. More study is currently underway to gain a better understanding of the relationship between PDEIs and ophthalmologic side effects.

A recently identified side effect of PDEIs is sudden hearing loss [46]. In some incidences, the loss was associated with vestibular symptoms such as tinnitus, vertigo, and dizziness. In almost all cases, the malady was unilateral. The hearing loss reported was temporary in about 1/3 of those affected, with uncertainty regarding the duration to resolution [46]. As with the ophthalmologic side effects, more study is currently underway to better characterize the relationship between PDEI use and hearing loss.

As previously mentioned, tadalafil selectively inhibits PDE-11. This has been concerning because high levels of PDE-11 are present in cardiac myocytes, pituitary gland, and the testes. Consequently, the possibility of adversely affecting cardiac function as well as reproductive and sexual-hormone axes cannot be dismissed. However, no data from clinical trials has suggested that tadalafil causes an increased risk of cardiac toxicity, and the clinical ramifications of PDE-11 inhibition are not clear at this time [32,47,48].

Contraindications and Warnings: All three agents are contraindicated if there is a known hypersensitivity. There is no indication for the use of PDEIs in children. The vasodilating effects of PDEIs may result in a small drop in arterial pressure. In healthy individuals this is rarely a problem, but in patients with cardiovascular disease who have low blood pressure at baseline, this could be concerning. PDEIs potentiate the hypotensive effects of organic nitrates. If used concurrently, the result may be a synergistic drop in blood pressure leading to profound hypotension. To avoid the possibility of prolonged hypotension, nitrates should be held for at least 24 hours before a PDE inhibitor can be given [32]. Further, nitrates should not be given within 24 hours of sildenafil or vardenafil, and 48 hours after tadalafil [32,39-41]. There is also a precaution for PDEI use with α-adrenergic blockers. It is well known that α-adrenergic blockers can cause orthostatic hypotension; consequently PDEIs can potentiate the hypotention [49-50]. The drug labeling for tadalafil, however, allows for concomitant use of the α-adrenergic blocker, tamsulosin, upto a dose of 0.4 mg once daily [41]. Despite contraindications and warnings, the concomitant use of PDEIs with various antihypertensive drugs has been reported to be reasonably safe [33,39,41].

An additional warning on the package label that is unique to vardenifil states: "Patients with congenital QT prolongation and those taking Class 1A (quinidine, procainamide) or Class III (amiodarone, sotalol) antiarrhythmics should avoid using Levitra." [40]. Unlike vardenafil, tadalafil and sildenafil do not carry this warning [39,41]. Although there have been no documented cases of Torsades de Pointes, small increases in QTc were observed in one study with vardenafil [50]. In a premarketing study of 59 healthy males, vardenafil 10mg resulted in mean QT corrected change of 4 msec. Consequently, vardenafil should be avoided in patients with congenital QT prolongation and patients taking class IA or class III antiarrythmic medications [40]. At recommended therapeutic doses, sildenafil has not shown significant electrophysiologic effects on the myocardium [39].

Drug Interactions: As previously mentioned, all three PDEIs are hepatically removed as cytochrome 3A4 (CYP 3A4) substrates [39-41]. Therefore, warnings exist for the use and the dosing of PDEIs in patients taking a plethora of agents known to be potent CYP 3A4 inhibitors (Table 2). Studies have shown that drugs such as ketoconazole, erythromycin, and sequinavir significantly increase the plasma levels of PDE inhibitor agents. In the case of sildenafil, these drugs increase the area under the curve (AUC) without affecting the half-life, which points to an inhibition of first pass metabolism leading to increased bioavailability. In one study with tadalafil, therapeutic doses of ketoconazole increased the tadafadil AUC by 4.1 fold, while increasing the peak plasma concentration slightly by 1.2-fold. Thus, PDEI potentiation by 3A4 inhibitors can result from either increased PDEI bioavailability, reduced PDEI elimination, or a combination of both mechanisms [33,37]. Conversely, drugs that induce the CYP 3A4 system can reduce the effectiveness of PDEIs. Bosentan, a potent CYP 3A4 inducer, reduces plasma sildenafil levels by about 50% when used concomitantly with sildenafil [37].

Both sildenafil and vardenafil have 2C isozymes listed as secondary pathways, but no warnings exist as to drug interactions with important 2C inhibitor drugs. More research is needed to better characterize the possibility of PDEI potentiation through medications known to inhibit the 2C9 and 2C19 pathways.

Use of PDEIs in Patients with CVD Heart Failure

Lack of exercise tolerance, a prevailing symptom of heart failure (HF), has been identified as a major predictor of patient prognosis [51,52]. Several studies have shown that PDEIs improve exercise capacity in patients with HF [53-55]. The benefits may be attributable to multiple mechanisms, including the alleviation of pulmonary hypertension and improvement of vascular endothelial function. Pulmonary hypertension, secondarily identified in 68-78% of patients with severe left ventricular systolic dysfunction, is often associated with concomitant right ventricular dysfunction [54]. In chronic left ventricular dysfunction, dysregulation of vascular smooth muscle tone frequently results in an elevation of pulmonary vascular resistance (PVR). Not surprisingly, PVR and right ventricular function are major predictors of both exercise tolerance and global prognosis in HF populations [54].

In one study, Lewis and colleagues[56] investigated the acute effects of a single 50 mg dose of sildenafil on cardiopulmonary exercise parameters and hemodynamic effects in 13 patients with stable New York Heart Association Class III HF. One hour after sildenafil administration, pulmonary arterial pressure was reduced by 14%; systemic and pulmonary vascular resistance was reduced by 19% and 21%, respectively. Resting and exercise cardiac index were increased by 20% and 12%, respectively ($p < 0.05$ for all parameters). However, there was no significant change in terms of arterial pressure, heart rate, or pulmonary capillary wedge pressure.

The same authors investigated the chronic effects of PDEIs [54]. Thirty-four patients with symptomatic HF and pulmonary hypertension received 12 weeks of treatment with sildenafil at doses of 25 to 75mg given orally three times daily. Again, at peak exercise, sildenafil significantly decreased pulmonary vascular resistance (PVR) by 23% (p=0.008) and increased cardiac output (CO) by 38%(p=0.004). Conversely, there was no effect on pulmonary capillary wedge pressure (PCWP), heart rate, arterial pressure, or systemic vascular reisistance(SVR) with longer term use. Commensurate with these findings, a four week study with sildenafil 50 mg given orally three times daily, conducted by Behling, [55] and a 6 month study using a 50mg twice daily regimen, conducted by Guazzi, [53] found significantly decreased systolic pulmonary artery pressure from baseline (p=0.004 for Behling, p <0.01 for Guazzi).

Patients with left ventricular assist devices (LVADs) have also benefited from sildenafil's ability to reduce pulmonary artery and systemic arterial pressures. The findings from a retrospective review of 10 consecutive LVAD patients concluded that sildenfil decreased pulmonary artery pressure and facilitated weaning from inhaled nitric oxide and inotropes without causing adverse hemodynamic effects [57].

PDEIs are also thought to improve endothelial dysfunction, a hallmark of hemostasis-gone-wrong in HF patients. The endothelium is involved in a number of physiologic processes, including growth of smooth muscle cells, regulation of vascular tone and permeability, and maintenance of the balance between coagulation and fibrinolysis. The development of endothelial dysfunction in HF is related to increased SVR and other adversely altered pulmonary hemodynamics [55]. Disruption in endothelial function causes reduced vascular nitric oxide release, impairs skeletal blood flow during exercise, and is associated with decreased functional capacity [58,59].

Katz and colleagues [60] investigated the possibility that PDE5 inhibition could have beneficial effects on endothelial function in HF patients. Using brachial artery ultrasound imaging to measure flow-mediated, endothelium-dependent vasodilation in response to transient arterial occlusion, the investigators found that, compared to placebo, the administration of sildenafil 25 and 50 mg resulted in a significant increase in brachial artery diameter after the release of 1, 3 and 5 min occlusions ($p < 0.05$). A study by Hryniewicz and colleagues[61] also utilized brachial artery ultrasound imaging and found that the concomitant doses of sildenafil and ACE-inhibitor ramipril had additive effects on brachial artery diameter at four hours after co-administration in HF patients.

The chronic effects of PDE5 inhibition on endothelial dysfunction have also been studied. In a four week trial, Behling and associates [55] assigned 11 patients to receive sildenafil 50 mg three times daily added to their current heart failure regimens. Patients in the placebo group showed a trend toward decreased forearm blood flow (FBF) (30% reduction, P = 0.07) after reactive hyperemia, while patients receiving the sildenafil regimen did not demonstrate any significant changes in FBF after reactive hyperemia from baseline. The investigators were unable to definitively state that there had been an improvement in endothelial function.

Guazzi and colleagues [53] found that HF patients receiving the same regimen for six months, again in addition to their current heart failure regimens, experienced significant increases in brachial artery flow-mediated dilatation (FMD) at 3 and 6 months compared to baseline (13.4% and 14.2% respectively, $P < 0.01$ for both). The findings suggest that chronic sildenafil administration is associated with improved long term endothelial function. Since there is thought to be a link between endothelial function and ergoreflex activity, the authors also sought to investigate the role of sildenafil in relief of abnormal skeletal muscle signaling due to muscle metabolic byproducts, a phenomenon known as ergoreflex. The study found that the ergoreflex effect on ventilation decreased significantly from baseline after 3 and 6 months of sildenafil treatment (67 and 72% respectively, $P < 0.01$ for both) suggesting that PDE5 inhibitors may have endothelium-mediated effects on muscle over-signaling that results in undesirable vasoconstriction [53].

Regardless of the underlying mechanism, patients with HF treated chronically with sildenafil have shown increased exercise capacity and improvement in quality of life [54]. Clinical trials have shown a significant increase in peak oxygen uptake, ventilator efficiency, Minnesota Living with Heart Failure Score, and fewer hospitalizations for HF [53-55]. However, there is reason for caution. For example, in patients with predominant right ventricular heart failure, cardiac output increases with sildenafil, suggesting that the drug has an inotropic effect [62]. Nagendran and colleagues [63] found that although PDE5 is not normally present in the right ventricular myocardium, in patients with a hypertrophied right ventricular myocardium, it is present [63]. If PDE5 is also present in diseased, hypertrophied left ventricular tissue, there is concern about the safety of long-term administration of PDEIs in patients with systolic heart failure. Indeed, the long-term use of milrinone, an inotropic PDE3 inhibitor, was found to increase morbidity and mortality in patients with severe chronic heart failure, and this could be a caveat regarding the use of PDEIs in this population [64,65].

HYPERTENSION

PDEIs produce mild systemic vasodilator effects without causing sympathomimetic-mediated increases in heart rate. Thus, they have the potential to lower blood pressure (BP) without inducing an increase in cardiac oxygen demand [66]. This desirable pharmacologic profile presents the opportunity for a new class of antihypertensive drugs. However, the acute effects of currently studied PDEIs, at least in terms of decreasing blood pressure, have thus far appeared relatively modest.

In a single-blind, four-way crossover trial by Jackson and colleagues, [67] eight healthy men aged 18-45 years received single doses of 100, 150, and 200 mg of sildenafil. BP was monitored at -1, 1, 3, 6, 9, and 12 hours after sildenafil administration. The result was a mean maximum reduction of 10 mm Hg systolic and 7 mm Hg diastolic BP. The BP reduction reached a peak at 3 hours post administration, and returned to baseline for most subjects 6 hours post-dose. In another study involving healthy volunteers receiving tadalafil 10 or 20 mg daily for 10 days, the drug did not significantly reduce systolic BP or have much of an effect on other BP parameters, but it did reduce diastolic pressure in the standing position by about 5 mm Hg compared to placebo by day 10 of therapy ($p < 0.05$) [68].

A study of the chronic effects of PDEIs on BP was conducted by Oliver and colleagues [69]. In a randomized, double-blind, two-way crossover study, 22 previously untreated hypertensive patients received either sildenafil 50 mg three times daily or placebo for 16 days. Both clinic and ambulatory BPs were measured. In the clinic, BPs decreased 5/4 mm Hg from baseline, similar to responses observed with other antihypertensive medications given as monotherapy. Meanwhile, ambulatory daytime BPs were reduced 8 /6 mm Hg, and nighttime pressures were reduced 5/4 mm Hg, compared to baseline ($p < 0.05$ for both parameters). Although sildenafil treatment decreased 24-hour, daytime, and nighttime pressures significantly, the magnitude of the BP-lowering effect was lower at nighttime. The findings suggest that the overnight dosing interval may be too long. This is an important observation because early morning surges in blood pressure are associated with increased cardiovascular morbidity and mortality, due in part to resultant silent ischemic events and cerebrovascular infarcts. Finally, patients with substantially elevated systolic BPs at baseline had greater decreases in BP than those with lower baseline BP, suggesting that sildenafil may be more useful in treating patients with more severe hypertension than those with milder disease [70,71].

In the aforementioned study, Oliver and colleagues [69] also investigated mechanisms other than systemic vasodilation through which PDEIs may exert beneficial effects in hypertension. By measuring carotid-femoral pulse wave velocity (CF-PWV), the authors assessed sildenafil's effects on arterial stiffness. They found no significant changes from baseline. However, there was a trend toward progressive reductions in CF-PWV, suggesting that sildenafil reduced arterial stiffness. The same authors also assessed sildenafil's effect on endothelial function through flow-mediated vasodilation (FMD) and did not find any significant changes in this parameter after 16 days. This study indicated that, contrary to findings reported in healthy and chronic heart failure subjects, sildenafil did not improve endothelial dysfunction in this particular venue. The authors hypothesized that hypertensive patients, unlike non-hypertensive patients, may rely on a vasodilatory pathway other than that involving nitric oxide. However, FMD is not significantly improved with a variety of other BP-lowering drugs, so sildenafil's potential as an antihypertensive drug should not be dismissed simply based upon this observation [69].

Interestingly, PDEIs may be useful as antihypertensive agents due to psychological as well as physiological effects. A retrospective cohort study by Scranton and colleagues found that treating ED with PDEIs for two years in 3,384 hypertensive men had a beneficial effect on BP [72]. Consistent with Oliver's aforementioned speculation, men with BP $\geq$ 160 mm Hg experienced the greatest BP reduction, with a mean decrease in systolic pressure of 17.8 mm Hg from baseline in the two year interval. The authors concluded that the beneficial benefits of starting a PDEI inhibitor therapy are likely multifactorial. For one, the benefits appear to be related to the intensification of an antihypertensive regimen, which involves an increase in the frequency of BP monitoring after a PDEI is prescribed [72]. Other theories are that patients are more likely to embark in more measures of good self-care, such as losing weight and exercising, when sexual activity is restored [73].

It has been observed that PDEIs have an additive effect with other BP-lowering medications. Webb and colleagues [74] reported that sildenafil, when administered to hypertensive patients taking amlodipine for one month, appreciated a modest maximal reduction of 8/7 and 10/8 mm Hg in sitting and standing BP, respectively. On the other hand a study by Zusman et al. [75] concluded that the additive effects of sildenafil, in combination with beta-blockers, diuretics, and ACE-inhibitors, was smaller than the effects found with amlodipine, and that the BP-lowering changes were unlikely to be clinically significant.

PDEIs have potential in treating patients with essential hypertension. However, further studies are needed. For example, an extended-release version of sildenafil, or the use of one of the longer acting drugs in its class, may result in a less fluctuant steady-state plasma concentration profile. The less fluctuant concentration-time curves would, of course, ameliorate or even eradicate nighttime or early morning decreases in BP-lowering [69].

PULMONARY HYPERTENSION

The previous section on PDEIs in HF addressed many studies that looked at the use of these agents in treating pulmonary hypertension (PH) secondary to HF. Outside of this disease state, the majority of studies with PDEIs have involved patients with idiopathic PH, or PH associated with connective tissue diseases.

The empiric use of PDEIs for PH seems to be logical. As discussed earlier, sildenafil, unlike vardenafil or tadalafil, shows a relatively high affinity for PDE 1c, a subtype PDE enzyme found in high concentrations in lung tissue [37]. Sildenafil has long been known to reduce pulmonary vascular resistance in a dose-dependent manner. In fact, the vasodilator effects appeared to be greater in the pulmonary circulation than in any other vascular bed within the human body. In addition, sildenafil has typically shown synergy with other commonly used agents, such as the inhaled prostacyclin analogue, iloprost. Sildenafil augmented and prolonged the therapeutic effect of iloprost [37]

In one study, all three PDEIs were assessed and compared for their hemodynamic influences over a two hour period in 60 consecutive PAH patients. All three agents induced significant pulmonary vasodilation, with peak effects occurring at 40-45 minutes for vardenafil, 60 minutes for sildenafil, and 75-90 minutes for tadalafil. Sildenafil and tadalafil caused a significant reduction in pulmonary SVR, whereas vardenafil did not. Significant improvement in arterial oxygenation only occurred with sildenafil. Thus, it is important to note that the three agents differ in terms of their pharmacokinetic properties, their selectivity for the pulmonary vascular beds, and their impact on arterial oxygenation. Of the three PDEIs, sidenafil exhibited the most desirable hemodynamic profile in this study [76].

In terms of chronic management, several small single center studies have reported beneficial effects of sildenafil for the long term treatment of PH [37]. However, the sentinel study that catapulted sildenafil into its new FDA indication was the SUPER-1 study [77]. This study involved 278 patients with symptomatic PH who were treated with either placebo or sildenafil at 20, 40, or 80 mg three times daily for 12 weeks. The primary endpoint was measurement of hemodynamic changes and total walking distance after a 6 minute walk distance test. The test was performed at baseline and at 12 weeks into treatment. All three sildenafil doses improved exercise capacity ($p < 0.001$ for all three doses) and WHO functional class rankings ($p=0.003$ for 20 mg, $p< 0.001$ for 40 and 80mg doses), as well as various hemodynamic markers, including mean arterial pulmonary pressure ($p=0.04$ for 20mg, $p=0.01$ for 40mg, and $p< 0.01$ for 80mg) over the placebo arm. However, despite apparent trends towards a dose-response relationship, there were no statistical differences found between the three dose regimens. In addition, the increase in the 6 minute walk distance achieved in the placebo controlled trial phase was sustained for up to 3 months when these patients were maintained on open label drug at the 80mg dose.

Because the dose-response curve appeared statistically flat in the SUPER-1 trial, the FDA decision was to license the drug at a fixed dose of 20mg administered three times daily. However, this single dose labeling has created a conundrum for clinicians treating PH with sidenafil [37]. If used with the known sildenafil inducer bosentan, the sildenafil dose is ostensibly only equivalent to about half, or 10mg three times daily, due to the metabolic induction elicited by bosentan [78,79]. Also, many clinicians feel that over time, as the disease progresses, larger doses may be needed. At least in one aspect, the Super-1 study supported a dose-response relationship, where 80mg given three times daily had a greater effect on PVR than did the lower doses [79].

Combination therapy with sildenafil has been studied, but currently there are only unblinded trials. Despite the aforementioned pharmacokinetic interaction, sildenafil with the endothelin-receptor antagonist bosentan has been found to arrest clinical deterioration [78,79]. Combination therapy with sildenafil and sitaxentan or ambrisentan, two newer endothelin receptor antagonists not known to be CYP-inducers, lacks the pharmacokinetic interaction, but pharmacodynamic data is currently lacking.[37] Finally, beneficial short and long term effects have been observed when sildenafil was combined with inhaled ilopros [80,81].

Sildenafil has also been effective in treating PH associated with HIV, [82,83] PH related to high altitude exposure, [84] PH in patients with non-operable chronic thromboembolism [85,86] and hypoxia-associated PH [87]. If sildenafil can improve parameters for hypoxia-associated PH, it may provide a modicum of hope for patients suffering from COPD, interstitial lung disease, and obstructive sleep apnea [37,88].

Continued interest in studying PDEIs for various types of PH prevails. For one, these agents are the only ones available that reduce PVR without compromising V'/Q'matching and subsequent oxygenation, which makes them more desirable in the treatment of patients who already have underlying lung disease. Secondly, these drugs may help improve right ventricular function by inhibiting PDE 5 found in the cardiac tissues of patients with right ventricular hypertrophy. The local PDE 5 inhibiting effect would enhance contractility and bolster CO, favorably changing two parameters that have already been linked to better outcomes in determining patient prognosis in those who have clinically succumbed to the adverse effects of PH [37].

DIABETES

ED and diabetes mellitus share many risk factors such as endothelial dysfunction, autonomic neuropathy, and vascular and hormonal abnormalities. Using a national managed care claims database Sun et al. [89] conducted a retrospective study to compare the prevalence rates of diabetes between men with ED (285,436) and men without ED (1,584,230). The findings showed that men with ED were more than twice as likely to have diabetes as men without ED (20.0% vs 7.5%). After adjusting for age and concurrent diseases, men with ED were still more likely to have diabetes than men without ED (odds ratio 1.60, $p < 0.001$). In the Massachusetts Male Aging Study (MMAS), [1] the prevalence of any degree of ED in diabetic men aged 40 to 70 years was estimated to be around 52%, and men with diabetes were three to four times more likely to have ED compared with those without diabetes.

ED may predate the clinical diagnosis of type 2 diabetes by years, and in fact, may be the first symptom of yet undiagnosed diabetes [90]. The United Kingdom Prevention of Diabetes Study (UKPDS) revealed that 20% of patients had ED at the time their diabetes was diagnosed [91]. Based on these findings, it has been suggested that ED can be used as an early, observable marker to detect diabetes earlier.

In men with silent ischemia and angiographic evidence of CHD, Gazzaruso et al. [92] reported that ED was significantly more prevalent than in men without silent ischemia (33.8% vs. 4.75, p=0.001). In fact, after adjustment for confounding variables, ED appeared to be the most efficient independent predictor of silent CAD. This suggests that ED in patients with diabetes can provide a rationale for screening for silent coronary artery disease.

The etiology of ED in the setting of diabetes is often complex and related to poor glycemic control, dyslipidemia, microvascular and macrovascular disease, autonomic neuropathy, and endothelial dysfunction. ED is often related to the duration and severity of diabetes and correlates with glycemic control [93]. It has been demonstrated that controlling blood sugar levels does improve erectile function [93].

Treatment with PDEIs is now considered first-line therapy because of convenience, effectiveness, and generally good tolerance to the drugs. Sildenafil, vardenafil, and tadalafil have not been directly compared in a head-to-head trial, but all three drugs significantly improve erectile function in patients with diabetes and ED.

In a 16-week randomized, double-blind, placebo-controlled, and fixed-dose study, 282 men (mean age, 46.4 years) with ED (mean duration, 3.6 years) and diabetes (mean duration, 11 years) were randomly assigned to receive 100 mg sildenafil or placebo approximately 1 hour before planned sexual activity [94]. The efficacy of the two treatments was assessed using responses to the International Index of Erectile Function (IIEF) questionnaire [95]. Positive clinical results were obtained in 68 (51%) of 134 patients in the sildenafil group compared with 14 (11%) of 128 patients in the placebo group ($p<0.003$). Boulton et al. [96] in a 12-week double blind, placebo-controlled randomized clinical trial, evaluated the effectiveness of sildenafil in 219 men with ED and type 2 diabetes. Primary criteria for efficacy included questions 3 (achieving an erection) and 4 (maintaining an erection) from the International Index of Erectile Function (IIEF, score range, 0-5). After 12 weeks, the mean scores for questions 3 and 4 had improved significantly in patients receiving sildenafil compared with placebo ($p < 0.0001$). In this study sildenafil was well tolerated and improved ED in men with type 2 diabetes independent of the degree of glycemic control or the presence of neuropathic and vascular complications. In a similar study, Rendel et al. [97] randomized 268 diabetic men with ED to receive either sildenafil or placebo for 12 weeks. In the sildenafil arm, 56% of the patients reported improved erections, compared to 10% in the placebo group ($p< 0.001$). A meta-analysis of 11 randomized, double-blind, placebo-controlled trials of sildenafil in patients with diabetes reported improved erections in 59% of patients with type 1 diabetes and 63% with type 2 diabetes [98]. Improvement has been noted regardless of age, race, severity and duration of ED [99]. However, the response rate in men with diabetes was less than the 83% improvement observed in men with ED who did not have diabetes. Randomized trials have also documented the effectiveness of tadalafil [100, 101] and vardenafil [42] in men with diabetes and ED. A multicenter, double-blind, placebo-controlled study assessed the effectiveness of tadalafil (10 or 20 mg) in 216 men with diabetes and severe ED.[100] Improved erectile function was reported in 22.2% and 22.6% of men receiving 10 and 20 mg respectively of tadalafil as compared with a decline of 4.1% for those patients receiving placebo.

Studies comparing response rates to PDEIs in diabetic versus non-diabetic men with ED have reported variable findings. In a multi-center study of 1,511 patients with ED, the response rates to sildenafil was lower for patients with diabetes (77.9%), as compared to those without diabetes (86.5%) ($p<0.01$). [102]. Patients with diabetes also required a higher dose of sildenafil as compared to those without diabetes. In another study with tadalafil, 76% of men with diabetes had improved erections, although only 58% of those receiving tadalafil (20 mg) reported erections sufficient for satisfactory intercourse [101]. In men without diabetes, the comparable rates were 81% and 75%, respectively. Similar findings have been observed with verdenafil [42]. The poorer efficacy of PDEIs in the diabetic population is thought to be related to poor vascular supply to the penile arteries resulting from macrovascular disease, [103] reduced production of nitric oxide as a result of advanced glycosylation product accumulation, [104] and impaired neurogenic and endothelium-dependent relaxation in penile arteries [105]. Many men with diabetes have subclinical neuropathy that may decrease the effectiveness of PDEIs.

Coronary Artery Disease

The relationship between CV disease and ED is well documented. In one study, 49% of patients who had acute chest pain and had angiographically documented CAD also had ED. [27]. Others have demonstrated a correlation between ED, the number of affected coronary vessels, and the severity of ischemic coronary disease. Recent findings from clinical trials suggest that ED may be an early marker of atherosclerosis, subclinical or undiagnosed CVD, and systemic vascular disease. The presence and recognition of ED, therefore provides a clinical tool to identify men at an early stage prior to the development of atherosclerosis or an adverse vascular event.

The PDEIs have been shown to be effective in men with known coronary artery disease [106,107]. Conti et al. [108] showed that sildenafil improved erections in 70% of men with known coronary artery disease compared with 20% in patients who received placebo. A recent analysis by DeBusk et al. [106] confirmed these results. Patients with ED and clinically stable coronary artery disease were randomized to sildenafil or placebo for 12 weeks. By 12 weeks, patients receiving sildenafil had significantly better improvements on question 3 and 4 of the International Index of Erectile Function than did patients receiving placebo ($n=72$; $p < 0.01$). Patients taking sildenafil were more likely to report improved erections (64%) and improved intercourse (65%) vs patients receiving placebo (21% and 19%).

Sildenafil, vardenafil, and tadalafil have not been associated with serious adverse cardiovascular events. Results from clinical trials do not indicate an increase in cardiac ischemia, MI, or mortality in patients taking PDEIs. [106-108]. It has been shown that when given to patients with stable CAD during exercise stress testing, PDEIs do not exacerbate ischemia compared with placebo [109, 110].

In a double-blind placebo-controlled crossover study of 105 men at high risk for CAD, the effects of sildenafil 50 mg and 100 mg were compared with placebo, using exercise echocardiography [109]. The findings showed no adverse effects on the left ventricular wall motion score with a similar hemodynamic response regarding heart rate, blood pressure, and exercise capacity. Fox et al. [111] tested sildenafil 100 mg in a study that included 108 men with stable angina. The primary end point was time to limiting angina, and secondary end points included time to angina, time to ST-segment depression, and exercise duration. All patients had ischemia at baseline and underwent exertion on a treadmill 1 hour after receiving sildenafil or placebo. In this study, sildenafil increased primary and secondary end points ($p<0.05$) and was generally well tolerated.

Mittleman et al. [112] pooled data from 124 double-blind clinical trials involving 5054 placebo-treated and 6896 sildenafil-treated patients and found that the overall incidence of MI and CV death were low and comparable between sildenafil and placebo treatments, $p = 0.801$. Studies that have extensively evaluated the use of tadalafil in patients with CVD have shown a similar safety profile compared to sildenafil with no adverse effects on cardiac function or ischemic threshold [49,113]. Because safety has not been established in patients with recent serious CV events, the use of PDEIs is not recommended in patients with unstable CAD, a recent history of MI and stroke (in the past 6 to 8 weeks or earlier), moderate to severe HF, cardiomyopathy and severe valvular heart disease.

The vasodilating effects of PDE inhibitors can be concerning, particularly in patients with CV disease, left ventricular outflow obstruction or aortic stenosis [114,115]. In the setting of angina, alternatives to nitrates should be considered after PDE inhibitor therapy. If a patient has taken sildenafil or vardenafil (half-life of 4 hours) and then develops angina, the recommendation from the American College of Cardiology/American Heart Association Consensus Committee is to withhold nitrates for 24 hours [114]. However, if a patient takes tadalafil (half-life of 17.5 hours) and then has angina, nitrates should be withheld for about 48 hours [115]. During the period of time in which nitrates should not be administered, other antianginal and anti-ischemic drugs may be used such as beta-blockers, calcium-channel blockers, aspirin, and others. Although nitrates are antianginal agents, they have not been shown to reduce adverse CV events or reduce cardiac mortality in the setting of an acute coronary syndrome.

Conclusion

ED is now considered both an early manifestation and an independent predictor of cardiovascular disease. In men presenting with ED, cardiovascular risk factors should be evaluated and managed in order to prevent future cardiac events. PDEIs provide a promising clinical therapeutic modality for improving not only the symptoms of ED, but also treating the underlying endothelial dysfunction that initially caused the ED. The PDEIs are now established as first- line therapy in the treatment for ED. All three agents appear equally effective in treating ED, but some differences in pharmacokinetics may drive physician and patient preferences towards one specific agent. Overall, PDEIs are well tolerated, and have been found safe in a wide array of patients, including those with comorbidities such as diabetes, hypertension, coronary artery disease, and heart failure.

References

[1] Feldman HA, Goldstein I, Hatzichristou DG, et al. Impotence and it medical psychosocial correlates: results of the Massachusetts Male Aging Study. *J. Urol.* 1994;151:54-61.

[2] KL, Bank AJ, Padma-Nathan H, et al. Erectile dysfunction is a marker for cardiovascular disease: results of the Minority Health Institute expert advisory panel. *J. Sex med* 2005;2:40-52.

[3] Speel TG, van Langen H, Meuleman EJ. The risk of coronary heart disease in men with erectile dysfunction. *Eur. Urol.* 2003;44:366-370.

[4] Jensen J, Lendorf A, Stimpel H et al. The prevalence and etiology of impotence in 101 male hypertensive outpatients. *Am. J. hypertens* 1999;12:271-275.

[5] Wei M, Macera CA, Davis DR et al. Total cholesterol and high density lipoprotein cholesterol as important predictors of erectile dysfunction. *Am. J. Epidemiol* 1994;140:930-937.

[6] Roumeguere T, Wespes E, Carpentier Y et al. Erectile dysfunction is associated with a high prevalence of hyperlipidemia and coronary heart disease risk. *Eur. Urol.* 2003;44:355-359.

[7] Bacon CG, Hu FB, Biovannucci E et al. Association of type and duration of diabetes with erectile dysfunction in a large cohort of men. *Diabetes Care* 2002;25:1458-63.

[8] Moulik PK, Hardy KJ. Hypertension, antihypertensive drug therapy and erectile dysfunction in diabetes. *Diabet Med* 2003;20:290-293.

[9] Rosen MP, Greenfield AJ, Walker TG et al. Cigarette smoking: an independent risk factor for atherosclerosis in the hypogastric-cavernous arterial bed of men with arteriogenic impotence. *J. Urol.* 1991;145:759-63.

[10] Fung MM, Bettencourt R, Barrett-Connor E. Heart disease risk factors predict erectile dysfunction 25 years later: the Rancho Bernardo study. *J. Am. Coll Cardiol.* 2004;43;1405-1411.

[11] Esposito K, Giugliano F, Martedi E et al. High proportions of erectile dysfunction in men with erectile dysfunction. *Diabetes Care* 2005;28:1201-1203.

[12] Solomon H, Man JW, Jackson G. Erectile dysfunction and the cardiovascular patient: endothelial dysfunction is the common denominator. *Heart* 2003;89:251-253.

[13] Virag R, Bouilly P, Frydman D. Is impotence an arterial disorder? A study of arterial risk factors in 440 impotent men. *Lancet* 1985;1:181-184.

[14] Jackson G. Erectile dysfunction and cardiovascular disease. *Int. J. Clin. Pract* 1999;53:363-368.

[15] Guay AT. ED2: erectile dysfunction = endothelial dysfunction. *Endocrinol. Metab Clin. North Am.* 2007;36:453-463.

[16] Sullivan ME, Thompson CS, Dashwood MR et al. Nitric oxide and penile erection: Is erectile dysfunction another manifestation of vascular disease? *Cardiovasc. Res.* 1999;43:658-665.

[17] Kaiser DR, Billups K, Mason C, et al. Impaired brachial artery endothelium-dependent and –independent vasodilation in men with erectile dysfunction and no other clinical cardiovascular disease. *J. Am. Coll Cardiol.* 2004;43:179-184.

[18] Tikkanen MJ, Jackson G, Tammela T, et al. Erectile dysfunction as a risk factor for coronary heart disease: implications for prevention. *Int. J. Clin. Pract* 2007;61(2):265-268.

[19] Miner M, Billups KL. Erectile dysfunction and dyslipidemia: relevance and role of phosphodiesterase type-5 inhibitors and statins. *J. Sex Med.* 2008;5:1066-1078.

[20] Kawashima S, Yokoyama M. Dysfunction of endothelial nitric oxide synthase and atherosclerosis. *Arterioscler. Thromb Vasc. Biol.* 2004;24:998-1005.

[21] Kirby M, Jackson G, Simonsen U. Endothelial dysfunction links erectile dysfunctiont to heart disease. *Int. J. Clin. Pract* 2005;59:225-229.

[22] Dhabuwala CB, Kumar A, Pierce JM. Myocardial infarction and its influence on male sexual function. *Arch. Sexual Behav.* 1986;15:499-504.

[23] Kloner RA, Mullin SH, Shook T, et al. Erectile dysfunction in the cardiac patient: how common and should we treat? *J Urol* 2003;170 (suppl):S46-S50.

[24] Blumentals WA, Gomez-Caminero A, Joo S, et al. Should erectile dysfunction be considered as a marker for acute myocardial infarction? Results from a retrospective cohort study. *Int. J. Impot. Res.* 2004;16:350-353.

[25] Thompson IM, Tangen CM, Goodman PJ, et al. Erectile dysfunction and subsequent cardiovascular disease. *JAMA* 2005;294:2996-3002.

[26] Billups KL. Erectile dysfunction as an early sign of cardiovascular disease. *Int. J. Impot. Res.* 2005;17 (suppl):S19-S24.

[27] Montorsi F, Briganti A, Salonia A et al. Erectile dysfunction prevalence, time of onset and association with risk factors in 300 consecutive patients with acute chest pain and angiographically documented coronary artery disease. *Eur. Urol.* 2003;44:360-5.

[28] Blumentals WA, Gomez-Caminero A, Joo S et al. Is erectile dysfunction predictive of peripheral vascular disease? *Aging Male* 2003;6:217-221.

[29] Pritzker MR. The penile stress tests: a window to the hearts of Man? *Circulation* 1999;100(suppl 1):350-353.

[30] Vlachopoulos C, Rokkas K, Iokeimides N, et al. Prevalence of asymptomatic coronary artery disease in men with vasculogenic erectile dysfunction: a prospective angiographic study. *Eur. Urol.* 2005;48:996-1003.

[31] Kloner RA. *Heart Disease and Erectile Dysfunction.* Humana Press Inc. Totowa, New Jersey. 2004.

[32] McCullough AR. An update on the PDE-5 inhibitors. *J. Androl.* 2003;24 (suppl):S52-S58.

[33] Salonia A, Rigatti P, Montorsi F. Sildenafil in erectile disfunction: A critical review. *Curr. Med. Res Opin* 2003;19:241-262.

[34] Jackson G. Hemodynamic and exercise effects of phosphodiesterase 5 inhibitors. *Am. J. Cardiol.* 2005; 96 (suppl): 32M- 35M.

[35] Hellstrom WJG, Kendirci M. Type 5 phosphodiesterase inhibitors: curing erectile dysfunction. *Eur. Urol.* 2006;49:942-945.

[36] Seftel AD. Challenges in oral therapy for erectile dysfunction *J. Androl* 2002;23:729-736.

[37] Wilkins MR, Wharton J, Grimminger F, Ghofrani HA. Phosphodiesterase inhibitors for the treatment of pulmonary hypertension. *Eur Respir J* 2008;32:198-209.

[38] Rakel: Textbook of Family Medicine on MD Consult, 7th Ed. Male Sexual Disorders. (2007). URL: http://www.mdconsult.com/das/book/body/93087398-3/698678431 /1481 /608.html Accessed: April 24, 2008.

[39] Sildenafil prescribing information. New York, NY:Pfizer;2007.

[40] Vardenafil prescribing information. Kenilworth, NJ:Schering-Plough;2007.

[41] Tadalafil prescribing information. Indianapolis, IN: Eli Lilly and Company; 2008.

[42] Porst H, Rosen R, Padma-Nathan H Golstein I, et al. The efficacy and tolerability of vardenafil, a new oral selective phosphodiesterasetype 5 inhibitor in patients with erectile dysfunction: the first at home clinical trial. *Int. J. Impot. Res.* 2001;13:192-199.

[43] Padma-Nathan H, McMurral JG, Pullman WE, et al. On-demand IC351(Cialis) enhances erectile function in patients with erectile dysfunction. *Int. J. Impot. Res.* 2001;13:2-9.

[44] Moreira SG, Brannigan RE, Sitz A, et al. Side effect profile of sildenafil citrate (Viagra) in clinical practice. *Urology* 2000;56:474-6.

[45] Sowka J, Neiberg L, Vollmer L. Optic atrophy after sildenafil use. *J. Am. Optometry Assoc* 2003;78:122-128.

[46] Waknine Y. Erectile dysfunction drugs linked to risk for hearing loss. Medscape Medical News 2007 http://www.medscape.com/viewarticle/564533.

[47] Baxendale RW, et al. Selectivity of sildenafil and other phosphodiesterase type 5 (PDE5) inhibitors against phosphodiesterase types 7-11. *J. Clin. Pharmacol.* 2001; 41:1015.

[48] Montorsi F, Nathan HP, McCullough A, et al. Tadalfil in the treatment of erectile dysfunction following nerve sparing radical retropubic prostectomy: a randomized, double blind placebo controlled trial. *J. Urol.* 2004;172:1036-41.

[49] Jackson G, Rosen RC, Kloner RA, et al. The second princeton consensus on sexual dysfunction and cardiac risk: new guidelines for sexual medicine. *J. Sex Med.* 2006;3:28-36.

[50] Kloner RA. Medscape: Erectile dysfunction and the cardiovascular disease connection: An update for clinicians. Accessed online: http://www.medscape.com/viewprogram /5895_pnt.

[51] De Groote P, Dagorn J, Soudan B, et al. B-type natriuretic peptide and peak exercise oxygen consumption provide independent information for risk stratification in patients with stable congestive heart failure. *J. Am. Coll Cardiol* 2004;43:584-1589.

[52] Bittner V, Weiner DH, Yusuf S. Prediction of mortality and morbidity with a 6-minute walk test in patients with left ventricular dysfunction SOLVD investigators. *JAMA* 1993;270 1702-1707.

[53] Guazzi M, Samata M, Arena R. Long-term use of sildenafil in the therapeutic management of heart failure. *J. Am. Coll Cardiol.* 2007;50:2136-2144.

[54] Lewis GD, Shah R, Shahzad K. Sildenafil improves exercise capacity and quality of life in patients with systolic heart failure and secondary pulmonary hypertension. *Circulation* 2007;116:1555-1561.

[55] Behling A, Rohde LE, Colombo FC. Effects of 5'-phosphodiesterase four-week long inhibition with sildenafil in patients with chronic heart failure: A double-blind, placebo-controlled clinical trial. *J. Cardiac Failure* 2008;14:189-196.

[56] Lewis GD, Lachmann J, Camuso J. Sildenafil improves exercise hemodynamics and oxygen uptake in patients with systolic heart failure. *Circulation* 2007;115:59-65.

[57] Klodell CT, Morey TE, Lobato ED. Effect of sildenafil on pulmonary artery pressure, systemic pressure, and nitric oxide utilization in patients with left ventricular assist devices. *Ann.* of *Thorac Surg* 2007;83: 68-71.

[58] Katz SD, Krum H, Khan T. Exercise-induced vasodilation in forearm circulation of normal subjects and patients with congestive heart failure: Role of endothelium-derived nitric oxide. *J. Am. Coll Cardiol.*1996; 28:585-590.

[59] Nakamura M, Ishikawa M, Funakoshi T, et al.. Attenuated endothelium-dependent peripheral vasodilation and clinical characteristics in patients with chronic heart failure. *Am. Heart J.* 1994;128:11641169.

[60] Katz SD, Balidemaj K, Homma S. Acute type 5 phosphodiesterase inhibition with sildenafil enhances flow-mediated vasodilation in patients with chronic heart failure. *J. Am. Coll Cardiol.* 2000;36:845-851.

[61] Hryniewicz K, Dimayuga C, Hudaihed A. Inhibition of angiotensin-converting enzyme and phosphodiesterase type 5 improves endothelial function in heart failure. *Clinical Science.* 2005;108:331-337.

[62] Michelakis E, Tymchak W, Lien D. Oral sildenafil is an effective and specific pulmonary vasodilator in patients with pulmonary arterial hypertension: Comparison with inhaled nitric oxide. *Circulation* 2002;105:2398-2403.

[63] Nagendran J, Archer SL, Soliman D. Phosphodiesterase type 5 is highly expressed in the hypertrophied human right ventricle, and acute inhibition of phosphodiesterase type 5 improves contractility. *Circulation* 2007;116:238-248.

[64] Goldsmith SR. Type 5 phosphodiesterase inhibition in heart failure: The next step. *J. Am. Coll Cardiol.* 2007;50:2136-44.

[65] Packer M, Carver JR, Rodeheffer RJ. Effect of oral milrinone on mortality in severe chronic heart failure. The PROMISE study research group. *N. Engl J. Med.* 1991;325:1468-1475.

[66] Ghiadoni L. Phosphodiesterase 5 inhibition in essential hypertension. *Current Hypertension Reports* 2008;10:52-57.

[67] Jackson G, Benjamin N, Jackson N, et al. Effects of sildenafil citrate on human hemodynamics. *Am. Cardiol.* 1999;83:13-19.

[68] Kloner RA, Mitchell M, Emmick JT. Cardiovascular effects of tadalafil. *Am. J. Cardiol.* 2003;92 (suppl):37M-46M.

[69] Oliver JJ, Melville VP, Webb DJ, et al. Effect of regular phosphodiesterase type 5 inhibition in hypertension. *Hypertension* 2006;48:622-627.

[70] Mancia G, De Backer G, Dominiczak A. 2007 guidelines for the management of arterial hypertension: The task force for the management of arterial hypertension of the European Society of Hypertension (ESH) and of the European Society of Cardiology (ESC) *Eur. Heart J.* 2007;28:1462.

[71] Giles TD. Circadian rhythm of blood pressure and the relation to cardiovascular events. *J. Hypertension* 2006;24 (suppl):S11-S16.

[72] Scranton RE, Lawler E, Botteman M, et al. Effect of treating erectile dysfunction on management of systolic hypertension. *Am. J. Cardiol.* 2007;100:459-463.

[73] Yao S, Messerle FH. Blood pressure control and sildenafil-carrot stick or sword of damocles? *Am. J. Cardiol.* 2007;100:552-553.

[74] Webb DJ, Freestone S, Allen MT. Sildenafil citrate and blood-pressure-lowering drugs: Results of drug interaction studies with an organic nitrate and a calcium antagonist. *Am. J. Cardiol.* 1999;83:21-28.

[75] Zusman RM, Prisant LM, Brown MJ. Effect of sildenafil citrate on blood pressure and heart rate in men with erectile dysfunction taking concomitant antihypertensive medication. Sildenafil study group. *J. Hypertension* 2000;18:1865-1869.

[76] Ghofrani HA Voswininckel E Reichenberger F, et al. Differences in hemodynamic and oxygenation responses to three different phosphodiesterse-5 inhibitors in patients with pulmonary arterial hypertension: a randomized prospective study. *J. Am. Coll Cardiol.* 2004;44:1488-1496.

[77] Galie N, Ghofrani HA, Torbicki A, et al. Sildenafil citrate therapy for pulmonary arterial hypertension. *N. Engl. J. Med.* 2005;353:2148-2153.
[78] Hoeper MM, Faulenbach C Golpon H, et al. Combination therapy with bosentan and sildenafil in idiopathic pulmonary hypertension. *Eur. Respir. J.* 2004;24:1007-1010.
[79] Mathai SC, Girgis RE, Fisher MR, et al. Addition of sidenafil to bosentan monotherapy in pulmonary arterial hypertension. *Eur. Respir. J.* 2007;29:469-475.
[80] Ghofrani HA, Wiedeman R, Rose F, et al. Combination therapy with oral sidenafil and inhaled iloprost for severe pulmonary hypertension. *Ann. Intern. Med.* 2002;136:515-522.
[81] Ghofrani HA, Rose F, Schermuly RT, et al. Oral sildenafil as long-term adjunct therapy to inhaled iloprost in severe pulmonary arterial hypertension. *J. Am. Coll Cardiol.* 2003;42:158-164.
[82] Carlsen J, Kjeldsen K, Gerstoft j. Sildenfil as a successful treatment of otherwise fatal HIV-related pulmonary hypertension. *AIDS* 2002;16:1568-1569.
[83] Schumacher YO, Zdebik A, Huonker M, et al. Sildenafil in HIV-related pulmonary hypertension. *AIDS* 2001;15:1747-1748.
[84] Ghofrani HA, Reichenberger F, Kohstall MG, et al. Sidenafil increases exercise capacity during hypoxia at low altitudes and at Mount-Everest base camp: a randomized, double-blind, placebo-controlled crossover trial. *Ann. Intern. Med.* 2004;141:169-177.
[85] Ghofrani HA, Schermuly RT, Rose F., et al. Sildenafil for long term treatment of non-operable chronic thromboembolic pulmonary hypertension. *Am. J. Resp. Crit Care Med.* 2003;167:1139-1141.
[86] Reichenberger F, Voswinckel R, Enke B, et al. .Long-term treatment with sidenafil in chronic thromboembolic pulmonary hypertension. *Eur. Respir. J.* 2007;30:922-927.
[87] Richalet JP, Gratadour P, Robach P, et al. Sildenafil inhibits altitude-induced hypoxemia and pulmonary hypertension. *Am. J. Respir Crit Care Med.* 2005;171:275-281.
[88] Higginbottam T. Pulmonary hypertension and chronic obstructive pulmonary disease: a case for treatment. *Proc. Am. Thorac. Soc.* 2005;2:12-19.
[89] un P, Cameron A, Seftel A, et al. Erectile dysfunction-An observable marker of diabetes mellitus? A Large national epidemiological study. *J. Urol.* 2006;176:1081-1085.
[90] Deutsh S, Sherman L. Previously unrecognized diabetes mellitus in sexually impotent men. *JAMA* 1980;244:2430-2.
[91] Manley SM, Meyer LC, Neil HAW et al. complications in newly diagnosed type 2 diabetic patients and their association with different clinical and biochemical risk factors. *Diabetes Res.* 1990;13:1-11.
[92] Gazzaruso C, Giordanetti S, De Amici E, et al. Relationship between erectile dysfunction and silent myocardial ischemia in apparently uncomplicated type 2 diabetic patients. *Circulation* 2004; 110:22-26.
[93] Romeo JH, Seftel AD, Madhun ZT, et al. Sexual function in men with diabetes type 2: association with glycemic control. *J. Urol.* 2000;163:788-791.
[94] Safarinejad MR. Oral sildenafil in the treatment of erectile dysfunction in diabetic men: a randomized double-blind and placebo-controlled study. *J. Diabetes and Its Complications* 2004;18:205-210.

[95] Rosen RC, Riley A, Wagner G, et al. The International Index of Erectile Function (IIEF): A multidimensional scale for assessment of erectile dysfunction. *Urology* 1997;49:822-830.

[96] Boulton AJM, Selam JL, Sweeney M, et al. Sildenafil citrate for the treatment of erectile dysfunction in men with type 2 diabetes mellitus. *Diabetologia* 2001;44:1296-1301.

[97] Rendell MS, Rajfer J, Wicker PA, et al. Sildenafil for treatment of erectile dysfunction in men with diabetes: a randomized controlled trial. *JAMA* 1999;281:421-426.

[98] Fink HA, Mac DR, Rutks IR, et al. Sildenafil for male erectile dysfunction: a systematic review and meta-analysis. *Arch. Intern. Med.* 2002;162:1349-60.

[99] Carson CC, Burnett AL, Levine LA, et al. The efficacy of sildenafil citrate (Viagra) in clinical populations: an update. *Urology* 2002;60 (suppl 2):12-27.

[100] Saenz de Tejada I, Anglin G, Knight JR, et al. Effects of tadalafil on erectile dysfunction in men with diabetes. *Diabetes Care* 2002;25:2159-64.

[101] Brock GB, Mcmahon CG, Chen KK et al. Efficacy and safety of tadalafil for the treatment of erectile dysfunction: results of integrated analyses. *J. Urol.* 2002;168:1332-1336.

[102] Ng KK, Lim HCP, Ng FC, et al. The use of sildenafil in patients with erectile dysfunction in relation to diabetes mellitus – A study of 1,511 patients. *Singapore Med. J.* 2002;43(8):387-390.

[103] Kadioglu A, Erdogru T, Karsidag K et al. Evaluation of penile arterial system with color Doppler ultrasonography in nondiabetic and diabetic males. *Eur. Urol.* 1995;27:311-314.

[104] Seftel AD, Vaziri ND, Ni Z et al. Advanced glycation end products in human penis: elevation in diabetic tissue, site of deposition, and possible effect through iNOS or eNOS. *Urology* 1997;50:1016-1026.

[105] Saenz de Tejada I, Goldstein I, Azadzoi K, et al. Impaired neurogenic and endothelium-mediated relaxation of enile smooth muscle from diabetic men with impotence. *N Engl J. Med* 1989;320:1025-1030.

[106] Deusk RF, Pepine CJ, Glasser DB, et al. Efficacy and safety of sildenafil citrate in men with erectile dysfunction and stable coronary artery disease. *Am. J. Cardiol.* 2004;93:147-153.

[107] Olsson AM, Persson CA. Efficacy and safety of sildenafil citrate for the treatment of erectile dysfunction in men with cardiovascular disease. *Int. J. Clin. Pract* 2001;55:171-176.

[108] Conti CR, Peine CJ, Sweeney M. Efficacy and safety of sildenafil citrate in the treatment of erectile dysfunction in patients with ischemic heart disease. *Am. J. Cardiol.* 1999;83:29C-34C.

[109] Arruda-Olson AM, Mahoney DW, Nehra A, et al. Cardiovascular effects of sildenafil during exercise in men with known or probable coronary artery disease: a randomized crossover trial. *JAMA* 2002;287:719-725.

[110] Thadani U, Smith W, Nash S, et al. The effect of vardenafil, a potent and highly selective phosphodiesterase-5 inhibitor for the treatment of erectile dysfunction on the cardiovascular response to exercise in patients with coronary artery disease. *J. Am. Coll Cardiol.* 2002;40:2006-2012.

[111] Fox KM, Thadani U, Ma PT, et al. Sildenafil citrate does not reduce exercise tolerance in men with erectile dysfunction and chronic stable angina. *Eur. Heart J.* 2003;24:2206-2212.

[112] Mitttleman MA, Glasser DB, Orazem J. Clinical trials of sildenafil citrate (Viagra) demonstrate no increase in risk of myocardial infarction and cardiovascular death compared with placebo. *Int. J. Clin. Pract.* 2003;57;597-600.

[113] Kloner RA, et al. Cardiovascular safety of vardenafil, a potent, highly selective PDE5 inhibitor in patients with erectile dysfunction: An analysis of five placebo-controlled trials. *Pharmacotherapy* 2002;22:1371.

[114] Cheitlin MD, Hutter AM, Brindis RG, et al. ACC/AHA expert consensus document use of sildenafil (Viagra) in patients with cardiovascular disease. *J. Am. Coll Cardiol.* 1999;33:272-281.

[115] DeBusk R, Drory Y, Goldstein I, et al. Management of sexual dysfunction in patients with cardiovascular disease: recommendations of the Princeton Consensus Panel. *J. Am. Coll Cardiol.* 2000;86:175-181.

[116] Kloner RA, Hutter AM, Emmick JT, et al. Time course of the interaction between tadalafil and nitrates. *J. Am. Coll Cardiol.* 2003;42:1855-1860.

INDEX

B

C

D

E

F

G

H

N

Q

R

S

T

U

V

W

Y